MEDICAL RADIOLOGY
Diagnostic Imaging

Editors:
A. L. Baert, Leuven
K. Sartor, Heidelberg

Foreword

It is my great pleasure and privilege to introduce another volume on modern musculo-skeletal imaging edited by A. M. Davies, K. Johnson and R. Whitehouse.

The hip joint and the bony pelvis are anatomical structures that are subject to frequent and various disease processes. Radiologists, orthopedic surgeons, and rheumatologists are confronted in their daily practice with many of these conditions. Due to the continuous progress in diagnostic imaging modalities and new insights into the pathophysiology and biomechanics of the hip joint and bony pelvis there is a need for regular updates of our knowledge in this field.

The concept of this book is based on a comprehensive coverage of both the imaging modalities and the applications of all these techniques to a specific anatomic area and all the pathologic conditions related to it.

The short preparation period of this volume – less than 15 months – ensures, as in the other volumes on musculoskeletal radiology in this series edited by A. M. Davies, that the most recent advances of hip joint and bony pelvis imaging are included.

I am greatly indebted to the three editors for their brilliant editorial work and their superb personal contributions. I congratulate them on their judicious choice of contributing authors, all well-known and internationally recognized experts in the field.

I am convinced that this excellent volume will be of great interest for radiologists in training and certified radiologists, and also for orthopedic surgeons and rheumatolo-gists.

It is my sincere wish that this work meets the same success as so many other volumes previously published in the series Medical Radiology – Diagnostic Imaging.

Leuven   ALBERT L. BAERT

Preface

As our understanding of the disease processes and the biomechanics of the hip joint and bony pelvis improves, there is a need to continuously update radiologists, orthopaedic surgeons and other professionals working in this field. This book, in common with several others published in this series, takes a dual approach to the subject.

The first section acquaints the reader with the full range of techniques available for imaging the hip joint and musculoskeletal pelvic pathology, emphasizing the indications and contraindications. The six chapters include contributions on radiography, computed tomography and CT arthrography, magnetic resonance imaging and MR arthrography, ultrasound, nuclear medicine and interventional techniques. The remaining 18 chapters discuss the optimal application of these techniques to specific pathologies, highlighting practical solutions to both common and uncommon clinical problems.

The discerning reader may note a few minor contradictions in the text (recommended gauge of needle, volume of contrast medium, use or not of local anaesthetics for arthrography, etc.) reflecting the different practices of the authors. The editors have deliberately not edited out these inconsistencies, thereby allowing the reader to appreciate that, even between centres of excellence, practices can and will vary.

The editors are grateful to the international panel of authors for their contributions to this book, which aims to provide a comprehensive overview of current imaging of the hip joint and musculoskeletal pelvis.

Birmingham   A. MARK DAVIES
Birmingham   KARL JOHNSON
Manchester   RICHARD W. WHITEHOUSE

Contents

Imaging Techniques and Procedures

1 Radiographic Evaluation

UGNE JULIA SKRIPKUS and AMILCARE GENTILI

CONTENTS

1.1
Radiographic Technique

For pelvic and hip pathology, radiographic evaluation can prove to be a relatively quick and inexpensive first line of imaging. In this chapter, basic imaging principles including patient positioning and radiographic projections will be discussed. For all imaging techniques discussed, gonadal shielding should be maximally utilized to decrease the amount of patient radiation exposure without compromising radiographic image quality.

1.2
Radiographic Projections of the Pelvis

Standard projections for the evaluation of the pelvis include AP, AP axial ("frogleg") and posterior oblique ("Judet").

U. J. SKRIPKUS, MD
Musculoskeletal Radiology Fellow, University of California, San Diego, 200 West Arbor Drive, San Diego, CA 92075, USA
A. GENTILI, MD
Professor, Department of Radiology, University of California, San Diego, 9300 Campus Point Drive, La Jolla, CA 92037, USA

1.2.1
Anteroposterior Projection of the Pelvis
(Bilateral Hips)

1.2.1.1
Technique: Supine

The patient is lying supine with the midsagittal plane of the pelvis centered with the midline of the long axis of the table. The pelvis should be in true AP position, with the distance from the table top to the anterior superior iliac spine on both sides of the pelvis being equal, to minimize rotation of the pelvis. Unless contraindicated, the feet are internally rotated approximately 15° to get the long axis of the femora parallel to the film. The feet may be gently taped together or a sandbag may be placed across the ankles to minimize movement during image acquisition. In the case of trauma, or when femoral neck fracture or dislocation is suspected, the feet should not be internally rotated. The elbows

should be flexed and the palms of the hands should rest gently on the chest or upper abdomen.

Alternatively, the arms may rest at the patient's sides. The shoulders should be in the same transverse plane as the pelvis. A pillow or other supporting structure should be placed behind the head and the knees. The central ray is directed perpendicularly to the midpoint of the film approximately 2 in. (5 cm) superior to the pubic symphysis or midway between the level of the anterior superior iliac spines and symphysis pubis. Respiration is suspended. If imaging is done as part of a hip evaluation, the centering should be performed approximately 2 in. (5 cm) caudad, to include more of the proximal femurs. Gonadal shielding should be used on all male patients. Ovarian shielding in female patients may obscure portions of the pelvis.

1.2.1.2
Radiographic Evaluation

On this projection, the entire pelvis, including L5, sacrum and coccyx, as well as the proximal femurs, including the greater trochanters, should be visualized. The lesser trochanters, if seen, should be demonstrated along the medial borders of the femurs. The femoral heads, which should be equal in size and position, should be well seen through the acetabula.

Fractures, dislocations, osseous lesions and degenerative changes are demonstrated. Congenital dislocation of the hip, evidenced by an abnormal relationship of the femoral head with the acetabulum can be visualized by two additional AP images of the pelvis, described by Martz and Taylor (1954). The first technique requires the central ray to be directed perpendicularly to the symphysis pubis to detect any lateral or superior displacement of the femoral head. The second technique is obtained with the central ray directed to the symphysis pubis at a cephalic angulation of 45° which will demonstrate anterior or posterior displacement of the femoral head.

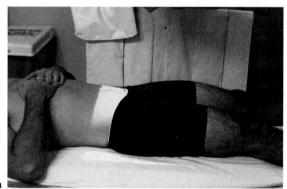

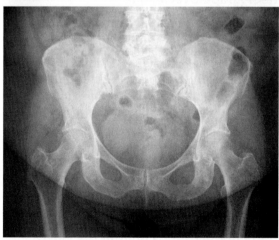

Fig. 1.1. **a** Patient positioning for anteroposterior (AP) pelvic radiograph. **b** AP pelvic radiograph

1.2.2
AP Axial Projection of the Pelvis
(Frogleg–Cleaves or Modified Cleaves Method)

This position is contraindicated in patients suspected of having a fracture, dislocation of the hip.

1.2.2.1
Technique

1.2.2.1.1
Modified Cleaves Method: Supine

The patient is in the supine position with the pelvis in true AP position. The midsagittal plane of the body is centered about the midline of the table. The elbows should be flexed and the palms of the hands should rest gently on the chest or upper abdomen. A pillow or other supporting structure should be placed behind the head. The shoulders should be in the same transverse plane as the pelvis. The hips are flexed bilaterally and the knees are bent to approximately 90° so as to draw the feet up as much as possible. The thighs are then abducted and the soles of the feet are apposed to one another for support and centered at the midline of the table. If possible, the thighs should be abducted approximately 40° from vertical to place the long axis of the femoral necks parallel with the plane of the film. Supports should be placed behind the legs as needed for stability. (The technique for a unilateral examination is adjusted so that the anterior superior iliac spine of the affected side is at the midline of the table. The ipsilateral hips and knee are then flexed and the foot is drawn up to the inner aspect of the contralateral knee. The thigh is then abducted to approximately 40° from vertical.) The central ray should be perpendicular to the film and centered approximately 1 in. (2.5 cm) superior to the pubic symphysis or 3 in. (7.5 cm) inferior to the anterior superior iliac spine. Respiration is suspended. Gonadal shielding should be used for both males and females without obscuration of a majority of pelvic structures.

1.2.2.1.2
Original Cleaves Method

The patient is positioned as described above for the modified Cleaves method. However, prior to abducting the thighs, the X-ray tube should be angled parallel with the long axes of the femoral shafts. The central ray should be angled approximately 40° cephalad to enter the symphysis pubis. Respiration is suspended. Gonadal shielding should be used for both males and females without obscuration of a majority of pelvic structures.

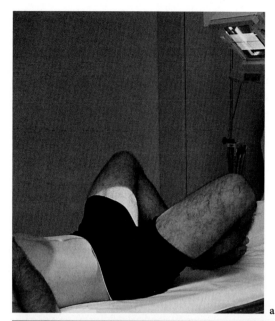

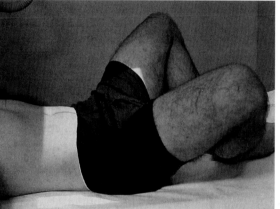

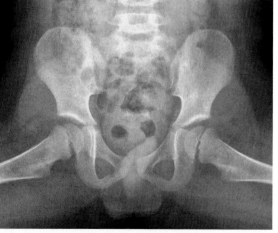

Fig. 1.2. a Patient positioning for original Cleaves frogleg pelvis radiograph. **b** Patient positioning for modified Cleaves frogleg pelvis radiograph. **c** Frogleg AP pelvis radiograph

1.2.2.2
Radiographic Evaluation

On this projection, the axial position of the femoral heads, necks and trochanters are visualized and direct comparison from one side to the other is possible. The acetabulum should also be well demonstrated. Symmetry of the pelvic bones should be appreciated if no rotation was present. The original Cleaves method demonstrates only a small part of the lesser trochanters on the posterior surface of the femurs.

1.2.3
Posterior Oblique Pelvis – Acetabulum ("Judet")

1.2.3.1
Technique

1.2.3.1.1
Judet Method: Semisupine

The patient is in a semisupine, 45° posterior oblique position, with the affected side superior or inferior, depending on anatomic structure of interest. The pelvis and thorax should be aligned with one another to avoid rotation. A pillow or other supporting structure should be placed behind the head and the back for support. The acetabulum and femoral head of interest should be positioned at the midline of the table. When anatomic structure of interest is inferiorly (dependently) positioned, the central ray should be perpendicular and centered 2 in. (5 cm) distal and 2 in. (5 cm) medial to ipsilateral anterior superior iliac spine. When anatomic structure of interest is superiorly positioned, the central ray should be perpendicular and centered 2 in. (5 cm) distal to ipsilateral anterior superior iliac spine. Respiration is suspended. Gonadal shielding should be done carefully to avoid obscuration of essential pelvic/acetabular structures.

1.2.3.2
Radiographic Evaluation

This technique is useful for evaluation of hip dislocation and acetabular fracture. For superiorly placed side of interest, the posterior rim of ipsilateral acetabulum and anterior ilioischial column, as well as the obturator foramen are well demonstrated. For inferiorly (dependently) placed side of interest, the ipsilateral anterior rim of the acetabulum as well as the posterior ilioischial column and iliac wing are well demonstrated.

1.3
Radiographic Projections of the Anterior Pelvic Bones

Standard projections for the evaluation of the anterior pelvic bones include PA axial "inlet" and AP axial "outlet."

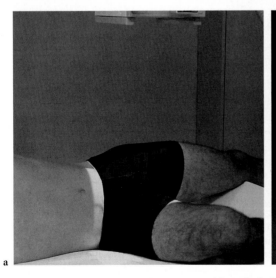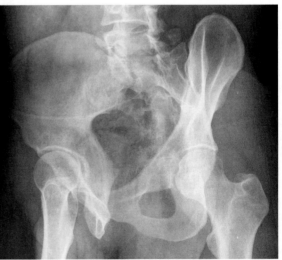

a   b

Fig. 1.3. a Patient positioning for posterior oblique "Judet" view of pelvis. **b** "Judet" view of pelvis, taken in RPO position

1.3.1
AP Axial "Outlet" Projection of the Anterior Pelvic Bones (Taylor)

1.3.1.1
Technique: Supine

The patient is supine on the table with the midsagittal plane of the patient's body centered about the midline of the table. The pelvis is in true AP position. A pillow or other supporting structure should be placed behind the head and the knees for comfort. For males, the central ray is directed approximately 20°–35° cephalad and centered at a point 2 in. (5 cm) distal to the upper border of the symphysis pubis. For females, the central ray is directed approximately 30°–45° cephalad and centered to a point 1–2 in. (2.5–5 cm) distal to the upper border of the symphysis pubis. Respiration is suspended. Gonadal shielding should be carefully applied to avoid obscuration of essential bony structures.

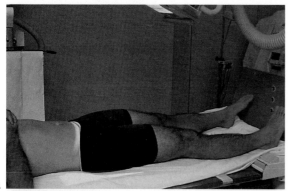

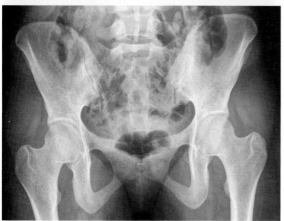

Fig. 1.4. a Patient positioning for AP axial "outlet" projection of the anterior pelvic bones. **b** "Outlet" radiograph of the anterior pelvic bones

1.3.1.2
Radiographic Evaluation

On this projection, the pubic and ischial bones will be magnified and only minimally superimposed on the sacrum and coccyx. The hip joints should also be included.

1.3.2
AP Axial "Inlet" Projection of the Anterior Pelvic Bones (Lilienfeld)

1.3.2.1
Technique: Seated Erect

The patient is seated erect on the table, with the knees flexed slightly and the feet resting on the table top. A supporting structure should be placed behind the knees. The midsagittal plane of the patient's body should be centered about the midline of the table. There should be no rotation of the pelvis. The arms should be extended behind the patient with the hands placed on the table top, supporting the torso in a position approximately 50° from vertical. A supporting structure should be placed behind the lower back and the back should be arched to place the pubic arch in a near-vertical position. The central ray is directed perpendicularly to the cassette and centered to a point 1.5 in. (3.8 cm) superior to the symphysis pubis. Respiration is suspended. Gonadal shielding for men should be carefully applied to avoid obscuration of essential bony structures.

1.3.2.2
Technique: Supine

The patient is supine on the table with the midsagittal plane of the patient's body centered about the midline of the table. The pelvis is in true AP position. A pillow or other supporting structure should be placed behind the head and the knees. The central ray is directed caudad 40° (approximately perpendicular to the plane of the pelvic inlet) and centered to the level of the anterior superior iliac spines. Respiration is suspended. Gonadal shielding for men should be carefully applied to avoid obscuration of essential bony structures.

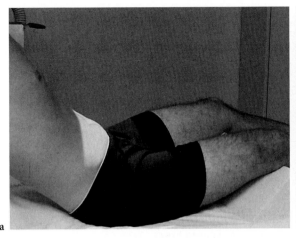
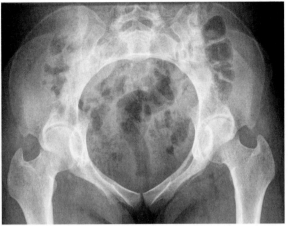

a   b

Fig. 1.5. a. Patient positioning for seated erect AP axial "inlet" projection of the anterior pelvic bones. **b** "Inlet" radiograph of the anterior pelvic bones

1.3.2.3
Radiographic Evaluation

On this projection, the ischial and pubic bones are visualized from a superoinferior approach, demonstrating the pelvic ring or inlet. The symphysis pubis should be centered to the radiograph. The medial third of the anterior superior and inferior pubic rami should be superimposed. The lateral two thirds should be nearly superimposed. The hip joints should also be included.

1.4
Radiographic Projections of the Sacroiliac Joints

Standard projection for the evaluation of the sacroiliac joints includes AP oblique.

1.4.1
AP Oblique Projection of the Sacroiliac Joints

1.4.1.1
Technique: Supine

The patient is lying supine on the table in posterior oblique position with the affected side elevated approximately 25°–30° and the body aligned such that the sagittal plane passing 1 in. (2.5 cm) medial to the anterior superior iliac spine of the elevated

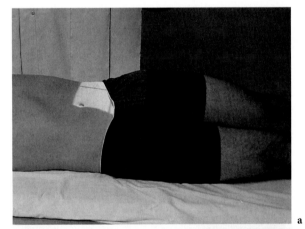

a

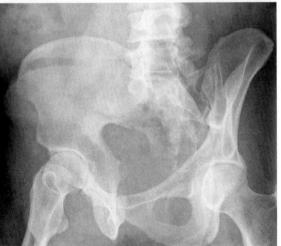

b

Fig. 1.6. a Patient positioning for AP oblique projection of the sacroiliac joints. **b** AP oblique projection of the sacroiliac joints

side is centered about the midline of the table. The anterior superior iliac spines should be in the same transverse plane. The head as well as the elevated shoulder, lower back and thigh should be supported by pillow wedges or by other means. With the central ray directed perpendicular to the plane of the film, it should enter 1 in. (2.5 cm) medial to the elevated anterior superior iliac spine. With the central ray at an angle of 25° cephalad, it should be centered 1 in. (2.5 cm) medial and 1.5 in. (3.8 cm) distal to the elevated anterior superior iliac spine. Alternatively, with the central ray perpendicular, it should be directed 1 in. (2.5 cm) medial to the elevated anterior superior iliac spine. Respiration is suspended. Gonadal shielding should be done carefully to avoid obscuration of essential bony structures. Shielding for women may be difficult to achieve without significant obscuration. Collimation should be close to the joint.

1.4.1.2
Radiographic Evaluation

On this projection, a profile view of the affected sacroiliac joint is seen. The adjacent structures are seen in an oblique position. Both sides should be evaluated for comparison.

1.5
Radiographic Projections of the Sacrum and Coccyx

Standard projections for the evaluation of the sacrum and coccyx include AP, PA, and lateral.

1.5.1
AP/PA Projection of the Sacrum and Coccyx

1.5.1.1
Technique: Prone or Supine

The patient can be positioned either in the supine or prone positions, depending upon physical ability and limitations. The pelvis should be place in true AP or PA position. The AP projection is preferred, as the sacrum and coccyx are positioned slightly closer to the film. The midsagittal plane of the body should be centered about the midline of the table. In the supine position, the elbows should be flexed and the palms of the hands should rest gently on the chest or upper abdomen or at the patient's sides. A pillow or other support structure should be placed under the head and the knees. In the prone position, the elbows should be flexed and the arms should be in a comfortable, bilaterally symmetrical position.

For evaluation of the sacrum: In the supine position, the central ray should be directed 15° cephalad and centered to the midpoint of the plane that passes midway between the symphysis pubis and the anterior superior iliac spines. In the prone position, the central ray should be directed 15° caudad and centered to the sacral curve. Respiration is suspended. Gonadal shielding should be done carefully in males to not obscure significant bony structures. Respiration is suspended. Shielding in women is not possible without significant image degradation. The urinary bladder should be empty. The lower colon should be free of gas for optimal image acquisition.

For evaluation of the coccyx: In the supine position, the central ray should be directed 10° caudad and centered to a point about 2 in. (5 cm) superior to the symphysis pubis. In the prone position, the central ray should be directed 10° cephalad and centered to the palpable coccyx. Respiration is suspended. Gonadal shielding should be done carefully in males to not obscure significant bony structures. Respiration is suspended. Shielding in women is not possible without significant image degradation. The urinary bladder should be empty. The lower colon should be free of gas for optimal image acquisition.

1.5.1.2
Radiographic Evaluation

On this projection, a true frontal projection of the sacrum and coccyx, free of superimposition is demonstrated. Evaluation of the sacrum should demonstrate neither foreshortening nor rotation. Fecal material should not overlap the sacrum. The sacroiliac joints and L5–S1 junction should be included. Evaluation of the coccyx should demonstrate no rotation and no segmental superimposition.

1.5.2
Lateral Projection of the Sacrum and Coccyx

1.5.2.1
Technique: Recumbent

The patient is recumbent with the affected side closest to the table and the hips and knees flexed to a

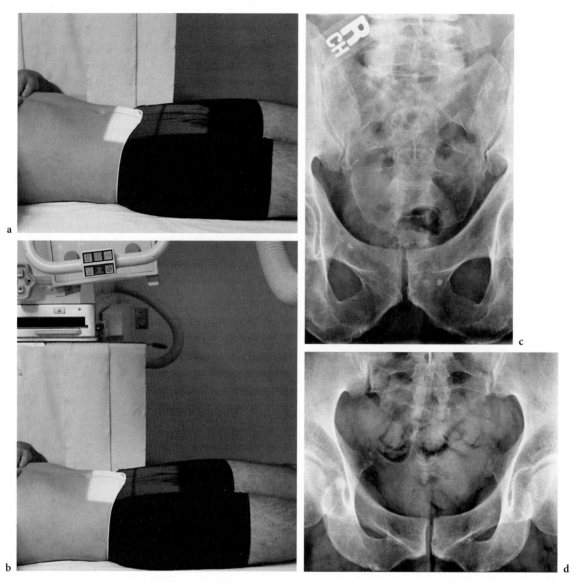

Fig. 1.7. a Patient positioning for anteroposterior (AP) view of sacrum. **b** Patient positioning for anteroposterior (AP) view of coccyx. **c** AP View of the sacrum. **d** AP view of the coccyx

comfortable position. For evaluation of the sacrum, the coronal plane passing 3 inches posterior to the midaxillary line is centered about the midline of the table. For evaluation of the coccyx, the coronal plane passing through the coccyx should be placed about the center line of the table either by palpation technique or by appreciating that the coccyx lies approximately 5 in. (12.7 cm) posterior to the midaxillary line. The vertebral column should be parallel to the tabletop. Therefore, a small support may be needed under the lower thoracic/upper lumbar spine. The arms should be positioned at right angles to the body, while allowing the patient to grasp onto the table for support. The pelvis should be in the true lateral

position with the bony landmarks, such as the anterior superior iliac spines, lying in the same vertical plane with respect to one another. Supports should be placed under the head, ankles and knees. The film should be positioned so that its midpoint is either at the level of the anterior superior iliac spines for the sacrum or at the level of the center of the coccyx. For evaluation of the sacrum, the central ray should be directed perpendicular to a coronal plane 3 in. (7.6 cm) posterior to the midaxillary line at the level of the anterior superior iliac spine. For evaluation of the coccyx, the central ray should be directed perpendicular to a coronal plane 3 in. (7.6 cm) posterior to the midaxillary line at the level of the coccyx.

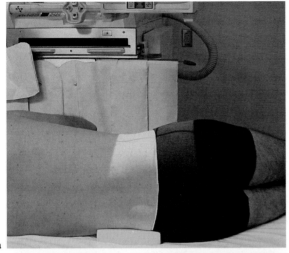

a

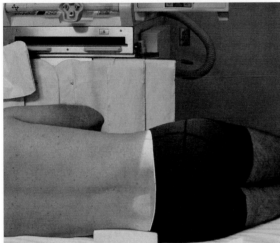

b

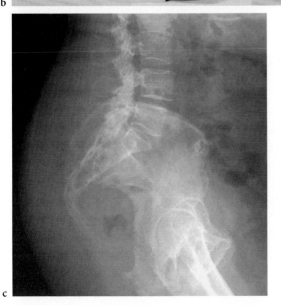

c

Fig. 1.8. a Patient positioning for lateral sacral radiograph. **b** Patient positioning for lateral coccyx radiograph. **c** Lateral sacral radiograph

1.5.2.2
Radiographic Evaluation

The lateral aspect of the sacrum or the coccyx is demonstrated. The sacrum and coccyx should be seen in their entirety. The posterior margins of the ischia and ilia should be closely superimposed.

1.6
Radiographic Projections of the Hip

Standard projections for the evaluation of the hip include AP, lateral (Lauenstein and Hickey), axiolateral (Danelius-Miller modification of Lorenz).

1.6.1
AP Projection of the Hip

1.6.1.1
Technique: Supine

The patient is supine with the pelvis in true AP position and the sagittal plane passing 2 in. (5 cm) medial to the anterior superior iliac spine centered about the midline of the table (placing the femoral neck at the midline of the table). The elbows should be flexed and the palms of the hands should rest gently on the chest or at the patient's sides. The feet, unless contraindicated, should be internally rotated approximately 15°–20° to position the long axes of the femora parallel to the plane of the film. In the case of trauma or when fracture or dislocation is suspected, the feet should not be rotated. Review of AP of the pelvis should be considered to assess for fracture or other derangement. The central ray should be directed perpendicular to the plane of the film and enter approximately 2.5 in. (6.4 cm) distal on a line drawn perpendicular to the midpoint of a line between the anterior superior iliac spine and the symphysis pubis. Alternatively, the central ray can be directed to a sagittal plane 2 in. (5 cm) medial to the affected side anterior superior iliac spine at the level just superior to the greater trochanter. Respiration is suspended.

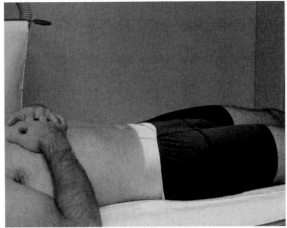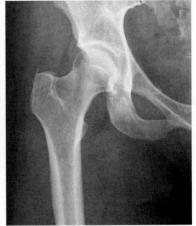

a   b

Fig. 1.9. a Patient positioning for anteroposterior (AP) hip radiograph. **b** AP hip radiograph

1.6.1.2
Radiographic Evaluation

On this projection, the head, neck, trochanters, and proximal third of the shaft of the femur is well demonstrated. The greater trochanter should be visualized in profile. The lesser trochanter may either not be seen or may minimally project beyond the medial border of the femur. The adjacent ilium, pubic bones, and symphysis pubis should also be included. Any orthopedic hardware should be completely visualized.

1.6.2
Lateral Projection of the Hip
(Lauenstein and Hickey)

This technique is not used in patients in whom fracture is suspected or in those who have sustained trauma.

1.6.2.1
Technique: Supine

The patient is supine and turned toward the affected side into a near lateral position. Care should be taken not to over-rotate and thereby allow for superimposition onto the affected side. The ipsilateral knee should be flexed to near 90° and the opposite thigh should be extended and supported at hip level. The head and elevated lower back should also be supported. The central ray should be directed perpendicularly (for the Lauenstein method) or at a cephalic

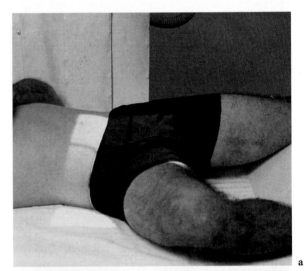

a

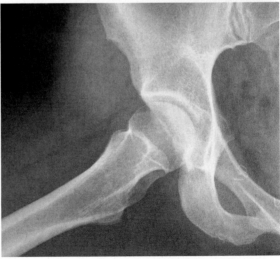

b

Fig. 1.10. a Patient positioning for lateral radiograph of the hip (Lauenstein method). **b** Lateral radiograph of the hip

angle of 20° (for the Hickey method) through the hip joint, located midway between the anterior superior iliac spine and the symphysis pubis.

1.6.2.2
Radiographic Evaluation

On this projection, the lateral position of the hip is optimized. The acetabulum, proximal femur and the relationship of the acetabulum with the articulating femur are demonstrated. In the Lauenstein method, the femoral neck will be overlapped with the greater trochanter.

1.6.3
Axiolateral Inferosuperior Projection of the Hip (Danelius–Miller)

1.6.3.1
Technique: Supine (Danelius–Miller Modification of Lorenz)

The patient is in the supine position and the pelvis is elevated slightly while maintaining a true AP position without rotation. The unaffected limb is elevated with the thigh placed in near vertical position. The leg should be supported at hip level with pillows or other supporting structures. The elevated extremity should be positioned so as to be outside of collimation field. To localize the long axis of the femoral neck, the center point of a line drawn between the anterior superior iliac spine and the superior border of the symphysis pubis should be connected to a point drawn approximately 1 in. (2.5 cm) distal to the most prominent lateral protrusion of the

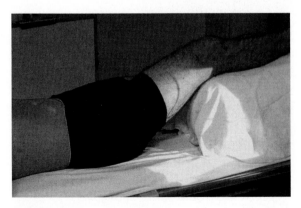

Fig. 1.11. Patient positioning for axiolateral inferosuperior radiograph of hip

greater trochanter. This will mark the axis of the femoral neck regardless of the position of the lower extremity. Unless contraindicated, the foot of the affected side should be internally rotated approximately 15°–20° and fixed in position with sandbags or other device. The elbows should be flexed and the palms of the hands should rest gently on the chest or upper abdomen. The cassette should be in the vertical position exactly parallel to the long axis of the femoral neck of the affected side. The central ray should be directed perpendicularly to the long axis of the femoral neck and centered approximately 2.5 in. (6.4 cm) below the point of intersection of the localization lines described above. Respiration is suspended. Gonadal shielding is not possible without obscuration of significant structures. Therefore, close collimation is essential.

1.6.3.2
Radiographic Evaluation

The proximal femur, including the head, neck, is well demonstrated in the lateral projection. The hip joint with the acetabulum should be well demonstrated. Any orthopedic hardware should be fully included.

1.7
Arthrographic Evaluation of the Hip

1.7.1
Technique: Supine

The patient is supine with the pelvis in true AP position. Unless contraindicated, the feet are internally rotated approximately 15° to get the long axis of the femora parallel to the film. The feet may be gently taped together or a sandbag may be placed across the ankles to minimize movement during image acquisition. In the case of trauma, or when femoral neck fracture or dislocation is suspected, the feet should not be internally rotated. The elbows should be flexed and the palms of the hands should rest gently on the chest or upper abdomen. Alternatively, the arms may rest at the patient's sides. The shoulders should be in the same transverse plane as the pelvis. A pillow or other supporting structure should be placed behind the head and the knees. Palpate the femoral artery and draw the course of the artery on the skin with a permanent marker. Mark the mid neck and the intertrochanteric line with a permanent marker. Sterilize the skin and drape the surrounding area. Under fluoroscopic guidance, enter the skin with 18–20 Gauge needle for aspiration or 20–22 Gauge needle for arthrogram at midpoint of the intertrochanteric line. Advance the needle anterolaterally toward the head/neck junction along the femoral neck. Confirm needle position within hip joint with < 1 cc of iodinated contrast material. Inject 12 cc of contrast material. A 1:200 dilution of gadolinium with contrast is to be used if MRI is to be performed after the arthrogram.

Variations of needle position include lateral oblique, inferior oblique, medial and lateral. Images should be obtained in AP, 20° posterior oblique, and abduction.

Fig. 1.12. a Needle positioning for lateral oblique approach for hip arthrography. **b** Needle positioning for inferior oblique approach for hip arthrography. **c** Needle positioning for medial approach for hip arthrography. **d** Needle positioning for lateral approach for hip arthrography ▽

1.7.2
Radiographic Evaluation

The hip joint should be outlined with contrast. Intra-articular bodies, fistula formation, labral pathologies, synovial processes and evidence of arthroplasty loosening are demonstrated on radiographic evaluation.

Suggested Reading

Ballinger WP, Frank ED (1999) Merrill's atlas of radiographic positions and radiologic procedures, 9th edn. Mosby, St Louis

Bontrager KL, Lampignano JP (2001) Radiographic positioning and related anatomy, 5th edn. Mosby, St Louis

Kreel L (1981) Clark's positioning in radiography, 10th edn. Yearbook Medical Publishers, Chicago

Martz CD, Taylor CC (1954) The 45 degree angle roentgenographic study of the pelvis in congenital dislocation of the hip. J Bone Joint Surg Am 36:528-532

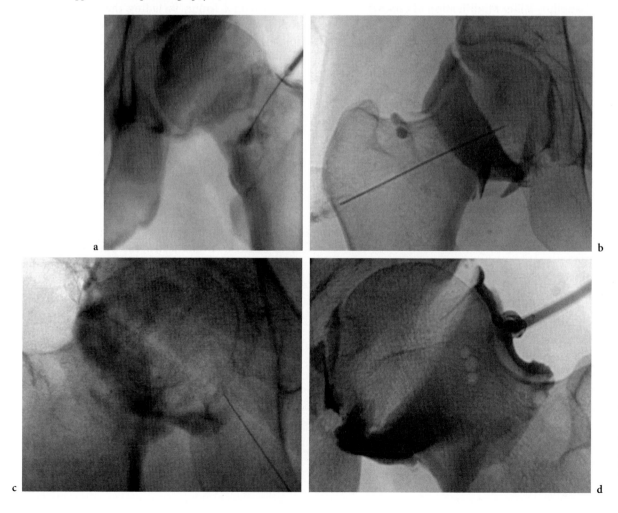

2 Computed Tomography (CT) and CT Arthrography

Richard William Whitehouse

CONTENTS

2.1
Introduction

Computed tomography (CT) and magnetic resonance (MR) imaging are now established methods of imaging investigation and both methods continue to develop. CT remains more suitable than MR in the assessment of acute trauma (e.g. acetabular fractures), but MR is considerably better for assessment of soft tissue injuries and tumours. The addition of arthrography further increases the specificity and sensitivity of both MR and CT for articular and acetabular labral lesions. CT remains essential in the assessment of patients in whom MR is contra-indicated (e.g. due to intracranial aneurysm clips or cardiac pacemakers). CT therefore continues to have a role in the diagnosis and management of many pathologies of the pelvis and hips. Having decided that CT is an appropriate investigation for an individual, the precise format of the examination will depend upon the suspected pathology and the equipment available. This chapter describes recent developments in CT scanners, considerations for pelvic and hip CT scanning, dose reduction strategies, CT hip arthrography and CT guided intervention. The main aim is to outline those considerations that should optimise the images obtained, whilst minimising the radiation dose to the patient, whatever CT scanner is used.

2.2
Developments in CT

A CT image is a Cartesian co-ordinate map of normalised X-ray attenuation coefficients, generated by electronically filtered computerised back projection of X-ray transmission measurements in multiple directions through a section of the object in question. Those areas where recent developments have been made include helical scanning, multislice acquisition and real time CT "fluoroscopy" (Dawson and Lees 2001). These developments have been made on the back of improving technology which includes slip-rings for power and data transmission to and from the gantry, higher heat loading and more rapid heat dissipation X-ray tubes, high efficiency solid state X-ray detectors, faster data transmission and processing abilities of the electronics.

R. W. Whitehouse, MD
Department of Clinical Radiology, Manchester Royal Infirmary, Oxford Road, Manchester, M13 9WL, UK

2.2.1
Slip Rings

The use of cables to supply power and take data from the rotating scanner gantry has now been superseded by slip rings. Replacing the cables with slip rings (large circumference electrically conducting rings) which encircle the X-ray tube path, and transferring power from the rings to the X-ray tube via conducting brushes on the X-ray tube gantry, allows the gantry to be continuously rotated in one direction. This has several advantages over the alternating wind up and unwind gantry rotation directions required by continuous cables. Rapid acceleration and deceleration of the gantry are no longer required yet a faster rotation speed can be achieved giving shorter scan acquisition times. The time delay between slices need be no longer than that required for table movement in conventional acquisition mode and the potential for acquiring continuously updated X-ray transmission data allows both helical scanning and CT fluoroscopy.

2.2.2
X-Ray Tubes

The development of slip rings resulted in a requirement for X-ray tubes to have both a higher heat capacity and a higher maximum tube current, as the mAs required for a single slice remained much the same but the time in which the slice was acquired was reduced. As an alternative to higher heat capacity, more rapid heat dissipation from the tube has been developed by one manufacturer. In addition, for helical scanning continuous X-ray output for up to 60 s may be required. The disadvantage of these X-ray tubes is the increased ease with which high radiation doses can be given to patients during CT investigations.

2.2.3
X-Ray Detectors

Xenon gas detectors, used in CT scanners for many years, have a conversion efficiency (X-rays to signal strength) of around 60%, which can diminish further if the detectors are not maintained. Solid state crystal detectors may have conversion efficiencies of nearly 100%, resulting in a 40% reduction in patient radiation dose for the equivalent scan appearances. The tendency for solid state detectors to continue emitting light after the X-rays had terminated (afterglow), and other technical problems with respect to the size of the front face of the individual detectors and the interspace material between adjacent detectors have been largely overcome.

The ease with which solid state detectors can be stacked in parallel adjacent channels has facilitated the development of multi-slice scanners. These scanners can acquire multiple sections simultaneously, which can be separately processed to give large numbers of thin sections, or recombined to give fewer thicker sections with lower noise.

2.2.4
Helical CT (Spiral or Volume Scanning)

The requirement for a break in the X-ray emission whilst the table is moved to the next slice position was overcome by the development of helical scanning. Helical scanning is performed by moving the table continuously during the exposure, from the first slice location to the last. Thus a helix of X-ray transmission data through the scan volume is acquired. To generate a CT image the data from adjacent turns of the helix are interpolated to produce transmission data which are effectively from a single slice location (KALENDER et al. 1990). This process can be performed at any location within the helix, (except the first and last 180°'s – where there is no adjacent helix of data for interpolation). In this way overlapping slices can be produced without overlapping irradiation of the patient. The relationship between the X-ray fan beam collimation and the table movement per rotation of the gantry is called the pitch ratio. Extended or stretched pitch scans are performed with pitch ratios greater than 1. Such extended pitches can be used to trade off between greater scan volumes; shorter scan acquisition times and lower scan radiation doses. Stretching the pitch ratio to 1.25 has little effect on the image appearances, but pitch ratios greater than 1.5 produce images with effective slice thickness' significantly greater than the nominal fan beam collimation thickness. Multislice scanners in particular may use pitch ratios of less than 1, this increases patient radiation dose and scan acquisition time but reduces image noise and some spiral scanner artefacts. By increasing the number of detector arrays ("multi-slice scanner") several interlaced helices can be acquired simultaneously with the table increment per gantry rotation increased proportionately (McCOLLOUGH and ZINK 1999). Initial developments in multi-slice scanners were aimed at reducing individual slice thicknesses, but once z-axis resolution is equivalent to in plane resolution, further reduction in slice thickness is of limited value. Adding further rows of detectors will then increase the total width of the detector bank. Whilst offering the potential for faster scan acquisition, the increasing divergence of the X-ray beam to the outer rows of detectors creates a "cone beam" geometry for the X-ray beam paths, requiring complex data corrections to reduce artefacts in the resultant images. Currently scanners offering up to 64 detector rows with up to 4 cm total detector width are available. Flat panel detectors, based on the Direct Digital Radiography technology, for CT data acquisition are under development. These detectors will allow both increased total detector width and variable effective slice thickness. The end result will be a scanner that can acquire the full examination data from a single gantry rotation without table movement. Whilst this offers significant reduction in acquisition time and total X-ray tube loading, recently developed radiation dose reduction techniques that modulate the X-ray tube current according to slice location will no longer be applicable.

Currently available individual detector widths of between 0.5 and 0.75 mm can achieve Y-axis resolution equivalent to in-plane resolution, giving true isometric voxels and consequent equivalent quality reformats in any plane.

The combination of multislice and helical scanning results in volume scan acquisition times which are many times faster than a single slice helical scanner with the same gantry rotation speed, and one or even two orders of magnitude faster than a non-spiral scanner. Multislice scanning reduces X-ray tube loading requirements as it acquires several slices simultaneously with the same tube loading as a single slice would require on a conventional scanner. The patient radiation dose however is not directly reduced and may be increased if greater volumes are scanned.

2.2.5
CT "Fluoroscopy"

In conventional CT transmission data from a 360° gantry rotation is required to generate an image. This is because two opposing beam paths then exist for each ray across the imaging volume. This produces improved signal to noise, corrections for the effects of divergent X-ray beams along each ray and beam hardening effects. Images can also be produced using 270°

or even 180° gantry rotation datasets. Such "partial scan" images have acquisition times proportionately shorter than full rotation scans. This can be useful for reducing movement artefacts in selected patients. For a 0.5 s per rotation scanner, the effective scan acquisition time will be one quarter of a second (250 ms). If the gantry continues to rotate and acquire data without table movement, continuously updated transmission data will be collected from which revised images can be generated. With extremely rapid processors and appropriate reconstruction algorithms, further delay for image reconstruction can be minimised and a continuously updated CT image displayed in "near real time" (Hsieh 1997). Such "CT fluoroscopy" imaging can be used for CT guided interventional procedures. As with all fluoroscopic procedures care should be taken to reduce fluoroscopy time to the minimum necessary and to avoid operator irradiation – instruments designed to keep the operators hands out of the CT section (Daly et al. 1998) and use of the lowest selectable tube current 50 mA is sufficient (Froelich et al. 1999) are advocated. To assist in maintaining short CT fluoroscopy exposure times, routine recording and auditing of fluoroscopy exposure times is advocated. An audible alarm after a preset exposure time may also assist in keeping exposures as short as possible. The use of a lead drape adjacent to the irradiated volume has been demonstrated to reduce operator exposure (Nawfel et al. 2000). High skin doses to patients and operators will occur if care is not taken.

2.2.6
Data Manipulation

The vast masses of image data acquired from a multislice spiral scanner produces problems of data storage and interpretation. It is no longer feasible to produce hardcopy images of every available section. With isometric voxels, reformatted images in any other image plane will have the same image quality as the acquisition images, potentially requiring even further hard copies.

Fast workstations, allowing rapid reformatting and display of examinations in the most appropriate plane for the pathology being demonstrated are therefore necessary, with hard copy restricted to representative images. Other image reconstruction methods (curved planes, surface rendered 3D images, minimum or maximum intensity projections, "transparent bone") can produce an array of visually stunning images (Fig. 2.1).

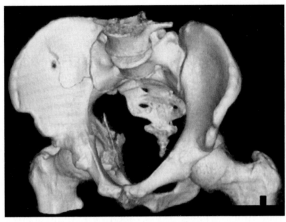 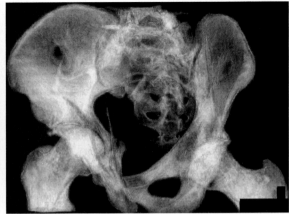

a   b

Fig. 2.1. a 3D surface shaded reconstruction, rotated to demonstrate a central fracture/dislocation of the hip. **b** "Transparent bone" reconstruction of the same CT data

The current state of the art device has a multislice helical scanner with solid state detectors, sub-second scan acquisition and image reconstruction times, CT fluoroscopy capability and a link to a powerful workstation with real time image manipulation software and a digital image data archive.

2.2.7
Reformatted Images

As spiral multislice scanning produces overlapping sections and thinner slice collimation (less than 1 mm), in plane and reformatted plane spatial resolutions are now similar, even for CT images from small fields of view. Volume acquisitions obtained in any plane can therefore be reformatted into other planes without loss of image quality (Fig. 2.2). For

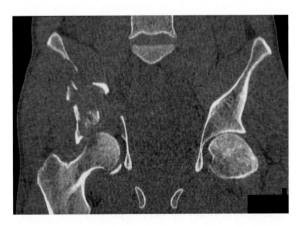

Fig. 2.2. Coronal reformatted image of a fracture/dislocation of the right hip

scanners not capable of such fine collimation, CT in the most appropriate plane for the expected pathology is still preferable if achievable. For non-helical scanners, overlapping transverse sections with a table increment of half the slice thickness will provide better z-axis resolution, but at twice the radiation dose to the patient.

2.3
Scan Image Quality

The amount of noise, beam hardening and streak artefacts in a CT image are dependent upon the following factors:

- Collimation slice thickness
- Partial or full rotation dataset
- Mass and distribution of tissue in the scan plane
- Scan time/movement
- High density extraneous material (e.g. contrast medium spills, surgical metalwork)
- KVp and mAs
- Field of view
- Matrix size
- Reconstruction algorithm
- Post-processing image sharpening or softening filters
- Viewing window width and level settings

Most of these factors are amenable to selection or modification by the scanner operator and can markedly affect the quality of the final image. The relationships between image noise, mAs and patient size are non linear, with a halving of patient size resulting in a quartering of image noise, whilst a fourfold increase in mAs is needed to half the image noise. For small patients, image noise is effectively low at all mAs settings and the absolute reduction in image noise achieved by quadrupling the mAs is small (Fig. 2.3).

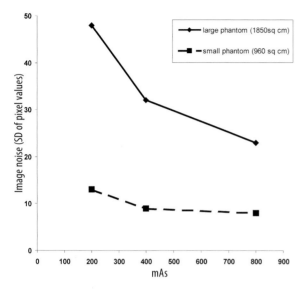

Fig 2.3. The influence of size and mAs on image noise for a CT scanner. Sections were performed through water density phantoms with 10 mm slice collimation

In addition, if the pathology being imaged is osseous, the width of the usual viewing window for bone renders noise less perceptible. As children are more radiation sensitive than adults as well as smaller, particular attention should be paid to reducing the mAs in this group of patients.

Streak artefacts can be generated by high density material within the scan plane but outside the field of view of the scanner. Tabletops, which contain edge grooves, tracks for the fixing of attachments or detachable mattresses can act as traps for spilt contrast media. Contrast droplets on the gantry window will also cause image artefacts. Scrupulous care to keep the tabletop and gantry clean is needed to remove these sources of artefact.

2.3.1
Internal Metalwork from Fixation Devices

The streak artefact generated from in-situ intramedullary rods is rarely excessive, and does not prevent adequate assessment of the bone cortex, making CT of value in assessing femoral fracture

union in selected cases. More intrusive streak artefact is seen when the CT plane is through locking screws in intramedullary rods, bone surface plates, hip joint replacements or fixation screws. Care in patient positioning (including decubitus positions where necessary), combined with gantry angulation in order to align the scan plane with the long axis of any screws present will reduce the number of sections degraded by streak artefact from the screws to a minimum and in the case of unilateral hip replacement may allow scanning of the contralateral hip without including the replacement metalwork in the scan plane at all. In scanners with operator selectable kVp, the use of the highest kVp setting will reduce streak artefact, as will the selection of a higher mAs (though the combination of increased kVp and mAs results in considerably greater tube loading and patient irradiation). Streak artefact also may appear visually less intrusive on volume rendered (3D) images (PRETORIUS and FISHMAN 1999). The streak artefact from modern titanium hip prostheses on multislice spiral scanners usually does not seriously degrade the images (Fig. 2.4).

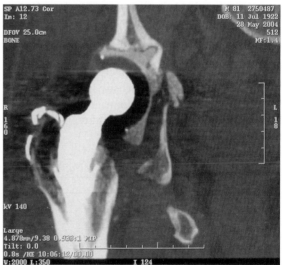

Fig 2.4. Coronal reformatted image through a hip replacement, demonstrating the bone-cement interface despite beam hardening and streak artefacts

2.3.2
CT Number, Hounsfield Units, Window Width and Levels

The scale of numbers used to define the greyscale in CT images is artificially limited by data storage constraints. The CT number scale runs from

–1000 for air, through 0 for water. The top end of the scale is usually constrained to fit into a 12-bit binary number (allowing number values from –1024 to +3072 to be stored). The Hounsfield unit (HU) is the true value which the CT number should represent. Scanner drift, calibration error, artefact or other limitation may render this inaccurate, which is why measurements made from scan images are best called CT numbers.

The Hounsfield unit value for any material is defined by formula 1:

$$HU_s = 1000 \, (\mu_s - \mu_w / \mu_w)$$

Where HU_s = The Hounsfield unit value for substance s

μ_s = Linear attenuation coefficient for substances
μ_w = Linear attenuation coefficient for water

This formula relates the HU value to the linear attenuation coefficients of the material being measured and water. As the linear attenuation coefficients of all materials change with X-ray beam energy, there are consequently only two fixed points on the Hounsfield scale. These are –1000, which is the HU value for no X-ray attenuation (i.e. a vacuum), and zero, which corresponds to the HU value for water (at the calibration pressure and temperature for the scanner). The HU scale is, in fact, open ended, with high atomic number, high density materials having values way in excess of the upper end of the usual scale (even on "extended scale scanners) (Table 2.1).

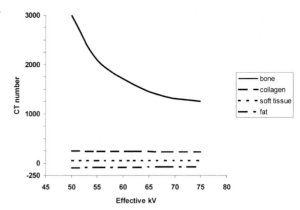

Fig. 2.5. The influence of scanner kV on CT numbers for bone and soft tissues

value for dense cortical bone is over 2000. Other high atomic number materials (contrast media, aluminium, and metal fixation devices) also show marked variation in HU value with beam energy. By contrast, the HU values of soft tissues, collagen and fat vary very little with effective beam energy as the linear attenuation coefficients for these materials closely follow those of water.

Consequently, in scanners which allow the operating voltage to be changed, the CT number for bone can be increased by using a low kVp (around 80 kVp). This increases the dependence of the CT number on the presence of bone or calcification and is particularly used for quantitative measurement of mineral density. A high kVp (usually around 140 kVp) can be selected to reduce the CT number of bone and metalwork, which has some effect in reducing streak artefacts.

For lower atomic number materials such as are present in soft tissues, the X-ray attenuation and consequent CT number is predominantly influenced by the electron density of the material, which is, in turn, closely related to the physical density of the material. Even the CT number of water is influenced by differences in temperature and differences in density exist between water at room and at body temperature. The presence of protein or high concentrations of salts will increase the CT number of body fluids. Measurement of the CT number of a region of interest in an image must therefore be considered only a guide to its composition. At an extreme not met in clinical practice, but potentially relevant to research, the CT number of ice at 0°C (approximately –80 HU) is lower than that of fat, the CT number of which increases as it cools (Whitehouse et al. 1993).

The visual impression of the density of a region of interest is influenced by the window and level set-

Table 2.1. Theoretical HU values for a variety of materials at 65 kV

Adipose tissue	–80
Water	0
Collagen	250
Dense cortical bone	1600
Aluminium	2300
Iron	34000
Iodine	141300
Lead	205000

The theoretical Hounsfield value for dense cortical bone calculated at an effective beam energy of 65 keV (equivalent to a scanner operating at around 120 kVp) is in the region of 1600 (Fig. 2.5). At lower energies (e.g. 55 kV – the approximate effective energy of a scanner operating at 80 kVp), the HU

tings of the image, the calibration of the display and the densities in the surrounding part of the image. Particularly within bone, the surrounding high density of bone can give a lytic lesion the visual impression of a lower density than actually exists. Consequently, measurement rather than estimation of any region of interest is essential, recording an image in which the CT numbers of important regions of interest are measured is a useful addendum to the hard copy.

The window width and level are calibrated contrast and brightness settings for image display. The most appropriate window level for cortical bone will be influenced by the bone density and the effective scan energy, whilst the window width may need to be quite narrow to demonstrate subtle intracortical density changes.

Reviewing images on the console prior to printing hard copies is recommended to obtain the best image settings for individual patients and to avoid overlooking pathology not demonstrated at "standard" settings.

2.3.3
Radiation Dose Reduction

CT of the pelvis typically gives an effective dose of 4 mSv for each acquisition in adults. Where soft tissue abnormality is being assessed, the combination of pre- and post contrast scans without excessive image noise will thus result in a dose of around 8 mSv. Beam hardening and streak artefacts from the dense bony ring of the pelvis are reduced by higher mAs and consequently even higher radiation doses. As regulatory authorities require medical exposure to ionising radiation to be both justified and minimised if performed, the relatively high radiation burden that CT of the pelvis delivers requires particular consideration. The increased ease with which CT scans can be obtained due to the speed and availability of multislice scanners is also generating debate about safety and dose reduction strategies (KALRA et al. 2004). For scans that are justified, use of the scout view to accurately identify the required limits of the scan should be mandatory, with rapid review of the top and bottom section to confirm adequate coverage. The mAs setting should be chosen to suit the size of the patient (JANGLAND et al. 2004), with particular care to select the lowest acceptable setting for children (FRUSH et al. 2003) and also the required image noise – images for high contrast structures such as bone or CT guided

biopsy needles are adequate at a much lower mAs than images for soft tissue lesions. Modern scanners offer tube current modulation, which varies the mAs during a scan, with the most sophisticated systems altering the mAs continuously to suit the attenuation of the patient in each projection. In the pelvis the markedly higher attenuation in the lateral projection compared to the AP projection results in a sinusoidal variation in mAs during scanning which can reduce the effective radiation dose by around 30% whilst not affecting or even improving image noise and streak artefacts (KALENDER et al. 1999). Where available such dose modulation should be the default scanner setting. Specific female gonad shielding is not possible on CT but encasement of the testicles by a "testis capsule" has been shown to reduce testicular radiation dose by 95% for abdominal CT scans (HIDAJAT et al. 1996). CT fluoroscopy systems may offer the option of turning off the tube current over an arc where the tube is above the patient. Whilst this is primarily intended to reduce operator exposure during interventional procedures, it will also reduce male patient testicular dose in pelvic procedures.

2.4
CT of the Hip and Pelvis

CT of the pelvis is a common component of abdominal CT scanning. Scanning of the pelvis for musculoskeletal disease is less frequent but remains the best investigation for pelvic fracture assessment. Other indications include CT measurement of femoral anteversion and some guided biopsy or ablation procedures. Most soft tissue pathologies around the pelvis and hips are better assessed by MR imaging.

2.4.1
Anatomy

Detailed knowledge of the anatomy and its appearances in all imaging planes is a prerequisite for adequate scan interpretation. Knowledge of anatomical structures not easily or consistently demonstrated on CT is still needed to assess the likelihood of their involvement by any pathology that is demonstrated. The anatomy of the region is best reviewed in appropriate detailed texts. Selected CT images are included here for comparative purposes (Fig. 2.6 and Table 2.2).

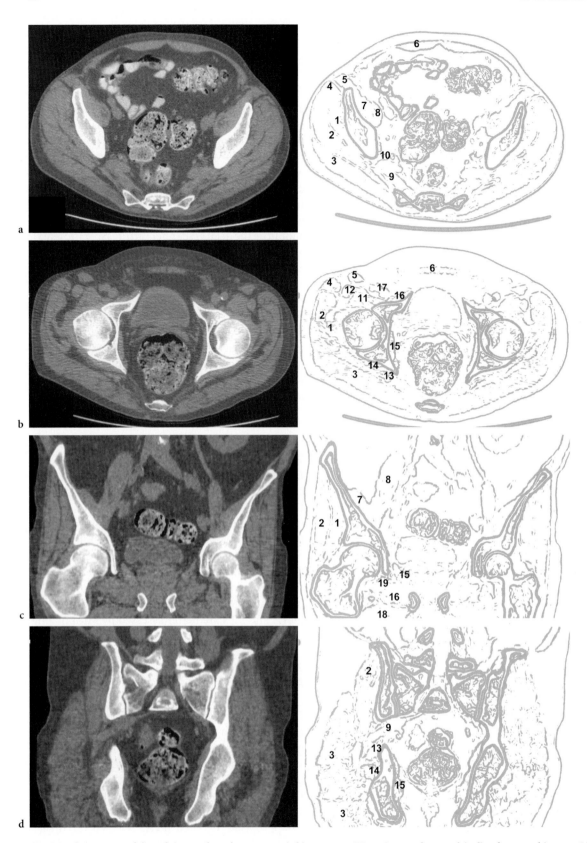

Fig. 2.6a–d. Anatomy of the pelvis on selected transverse (**a,b**) 1.25 mm CT sections and coronal (**c,d**) reformatted images. Line drawings of each section identify structures as enumerated in Table 2.2

Table 2.2. Anatomical structures shown in Fig. 2.6

1	Gluteus minimus
2	Gluteus medius
3	Gluteus maximus
4	Tensor fascia lata
5	Sartorius
6	Rectus abdominis
7	Iliacus
8	Psoas
9	Piriformis
10	Superior gluteal vessels
11	Ilio-psoas
12	Rectus femoris
13	Sciatic nerve with vessels
14	Gemellus muscles and obturator internus tendon
15	Obturator internus
16	Pectineus
17	Femoral vessels
18	Adductor brevis
19	Obturator externus

For the clearest depiction of articular surfaces and fractures, images perpendicular to the plane of the articulation or fracture are usually best, whilst for tendons and ligaments an imaging plane perpendicular to the long axis of the structure is useful, this may require thin section scanning with reformats.

2.4.2
Immobilisation

Gross patient movement artefact is not common in pelvic scanning. Bowel peristalsis and respiratory movements also usually have negligible effects on pelvic CT. Polytrauma patients may be immobilised on a spinal board, these are usually designed to be relatively radiolucent and do not interfere with scanning.

2.4.3
Patient Positioning

AS described above, volume acquisitions obtained in any plane can be reformatted into other planes without marked loss of image quality. For scanners not capable of such fine collimation, CT scanning in the most appropriate plane for the expected pathology is still preferable. Care in positioning the patient on the scanner table in supine or decubitus positions and judicious use of gantry angulation to avoid orthopaedic metalwork are the commonest modi-

fications to pelvic CT scanning (Fig. 2.7), though not all scanners can perform multislice acquisitions with an angled gantry.

2.5
Indications

CT of the pelvis and hips is particularly suited to the demonstration of complex bony anatomy such as the evaluation of bony morphological abnormalities and fractures. Intraosseous tumours are well demonstrated, for example the nidus of an osteoid osteoma, which can be overlooked on MR imaging, is characteristic and clearly demonstrated on CT. The presence of tumour matrix ossification or calcification is also clear on CT. In osteomyelitis, the presence and location of sequestra are revealed. With the addition of arthrography, osteochondral and acetabular labral lesions will be well demonstrated. Soft tissue pathology is less well demonstrated than with MR and intravenous contrast medium injection provides less satisfactory contrast enhancement than the equivalent MR examination but valuable information on soft tissue lesions is still obtainable from CT (for example, size, extent, tumour calcification, enhancement, articular involvement). CT can be used to guide biopsy and aspiration procedures.

The accurate three dimensional localisation of the bone anatomy with CT can be used to calculate the mechanical axes of long bones and the relationships of the joints. This can then be used in the preoperative planning of joint replacements. The CT scanogram, usually used to identify the start and finish points for a CT investigation, can also be used for limb length measurements.

The limitations of CT are usually described in relationship to MR, and consequently the poorer soft tissue contrast of CT is top of the list. Where MR is available and not itself contra-indicated, it is the most appropriate modality for imaging soft tissue lesions. The other limitations of CT in relation to MR are the direct multiplanar capability of MR and the use of ionising radiation with CT.

2.5.1
Trauma

In the acutely traumatised patient, speed and patient safety are important requirements for a satisfactory examination. This gives limited scope for scan

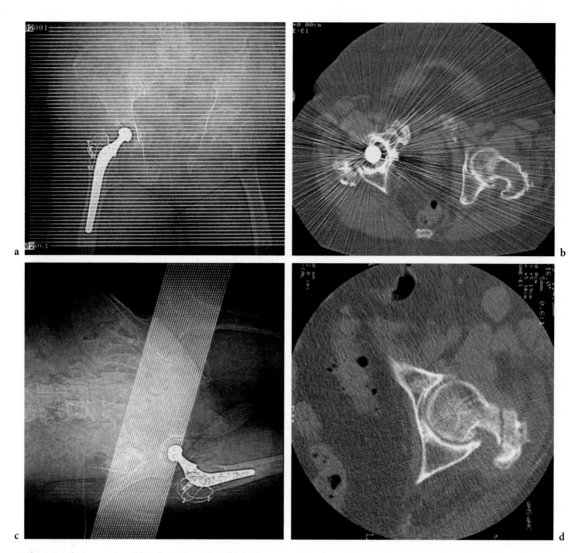

Fig. 2.7a–d. Scout view (**a**)and axial section (**b**) with conventional positioning demonstrate streak artefact from hip replacement, whilst a decubitus position and angled gantry avoids the hip replacement (**c**) and no streak artefact occurs over the contralateral hip (**d**)

technique modifications. As the primary aim of the examination is to determine the size and disposition of fracture fragments and joint alignments, the aim is to ensure adequate coverage of the injured region in a single helical acquisition with effective slice thickness appropriate to the size of the fracture fragments. For osseous detail, even in the pelvis, a low mAs is sufficient, but haematomas may still being evident (Fig. 2.8). An AP scout view to determine appropriate start and end points for the acquisition should be routine. The smaller the collimation thickness, pitch, and reconstruction interval, the better the quality of reformatted planar and 3D images, giving overlapping helical acquisition sections a small advantage over conventional contiguous transverse sections for fracture classification.

If helical scanning is not available, a mixed protocol of thicker sections to cover the extent of the fracture, with thinner sections through the region of the articular surface injury can also be used. Three-dimensional surface reconstructions provide an easily interpreted overview of fracture fragment disposition, particularly useful in badly comminuted injuries (Pretorius and Fishman 1999).

2.5.2
Articular Cartilage

Thin section CT (particularly multislice helical) combined with arthrography (see Sect. 2.6) has been used as the gold standard for measuring articular

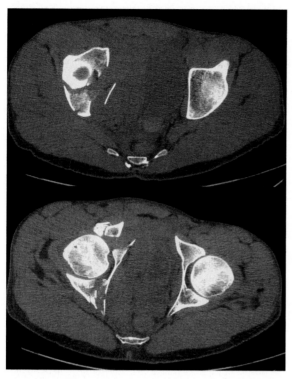

Fig. 2.8. Axial CT sections of a central fracture/dislocation of the hip. Note the haematoma in the pelvis, displacing the bladder

cartilage thickness and volume in the knee. These techniques are probably equally applicable to the hip, though there is little published literature on CT hip arthrography.

These measurements are of increasing clinical importance as targeted treatments for osteoarthritis are being developed (HANGODY et al. 1998). Many of these studies are aimed at validating MR methods of cartilage measurement in the knee, rather than advocating the use of CT arthrography (ECKSTEIN et al. 1997, 1998; HAUBNER et al. 1997). Nevertheless, CT arthrography currently remains more sensitive than non-arthrographic MR for subtle cartilage defects (DAENEN et al. 1998) and the minimally invasive technique allows accurate measurement of capsular volume, fluid aspiration for laboratory studies and injection of therapeutic agents as required (BERQUIST 1997).

2.5.3
Femoral Anteversion

Femoral anteversion is a measure of the angle of the femoral neck, relative to a line across the back of the femoral condyles, as viewed down the long axis of the femur (Fig. 2.9). The degree of femoral anteversion is often increased in conditions such as cerebral palsy. Surgical correction of this rotational deformity of the femur is considered to be of value in improving lower limb function in these patients. Methods of measuring femoral anteversion have been described using plain film, CT, MR and US. The CT measurement is probably most widely used and robust (KUO et al. 2003). Both two- and three-dimensional CT techniques have been described, the three-dimensional methods being particularly valuable when the femur is not aligned with the z-axis of the scanner – for example if the hip is flexed and adducted. The 3D technique scans the entire femur and a 3D surface render of the femur is then rotated on the workstation to generate a true axial view from which the measurement can be made. Whilst more accurate in this situation than a 2D method, the accuracy is still sub-optimal, with errors of over 5° in 86% of in vitro test objects in one series (DAVIDS et al. 2003). 2D methods require a pair of single sections through the femoral neck and femoral condyles, though more than one section at each site may be required, particularly if the femoral neck has a valgus deformity. Normal adult value for femoral anteversion is 12–15° (DELAUNAY et al. 1997).

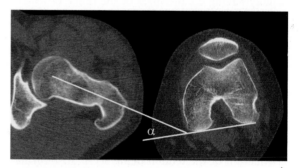

Fig. 2.9. Axial CT images of the femoral neck and condyles, presented side by side for clarity. The angle (á) between a line along the femoral neck and the posterior margins of the condyles is the femoral anteversion

2.5.4
Soft Tissues

The imaging examination of soft tissue masses and synovial diseases of the hip is best undertaken by MR (with or without Gd-DTPA enhancement), augmented by radiographs and possibly specialist US examination. CT has a limited role where these methods are contra-indicated or unavailable but some pathologies (e.g. fatty tumours such as lipoma arborescens, calcified lesions — synovial osteochondromatosis, gouty tophi and dense lesions such as pigmented villonodular synovitis) may have characteristic appearances on CT (CHEN et al. 1999; LIN et al. 1999). CT is unreliable for follow-up scanning of the resection site of soft tissue sarcoma (HUDSON et al. 1985).

Contrast enhancement can be used with volume rendering to demonstrate arterial and graft stenosis and obstructions after vascular surgery down to the popliteal vessels (ISHIKAWA et al. 1999) and other vascular lesions. Similarly, soft tissue enhancement in masses or synovium can be demonstrated but timing is critical, with peak enhancement being later, less marked and more variable in onset than in the abdomen. CT scanner software which pre-scans at low mA to detect the onset of enhancement and triggers the study at that point may have a role.

2.5.5
Tendons

The tendons around the pelvis and hips are clearly depicted by CT. In cross section, tendons appear as homogeneous, well circumscribed, rounded densities of higher attenuation than other soft tissues, usually having CT numbers in the range of 75–115 and thus being visible within their muscles of origin as well as when surrounded by fat in their more distal courses. Tendons are therefore best demonstrated with sections perpendicular to their courses. Fluid around the tendon may be identified on CT as a ring of lower attenuation surrounding the tendon, though with less sensitivity to small quantities of fluid than MR. Tendinosis and tendon rupture can also be demonstrated on CT, with thickening and reduction in attenuation of the tendon being seen. 3D reformations from multiple thin sections can provide exquisite demonstration of tendon and osseous anatomy. Thus whilst CT can be used to demonstrate gross tendon pathology and associated osseous abnormality, MR is more sensitive and more specific for the tendon lesion. Scar tissue, oedema, early tendon degeneration and small amounts of inflammatory fluid are difficult to differentiate on CT.

2.6
Arthrography

CT arthrography can be performed as an adjunct to conventional hip arthrography. With double contrast arthrography, CT can be performed immediately after the conventional examination as only a small amount of iodinated contrast medium is injected (3–6 ml of 300 mgI/ml). If single contrast arthrography is performed with larger quantities of dense contrast, an interval of 2–3 h between the conventional technique and the CT examination allows the contrast medium density to dilute to a level appropriate for CT. If an immediate CT arthrogram is planned, appropriate reduction in contrast medium concentration is needed e.g. 150 mg I/ml non-ionic water-soluble contrast medium.

Indications for CT arthrography in any joint are the demonstration of intra-articular loose bodies (TEHRANZADEH and GABRIELLE 1984), chondral lesions and osteochondral defects. In the hip, CT arthrography may also be used for the evaluation of labral tears, assessment of severe proximal femoral focal deficiency in neonates (COURT and CARLIOZ 1997) and in the investigation of anterior hip pain (MANSOUR and STEINGARD 1997). Arthrography can be combined with diagnostic joint aspiration. Posterior capsule redundancy in patients with recurrent posterior hip dislocation has also been demonstrated (GRAHAM and LAPP 1990).

2.6.1
Technique

Fluoroscopy screening is used for needle placement and confirms correct location during injection of contrast medium. Local anaesthetic should not be necessary, though preparation of the skin with topical anaesthetic cream may be useful in children. Using an aseptic technique, a small gauge, adequate length needle (e.g. a 23-G "spinal" needle) is introduced into the hip joint from an anterolateral approach, avoiding the femoral vessels and aiming to hit the femoral neck at the junction with the femoral head, this part of the femoral neck still being intracapsular. A slightly inferior skin entry point with mild cephalad angulation of the needle assists in accurate needle placement. A single contrast technique with 3–6 ml of 150 mg/ml I contrast is satisfactory for a CT arthrogram and avoids the streak artefact that may occur at air/fluid interfaces. AP fluoroscopy during injection confirms correct needle location as contrast should flow rapidly away from the needle tip into the joint. A misplaced needle results in focal accumulation of contrast at the needle tip. After removing the needle, gentle manipulation ensures the contrast extends throughout all the joint capsular recesses. After conventional arthrographic films if required, axial CT through the hip is performed (Fig. 2.10).

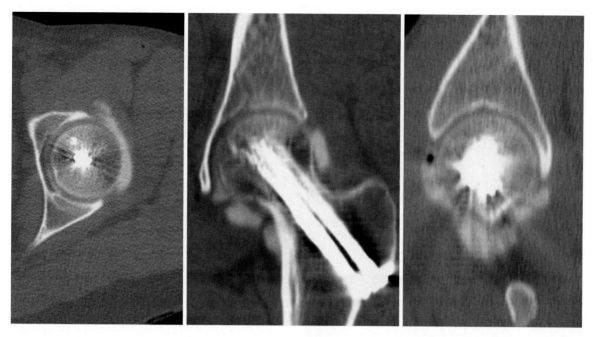

Fig. 2.10. Axial, coronal and sagittal images from a CT hip arthrogram. Performed to investigate pain and "clicking" after pinning of a stress fracture of the femoral neck. CT arthrography was performed as it was anticipated that the internal fixation would interfere with MR imaging. (Images courtesy of Dr W. Bhatti, Consultant Musculoskeletal Radiologist, Wythenshawe Hospital, UK)

2.7
CT Guided Interventions

CT is being increasingly used to guide interventional procedures, recently encouraged by the development of CT fluoroscopy which enables more rapid and accurate placement of needles and interventional devices (DE MEY et al. 2000). As described above (Sect. 2.2.5) care needs to be taken to minimise operator and patient X-ray exposure during CT guided biopsy. CT fluoroscopy times of around 10 s should suffice for most biopsy procedures (GOLDBERG et al. 2000). Limiting the fluoroscopy to identification of the needle tip rather than the entire needle will also reduce operator and patient radiation dose (SILVERMAN et al. 1999). The CT section thickness should be appropriate to the size of the lesion, otherwise partial volume averaging may include both the needle tip and the lesion in the same section, erroneously suggesting an accurate needle location. CT can be used to guide biopsy of bone and soft tissue lesions. Where primary malignancy is present then the course of the biopsy track and the compartment(s) through which it passes may need excision with the tumour at the time of definitive surgery. Biopsy of such lesions must therefore only be performed after consultation and agreement of

the approach with the surgeon who will carry out the definitive treatment. Accuracy of CT guided biopsy is increased if specimens are obtained for both cytology and pathology, overall accuracy of around 80% should be achieved (HODGE 1999).

Percutaneous treatment of osteoid osteoma can also be performed with CT guidance. A preliminary diagnostic scan is usually performed (Fig. 2.11). For the procedure a planned approach avoiding vascular structures is required, the femoral vessels are usually clearly visible on non-enhanced CT but a preliminary contrast enhanced scan to identify the vessels can be performed if necessary. It is possible to treat osteoid osteomas by complete removal via CT guided biopsy (VOTO et al. 1990), this may be difficult to achieve with biopsy needles unless a large bore needle is used and several passes are made through the lesion. More recently techniques aimed at destroying the tumour with heat, either from a radiofrequency ablation probe or a laser heated probe, both of which are available with fine probes for passage down a biopsy needle have been used (Fig. 2.12). In either case, to avoid complications the lesion to be treated should be more than a centimetre from neurovascular or other critical structures. A preliminary biopsy for histological confirmation of the diagnosis is necessary as in one series, 16% of

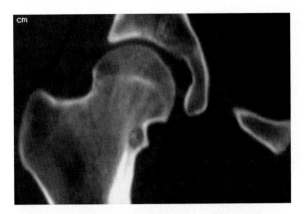

Fig. 2.11. Coronal reformatted image demonstrating an osteoid osteoma in the femoral neck

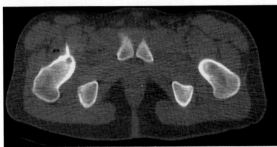

a

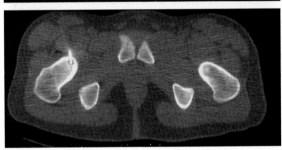

b

Fig. 2.12a,b. a Axial low mAs image demonstrates a biopsy drill placed down to the superficial surface of an osteoid osteoma, without transfixing the nidus – allowing a bone biopsy needle to be passed through the lesion for histological confirmation. **b** Radiofrequency ablation probe placed across the nidus through the biopsy track

lesions were not osteoid osteomas (SANS et al. 1999). Osteoid osteomas can cause severe pain when biopsied, although some series report the use of local anaesthesia, epidural or general anaesthesia may be necessary. Although the bulk of CT guided interventional procedures are performed by radiologists in the radiology department, the development of mobile CT scanners has allowed the use of CT guidance for procedures performed in theatre, allowing the orthopaedic surgeon to make greater use of CT guidance for minimally invasive procedures.

2.8
Conclusion

With appropriate attention to technique, CT continues to have a role in the diagnosis and management of many conditions in and around the pelvis and hips. Some pathologies will however, only be adequately demonstrated using CT arthrography and/or a scanner capable of sub-millimetre resolution in the y-axis.

References

Berquist TH (1997) Imaging of articular pathology: MRI, CT, arthrography. Clin Anat 10:1–13

Chen CK, Yeh LR, Pan HB, Yang CF, Lu YC, Wang JS, Resnick D (1999) Intra-articular gouty tophi of the knee: CT and MR imaging in 12 patients. Skeletal Radiol 28:75–80

Court C, Carlioz H (1997) Radiological study of severe proximal femoral focal deficiency. J Pediatr Orthop 17:520–524

Daenen BR, Ferrara MA, Marcelis S, Dondelinger RF (1998) Evaluation of patellar cartilage surface lesions: comparison of CT arthrography and fat-suppressed FLASH 3D MR imaging. Eur Radiol 8:981–985

Daly B, Templeton PA, Krebs TL, Carroll K, Wong You Cheong JJ (1998) Evaluation of biopsy needles and prototypic needle guide devices for percutaneous biopsy with CT fluoroscopic guidance in simulated organ tissue. Radiology 209:850–855

Davids JR, Marshall AD, Blocker ER, Frick SL, Blackhurst DW, Skewes E (2003). Femoral anteversion in children with cerebral palsy. Assessment with two and three-dimensional computed tomography scans. J Bone Joint Surg Am 85A:481–488

Dawson P, Lees WR (2001) Multi-slice technology in computed tomography. Clin Rad 56:302–309

Delaunay S, Dussault RG, Kaplan PA, Alford BA. (1997) Radiographic measurements of dysplastic adult hips. Skeletal Radiol 26:75–81

De Mey J, Op de Beeck B, Meysman M, Noppen M, de Maeseneer M, Vanhoey M, Vincken W, Osteaux M (2000) Real time CT-fluoroscopy: diagnostic and therapeutic applications. Eur J Radiol 34:32–40

Eckstein F, Adam C, Sittek H, Becker C, Milz S, Schulte E, Reiser M, Putz R (1997) Non-Invasive determination of cartilage thickness throughout joint surfaces using magnetic resonance imaging. J Biomech 30:285–289

Eckstein F, Schnier M, Haubner M, Priebsch J, Glaser C, Englmeier KH, Reiser M (1998) Accuracy of cartilage volume and thickness measurements with magnetic resonance imaging. Clin Orthop 352:137–148

Froelich JJ, Ishaque N, Saar B, Regn J, Walthers EM, Mauermann F, Klose KJ (1999) Steuerung von perkutanen Biopsien mittels CT-Fluoroskopie. [Control of percutaneous biopsy with CT fluoroscopy.] Rofo Fortschr Geb Rontgenstr Neuen Bildgeb Verfahr 170:191–197

Frush DP, Donnelly LF, Rosen NS (2003) Computed tomography and radiation risks: what pediatric health care providers should know. Pediatrics 112:951–957

Goldberg SN, Keogan MT, Raptopoulos V (2000) Percutaneous CT-guided biopsy: improved confirmation of sampling site and needle positioning using a multistep technique at CT fluoroscopy. J Comput Assist Tomogr 24:264–266

Graham B, Lapp RA (1990) Recurrent posttraumatic dislocation of the hip. A report of two cases and review of the literature. Clin Orthop 256:115–119

Hangody L, Kish G, Karpati Z, Udvarhelyi I, Szigeti I, Bely M (1998) Mosaicplasty for the treatment of articular cartilage defects: application in clinical practice. Orthopedics 21:751–756

Haubner M, Eckstein F, Schnier M, Losch A, Sittek H, Becker C, Kolem H, Reiser M, Englmeier KH (1997) A non-invasive technique for 3-dimensional assessment of articular cartilage thickness based on MRI, part 2. Validation using CT arthrography. Magn Reson Imaging 15:805–813

Hidajat N, Schröder RJ, Vogl T, Schedel H, Felix R (1996) Effektivität der Bleiabdeckung zur Dosisreduktion beim Patienten in der Computertomographie. [The efficacy of lead shielding in patient dosage reduction in computed tomography.] Rofo Fortschr Geb Rontgenstr Neuen Bildgeb Verfahr 165:462–465

Hodge JC (1999) Percutaneous biopsy of the musculoskeletal system: a review of 77 cases. Can Assoc Radiol J 50:121–125

Hsieh J (1997) Analysis of the temporal response of computed tomography fluoroscopy. Med Phys 24:665–675

Hudson TM, Schakel M, Springfield DS (1985) Limitations of computed tomography following excisional biopsy of soft tissue sarcomas. Skeletal Radiol 13:49–54

Ishikawa M, Morimoto N, Sasajima T, Kubo Y (1999) Three-dimensional computed tomographic angiography in lower extremity revascularization. Surg Today 29:243–247

Jangland L, Sanner E, Persliden J (2004) Dose reduction in computed tomography by individualized scan protocols. Acta Radiol 45:301–307

Kalender WA, Seissler W, Klotz E, Vock P (1990) Spiral volumetric CT with single-breathhold technique, continuous transport and continuous scanner rotation. Radiology 176:181–183

Kalender WA, Wolf H, Suess C (1999) Dose reduction in CT by anatomically adapted tube current modulation. II. Phantom measurements. Med Phys 26:2248–2253

Kalra MK, Maher MM, Saini S (2004) Radiation exposure and projected risks with multidetector-row computed tomography scanning: clinical strategies and technologic developments for dose reduction. J Comput Assist Tomogr 28 [Suppl 1]:S46–S49

Kuo TY, Skedros JG, Bloebaum RD (2003) Measurement of femoral anteversion by biplane radiography and computed tomography imaging: comparison with an anatomic reference. Invest Radiol 38:221–229

Lin J, Jacobson JA, Jamadar DA, Ellis JH (1999) Pigmented villonodular synovitis and related lesions: the spectrum of imaging findings. AJR 172:191–197

Mansour ES, Steingard MA (1997) Anterior hip pain in the adult: an algorithmic approach to diagnosis. J Am Osteopath Assoc 97:32–38

McCollough CH, Zink FE (1999) Performance evaluation of a multi-slice CT system. Med Phys 26:2223–2230

Nawfel RD, Judy PF, Silverman SG, Hooton S, Tuncali K, Adams DF (2000) Patient and personnel exposure during CT fluoroscopy-guided interventional procedures Radiology 216:180–184 (and comments pp 9–10)

Pretorius ES, Fishman EK (1999) Volume-rendered three-dimensional spiral CT: musculoskeletal applications. Radiographics 19:1143–1160

Sans N, Morera-Maupome H, Galy-Fourcade D, Jarlaud T, Chiavassa H, Bonnevialle P, Giron J, Railhac JJ (1999) Resection percutanee sous controle tomodensitometrique des osteomes osteoides. [Percutaneous resection under computed tomography guidance of osteoid osteoma. Mid-term follow-up of 38 cases.] Suivi a moyen terme de 38 cas. J Radiol 80:457–465

Silverman SG, Tuncali K, Adams DF, Nawfel RD, Zou KH, Judy PF (1999) CT fluoroscopy-guided abdominal interventions: techniques, results, and radiation exposure. Radiology 212:673–681

Tehranzadeh J, Gabrielle OF (1984) Intra-articular calcified bodies: detection by computed arthrotomography. South Med J 77:703–710

Voto SJ, Cook AJ, Weiner DS, Ewing JW, Arrington LE (1990) Treatment of osteoid osteoma by computed tomography guided excision in the pediatric patient. J Pediatr Orthop 10:510–513

Whitehouse RW, Economou G, Adams JE (1993) The influence of temperature on quantitative computed tomography: implications for mineral densitometry. J Comp Assist Tomogr 17:945–951

3 MR and MR Arthrography

Josef Kramer, Gerhard Laub, Christian Czerny, and Michael P. Recht

CONTENTS

J. Kramer, MD, PhD
Röntgeninstitut am Schillerpark, Reanerstrasse 6–8, 4020 Linz, Austria
G. Laub, PhD
Siemens Cardiovascular Center, Peter V. Ueberroth Bldg. Suite 3371, Los Angeles, CA 90095-7206, USA
C. Czerny, MD
General Hospital/University Medical School Vienna, Währinger Gürtel 18–20, 1090 Vienna, Austria
M. P. Recht, MD
The Cleveland Clinic Foundation, Diagnostic Radiology/Musculoskeletal Section, 95 Euclid Avenue, Cleveland, OH 44195-5145, USA

3.1 Introduction

During the past decade MR imaging of the hip joint has gained high value. Nowadays, this method plays an important role in the evaluation of hip disorders. Scanning techniques have improved dramatically and provide MR images with excellent quality. However, an optimal MR examination obtains a maximum amount of information in a given time period. Local practices and other factors dictate certain aspects of the examination. In every clinical setting there must always be a compromise between a long examination, which may be unnecessarily thorough, and a cursory study, which leaves major questions unanswered. Normally, most institutions use a routine protocol which provides adequate visualization of the hip joint and demonstrates the majority of pathologic changes. Additional protocols may be tailored to specific clinical problems. The demonstration of most pathology within the hip requires pulse sequences that provide optimal visualization of mobile water-bound protons. Increased water content is seen in joint effusions, and in ligaments, tendons and muscles following injury. It is also present in inflammatory changes, in soft tissues, and in bone marrow edema following contusions. However, some questions can only be answered with sufficient accuracy by using intraarticular administration of contrast agents. A high spatial resolution is a further requirement for imaging of the hip joint, especially if subtle pathologic changes are suspected.

3.2 General Considerations

Many factors contribute to image quality. In addition to the hardware employed, these include the signal to noise ratio (SNR), contrast to noise ratio (CNR), spatial resolution, pulse sequences, and scan time. The field strengths of the main magnet field vary from low to high (0.2–1.5 T). More recently, whole body 3 T magnets have become commercially available, and are used for routine clinical imaging. The field strength influences directly the SNR. In a first approximation, the MR signal increases linearly with the main magnetic field, and, therefore, a higher field strength magnet offers a better SNR and, consequently, a shorter examination time may be expected or the spatial resolution can be increased without the drawback of loss of signal to noise difference. Because of claustrophobia in a some patients, there is increasing interest in open MR units operating at magnetic field strengths of 0.2–0.7 T for use in body imaging. The advantages of these systems are that they are easier to install and cheaper to maintain than whole body imaging systems operating at higher field strengths. Recent studies employing ultra-high field strengths of 3.0 T are very promising in producing higher resolution images (Niitsu et al. 2000; Peterson et al. 1999). In fact, musculoskeletal imaging is considered to be one of the major reasons for continued developments of 3.0 T systems. Besides the main magnetic field, there are many other technical factors which influence the SNR. Most importantly, dedicated coils are essential for optimal signal. However, simultaneously phased array coils have demonstrated certain advantages in hip examinations, as well as offering the possibility to image both hip joints with reasonable spatial resolution (Fig. 3.1).

3.2.1
Contrast-to-Noise Ratio

The contrast-to-noise ratio describes the system's ability to differentiate two tissues under consideration. The contrast-to-noise ratio (CNR) depends on the difference in signal strength between both tissues, and the SNR. Pulse sequence type and sequence parameters need to be selected carefully to obtain optimal contrast, and SNR. In some situations where the intrinsic tissue contrast is inadequate, the administration of MR contrast agents can be very helpful to provide excellent tissue contrast.

3.2.2
Signal-to-Noise Ratio

The signal-to-noise ratio is influenced by many factors (non-operator-dependent factors: magnetic

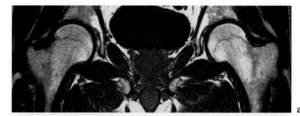
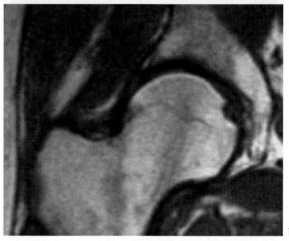

Fig. 3.1a,b. T1-weighted spin echo images of both hips (**a**) and the right hip (**b**). Normal bone marrow shows hyperintense signal intensity, musculature is low to intermediate signal

field strength, molecular structure of the tissue, proton density, and T1 and T2 relaxation times; operator-dependent factors: coil design, field of view, number of excitations, sampling bandwidth, matrix size, slice thickness, TR, TE, and flip angle). Changes in TR influence the degree of T1 weighting and hence the signal attenuation. In T2-weighted images, variations in the TE influence the T2 weighting and consequently the signal attenuation. Proton density-weighted images are only slightly attenuated by T1 or T2 relaxation and thus have a higher SNR than either T1-weighted or T2-weighted images (Heron and Hine 2002).

Voxel size is one of the most important determinants of the SNR. Larger voxels have a higher SNR than small voxels because they contain more protons to produce signals. The SNR is influenced by any change in parameter which alters the voxel size. It can be appreciated, for instance, that doubling the field of view results in a doubling in the length of two sides of the voxel and hence a fourfold increase in the SNR, whereas doubling the slice thickness doubles the length of only one side of the voxel and hence only doubles the SNR. Both matrix size and number of acquisitions affect the SNR. Doubling the matrix size in both the phase encoding and frequency encoding directions for a fixed field of view results in the SNR being reduced by a factor of the square root of 2, but the scan time is doubled because there are twice as many phase encoding steps to sample. Doubling the number of acquisitions doubles the scan time but only increases the SNR by a maximum of the square root of 2 (about 1.4). In cases where SNR is not sufficient, repeating excitations at any phase encode setting is recommended. The number of repetitions is referred to as Nex, and SNR increases with the square root of Nex.

In the frequency encoding axis the sampling bandwidth determines the range of frequencies sampled. Reducing the sampling bandwidth results in less high frequency noise being sampled and consequently, as the signal remains unaltered, there is an increase in the SNR. In general, the SNR scales inversely proportional to the sampling bandwidth. Therefore, from a SNR perspective, a lower bandwidth is preferable. Other factors, in particular the chemical shift effects, will usually set a limit for the bandwidth which is applied. Furthermore, a lower sampling bandwidth usually increases the minimum TE that can be employed in the sequence, as the readout period becomes longer with a smaller sampling bandwidth.

The choice of pulse sequence also influences the SNR. In spin echo sequences all of the longitudinal magnetization is converted into transverse magnetization, but in gradient echo pulse sequences only a proportion of the longitudinal magnetization is converted into transverse magnetization as in this case the flip angle is less than 90°. As a result of this, the signal is generally greater in spin echo sequences. In summary, SNR can be increased by using a large field of view, a coarse matrix and a large slice thickness. Spin echo sequences, and in particular those with proton density weighting, produce the highest SNR. Additionally, the number of acquisitions should be as high as possible.

3.2.3
Spatial Resolution

The spatial resolution is the ability to distinguish between two points and it improves as voxel size decreases. Separate tissues within the same voxel are not separately visualized on the MR image but separate tissues in adjacent voxels are differentiated. When a voxel contains more than one type of tissue, the signal intensity of that voxel is the average of the signal intensities of the individual tissues and this results in partial volume averaging. There is a direct relationship between the size of the voxel and the resolution, with a small voxel size resulting in better resolution. Therefore, the voxel size in an imaging sequence needs to be adjusted to the anatomic structures which need to be resolved.

The voxel size is a volume of sampled tissue within the patient, and the relationship between voxel size and field of view is indicated in the following equation:

$$\text{Voxel size} = \frac{(\text{FOVread} \times \text{FOVphase} \times \text{slice thickness})}{\text{matrix size} / \text{Nphase}} \quad (1)$$

where FOVread and FOVphase refers to the field of view in the read, and phase encode directions, respectively. The matrix size is usually referred to as the number of frequency encodings, and Nphase refers to the number of phase encodings. In most imaging systems the matrix size is limited to a power of 2, or multiples of 64. The number of phase encodings is flexible, and can be given any number equal or less to the matrix size. Based on Eq. 1 any desired resolution can be achieved (Fig. 3.2). For practical reasons, however, limitations exist with respect to the selection of the parameters which are described in the following:

- FOVread: the field of view in the read direction must be selected to cover the region of interest. Due to the low-pass filtering properties in the frequency encoding direction there is no wraparound artifact even if the object is larger than the FOV. This is the reason why the read direction is always selected to view along the longest dimension along the body.
- FOVphase: the field of view in the phase direction usually corresponds to the FOV in the read direction. A partial FOV can be selected on state-of-the art imaging systems, i.e. the FOV in the phase direction is a fraction of the FOV in the read direction. Partial FOV is useful for saving scan time as fewer phase encode steps are necessary to achieve the same spatial resolution. However, one must be careful in selecting a sufficiently large FOVphase to avoid wrap around artifacts. Unlike in the frequency encoding direction, there is no cutoff of signal intensities outside the dimension of the FOV in the phase encode direction. If the object is larger than the FOVphase, it will be wrapped to the other side, and may obscure important information.

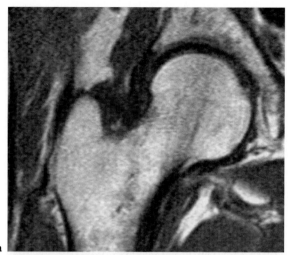

a

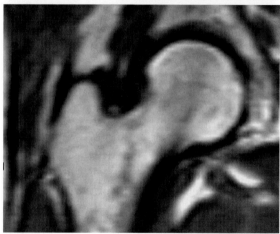

b

Fig. 3.2a,b. The effect of FOV on image quality can be observed. A FOV of 180 cm in (**a**) and 500 cm in (**b**) was used. Large FOV (**b**) causes a decrease of spatial resolution and blurring of image details

Nphase: The number of phase encodes determines the spatial resolution in the phase encode direction. On most commercial imaging systems, the number of phase encodes can be selected independently of the matrix size. A larger Nphase results in a better spatial resolution due to a smaller voxel size. However, the scan time increases as only one phase encode value is acquired per TR interval. Also, SNR decreases with the smaller voxel size.

3.2.4
Scan Time

The scan time Ts of a sequence is given by:

$$Ts = TR \times Nphase \times Nex \tag{2}$$

where TR denotes the pulse repetition time of the sequence and matrix size and Nphase denote the number of frequency and phase encodes, respectively. Nex refers to the number of excitations per each phase encode setting (Nex is also referred to as the number of acquisitions). Ideally, the data acquisition should be completed in the shortest possible time without compromising image quality. Nphase needs to be selected with respect to the necessary spatial resolution in the phase encode direction. As shown before, there are situations where one excitation does not provide sufficient SNR, and multiple repetitions are necessary (Nex > 1). The SNR increases with the square root of Nex, but scan time increases accordingly.

3.2.5
Image Contrast

The matrix size should be selected large enough to obtain sufficient spatial resolution. A larger matrix size will show more details in the object because of the improved spatial resolution (Fig. 3.3). However, the SNR in the image will be correspondingly smaller as shown before. A compromise needs to be made between spatial resolution and SNR based on sequence characteristics, system performance, and clinical needs. The scan time is not primarily affected by the matrix size, as each frequency read-out is acquired during one TR interval. However, on most imaging systems, the number of phase encodes is correlated to the matrix size, i.e. doubling the matrix size will also double the phase encodes which will double the scan time as will be shown later.

All imaging sequences are based on the idea of generating a spin echo which is frequency and phase encoded to create the spatial information. Two major methods are commonly employed to generate the echo following the initial excitation. Each method has specific characteristics which are important for musculoskeletal imaging. In the so-called spin echo technique, a second radio-frequency (RF) pulse is used to reverse the magnetization and form an echo at a time equal to the interval between the two RF pulses. In addition to refocusing of the magnetization, this second RF pulse also reverses the dephasing of magnetization which has occurred due to field inhomogeneities (T2* relaxation). The signal intensity in this pulse sequence decays with a time equal

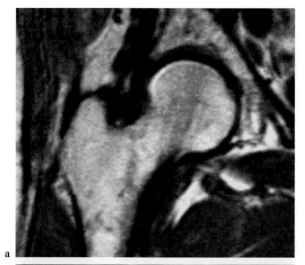

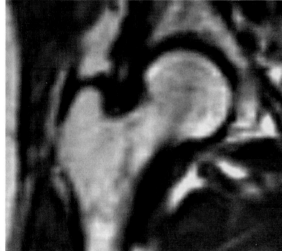

Fig. 3.3a,b. A body array coil was used. Images (**a**) and (**b**) show the effect of the matrix on image quality. In (**a**) the matrix was 320×320 and in (**b**) 103×128. There was no change of further image parameters. Image quality in (**b**) is definitely worse compared to (**a**)

gradient. Due to the absence of an 180° refocusing pulse the dephasing of the transverse magnetization due to magnetic field inhomogeneities cannot be compensated for, and the signal decays with T2* (T2* relaxation). T2* relaxation is generally shorter than T2 relaxation time, and can be much shorter depending on the actual field inhomogeneities. The longer the echo time (TE), the stronger the signal attenuation due to T2* will be. A good homogeneity is required to obtain optimal results. In a gradient echo sequence the flip angle can be smaller than 90°, as the echo is created by gradients, not a refocusing RF pulse. Therefore, much shorter TR times can be applied without saturation of the spins. This allows new applications such as 3D imaging which is not possible with the spin echo sequences due to excessive scan time because of the long TR times.

3.3
Pulse Sequences

3.3.1
T1-Weighted Spin Echo Sequence

TI-weighted spin echo images (T1-SE) are obtained with a relatively short TR. The echo time TE is chosen to be as small as possible to minimize T2 signal decay, and keep a pure T1 contrast. As a result of the short TR, structures with a long T1 relaxation time become progressively saturated and demonstrate low signal intensity (e.g. muscles and fluid-containing structures). Fat, however, which has a very short T1, demonstrates high signal intensity. T1-SE in the hip is used primarily for evaluation of bone marrow disorders such as avascular necrosis and detecting fractures or overuse syndromes (Fig. 3.4).

3.3.2
T2-Weighted Spin Echo Sequence

T2-weighted spin echo images (T2-SE) are obtained with a relatively long TR to minimize T1 saturation effects. The echo time TE is chosen to show differences in the T2 relaxation times. This occurs at echo times of around 60–100 ms. At this TE all body fluids produce a high signal intensity due to its T2 relaxation characteristics. Muscle, however, is of relatively low signal intensity and fat is of intermediate signal intensity. The SNR in these images is inferior to the SNR in proton density-weighted

to the T2 relaxation time, and the T2* decay has been eliminated by the refocussing process. As a result of the 180° refocusing pulse, the contrast in spin echo images is related to the T1 and T2 relaxation times of the tissues and to the chosen TR and TE. As a result of the 90° excitation pulse in the spin echo sequence, the TR must be relatively long in the order of the T1 times of the tissue to make sure that the spins have sufficiently recovered between TR intervals to produce enough magnetization.

The other method, gradient echo imaging, simply uses gradient pulses to generate a gradient echo. A negative dephasing pulse is followed by the positive readout gradient, and an echo is formed right when the dephasing is compensated for by the readout

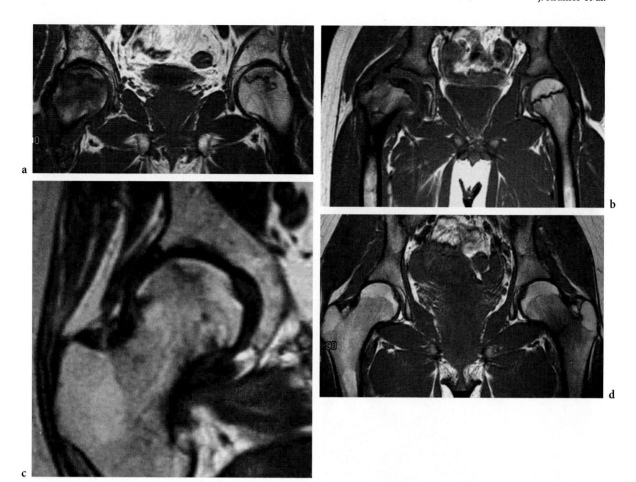

Fig. 3.4a–d. T1-weighted SE images. **a** Bilateral avascular necrosis of the femoral head. The necrotic area is clearly delineated from adjacent bone. On the right side concomitant bone marrow edema is visible. **b** Perthes disease of the right hip. In contrast to the normal fatty marrow of the epiphysis of the left hip on the right side signal alterations due to edema, granulation tissue, and sclerosis can be observed. **c** In the weight-bearing zone of the femoral head a fine fissure almost imitating an early change of necrosis can be seen. **d** A typical stress fracture at the medial aspect of the left femoral neck is evident

images, but the pathology, which is characterized by an increased fluid content, is accentuated. T2-SE are rarely used in evaluation of the hip because of the advantages of fast (turbo) spin echo T2 weighted images.

3.3.3
Proton Density-Weighted Spin Echo Images

Proton density-weighted spin echo images (PD-SE) are obtained with a long TR and short TE and provide signal which reflects the density of protons within the imaging field. The TR must be long enough to make sure that all tissues have sufficiently recovered during the TR interval. In

general, the choice of the TR also depends on the field strength as the T1 relaxation times tend to increase with higher field strengths. Similar to the T1-weighted sequences, the echo time TE is chosen to be as small as possible to minimize T2 signal decay. Because the T1 and T2 effects are minimized the PD-SE images have a high SNR and are useful for providing anatomical detail. In an effort to keep the scan time relatively short, the TR is not always used as long as it should be to reduce T1 saturation effects. The choice of TE is also subject to some constraints. For bandwidth and gradient performance considerations the minimum TE is usually around 10–20 ms. Therefore, some T1 and T2 effects are still noticeable in the image contrast of a PD-SE imaging sequence.

3.3.4
Fast Spin Echo Sequences

One of the time-limiting factors with the spin echo sequences is the fact that only one echo is generated per TR interval. In a modification called fast SE (FSE), or turbo SE (TSE) several echoes are generated using multiple 180° refocusing pulses. Each echo is individually phase encoded, and scan time is reduced proportionally. The number of echoes produced after one excitation pulse is called echo train length (ETL). Using the fast spin echo technique, proton density, T2-weighted, and T1-weighted SE images can be obtained in a fraction of the time required for conventional spin echo sequences. The downside of the fast spin echo technique is related to the signal variation of the individual echoes due to T2 decay. As a result fast spin echo images are susceptible to blurring and edge artifacts which is particularly noticeable for very long echo trains. In practice, these artifacts can be minimized by using a short echo train length and a long effective TE. Another difference to the conventional spin echo sequence is the appearance of fat. Due to the many refocusing pulses applied in the fast spin echo technique, fat appears of higher signal intensity, while solid structures are of lower signal intensity than in conventional spin echo images. FSE sequences are routinely used in the evaluation of the hip, often with the addition of fat suppression. These sequences are excellent at detecting bone marrow edema as well as soft tissue pathology such as masses, infection, or muscle injuries (Fig. 3.5).

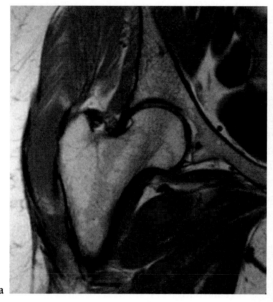

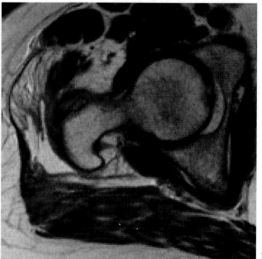

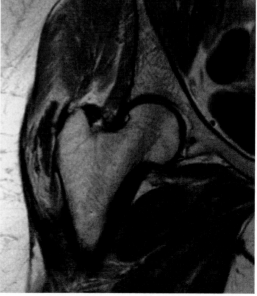

Fig. 3.5a–c. a T1-weighted SE (spin echo) image; **b** fast T2-weighted SE image; **c** T1-weighted SE after intravenous contrast administration. Adjacent to the major trochanter a fluid collection (bright on T2-weighting, rim enhancement after contrast can be seen due to bursitis)

3.3.5
Gradient Echo Sequences

In a gradient echo sequence the transverse magnetization is generated by a flip angle which is smaller than 90°. Magnetic field radiant pulses are used to dephase and rephase the transverse component of the magnetization, and generate an echo. Any magnetic field inhomogeneities will effect the amount of signal at the echo. This is known as the T2* effect.

Some institutions use gradient echo images to assess hyaline cartilage, particularly in conjunction with fat suppression. Gradient echo images do not provide adequate visualization of bone marrow edema and they are not recommended for the evaluation of bony pathology (Fig. 3.6). However, they may be useful if assessment of lesions of the hyaline cartilage has to be performed.

Similar to spin echo sequences the tissue contrast can be adjusted by proper selection of the imaging parameters. T1-weighted gradient echo images are obtained by the combination of a large flip angle, short TR and short TE. T2*-weighted images can be generated by a small flip angle and a TR which is relatively long in order to permit sufficient recovery of the longitudinal magnetization of the spins. Gradient echo images have scan times which can be significantly shorter than spin echo images. This is due to the shorter TR which is associated with the smaller excitation angle. The main disadvantage is their susceptibility to magnetic field inhomogeneities.

Gradient echo sequences are frequently used to obtain volume, or 3D acquisitions. This technique is particularly useful for the detection of subtle alterations of joint structures. With volume acquisitions a sub-millimeter, isotropic resolution can be obtained. The small voxels also help to minimize susceptibility-related signal intensity losses which are associated with gradient echo sequences. An entire volume of tissue is imaged and the volume is subdivided into thin sections using a second phase encoding gradient along the slice selection gradient. The scan time in the volume acquisition is defined as:

$$Ts = TR \times Nphase1 \times Nphase2 \times Nex \qquad (3)$$

where Nphase1 and Nphase2 refer to the number of phase encodings in the conventional phase encode direction, and in the slice select direction, respectively. Nex is usually set to be 1 to keep the scan time within an acceptable range. Unlike in multi-slice 2D imaging, there is no inter-slice gap and no cross-talk between individual slices which enables a perfect means of postprocessing. In order to be able to reconstruct the object in multiple planes without a reduction in image quality it is essential that the voxels are isotropic, or nearly isotropic.

Volume imaging generates large datasets with a requirement for considerable storage capacity. Obtaining hardcopy of all available images is impractical. Images are typically viewed on image processing workstations which allow quick and easy multi-planar reconstructions. The isotropic three-dimensional resolution is particularly useful for visualizing very small structures and for reformatting images of structures which do not lie in a single anatomical plane, such as ligaments or the labrum.

3.3.6
Echo Planar Imaging

Echo planar imaging (EPI) is a fast imaging technique in which multiple gradient echoes are acquired for each excitation. In effect, EPI is the gradient echo equivalent of fast spin echo imaging. There is only one excitation pulse and all of the echoes are obtained from this using gradient reversal. Therefore, movement artifacts do not occur with these very fast imaging times. However, due to the long echo readout most of the signal is lost by T2* decay, and, therefore, single-shot EPI techniques are

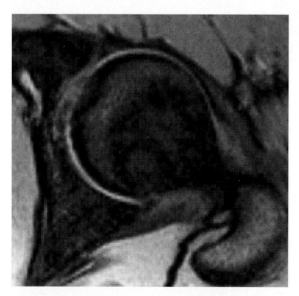

Fig. 3.6. T1-weighted two-dimensional gradient echo (2D GE) image in axial orientation. Hyaline cartilage appears bright and can be differentiated from adjacent bony structures

not used for imaging of the hip. The T2* sensitivity is reduced considerably when using only a small number of echoes after the excitation pulse. In a so-called multi-shot approach all of the raw data are acquired in repeated excitations with different phase encoding values. In the future it may play a role in dynamic studies of the hip joint during movement and in MR fluoroscopy for the assessment of the containment of joint structures and for guiding interventional procedures.

3.3.7
Steady State Free Precession Sequences

For steady state free precession (SSFP) sequences, the pulse sequence is designed so that the phase coherence of the transverse magnetization is maintained from repetition to repetition. This is different from the gradient echo sequences where the transverse magnetization is spoiled after each repetition using spoiler gradient and RF spoiling techniques. Thus the transverse magnetization generated by a given excitation RF pulse may contribute to the signal measured in many succeeding echo periods. Because phase coherence is maintained, the complete magnetization vector is in a steady state from repetition to repetition during the free precession between RF pulses.

The SSFP pulse-sequence configuration of the two signal components generated by a train of equally spaced RF pulses. Images can be formed from the FID component (fast imaging with steady state precession, FISP), from the echo component (time-reversed FISP, i.e. PSIF), or from a combination of the two components. Because both the FID and echo signals represent a superposition of many individual coherent pathways, the equations describing the signal behavior for these two components are much more complicated than those for a spin echo, or gradient echo sequence. In general, the signals depend on both T1 and T2 in a complex and mathematically inseparable way. Nonetheless, some statements can be made concerning the general contrast properties for FISP-type pulse sequences: first, contrast weighting that depends on T1 and T2 occurs at short TR and high flip angle. Second, proton-density weighting occurs at low flip angle and short TE, and third, T2* weighting occurs at low flip angle and long TE.

In summary, imaging with SSFP sequences is a flexible technique for the rapid acquisition of MR images that can provide a wide variety of image contrast behaviors. However, the SNRs obtained with SSFP sequences are often lower than those obtained for SE-based techniques. In addition, true T2 weighting cannot be obtained, because the signal decay for long echo time GRE and SSFP sequences includes the effect of field inhomogeneities. In some applications this sensitivity to field inhomogeneities is an important contrast mechanism, but in imaging of the hip joint it mostly degrades the image quality.

3.3.8
Dual Echo in Steady State Sequences

A modification of the basic SSFP sequence produces the so-called dual echo in steady state (DESS) sequence. In this sequence a dual echo readout is applied to collect both the FISP and the PSIF signal simultaneously. Both images show the identical anatomical structures with different contrast. The overlay of both images creates an unusual contrast in which anatomical structures are displayed with good overall contrast, and fluids are shown with very high signal intensity. With the inherently high SNR the DESS technique can provide for tissues with long T1 and T2 relaxation times, the DESS sequence is well suited for applications that benefit from high contrast between fluid and surrounding tissue (Fig. 3.7).

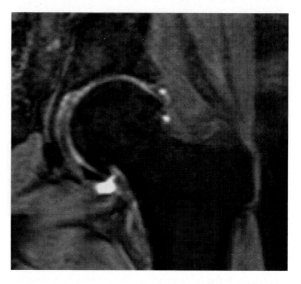

Fig. 3.7. DESS image. Fluid shows high signal intensity and thus enables differentiation from hyaline cartilage

3.3.9
Fat Suppression Techniques

Three methods of fat suppression are in use (DEL-FAUT et al. 1999). These are fat saturation, inversion recovery technique and opposed phase imaging. The last-mentioned technique is principally used for the detection of small amounts of fat in lesions, e.g. adrenal gland tumors. It may also be used for the evaluation of bone marrow diseases (DISLER et al. 1997).

In the selective fat saturation technique an RF pulse with the same resonance frequency as fat is preceding every slice-selection RF pulse. The magnetization from fat is dephased using a spoiling gradient pulse to remove all signal from lipid structures. This technique is referred to as CHESS (chemical selective saturation) as it saturates tissues according to their chemical nature (which is related to the resonance frequency). Consequently, no signal from fat is visible on MR images. The advantages of this technique are that only fat is suppressed and all other tissues are not affected, and it may be combined with any imaging sequence. It is useful in post-contrast scanning, e.g. following intravenous contrast enhancement and MR arthrography. The fat saturation technique has a number of disadvantages, however. Fat saturation may be unreliable due to inhomogeneities in the static magnetic field. These inhomogeneities result in imperfect fat saturation, and partial saturation of other tissues. State-of-the

art imaging systems provide adequate field homogeneity to get good fat saturation, and, if necessary, the homogeneity can be further improved by shimming techniques. The water component of fat and some fatty acids are not suppressed and can result in inadequately fat-suppressed images. Fat suppression may be poor with magnets of low field strength because the chemical shift between lipid and water increases with the magnetic field strength. Another disadvantage of the CHESS technique is that the fatsat pulse requires extra time. This results in fewer slices in a multi-slice imaging sequence (assuming the TR is kept constant), or requires an increase in the TR in an effort to keep the same number of slices with a corresponding increase in scan time.

The inversion recovery sequence (short T1 inversion recovery – STIR – sequence uses the differences between the T1 of fat and water. Following a 180° inversion pulse the magnetization of fat recovers much faster than that of water. By applying the 90° pulse at the null point of fat (the point at which the longitudinal magnetization equals zero), the signal from fat is completely suppressed. One advantage of this technique is that it can be employed on low field strength magnets and it is not affected by main magnetic field inhomogeneities. The T2 and T1 differences are combined, resulting in high tissue contrast (water appears very bright). Therefore, edema in soft tissues as well as in bone marrow is detected with high sensitivity (Fig. 3.8). However, there are several disadvantages of this technique. SNR is relatively

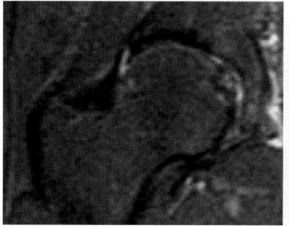
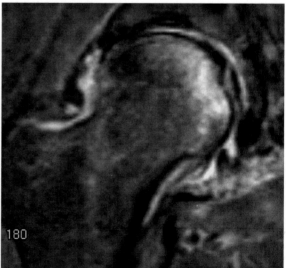

Fig. 3.8.a,b. Turbo inversion recovery sequence. In a normal hip (**a**) the signal from fatty marrow is suppressed. Minimal joint fluid (hyperintense signal) is visible. **b** Patient had suffered a hip trauma. Moderate hyperintense signal alteration in the femoral head (typical for bone contusion) is visible

low, which influences the spatial resolution directly. Tissues with a similar T1 to fat are also suppressed, for example mucoid tissue, hemorrhage, proteinaceous fluid, melanin and gadolinium. For this reason inversion recovery images are not suitable for MR arthrography or examinations after intravenous application of contrast material. Second, tissues with a short T1 and long T1 may have the same signal on inversion recovery images, and cannot be distinguished from each other. Spin echo and fast spin echo sequences are the only sequences which are suitable for use with inversion recovery techniques. Fat suppression techniques are employed in the hip for improvement of sensitivity of bone marrow edema and the suppression of normal fat in post-gadolinium imaging. This may either be in MR arthrography or following intravenous gadolinium. The fat saturation technique (CHESS) is most effective for post-gadolinium scanning. Fat suppression techniques are also used to assist tissue characterization. This is especially true for the detection of bone marrow edema and demonstration of the extent of infiltration by tumor. Either fat saturation or inversion recovery techniques may be employed for these purposes and these sequences are a mainstay of hip MR imaging.

3.3.10
Magnetization Transfer Technique

In tissues the hydrogen being imaged consists of two exchanging pools: freely mobile water protons and restricted motion macromolecular protons. Magnetization transfer contrast makes use of the fact that protons bound in macromolecules do not participate directly in the production of the MR signal whereas free protons in water do. Although the center frequencies of these two groups are the same, the restricted protons have a much shorter T2 and thus a much broader resonance. With magnetization transfer contrast sequences, low-power radiofrequency irradiation is applied off resonance to selectively saturate protons with a short T2. Consequently, the partially saturated protons emit less signal and therefore tissues which contain bound water demonstrate lower signal intensity on magnetization contrast images (WOLF et al. 1991; BALABAN and CECKLER 1992). In this way the contrast generally resembles that of T2-weighted images and considerable signal is lost in solid tissues but this does not occur in fluid or adipose tissue. Magnetization contrast, therefore, provides unique information regarding the interaction between water and macromolecules.

3.4
MR Arthrography

3.4.1
Introduction

MRI has been shown to be very useful in the diagnosis of several joint disorders. The use of MR arthrography is increasing due to its improved accuracy compared with conventional MRI for the diagnosis of several intra-articular disorders.

3.4.2
Techniques for MR Arthrography of the Hip

In our institution MR arthrography of the hip is performed as a two-step procedure. Joint injection is usually performed under fluoroscopy followed by MR imaging. The patient is in supine position with the leg extended and slightly internally rotated. The puncture site is marked on the skin between the subcapital and transcervical portions of the femoral neck. This point is lateral to the femoral artery and below the inguinal ligament. Under sterile conditions, a 20-gauge disposable needle is directed straight onto the femoral neck (Fig. 3.9). A few drops of iodinated contrast agent are injected through an extension tube (to avoid radiation exposure to the hands) to confirm intra-articular location; following this 10–20 ml of the Gd-DTPA solution is injected into the joint.

An alternative method of streamlining intra-articular injections when performing conventional MR imaging prior to the MR arthrographic portion of the examination was reported recently (MILLER 2000). By this technique the total MR examination time can be shortened by eliminating a visit to the fluoroscopy suite in the middle of the MR study. The lower extremity is held in neutral or slight internal rotation by tapering the feet together. A metal marker is placed over the middle of the femoral neck, and the skin is marked. If contrast is needed, the injection can be performed on the MR table. An MR-compatible plastic cart with drawers containing arthrography supplies is used. The feet are taped together as they were in the fluoroscopy suite, and a 22-gauge needle is placed straight down until bone is reached.

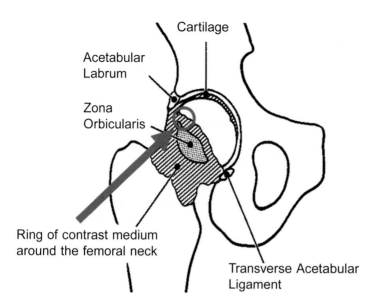

Cartilage

Acetabular
Labrum

Zona
Orbicularis

Ring of contrast medium
around the femoral neck

Transverse Acetabular
Ligament

Fig. 3.9. A schematic drawing of the right hip joint with the *arrow* pointing to the injection site (*circle*). The *dark area* shows the distribution of contrast material initially after injection

Low resistance to the injection confirms the needle position. Although this technique uses fluoroscopy to landmark the joint of interest, the fluoroscopy portion of the procedure can be performed at any time prior to the MR examination, thus uncoupling the fluoroscopy and MR schedules from each other and allowing the arthrographic portion of the study to be performed in the MR suite immediately after the conventional MR portion.

Because of the spherical nature of the hip, imaging in all three planes is necessary to evaluate joint and in particular labrum. T1-weighted imaging is used to visualize the high signal of the intra-articular contrast solution. Fat saturation increases contrast between the intra-articular gadopentetate dimeglumine and the adjacent soft tissues. Fat suppression is crucial in MR arthrography because fat and contrast medium have similar signal intensities on T1-weighted images. The combination of MR arthrography and three-dimensional gradient recalled echo-imaging shows a higher sensitivity for subtle lesions than MR arthrography with spin echo sequences (KRAMER et al. 1992).

MR arthrography is performed by injecting a gadolinium-diethylenetriamine pentaacetic acid (Gd-DTPA) mixture into the joint. A Gd-DTPA mixture consisting of 0.2 ml of a standard Gd-DTPA solution (469.01 mg/ml, Magnevist, Schering AG, Germany) mixed with 50 ml of saline (2 mmol/l Gd-DTPA solution) allows excellent delineation of contrast medium and the intra-articular structures or abnormalities (ENGEL et al. 1990). No side effects have been reported to date that are attributable to intra-articular Gd-DTPA. Imaging should be per-

formed immediately after the intra-articular injection of contrast medium, to prevent absorption of contrast solution and guarantee the desired capsular distention, although imaging delays of up to 1–2 h are tolerated (WAGNER et al. 2001). Gd-DTPA and iodinated contrast material can be mixed before MRI without any release of free gadolinium and is safe for confirming the intra-articular placement of contrast material (BROWN et al. 2000).

It has been shown that intravenous administration of Gd-DTPA also leads to an enhancement effect of the joint cavity (indirect MR arthrography). This technique has been proposed as an alternative to direct MR arthrography (VAHLENSIECK et al. 1995, 1996, 1997; WINALSKI et al. 1991; KRAMER et al. 1997; PEH et al. 1999). The enhancement effect, however, is only mild and often heterogeneous, although exercise improves both the homogeneity and amount of enhancement in the joint. However, there are several drawbacks of this technique. The main limitation is the relative lack of joint distention, which is frequently necessary to accurately diagnose capsular trauma and soft tissue injury. A further drawback of indirect MR arthrography is that juxta-articular structures, such as vessels, and the synovial membranes of bursae and tendon sheaths also demonstrate enhancement, which may lead to confusion with extravasation of contrast medium or the presence of abnormal joint recesses. Patients who have undergone MR arthrography reported discomfort to be less than expected (ROBBINS et al. 2000). Arthrography-related discomfort was well tolerated and rated less severe than MRI-related discomfort.

3.4.3
Anatomy of the Hip Joint

The hip is a ball-and-socket joint, which exhibits a wide range of motion in all directions. The spherical acetabular socket covers the femoral head nearly completely except for its inferior medial aspect, known as the acetabular notch, where the socket is deficient. The transverse acetabular ligament spans this deficient portion of the acetabulum. The fibrocartilaginous labrum rims the acetabulum and is triangular in cross section. The labrum is thicker posterosuperiorly and thinner anteroinferiorly (KEENE and VILLAR 1994; TSCHAUNER et al. 1997). The acetabular labrum consists of fibrocartilaginous tissue with fibrovascular bundles. This fibrocartilage lacks the highly organized structure seen within the fibrocartilaginous meniscus of the knee. The labrum is attached directly to the osseous rim of the acetabulum. It blends with the transverse ligament at the margins of the acetabular notch. Contrary to the shoulder, the acetabular labrum increase the depth of the joint rather than increasing its diameter (ENGEL et al. 1990). Clinical and arthroscopic studies have documented the importance of the acetabular capsular-labral complex as a biomechanical component of the hip joint (SUZUKI et al. 1986; UEO et al. 1990). The joint capsule inserts onto the acetabular rim. Along the anterior and posterior joint margins, the capsule inserts directly at the base of the labrum; a small perilabral recess is created between the labrum and joint capsule. The iliopsoas bursa, directly anterior to the hip joint, communicates with the joint in 10%–15% of normal anatomic specimens and may be involved in patients with synovitis (WILLIAMS and WARWICK 1980).

3.4.4
Labral Lesions

Among several possible causes for chronic hip pain acetabular labral tears are a relatively rare entity. Labral lesions may be observed in patients with developmental dysplasia of the hips, and in patients with a history of hip trauma (DAMERON 1959; DORELL and CATTERALL 1986; FITZGERALD 1995; KLAUE et al. 1991; McCARTHY and BUSCONI 1995a,b). In patients suffering from hip dysplasia, the increased stress on the acetabulum and on the superior labrum as it assumes more of the weight-bearing function is believed to contribute to development of the tears (KLAUE et al. 1991). Posttraumatic labral tears may occur following minor or major trauma particularly hip dislocations. Degenerative tears may also occur. Early recognition and debridement can result in substantial pain relief and may prevent development of degenerative disease (ALTENBERG 1977). Conventional MR imaging is not accurate for the diagnosis of labral tears (CZERNY et al. 1996, 1999; LEUNIG et al. 1997; PETERSILGE et al. 1996; PETERSILGE 1997, 2000, 2001; KRAMER et al. 2002; STEINBACH et al. 2002). There are several causes for this, the most important being inadequate joint distention that prevents separation of the labrum and capsule.

A classification system for the evaluation of acetabular labral lesions by MR arthrography was established by CZERNY et al. (1996). Normal labra (stage 0), are of homogeneous low signal intensity, triangular shaped, and a continuous attachment to the lateral margin of the acetabulum without a notch or a sulcus is visible. A recess between the joint capsule and the labrum, a so-called labral recess, is observed. Stage 1A lesions are characterized by an area of increased signal intensity within the center of the labrum that does not extend to the margin of the labrum, a triangular shape, and a continuous attachment to the lateral margin of the acetabulum and a labral recessus (Fig. 3.10). Stage 1B is similar to stage 1A, but the labrum is thickened and in most patients no labral recessus can be observed. These findings are similar to the mucoid degeneration seen in low-grade meniscal lesions. In stage 2A lesions an extension of contrast material into the labrum without detachment from the acetabulum is visible (Fig. 3.11). In this stage the labrum is triangular, and has a labral recessus. Stage 2B are the same as stage 2A except the torn labrum is thickened (Fig. 3.12). Stage 2 findings are consistent with partial labral tears. Stage 3A labra, complete labral tears, are detached from the acetabulum but are of triangular shape, whereas stage 3B labra are thickened and detached from the acetabulum (Fig. 3.13).

Contrast material enables the visualization of the labral recessus and the clear delineation of the capsular-labral complex (HODLER et al. 1995). However, labral lesions may be staged incorrectly even with MR arthrography if only a small volume of contrast material is injected or there is a scarred, shrunken joint capsule caused by previous surgical interventions.

A wide spectrum of appearances has been described for the labrum in asymptomatic individuals. However, the majority of these findings have been based on studies performed without joint distention. It is unclear whether the described appearances represent variations in normal anatomy or

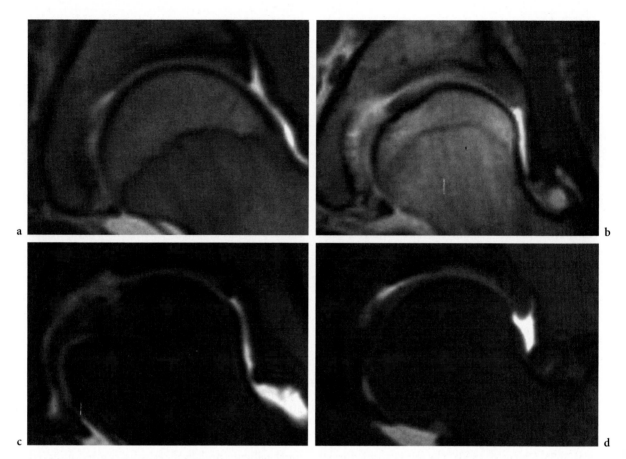

Fig. 3.10a–d. After administration of contrast material. T1-weighted SE (**a,b**) and T1-weighted SE sequence with fat suppression (**c,d**). **a,c** Normal labrum (type 0). **b,d** Labrum is enlarged (type 1B). No tear is visible. The contrast material is delineating the intraarticular joint structures very well

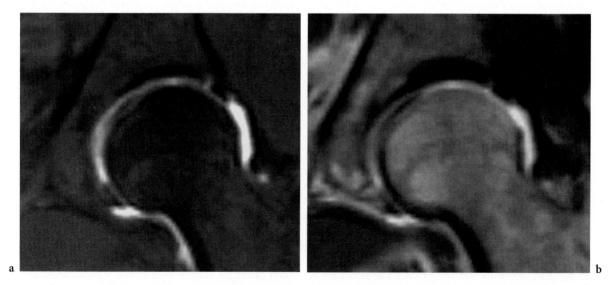

Fig. 3.11a,b. T1 weighted (SE sequence) MR arthrogram with and without fat suppression. A small tear is visible in the craniolateral portion of the labrum (type 2A)

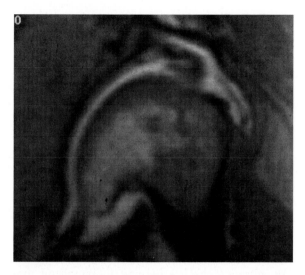

Fig. 3.12. T1-weighted SE image after intraarticular instillation of a Gd-DTPA solution. A patient with severe hip dysplasia. The labrum shows signal alterations and it is enlarged. A horizontal tear is visible (type 2B)

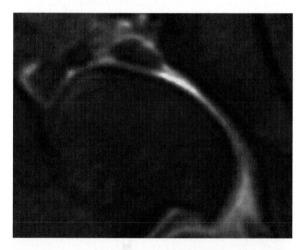

Fig. 3.13. Fat suppressed T1-weighted MR arthrogram. Patient suffering from hip dysplasia shows a completely torn labrum which is slightly detached from the acetabular rim (surrounded by contrast material) (type 3B)

asymptomatic abnormalities. Controversy remains regarding the reality of a sublabral sulcus of the anterosuperior aspect of the labrum. The presence of a sublabral sulcus has been raised as the possibility of a potential pitfall in the diagnosis of acetabular labral abnormalities with MR imaging (LECOUVET et al. 1996). However, the clinical implications of an absent labrum and of a sulcus between the labrum and the acetabulum anterosuperiorly are not known. Such a sulcus has been described in histologic specimens of fetal hips, however, although the possibility that its existence is artifactual because of fixation techniques

has been raised (WALKER 1981). It is believed that any intralabral collection of contrast material should not be mistaken for a normal sublabral sulcus but, rather, should be suspected to be a tear or detachment (CZERNY et al. 2002). In contrast PETERSILGE (2000) observed such a sulcus commonly on MR arthrographic images, located consistently at the anterosuperior aspect of the joint. Because of the consistent location of this finding and the well-defined margins of the sulcus as well as the presence of a well-defined insertion onto the subchondral bone some believe that this appearance is likely an anatomic variant.

Another potential pitfall with MR arthrography is a groove separating the acetabular labrum from acetabular articular cartilage in the region of the acetabular fossa (KEENE and VILLAR 1994). This groove should not be confused with a labral tear because its location is different from that of labral tears, which occur most frequently anterosuperiorly. No instances of absent labra are reported (LECOUVET et al. 1996). Sensitivity, specificity, and accuracy for detection and correct staging of labral lesions with MR arthrography has been reported to be 91%, 71%, and 88% respectively, while the sensitivity and accuracy of conventional MR imaging was 30% and 36% (CZERNY et al. 1996, 1999). Because labral abnormalities are believed to be a precursor of osteoarthritis, early interventions is thought to be critical in the treatment of labral abnormalities. The determination of the type, extension, and location of labral abnormalities as shown with MR arthrography is helpful in such treatment (HODLER et al. 1995).

3.4.5
Loose Bodies

Loose bodies in the hip joint are rare but may cause chronic joint pain, locking, and limited range of motion and may occur with or without associated osteochondral defects. In patients with suspected intra-articular loose bodies, the value of an imaging examination is determined by its capabilities for excluding the presence of loose bodies and decreasing the need for diagnostic arthroscopy (HAIMS et al. 1998; PALMER 1998). Frequently, intra-articular loose bodies cannot be differentiated from surrounding tissues on conventional MR imaging. If there is joint fluid present conventional T2-weighted sequences may help to differentiate loose bodies from surrounding structures. In some patients specificity may be decreased, however, because of the difficulty in differentiating true loose bodies from osteophytes, synovial folds, and hypertrophic synovitis. Characteristically, on MR arthrography loose bodies are surrounded by contrast material, which improves their detection and enables an accurate determination of their number and topography. Arthroscopic techniques offering the least traumatic method of removing loose bodies of foreign bodies from the hip joint are preferred to open arthrotomy, although arthroscopy of the hip is still not widely practiced (Die et al. 1991). Only the accurate detection of these lesions may allow early therapeutic intervention, however, and relief of pain, and prevent or delay the development of osteoarthritis (Czerny et al. 1996, 1999, 2001). In addition, the diagnostic sensitivity and specificity of MR arthrography in detecting intra-articular bodies is improved because contrast solution separates loose bodies from the capsule and completely surrounds them, whereas osteophytes and synovial projections are only partially outlined.

3.4.6
Cystic Lesions

Ganglion cyst have been reported in association with labral tears (Haller et al. 1989; Czerny et al. 1999; Petersilge et al. 1996; Klaue et al. 1991; Magee and Hinson 2000; Schnarkowski et al. 1996). These cysts typically start out as extra-articular soft tissue collections and may eventually erode into the adjacent acetabulum. The erosion created in the acetabulum may be visible on plain films and may be a clue to labral pathology as the underlying cause of hip pain. Additionally it has been suggested that when perilabral cysts are identified a search for an underlying labral tear should be undertaken. These cysts appear to have an increased frequency in those patients with associated developmental dysplasia (McCarthy and Busconi 1995b).

3.4.7
Cartilage Lesions

On MR images and at histologic analysis hyaline cartilage of the hip joint has shown a thickness of 1–2 mm (Hodler et al. 1992). In contrast, articular cartilage of the knee may be up to 7 mm in diameter, with the highest values in the patella (Ahn et al. 1998). Cartilage lesions of the hip are not uncommon in young and middle-aged patients who are suspected of having femoroacetabular impingement and/or labral abnormalities (Schmid et al. 2003)

(Fig. 3.14). These defects are mostly found in the anterosuperior part of the acetabulum. The diagnostic performance of MR arthrography in the detection of articular cartilage damage in the hip joint is inferior to that in the knee joint with sensitivities and specificities of MR arthrographic detection of cartilage damage slightly below 80%. This may be due to the relatively thin cartilage in the hip leading to volume averaging of the cartilage layer with adjacent bone, and intraarticular contrast material due to the spherical shape of the femoral head.

3.4.8
Conclusions

MR arthrography has become an important tool for the evaluation of a variety of articular disorders providing new insights into the lesions underlying mechanical hip pain. Although not necessary in all patients, MR arthrography may facilitate the evaluation of patients with suspected intra-articular pathology in whom conventional MR imaging is not sufficient for an adequate therapy planning. This technique combines arthrographic advantages, like joint distention and delineation of intra-articular structures, with the high quality of MR imaging. Diagnostic confidence can frequently be improved by MR arthrography, particularly in the assessment of subtle lesions and complex anatomic structures. MR arthrography has been proven especially useful in patients with suspected acetabular labral lesions, osteochondral defects or loose bodies.

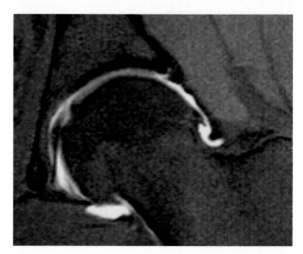

Fig. 3.14. Fat suppressed T1-weighted image after intra-articular contrast application. At the lateral aspect of the femoral head a severe cartilage thinning and a small osteophyte is visible. The labrum appears torn craniolaterally

References

Ahn JM, Kwak SM, Kang HS et al (1998) Evaluation of patellar cartilage in cadavers with a low-field-strength extremity-only magnet: comparison of MR imaging sequences, with macroscopic findings as the standard. Radiology 208:57–62

Altenberg AR (1977) Acetabular labrum tears: a cause of hip pain and degenerative arthritis. South Med J 70:174–175

Balaban RS, Ceckler TL (1992) Magnetization transfer contrast in magnetic resonance imaging. Magn Reson Q 8:116

Brown RR, Clarke DW, Daffner RH (2000) Is a mixture of gadolinium and iodinated contrast material safe during MR arthrography? AJR Am J Roentgenol 175:1087–90

Czerny C, Hofmann S, Neuhold A et al (1996) Lesions of the acetabular labrum: accuracy of MR imaging and arthrography in detection and staging. Radiology 200:225–230

Czerny C, Hofmann S, Urban M et al (1999) MR arthrography of the adult acetabular capsular-labral complex: correlation with surgery and anatomy. AJR Am J Roentgenol 173:345–349

Czerny C, Kramer J, Neuhold A, Urban M, Tschauner C, Hofmann S (2001) Magnetresonanztomographie und Magnetresonanzarthrographie des Labrum acetabulare: Vergleich mit operativen Ergebnissen. Fortschr Röntgenstr 173:702–707

Czerny C, Oschatz E, Tschauner C, Hofmann S, Kramer J (2002) MR-Arthrographie des Hüftgelenks. Radiologie 42:451–456

Dameron TB (1959) Bucket-handle tear of acetabular labrum accompanying posterior dislocation of the hip. J Bone Joint Surg Am 41:131–134

Delfaut EM, Beltran J, Johnson G et al (1999) Fat suppression in MR imaging: techniques and pitfalls. Radiographics 19:373–382

Die T, Akamatsu N, Nakajima I (1991) Arthroscopic surgery of the hip joint. Arthroscopy 7:204–211

Disler DG, McCauley TR, Ratner LM et al (1997) In-phase and out-of-phase MR imaging of bone marrow: prediction of neoplasia based on the detection of coexistent fat and water. AJR 169:1439–1447

Dorell JH, Catterall A (1986) The torn acetabular labrum. J Bone Joint Surg Br 68:400–403

Engel A, Hajek PD, Kramer J (1990) Magnetic resonance knee arthrography. Acta Orthop Scand 61 [Suppl 240]:1–47

Fitzgerald RH (1995) Acetabular labrum tears. Clin Orthop 311:60–68

Haims A, Katz LD, Busconi B (1998) MR arthrography of the hip. Magn Reson Imaging Clin North Am 6:871–883

Haller J, Resnick D, Greenway G et al (1989) Juxtaacetabular ganglionic (or synovial) cysts: CT and MR features. J Comput Assist Tomogr 13:976–983

Heron C, Hine A (2002) Magnetic resonance imaging. In: Imaging of the knee – technique and applications. Davies AM, Cassar-Pullicino VN (Editors) Springer, Berlin Heidelberg New York, pp 41–63

Hodler J, Trudell D, Pathria MN, Resnick D (1992) Width of the articular cartilage of the hip: quantification by using fat-suppression spin-echo MR imaging in cadavers .Am J Roentgenol 159:351–355

Hodler J, Yu JS, Goodwin D et al (1995) MR arthrography of the hip: improved imaging of the acetabular labrum with histologic correlation in cadavers. Am J Roentgenol 165:887–891

Keene GS, Villar RN (1994) Arthroscopic anatomy of the hip: an in vivo study. Arthroscopy 10:392–399

Klaue K, Durnin CW, Ganz R (1991) The acetabular rim syndrome. J Bone Joint Surg Br 73:423–429

Kramer J, Recht MP (2002) MR arthrography of the lower extremity. Radiol Clin North Am 40:1121–1132

Kramer J, Stiglbauer R, Engel A et al (1992) MR contrast arthrography (MRA) in osteochondrosis dissecans. J Comput Assist Tomogr 18:254–260

Kramer J, Scheurecker A, Engel A et al (1997) Magnetic resonance arthrography: benefits and indications. Adv MRI Contrast 4:104–119

Lecouvet FE, Vande Berg BC, Malghem J et al (1996) MR imaging of the acetabular labrum: variations in 200 asymptomatic hips. AJR Am J Roentgenol 167:1025–1028

Leunig M, Werlen S, Ungerböck A et al (1997) Evaluation of the acetabular labrum by MR arthrography. J Bone Joint Surg Br 79:230–234

Magee T, Hinson G (2000) Association of paralabral cysts with acetabular disorders. Am J Roentgenol 174:1381–1384

McCarthy JC, Busconi B (1995a) The role of hip arthroscopy in the diagnosis and treatment of hip disease. Can J Surg 38:13

McCarthy JC, Busconi B (1995b) The role of hip arthroscopy in the diagnosis and treatment of hip disease. Orthopedics 18:573–576

Miller TT (2000) MR arthrography of the shoulder and hip after fluoroscopic landmarking. Skeletal Radiol 29:81–84

Niitsu M, Nakai T, Ikeda K et al (2000) High-resolution MR imaging of the knee at 3 T. Acta Radiol 41:84–88

Palmer WE (1998) MR arthrography of the hip. Semin Musculosk Radiol 2:349–361

Peh WC, Cassar-Pullicino VN (1999) Magnetic resonance arthrography: current status. Clin Radiol 54:575–587

Petersilge CA (1997) Current concepts of MR arthrography of the hip. Semin Ultrasound CT MR 18:291–301

Petersilge CA (2000) Chronic adult hip pain: MR arthrography of the hip. Radiographics 20:S43–S52

Petersilge CA (2001) MR arthrography for evaluation of the acetabular labrum. Skeletal Radiol 30:423–430

Petersilge CA, Haque MA, Petersilge WJ et al (1996) Acetabular labral tears: evaluation with MR arthrography. Radiology 200:231–235

Peterson DM, Carruthers CE, Wolverton BL et al (1999) Application of a birdcage coil at 3 Tesla to imaging of the human knee using MRI. Magn Reson Med 42:215–221

Robbins MI, Anzilotti KF Jr, Lange RC (2000) Patient perception of magnetic resonance arthrography. Skeletal Radiol 29:265–269

Schmid MR, Nötzli HP, Zanetti M, Wyss TF, Hodler J (2003) Cartilage lesions in the hip: diagnostic effectiveness of MR arthrography. Radiology 226:382–386

Schnarkowski P, Steinbach LS, Tirman PF et al (1996) Magnetic resonance imaging of labral cysts of the hip. Skeletal Radiol 25:733–737

Steinbach LS, Palmer WE, Schweitzer ME (2002) MR arthrography. Radiographics 22:1223–1246

Suzuki S, Awaya G, Okada Y et al (1986) Arthroscopic diagnosis of ruptured acetabular labrum. Acta Orthop Scand 57:513–515

Tschauner C, Hofmann S, Czerny C (1997) Hüftdysplasie: Morphologie, Biomechanik und therapeutische Prinzipien unter Berücksichtigung des Labrums Acetabulare. Orthopade 26:89–108

Ueo T, Suzuki S, Iwasaki R et al (1990) Rupture of the labra acetabularis as a cause of hip pain detected arthroscopically, and partial limbectomy for successful pain relief. Arthroscopy 6:48–51

Vahlensieck M, Wischer T, Schmidt A et al (1995) Indirekte MR-Arthrographie: Optimierung der Methode und erste klinische Erfahrung bei frühen degenerativen Gelenksschäden am oberen Sprunggelenk. Fortschr Röntgenstr 162:338–341

Vahlensieck M, Peterfy GG, Wischer T et al (1996) Indirect MR arthrography: optimization and clinical applications. Radiology 200:249–254

Vahlensieck M, Lang P, Sommer T et al (1997) Indirect MR arthrography: techniques and applications. Semin Ultrasound CT MR 18:302–306

Wagner SC, Schweitzer ME, Weishaupt D (2001) Temporal behavior of intra-articular gadolinium. J Comput Assist Tomogr 25:661–670

Walker JM (1981) Histologic study of the fetal development of the human acetabulum and labrum: significance in congenital hip disease. Yale J Biol Med 54:255–263

Williams PL, Warwick R (eds) (1980) Arthrology: the joints of the lower limb-the hip (coaxial) joint. In: Gray's anatomy. 36th edn. Saunders, Philadelphia, pp 477–482

Winalski CS, Weissmann BN, Aliabadi P et al (1991) Intravenous Gd-DTPA enhancement joint fluid: a less invasive alternative for MR arthrography. Radiology 181:304

Wolf SD, Eng J, Balaban RS (1991) Magnetization transfer contrast: method for improving contrast in gradient-recalled-echo images. Radiology 179:133

4 Ultrasound

STEFANO BIANCHI and CARLO MARTINOLI

CONTENTS

4.1
Introduction

In the past ultrasound examinations of the hip were largely performed in infant hips to rule out developmental hip dysplasia. Improvement of new transducers and the widespread awareness of the usefulness of US for assessing musculoskeletal disorders have resulted in a growing number of hip examinations. Due to its recognized increased capacity to image this region, US is increasing used mainly to detect intraarticular joint fluid, and to evaluate of para-articular masses and tendon disorders. As in other areas of the body, accurate knowledge of the normal and abnormal US anatomy is a definite prerequisite for a successful US assessment. This chapter describes the examination technique and normal US appearance of the hip region. Since the US examination technique for the adult hip differs significantly from that of the pediatric hip, this will be described in chapter 8.

S. BIANCHI, MD
Institut de Radiologie, Clinique des Grangettes, 7 Chemin des Grangettes, 1224 Chêne-Bougeries, Switzerland
C. MARTINOLI, MD
Professor of Radiology, Istituto di Radiologia, Università di Genova, Largo Rosanna Benzi 1, 16100 Genova, Italy

4.2
Technique of Examination and Normal US Appearance

Prior to a US examination, two steps are fundamental. Firstly, a basic history must be obtained and a physical examination carried out since these are important to accurately target the US examination. This usually takes no more then a couple of minutes and can be performed with the patient on the examining bed. Location, type and intensity of pain, as well as worsening during the night or when performing daily activities must be investigated, followed by an assessment of range of movements and palpation of the periarticular region to identify joint stiffness and pinpoint tenderness. Specific maneuvers are only performed if a definite diagnosis is suspected. For example, if a tendinopathy of the gluteus medius is assumed, resisted abduction of the lower extremity with the knee extended can corroborate the suspicion by showing local peritrochanteric pain. Secondly, a careful review of the previous imaging examinations must be performed. The opportunity to review a recent, well performed pelvis radiograph and oblique view of the affected hip is a prerequisite for a correct US examination. Standard radiographs can show bones, coxofemoral, sacroiliac and symphysis pubis joints, as well as calcific deposits located within the periarticular areas. CT scan and MR imaging are rarely available before US.

The patient is examined lying supine on the examining bed. Adequate exposure of the hip region is essential. A description of the US examination technique is simpler, particularly for the novice sonographer, if the region is divided into several areas. We usually start a routine examination with the anterior region, with the patient lying supine. Then the lateral region is studied while the patient turns on the opposite side. Finally the posterior structures are investigated in the prone position.

4.2.1
Anterior Aspect

The examination can be divided in different regions that are first examined by transverse images, well suited for a panoramic view, and then by longitudinal sonograms. A standardized examination is performed by examining the different regions, from cranial to caudal.

Transverse images of the anterosuperior iliac spine (ASIS) region show the spine as a regular hyperechoic line with posterior shadowing (Fig. 4.1). Since the spine is located very superficial and close to the skin, an adequate amount of gel must be deployed in thin patients for its proper assessment. The thin sartorius muscle (SA) can be detected medially, while the larger tensor fascia lata muscle (TFL) is found laterally. Both have short triangular-shaped tendons that are best evaluated by tilting the transducer in the sagittal plane. Longitudinal sonograms over the tendons show them as hyperechoic structures inserting into the hyperechoic outline of the ASIS (Fig. 4.2). The mean thickness of the TFL tendon was 2.1 mm in a group of 40 healthy asymptomatic subjects with no difference between the right and left side (Bass and Connel 1992). Both tendons must be accurately examined since they can be affected by

tendinopathy in sportsmen and lead to unexplained anterior groin pain (Bass and Connel 1992). The SA and TFS muscles are then imaged by more distal scanning. Both are located superficially under the fascia. The most internal SA directs medially to reach the internal aspect of the thigh. After a few centimeters it can be seen overlying the rectus femoris muscle (RF). The TFL extends laterally and inferiorly to insert into the anterior border of the fascia lata (FL). Compared to the adjacent muscles, its distal portion contains a larger amount of fat deposited among muscle fascicles which is responsible for its more echogenic appearance (Bass and Connel 1992). The distal insertion can be easily evaluated by longitudinal scans and presents a pointed appearance due to gradual distal tapering of the muscle. This appearance resembles that of the distal insertion of the rectus femoris and gastrocnemius medial head. A globular appearance, even if localized, must be interpreted as a distal myotendinous avulsion.

The transducer is then moved to a more medial location where transverse sonograms reveal the intrapelvic portion of the iliopsoas (IP) muscle lying over the anterior face of the iliac wing (Fig. 4.3). In thin subjects US can detect the intramuscular tendon as a hyperechoic structure surrounded by the muscle fibers. This region must always be ana-

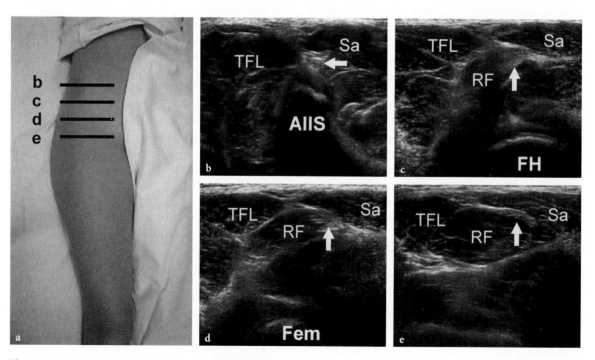

Fig. 4.1a–e. Anterior aspect. **a** Probe positioning for transverse examination. **b–e** Corresponding sonograms obtained from cranial to caudal. *TFL*, tensor fascia lata muscle; *Sa*, sartorius muscle; *RF*, rectus femoris muscle; *arrow*, tendon of the rectus femoris muscle; *AIIS*, anterior inferior iliac spine; *FH*, femoral head; *Fem*, femur

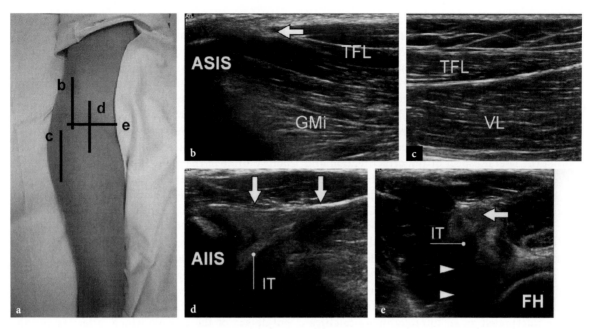

Fig. 4.2a–e. Anterior aspect. **a** Probe positioning for transverse examination. **b–e** Corresponding sonograms. **b,c** Sagittal sonograms obtained over the tensor fascia lata muscle (*TFL*). *GMi*, gluteus minimus muscle; *VL*, vastus lateralis muscle; *ASIS*, anterior superior iliac spine. **d,e** Sagittal and transverse sonograms obtained over the rectus femoris tendon. *IT*, indirect tendon; *arrowheads*, posterior shadowing of the indirect tendon; *arrows*, direct tendon; *FH*, femoral head; *AIIS*, anterior inferior iliac spine

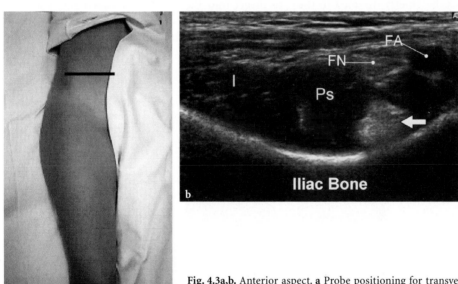

Fig. 4.3a,b. Anterior aspect. **a** Probe positioning for transverse examination. **b** Corresponding sonogram. *I*, iliac muscle; *PS*, psoas muscle; *FA*, femoral artery; *FN*, femoral nerve; *arrow*, iliopsoas tendon

lyzed in case of IP bursa fluid enlargement since in these cases the bursa can continue inside the pelvis and present as a pelvic mass (BIANCHI et al. 2002a). The internal echostructure of the IP muscle must be carefully examined, particularly in patients with total hip replacement. Any anomaly of the IP muscle due to partial tears and associated hematoma can be

seen in symptomatic patients if the posterior face of the muscle impinges against a protruding acetabular cup (REZIG et al. 2004).

After completing examination of the cranial part of the anterior aspect, the transducer is then moved distally to image the anteroinferior iliac spine (AIIS). The spine can be easily detected as a hyperechoic structure that, with respect to the ASIS, appears to be located in a deeper position. The only structure that inserts into the AIIS is the direct tendon of the RF. This is the strongest of the three tendons that constitutes the proximal attachment of this muscle. The other two tendons are made by the indirect tendon that can be appreciated by careful axial examination as a hyperechoic band arising from the superior aspect of the acetabulum and joining the lateral aspect of the direct tendon and the reflex tendon that is directed upward and medially to merge with the hip anterior capsule. While the reflex tendon is not detectable on US, the main direct tendon is easily assessed by transverse and sagittal sonograms obtained just distal of the AIIS (Figs. 4.1, 4.2). It appears as a thick, hyperechoic, oval structure. The sonographer must be aware that the normal tendon can display a posterior shadowing, particularly in transverse images, and this must not be interpreted as an intratendinous calcification. The reason for this phenomenon is unknown although we believe that it can be related to changes in fiber direction due to joining of the indirect and direct tendon. It must be noted that, although in adults scanning must be chiefly directed to the tendons inserting into the iliac spines, in children attention must be paid to the bone during examination since apophyseal avulsions are mainly found in the pediatric population.

Images are then obtained at the level of the hip joint (Fig. 4.4). This is best evaluated by transverse oblique images obtained over the femoral neck and by sagittal sonograms. To obtain accurate imaging of the anterior synovial cavity once the femoral head is detected by transverse images the lateral corner of the transducer is rotated inferiorly until the typical bone outline of the femoral neck is evident. Images obtained in this plane are well suited to image the anterior synovial recess and detect intraarticular effusion. The anterior hip synovial recess has been well described by Robben et al. (1999) who correlated US appearance with anatomic and histological appearance in cadavers. The anterior recess lies between the deep fascia of the IP muscle and the femoral neck and is composed by an anterior and a posterior layer. The two layers correspond to the cul-de-sac of the capsule which, after leaving the anterior border of the acetabulum, runs inferolaterally to reach the intertrochanteric line. At this level the most superficial fibers continue with the periosteum while the deepest reflect and travel upward to insert into the junction between the head and the neck at the caudal edge of the articular cartilage. Each layer is made up of a thick fibrous and a

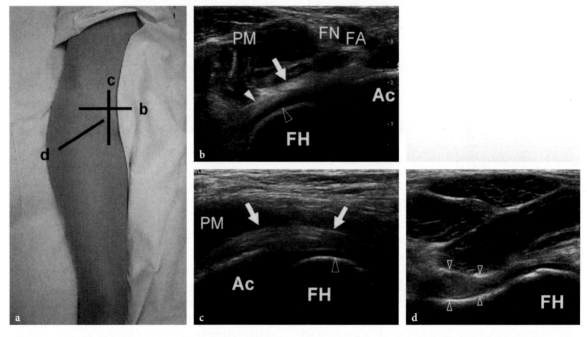

Fig. 4.4a–d. Anterior aspect. **a** Probe positioning for examination of the psoas muscle and tendon (**b,c**) and of the anterior joint recess of the hip joint (**d**). **b,c** Corresponding sonograms. *PM*, psoas muscle; *arrow*, psoas tendon; *white arrowhead*, anterior joint capsule; *void arrowhead*, cartilage of the femoral head; *FH*, femoral head; *Ac*, acetabulum. **d** *FH*, femoral head; *FN*, femoral nerve; *FA*, femoral artery; *arrowheads*, anterior joint recess

thin synovial component. The fibrous component, composed histologically of collagen fibers, appears on US as a 2 to 4 mm hyperechoic band while the normal one- to three-cell thick synovial lining is too thin to be detected. The anterior fibrous layer is thicker then the posterior layer, probably because the anterior capsule is reinforced by the iliofemoral ligament. The two layers are separated, in the absence of intraarticular effusion, by a hyperechoic line that represents an interface between the layers corresponding to the collapsed recess. This sign has been referred by to by ROBBEN et al. (1999) as the stripe sign. In adults the diagnosis of adult hip effusion is made when the anterior synovial recess is distended by greater then 7 mm (KOSKI et al. 1989). Nevertheless it must be noted that differentiation of the two layers with US is easier in infant hips and can be more difficult, if at all possible, in adults (WEYBRIGHT et al. 2003). Obese patients are particularly difficult to examine because of the deeper position of the joint and use of lower frequency transducers can be of only partial aid. Attention must be made not to confuse the anterior and posterior capsule layers with an effusion since the capsule can appear hypoechoic when imaged not perpendicularly to the US bean. The fibrocartilaginous acetabular labrum can be detected as a hyperechoic homogeneous triangle that present the same aspect of the glenoid labrum or knee menisci. Its assessment requires accurate positioning of level of focalization and seldom utilization of 5 MHz transducers.

Transverse sonograms can accurately disclose the structures superficial to the articular plane. The muscles are best imaged by transverse and longitudinal scans. The muscles detected at this level from lateral to the medial are: the TFL, RF, SA, IP and the pectineus (PE) muscles.

Overlying the joint space the IP muscle is found lying in a lateral position while the femoral nerve, artery and vein are found in a more medial position (Fig. 4.4). The IP muscle lies just superficial to the capsule plane. Its posterior fascia is closely related with the anterior hip capsule and the two structures are barely discernible at US. The hyperechoic tendon is located inside the posterior part of the muscle and can be detected at both at transverse and sagittal plane running anteriorly to the acetabular labrum. A synovial bursa, the IP bursa, is located between the tendon and the anterior capsule. The main function of the bursa is reduction of IP tendon friction over the hip joint during muscle activation and joint movements (GINESTY et al. 1998). With respect of the anatomic situation the IP bursa is similar to the gastroc-

nemius-semimembranous synovial bursa. Both are located close to the joint capsule and separate it from a paraarticular tendon. In both cases a communication with the joint space can be found particularly in adult. Communication with the hip joint is found in 15% of subjects and can be congenital or acquired. In pathologic cases in which large joint effusions rise the intraarticular pressure the two bursae can be filled by fluid and lessen tension on the adjacent joint. Like the majority of other bursae, the IPB is normally collapsed and can not be detected by US. On the other hand, US has proved to be an efficient and easy modality to detect and evaluate intrabursal effusion and synovial hypertrophy (BIANCHI et al. 2002a). Once the IP muscle and tendon are examined, the transducer is displaced medially to image the femoral neurovascular pedicle (Fig. 4.5). The femoral nerve, artery, and vein are then imaged from lateral to medial. The femoral nerve presents the typical internal fascicular pattern that can only be well imaged proximally since it divides into the terminal branches just after leaving the pelvic cavity. The normal femoral vein is of larger diameter than the artery and collapses under the pressure of the transducer. This maneuver must be part of all hip US examinations. Calcific plaques inside the artery wall are frequently noted in elderly patients. Detailed evaluation of internal flow necessitates use of the color Doppler technique.

A more distal assessment of the cranial aspect of the RF muscle clearly depicts its peculiar internal architecture made by a central tendon continuing the indirect tendon and a superficial tendon lamina arising from the direct tendon (BIANCHI et al. 2002b). This US appearance correlates well with cadaver studies and MR imaging data (BIANCHI et al. 2002; HASSELMAN et al. 1995) and can explain the occurrence of intrasubstance incomplete tear (HUGHES et al. 1995).

4.2.2
Lateral Aspect

The superficial gluteus medius muscle (GMe) and the deep gluteus minor (GMi) are found in the lateral hip region (Figs. 4.6–4.8). The GMi originates from the anterior portion of the lateral aspect of the iliac wing to extend inferiorly. The GMe has a wider surface of insertion originating from the posterior two thirds of the iliac wing and covers most of the GMi. Both muscles act as abductors and in addition flexors (posterior part of the GMe) and extensors (GMi) of the lower extremity. They insert in the

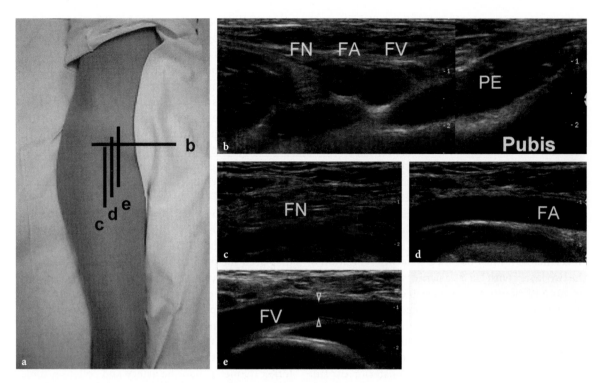

Fig. 4.5a–d. Anterior aspect. **a** Probe positioning for examination of the anterior vessels and nerves. **b** Transverse sonogram. **c–e** Sagittal sonograms. **b–e** Corresponding sonograms. *PE*, pectineus muscle; *FN*, femoral nerve; *FA*, femoral artery; *FV*, femoral vein; *arrowheads*, parietal valves

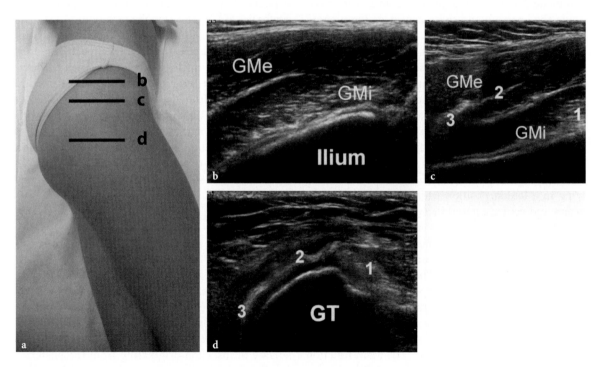

Fig. 4.6a–d. Lateral aspect. **a** Probe positioning for transverse examination. **b–d** Corresponding sonograms obtained from cranial to caudal. *GMe*, gluteus medius; *GMi*, gluteus minimus; *1*, GMi tendon; *2*, GMe anterior tendon; *3*, GMe posterior tendon; *GT*, greater trochanter

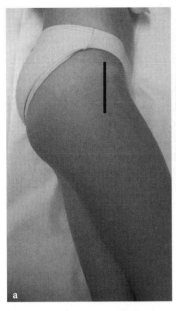
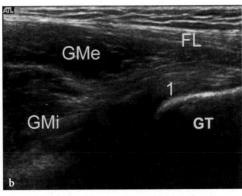

Fig. 4.7a,b. Lateral aspect. **a** Probe positioning for coronal examination. **b** Corresponding sonogram. *GMe*, gluteus medius; *GMi*, gluteus minimus; *1*, GMi tendon; *FL*, fascia lata; *GT*, greater trochanter

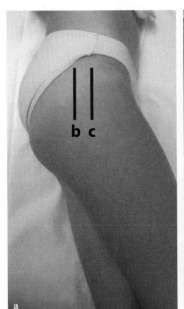
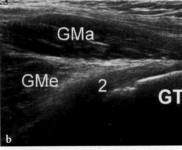
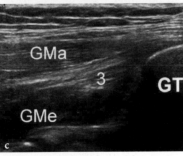

Fig. 4.8a–c. Lateral aspect. **a** Probe positioning for coronal examination. **b,c** Corresponding sonograms. *GMa*, gluteus maximus; *GMe*, gluteus medius; *2*, GMe anterior tendon; *3*, GMe posterior tendon; *GT*, greater trochanter

greater trochanter (GT), a large apophysis located at the superolateral aspect of the femoral proximal metaphysis that presents an anterior, a lateral, and a superoposterior facet. The GMi muscle continues in a strong tendon that is directed downward to insert into the anterior facet. The posterior portion of the GMe muscle continues into a strong tendon that inserts into the superolateral facet. The anterior and middle part continues into a thin tendinous lamina that inserts, together with muscle fibers, into the inferior aspect of the lateral facet (Pffirmann

et al. 2001). The fascia lata (FL) is a thick fibrous band located superficial to the GMe cranially and to the lateral aspect of the trochanter distally. The anterior portion of the GMa and the TFL insert into the FL. Several synovial bursae found in the region allow smooth gliding among the tendons and fascia lata and the GT. The most common bursa is the trochanteric, followed by the GMe and the GMi bursae. The first is located between the under-surface of the GMa and the posterior facet of the GT and the lateral aspect of the GMe tendon. The GMe bursa is located between the anterosuperior aspect of the lateral facet and the medial aspect of the GMe tendon while the GMi bursa is located anteromedially to the GMi insertion.

For proper examination of the lateral aspect of the hip the patient is then asked to turn on to the contralateral hip. The lateral face is scanned by transverse and coronal images. Transverse images obtained cranial to the greater trochanter show the GMe and GMi muscles whose anterior margins blend together. To localize the anterior portion of the GMi the sonographer must first visualize the TFS, then, by moving the transducer posteriorly, the anterior margins of both muscles can be recognized. Similarly, posterior images over the anterior portion of the large GMa are first obtained to help identification of the posterior part of the GMe. In a more superficial location the thick hyperechoic FL is detected as a hyperechoic band that joins the anterior portion of the GMa and the posterior part of the TFS and lies on the lateral aspect of the GMe. Deep to the muscle plane the hyperechoic line corresponding to the lateral aspect of the iliac bones is found. Once the muscle bellies have been evaluated the transducer is moved inferiorly at the level of the GT. Due to the different orientation of the GMe and GMi muscles an optimal assessment of their tendons can be obtained only by evaluating each tendon separately. The GMi tendon can be seen at the anterior level as a hyperechoic structure that arises from the deep part of the muscle and inserts into the anterior GT facet. Images obtained over the lateral facet shows the lateral tendon of the GMe tendon as a curvilinear band. Moving the transducer more posteriorly allows visualization of anterior part of the GMa muscle covering the oval posterior component of the GMe tendon. Images are then obtained at the supratrochanteric and trochanteric region by tilting the transducer in the coronal plane. The more superficial distal tendons are more easily evaluated. Moving the probe from anterior to posterior enables assessment of the GMi, as well as the lateral portion and posterior part of the GMe. The tendons can be properly evaluated by tilting the probe parallel to their long axis in order to avoid anisotropy. The bone attachment into the different GT facets can be detected. Because of the small amount of synovial fluid, the peritrochanteric bursae are not visualized by US in normal conditions.

Coronal images are the best suited to demonstrate the FL that appears as a uniform hyperechoic band with smooth borders overlying the GMe muscle cranially, and the lateral GMe tendon distally.

4.2.3
Posterior Aspect

The posterior hip is more rarely examined due to infrequent disorders. An adequate study in an adult usually requires a 5 MHz transducer due to the thickness of the subcutaneous tissues and of the GMa muscle. The GMa is examined by images obtained in the transverse and sagittal oblique plane. The entire muscle can be imaged from its medial origin to its lateral insertion into the femur and FL.

The deeper structures are more difficult to evaluate (COHEN 2002) (Figs. 4.9–4.11). First the medial

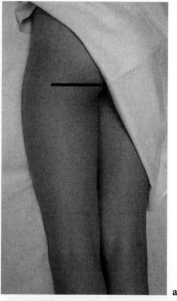

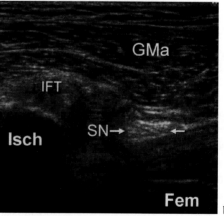

Fig. 4.9a,b. Posterior aspect. a Probe positioning for transverse examination. b corresponding sonogram. *GMa*, gluteus maximus; *IFT*, ischiofemoral tendons; *SN*, sciatic nerve; *Isch*, ischiatic tuberosity; *Fem*, femur

structures are examined. For this purpose the most useful landmark is the hyperechoic ischial tuberosity. Once detected the cranial part of the ischiocrural tendons can be demonstrated inserting on its lateral aspect. Usually the different tendons, the semimembranosus (SM) and the semitendinosus-biceps (ST-B) tendon cannot be distinguished. In a more lateral location, surrounded by fat, the sciatic nerve can be seen lying between the deep quadratus femoris and the superficial GMa muscle. The nerve has an oval to flattened appearance and presents the typical internal fascicular echotexture. More caudally the conjoined tendon of the ST-B can be seen in a more superficial and lateral position with respect to the SM tendon. The two hyperechoic tendons, together with the lateral sciatic nerve, form a hyperechoic triangle known as the "Cohen triangle" from the author that first described it (COHEN 2002). Detection of the triangle is very helpful since it allows a correct individualization of the main anatomic structure of the area. More caudally the ST-B appears as a comma shaped structure located between the medial ST muscle, the fibers of which originate more cranial than those of the B muscle, and the lateral SM muscles. The SM tendon continues in a large aponeurosis that directs medially and posteriorly. No fibers of

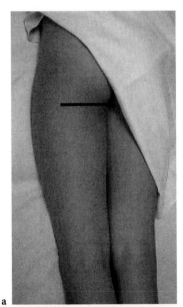

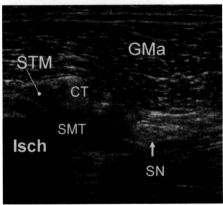

Fig. 4.10a,b. Posterior aspect. a Probe positioning for transverse examination. b Corresponding sonogram. *GMa*, gluteus maximus; *STM*, semitendineus muscle; *CT*, common tendon of the biceps tendon and semitendinosus tendon; *SMT*, semimembranosus tendon; *SN*, sciatic nerve; *Isch*, ischiatic tuberosity

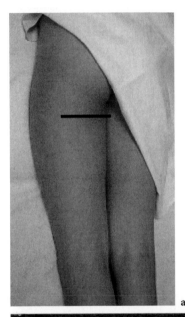

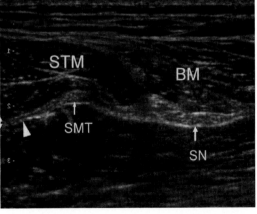

Fig. 4.11a,b. Posterior aspect. a Probe positioning for transverse examination. b Corresponding sonogram. *STM*, = semitendinous muscle; *BM*, biceps muscle; *SMT*, semimembranous tendon and tendon lamina (*arrowhead*); *SN*, sciatic nerve

the SM muscle are present at this level. Lower down, sonograms allow detection of ST and B muscles and the more internal triangular-shaped SM muscle. The sciatic nerve can be easily detected at this level since it runs just posterior to the B muscle. To summarize the organization of the ischiocrural muscles it must be noted that the ST and B muscle arise from a common tendon located superficial to the SM tendon. These tendons insert into the lateral aspect of the ischial tuberosity rather then into the inferior face. Transverse caudal images show that the first muscle that appears is the ST followed by the lateral B and in a more distal location by the medial SM. The sciatic nerve is always located laterally to the tendons. Cranially it forms the anterolateral corner of the Cohen triangle, in a more distal location it can be detected just below the biceps muscle. The posterior aspect of the hip joint and deep muscles are very difficult to assess and differentiate.

References

Bass CJ, Connel DA (2002) Sonographic findings of tensor fascia lata tendinopathy: another cause of anterior groin pain. Skeletal Radiol 31:143–148

Bianchi S, Martinoli C, Keller A et al (2002a) Giant iliopsoas bursitis: ultrasound findings with MRI correlations. J Clin Ultrasound 30:437–441

Bianchi S, Martinoli C, Peiris Waser N et al (2002b) Rectus femoris central tear. Skeletal Radiol 31:581–586

Cohen M (2002) Echoanatomie des ischio-jambiers. Gel contact 9:4–8

Ginesty E, Dromer C, Galy-Fourcade D (1998) Iliopsoas bursopathies. A review of twelve cases. Rev Rhum Engl Ed 65:181–186

Hasselman CT, Best TM, Hughes C 4th, Martinez S, Garrett WE Jr (1995) An explanation for various rectus femoris strain injuries using previously undescribed muscle architecture. Am J Sports Med 23:493–499

Hughes C 4th, Hasselman CT, Best TM, Martinez S, Garrett WE Jr (1995) Incomplete, intrasubstance strain injuries of the rectus femoris muscle. Am J Sports Med 23:500–506

Koski JM, Anttila PJ, Isomaki HA (1989) Ultrasonography of the adult hip joint. Scand J Rheumatol 18:113–117

Pffirmann CWA, Chung CB, Theumann NH et al (2001) Greater trochanter of the hip: attachment of the abductor mechanism and a complex of three bursae-MR imaging and MR bursography in cadavers and MR imaging in asymptomatic volunteers. Radiology 221:469–477

Rezig R, Copercini M, Montet X et al (2004) Ultrasound diagnosis of anterior iliopsoas impingement in total hip replacement. Skeletal Radiol 33:112–116

Robben SGF, Lequin MH, Diepstraten AFM et al (1999) Anterior joint capsule of the normal hip in children with transient synovitis: US study with anatomic and histology correlation. Radiology 210:499–507

Weybright PN, Jacobson JA, Murry KH et al (2003) Limited effectiveness of sonography in revealing hip joint effusion: preliminary results in 21 adult patients with native and postoperative hips. AJR 181:215–218

5 Nuclear Medicine

Sharon F. Hain and Ignac Fogelman

CONTENTS

5.1 Introduction

Nuclear medicine techniques can be of enormous value in the assessment of the hip and bony pelvis. The most widely used technique is the isotope bone scan, which provides a wealth of diagnostic information in both benign and malignant bone disease. A knowledge of the normal pattern of tracer uptake throughout the skeleton as well as normal anatomical variants and conditions causing specific changes

S. F. Hain, MD
The Institute of Nuclear Medicine, The Middlesex Hospital, UCH, London, UK and Charing Cross Hospital, Hammersmith Hospitals NHS Trust, London, UK
I. Fogelman, MD
Kings College and Guy's and St Thomas' NHS Trust, London, UK

are necessary in order to use the bone scan appropriately. When used in this way it is a highly sensitive technique. Where questions of specific abnormalities such as infection, infarction or loosening of prosthesis are raised other nuclear medicine procedures are useful. These include white cell imaging, gallium scintigraphy and, more recently, positron emission tomography. Each technique has specific technical requirements and potential pitfalls which should be understood and accounted for in order to correctly interpret the images. Then these studies, often together with the bone scan, provide valuable diagnostic information.

5.2 Bone Scintigraphy

5.2.1 Technique

The commonest nuclear medicine examination in the evaluation of the hip and bony pelvis is the planar bone scan. This is not merely an adjunct to radiographs as fundamentally different information is obtained with each technique and the two often work in symbiosis. The radiograph reflects anatomical change in the bone often due to changes in the bone mineral whereas the bone scintigraph is a reflection of abnormal metabolism in the bone due to changes in vascularity and osteoblastic activity. The bone scintigraph is often abnormal before the radiograph. It may also indicate if a lesion identified on radiograph is clinically significant or provide confirmation or disproof of the radiographic diagnosis (Fig. 5.1). The most frequently used compounds for bone scintigraphy are the diphosphonates such as methylene diphosphonate (MDP). These are adsorbed onto bone surfaces (Fogelman 1980) and have a particular affinity for sites of new bone formation. They are labelled with technetium-99m (99mTc) at doses of 500–1000 MBq. This isotope

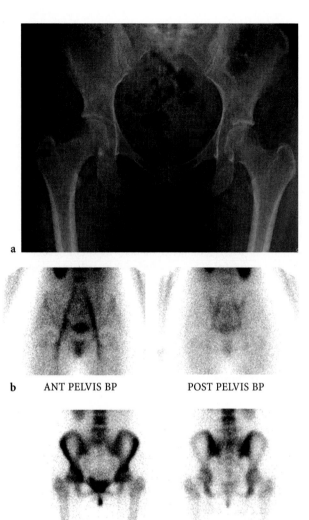

Fig. 5.1a. Plain radiograph of the pelvis showing small lesion in the right neck of femur reported as possible osteoid osteoma. **b** Corresponding bone scintigraph to (**a**). The early blood pool images (*top row*) show normal vascularity and the delayed images (*bottom row*) are normal. This shows that the lesion is not an osteoid osteoma as this would have increased vascularity and increased uptake on delayed imaging

is readily available and has physical properties that make it ideal for routine patient studies. The bone scintigraph is highly sensitive for detecting skeletal abnormalities but does lack specificity. This is balanced by a knowledge of recognisable patterns of uptake which will often suggest a specific diagnosis.

The planar bone scintigraph may be performed as a single delayed image or as a 2–3 phase scan. In patients with a localised problem, e.g. fracture or infection the three or two phase bone scan with

evaluation of vascularity (in the early phases) may be useful. The dynamic flow or first phase involves the patient being injected whilst lying under the camera with images collected for the first minute or so. The blood pool phase (2nd phase) occurs between 2 and 5 min. The final delayed imaging is performed 2–4 h following injection depending on the radiopharmaceutical. These delayed times have been chosen as they provide the best quality images with maximum bone to soft tissue ratio. At this time most of the unbound radiopharmaceutical will have been excreted by the kidneys and there will not have been significant physical decay of the 99mTc. Nowadays, the modern gamma cameras provide rapid single sweep whole body images. On some occasions extra views following the whole body sweep may be helpful to clarify a possible abnormality or more accurately localise it. The 99mTc-MDP is normally excreted through the renal tract and the kidneys are normally visualised with high uptake seen in the bladder. Thus, in the pelvis difficulties can be encountered examining the pubic bones due to radioactive urine in the bladder. Squat or subpubic views (where the patient literally sits on the camera head) or oblique images can overcome this problem. Pin hole collimators can be used to increase the detection rate of small and difficult to visualise lesions such as Perthes disease or tendon avulsion.

Single photon emission computed tomography (SPECT) is an additional technique undertaken that provides three-dimensional imaging enabling improved anatomical localisation. It provides further improved contrast between bone and soft tissue and hence greater sensitivity. It is performed at 2–4 h post-injection usually after the whole body images. Its most common use is in the spine but it can be of use in the hip and pelvis particularly for the evaluation of avascular necrosis of the hip. It is generally considered to be of less value in the pelvis due to attenuation artefact and image degradation from the very active bladder.

5.2.2
Normal Variants and Pattern Recognition

It is important to understand the appearance of the normal bone scintigraph in order to accurately assess any abnormality. The positive bone scan typically shows an area of increased uptake resulting from an osteoblastic reaction to local insult. Such areas will often be seen as sclerotic on X-ray. Rarely with excess osteoclastic activity (lesion seen as lytic on X-ray) these will be visualised on bone scan as areas of decreased uptake or 'cold' lesions. In most cases there will be increased uptake representing a local osteoblastic response. Some alterations on the bone scan may be subtle and involve both decreased vascularity and uptake, e.g. reflex sympathetic dystrophy syndrome in children. Therefore, knowledge of the particular clinical problem and any relevant patient history and normal appearance is vital.

The most important feature in a normal bone scintigraph is symmetry about the midline. Asymmetry can be assessed quickly which may point to pathology. Uptake of tracer should be uniform throughout the skeleton. The highest uptake is seen normally in the most metabolically active bone, usually that with a high trabecular component and which is subject to most stress, e.g. the spine with its weight bearing role. Ideally while being imaged patients should be lying flat with the pelvis square although this is not always achieved. Particularly in the pelvis, rotation of the patient must be looked for and assessed on the final images or else one side may be wrongly reported as abnormal. Normally, the sacroiliac joints have increased uptake compared to the rest of the pelvis and hip joints due to weight bearing load. Where altered weight bearing has changed the load, e.g. scoliosis or acute conditions such as fracture in the lower limb asymmetry may occur. In women, a knowledge of a history of recent pregnancy will prevent increased pubic uptake due to diastasis from delivery being diagnosed as osteitis pubis (another cause of increased pubic bone uptake on the bone scintigraph).

Children pose a particular problem as in the bone scintigraph there is normal increased uptake in the metaphyseal-epiphyseal area of the long bones. As areas of intense metabolic activity these regions would be expected to have increased uptake with the intensity decreasing with age and until fusion in adolescence. Any alteration in the normal appearance of the growth plate may suggest abnormal growth or development. Knowledge of the age defined normals is vital for interpretation. The shape of the growth plate is also important. Non-ambulatory infants have globular growth plates due to the absence of weight bearing. In a normal ambulatory child/adolescent the edge of the growth plate should be well demarcated and this becomes more marked towards skeletal maturity. Any blurring would arouse suspicion of pathology. Evaluation of each component of the growth complex should be undertaken and each side compared. It is necessary then that the child must be lying straight and the pelvis and legs in the same position on each side to avoid mistakes due to rotation and positioning whilst imaging. Conditions such as renal failure or steroids may cause decreased uptake in the normal growth plates and delayed ossification. Radiotherapy will cause this as well in the radiotherapy field. At fusion there can be intense increased uptake of tracer in the growth plates as a normal variant, e.g. ischiopubic synchondrosis (CAWLEY et al. 1983) which should not be confused with pathology.

To evaluate the abnormal bone scan in addition to an understanding of normal variants it is necessary to be fully aware of any relevant clinical history. Beyond this recognisable patterns of increased activity are often seen which may suggest a specific diagnosis, despite the apparent lack of specificity of the bone scintigraph. These will be discussed below.

5.2.3
Extra-Osseous Uptake on the Bone Scintigraph and Artefacts

There are many examples of diphosphonate uptake being described outside of the bone itself. In general this will be explained by the presence of microcalcification in the lesion. In the pelvis and hip any tumour and local metastases may potentially have uptake and if any unsuspected areas are seen within the pelvis further imaging should be performed and a cause elucidated. Nearly all soft tissue tumours (including sarcoma and neurofibroma) take up diphosphonates and it has been suggested that bone scanning could be used to assist in surgical planning of sarcomatous tumours by showing the relationship between the tumour and local bone (CHEW et al. 1981). MR imaging nowadays makes this much less useful.

Extra-osseous uptake in muscle may also be seen and is most commonly due to myositis ossificans or heterotopic bone formation which occurs after trauma, hip surgery or due to prolonged immobility (ORZEL et al. 1984). Benign abnormalities can be associated with extra-osseous uptake including the sites of drug injection (BROWN and MILLER 1994) and calcifying haematoma and scars. Diffuse accumulation of soft tissue uptake can be seen in the affected limb in lymphoedema (Fig. 5.2) and in chronic DVT (ZUCKIER et al. 1990; TRUIT et al. 1998). Although uptake is generally seen in organs outside the pelvis occasionally amyloid will result in MDP accumulation in bowel lying inside the pelvis (JANSSEN et al.

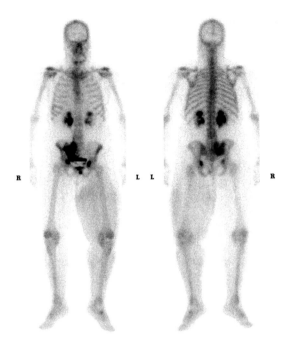

As tracer is excreted through the bladder contamination following micturition can cause false positive findings on the bone scintigraph. The pattern is often typical and away from bone but where doubt exists, e.g. the uptake is directly in the line of bone on the planar image the patients should have the area washed and further imaging performed. Ileal conduits following cystectomy result in high uptake in the bowel and may obscure the pelvic bones (Fig. 5.3). Catheter bags should be placed away from the pelvis and hip during imaging to prevent obscured views (Fig. 5.4)

Foreign objects including metal such as zips and belt buckles as well as coins in the pockets can cause attenuation artefacts on 99mTc. These areas are readily identified by their non-anatomical site and shape and photopaenic/'cold' appearance (Fig. 5.5). Professional radiographers ensuring removal of such objects before imaging should mean that the incidence of this is low.

Fig. 5.2. Bone scintigraph in a patient with a pelvic tumour. The scan shows uptake in the soft tissues of the left leg in the known lymphoedema

1990). Although rare soft tissue metastases do have uptake of tracer (HAIN et al. 1999). An accurate clinical history will prevent any inappropriate reporting, and knowledge of these patterns will encourage the reporting physician to seek a history if this has not been forthcoming.

5.3
Other Techniques – Infection Imaging

Several other nuclear medicine tracers and procedures may be of value in assessing the hip and pelvis. These may often be assessed with and in addition to the bone scan. In assessing infection generally either gallium or white cell imaging is performed and the results often compared with the bone scintigraph.

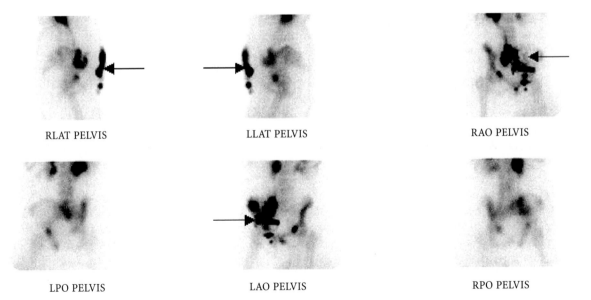

| RLAT PELVIS | LLAT PELVIS | RAO PELVIS |

| LPO PELVIS | LAO PELVIS | RPO PELVIS |

Fig. 5.3. Local pelvic views on bone scintigraph in a patient with ileal conduit (*arrow*). The scan indicates that lateral oblique views provide adequate imaging to view the pelvic bones despite the presence of uptake in the ileal conduit

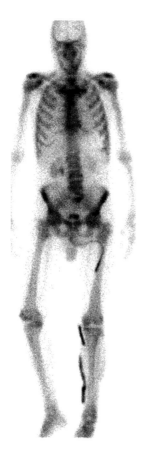

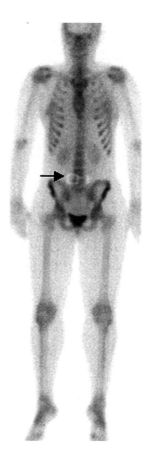

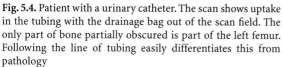

Fig. 5.4. Patient with a urinary catheter. The scan shows uptake in the tubing with the drainage bag out of the scan field. The only part of bone partially obscured is part of the left femur. Following the line of tubing easily differentiates this from pathology

Fig. 5.5. Cold area (*arrow*) seen on bone scintigraph caused by belt buckle

5.3.1
Gallium Scintigraphy

Gallium 67 citrate (Ga-67) is an isotopic tracer that is taken up at sites of infection. Generally 100 MBq is administered and imaging performed 48 h post injection. Uptake at sites of infection is due to leakage of gallium bound to lactoferrin through abnormally permeable capillaries. It also demonstrates uptake in abnormal bone at non-specific and non-infected sites. This is at the same places where diphosphonate uptake may occur on bone scintigraph. Thus, the gallium must always be evaluated with a recent bone scan. If gallium uptake is greater than that seen with MDP on the bone scan then infection is considered likely and this is referred to as incongruous uptake. The bone scan should always be performed first as a normal bone scan precludes infection and avoids the need for Gallium and extra exposure to

radiation. As gallium is imaged 48 h after injection, assessment of the bone scan as abnormal will allow the gallium injection to be given on the same day that the bone scintigraph is performed, enabling the patient to return and complete the investigation in the minimal amount of time.

5.3.2
Labelled Leucocytes

Radioactively labelling the patients own leucocytes is an effective method of assessing infection. The common radioactive labels used are either technetium using exametazime (HMPAO) as the carrier or indium-111 using oxime (In-111). To perform the procedure the patients blood is collected from a vein and the whole blood spun to separate the white cells. The white cell component is labelled with the radioactive isotope and this mixture reinjected intravenously into the patient. If technetium is used the images have to be performed on a different day to the bone scintigraph as the isotope is the same. 99mTc white cell scanning requires imaging at 1 and 3 h post reinjection of the labelled cells. For indium, technically, the cell labelling and reinjection process can be performed on the same day as the bone scan due to the different isotope and higher energy and different photopeak windows of the In-111. The patient must still return on the following day as 24-h images are performed. There is some crossover in the energy window between In-111 and 99mTc leading to some potential problems and many departments prefer to delay the white cell component. This technique, whether with In-111 or 99mTc, is labour intensive and requires special laboratory facilities which make it expensive and impossible for some smaller departments to perform. Other methods using phagocytic labelling have been developed which avoid the necessity to remove and label the white cell content thus avoiding expensive and specialised equipment. As the leucocytes in this technique are not activated, which occurs with labelling, they do not behave physiologically. This may affect the accuracy of the technique although good results can be obtained.

5.3.3
Positron Emission Tomography

The development of PET scanning has introduced a new imaging technique for infection. With uptake of glucose and therefore the glucose analogue 2 fluoro-deoxyglucose labelled with the positron emitter F-18 in metabolically active tissue, including infection, PET scanning provides the newest technique in the armamentarium of infection imaging.

5.4
Nuclear Medicine Techniques in the Hip and Pelvis for Clinical Conditions

With the background of normal tracer distribution and normal patterns of uptake in various conditions the nuclear medicine techniques are potentially of enormous value in evaluating the hip and bony pelvis. Several difficulties and specific changes can occur which must be recognised in order to accurately assess clinical conditions.

5.4.1
Diagnosis of Infection and Elucidation of the Cause of Pain in Hip Prosthesis

Two of the commonest reasons for performing nuclear medicine studies in the hip and pelvis are for the evaluation of possible osteomyelitis or hip pain in a patient with a total hip prosthesis. Pain related to a prosthesis can be due to many causes including loosening or infection and a knowledge of the expected pattern of change in appearance on scintigraphy over time is important.

Where there is a question of osteomyelitis in the hip and bony pelvis the three phase bone scintigraph is the first test that should be performed. It is generally recognised that bone scintigraphy will be abnormal several days to weeks before conventional radiographs (HANDMAKER and LEONARDS 1976). Increased uptake in the early blood pool images with uptake in the bone at 3 h makes osteomyelitis highly likely. It is important to scan the whole body as infection may be multifocal, especially in children. With the modern gamma camera and whole body sweeps this procedure is easy to perform, even in children. Uptake seen only on the early images with no abnormal bone uptake on the later images suggests inflammation in the soft tissues only and this is typically seen in cellulitis. The use of recent antibiotic therapy must be known as it may lead to a false negative result.

Other tracers may be necessary to diagnose infection, particularly as the bone scan may not be specific enough for accurate diagnosis. Gallium was for many years the procedure of choice although white cell scanning has replaced this to a large extent. If Gallium uptake is greater than that seen with MDP on the bone scan then the scans have 'incongruous uptake' and infection is considered likely. As Gallium is taken up into any abnormal bone, uptake similar to that seen on the bone scintigraph is 'congruous' and unlikely to be infection. In addition, bone scintigraphy plus or minus gallium can be of use in patients with sickle cell disease where the query is to differentiate between infarction, sickle crisis or infection. Early on, X-ray is usually normal and a bone scan is a quick, simple procedure. Normal or reduced uptake is seen in sickle crisis whereas increased uptake is seen in infection and infarction. Gallium can then be used to differentiate infection (positive) from infarction (negative).

An important clinical problem in the hip is to clarify the cause of pain in a femoral prosthesis that could be due to infection or perhaps loosening. The three phase bone scan combined with infection

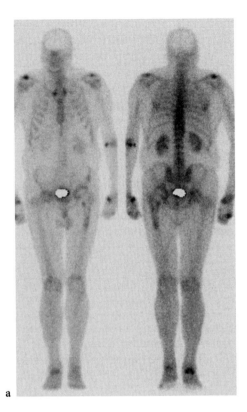

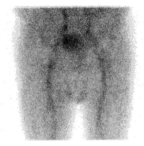

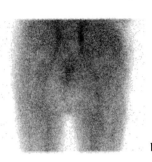

a

b

Fig. 5.6a,b. A patient with a 5-year-old left total hip prosthesis presented with pain. **a** Early blood pool images (*anterior on left, posterior on right*) show normal vascularity. **b** Delayed images show increased uptake in the hip prosthesis. This is greater than expected at 5 years and is focal in the acetabulum, tip and lesser trochanter. With no significant vascularity the likely cause is loosening

imaging is very useful. Even where the only relevant issue is whether infection is present or not the bone scan should be performed before specific infection imaging. A normal bone scan will effectively exclude any pathology. One problem in patients with painful hips following prosthesis is that only 37% may have a normal scan appearance but not all of these will have significant pathology which will require surgery (MILES et al. 1992). This is because when a prosthesis is inserted there are significant changes to load distribution and the biomechanical forces in the joint which cause changes in the bone and hence on the very sensitive bone scintigraph. Depending on the type of prosthesis, in particular cemented versus non-cemented, the appearance on bone scintigraphy will be affected. For older cemented prosthesis the changes on bone scan are well described. These have persistent uptake equal to the SI joint for at least 2 years post surgery and this uptake only diminishes at 3 years. Focal uptake at the tip of the femoral prosthesis is increased in 10% and that in the acetabulum in 12% at 2 years reducing slightly thereafter (UTZ et al. 1986). In cementless prosthesis it is common to see uptake at the tip persisting for more than 2 years (OSWALD et al. 1989). Loosening is classically described as having focal uptake on bone scan especially at the tip but, since this can be

a common finding for several years, false positive results can occur. In fact, on bone scan a loose prosthesis may have focal or diffuse uptake and since diffuse uptake is also seen with infection a further test, e.g. white cell scan may be necessary to differentiate the two conditions. Pattern recognition of specific areas of uptake is important. Uptake in the greater trochanter is extremely common and due to the osteotomy and on its own unlikely to represent either infection or loosening. Uptake in more than one site and especially the lesser trochanter combined with the femoral tip is far more significant and likely to indicate loosening (Fig. 5.6). Where infection must be excluded leucocyte imaging with In-111 is regarded as the first choice of infection agent in this case. Cross talk can occur with the 99mTc window from the bone scan if these are done on the same day. If this protocol is used then it is foreseeable that an abnormality seen on the In-111 will really be a persisting abnormality from the bone scintigraph and therefore only incongruous lesions can be defined with certainty. This can be avoided by performing the indium white cell scan on a different day which would also allow the use of technetium white cell labelling, which is cheaper and more widely available but less sensitive for identifying low grade infection.

False positives can occur and in particular are seen in non-cemented prostheses. This is due to displacement of activated marrow during surgery which may form bone islands and will be positive on both bone and leucocyte scanning. A further scan with a bone marrow seeking agent such as nano-colloid, labelled with 99mTc, should be performed and compared with the others. Concordant scans (bone marrow uptake in the same place) indicates bone marrow displacement whereas normal marrow uptake in the presence of high bone and leucocyte uptake indicates infection. This combined technique reduces the number of false positive results seen with In-111 (SEABOLD et al. 1991).

False negatives can be seen in chronic infection where there is insufficient influx of white cells into the area. In this case Ga-67 would be a more useful infection imaging agent. Gallium, as previously mentioned, is taken up at the site of abnormal bone metabolism and MDP accumulation. Thus, congruity of uptake between the bone and gallium may not indicate infection. On the other hand, incongruity, i.e. uptake in excess of that which would be anticipated from the bone scintigraph imaging indicates infection. The results with Gallium are good showing a sensitivity of 83% and specificity of 81% (HARRIS and BARRACK 1993). Generally, white cell scanning would be regarded as better than Gallium with a sensitivity of 88% and specificity of 90% (HARRIS and BARRACK 1993).

Most recently FDG-PET has shown promise in differentiating loosening and infection in the hip by identifying increased uptake in infection at the bone-prosthesis interface (ZHUANG et al. 2001).

5.4.2
Trauma – Defining Fracture, Complications and Assessment of Fracture Risk

In the presence of a suggestive clinical history a plain radiograph usually shows a fracture within 24 hours of injury in 95% of patients less than 65 years of age (MARTIN 1979). In older patients the radiograph may not be abnormal until up to 72 hours. Where the initial radiograph is negative three phase bone scintigraphy is valuable in confirming or excluding fracture. A particular area of difficulty in the hip and pelvis is the elderly patient with a suspected fractured neck of femur (DEUTSCH et al. 1989). Occasionally the bone scan may also be negative early on. In such cases it is worth repeating the bone scan several days later as it will still be abnormal before the radiograph.

Bone scintigraphy may also be useful in pelvic fracture which again can be difficult to define on radiograph. On bone scintigraphy a sacral fracture typically appears as a styled 'H' across the sacrum and vertically down the SI joints, referred to as the Honda sign because of it similarity to the Honda Company trademark. In assessment of pelvic fracture, where a sacral fracture is seen, contra-coup injury should always be assessed especially in the pubic rami. Due to excretion of tracer through the bladder this may be difficult to define. In this case an extra view, a subpubic, should be performed which allows good visualisation of the pubic rami. This requires the patient to sit on the camera head and if the patient is infirm or in pain this may not be possible. Alternatively a late view at 24 hours after bladder emptying will give the same information.

Where there is a known fracture, e.g. in the proximal femur continued symptoms may suggest non-union. This can be difficult to diagnose clinically and radiologically. A bone scintigraph may be helpful as reduced uptake at the fracture site will confirm atrophic non-union.

5.4.3
Avascular Necrosis and Infarction

As mentioned previously bone scintigraphy is useful in sickle cell disease to differentiate infarct from infection. In other forms of infarction, e.g. Perthes disease and avascular necrosis, it may also be helpful. Avascular necrosis may occur after fracture, especially in the neck of femur, or may be spontaneous as a complication of treatment with corticosteroids. The early diagnosis can be difficult as the radiograph is usually normal. In the case of previous fracture and surgery MR imaging cannot be performed due to the metal implants. In both infarction and avascular necrosis the pathological bone process is ischaemia and the bone scintigraph will be abnormal very early on with decreased uptake in the affected area. With time the bone scintigraph shows an area of increased uptake which is due to the reaction of surrounding normal bone to the infarcted area. Classically in avascular necrosis of the hip planar imaging should show a bull's eye lesion, i.e. a rim of increased uptake surrounding a photopaenic/cold centre. This is not always seen and SPECT imaging can be particularly helpful. This will usually identify the central photon deficient lesion (COLLIER et al. 1985).

5.4.4
Malignancy

The standard planar whole body bone scan remains extremely important in the evaluation of bony metastatic disease both in the pelvis and beyond. Compared to plain radiography a bone scan provides a simple relatively low radiation dose method for examining the entire skeleton in one examination. In addition, an abnormality on bone scan representing a metastatic deposit may precede that on radiograph in some cases by several months (TOFE et al. 1975; PISTENMA et al. 1975; CITRIN et al. 1977). Many tumours will have management alteration depending on the presence of metastatic bone lesions and the bone scintigraph is therefore very important in early staging of the malignancy as well as defining the extent of bone metastases at any stage of the disease. The pelvis and proximal femur along with the spine, ribs, proximal humerus are the commonest sites for metastatic lesions (Fig. 5.7). Typically, a metastasis appears as a focal area of uptake not corresponding to a defined anatomical area. Osteolytic metastases appear as cold areas and can be seen in certain tumours, e.g. renal and thyroid (Fig. 5.8).

Such lesions should not be overlooked. Metastatic involvement of the skeleton by myeloma will often be negative on bone scintigraphy and generally the bone scan under-represents the extent of disease when compared to radiographs.

A potential pitfall in interpreting a bone scan in malignancy is recognising the superscan (CONSTABLE and CRANAGE 1981) (Fig. 5.9). This is a scan that looks like an excellent quality study with increased uptake into all the bone and little in the soft tissue. It occurs because the focal lesions in the skeleton are so extensive that they coalesce to produce an image of diffuse increased uptake. There is usually no or little kidney and soft tissue uptake due to less tracer being free to be taken up into soft tissue or excreted and hence also because of increased contrast. To aid with interpretation it is often possible to identify some focal lesions especially in the ribs.

Where abnormalities are visualised on bone scintigraphy and treatment is initiated it is possible to use periodic scintigraphic examination to assess response of the disease to therapy. It is important that such scans are performed with a reproducible technique especially with regard to image contrast. In general, a decrease in size and intensity of lesions

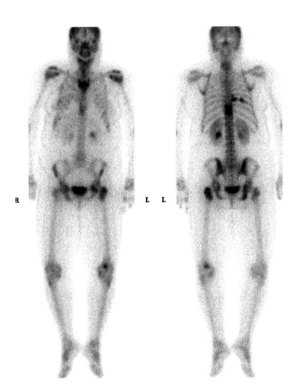

Fig. 5.7. Bone scintigraph showing uptake consistent with bone metastases in the common sites of the left proximal femur, thoracic spine and right rib

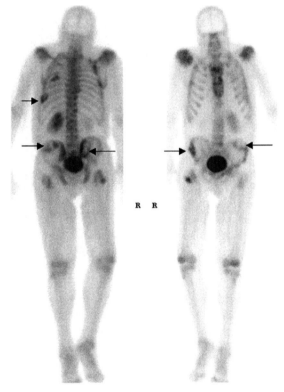

Fig. 5.8. Bone scintigraph in a patient with renal cancer. The scan shows multiple areas with a rim of increased uptake and a photopaenic centre (*arrows*) typical of osteolytic metastases

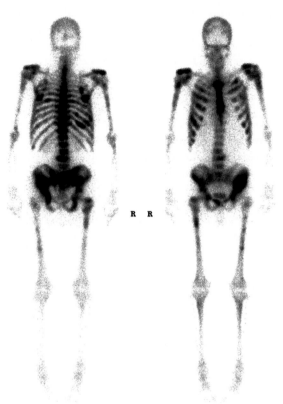

Fig. 5.9. A superscan of malignancy with increased uptake in the bone marrow with more focal lesions seen in the ribs and pelvis

represents response to treatment, whereas new lesions or increase in size demonstrates progressive disease. Some caution in interpretation is needed though as in the first few months following initiation of successful therapy a flare response (ROSSLEIGH et al. 1982, 1984) will invariably occur, where there is a short-term worsening of the scan findings including increase in the intensity of lesions and occasionally new lesions. This process is due to osteoblastic activation as part of the healing process. Thus, care must be taken in reporting a bone scan within the first few months after initiation of treatment although this is not a problem after 6 months.

At a site of metastatic bone disease a pathological fracture may occur. The most worrying of these is in the proximal femora and if present these may be treated surgically or with radiotherapy thereby preventing fracture. The bone scan is therefore useful to define these lesions. Although it cannot predict the risk of fracture, by identifying the presence of a lesion, other investigations may be performed and appropriate and preventive action, with consequent decreases in morbidity, may be undertaken.

With the expansion of PET in oncology it is not surprising that its potential to identify bony metastases has been evaluated. The commonest PET tracer, F-18 FDG is taken up into tumour cells including those in bone. Generally, PET identifies bony metastatic disease as well as the bone scan in most tumours with some reports of improved sensitivity in lung and breast cancer (COOK et al. 1998; CHERAN et al. 2004). One potential pitfall is in sclerotic lesions where COOK et al. (1998) found PET is falsely negative although interestingly these patients had a longer survival than those with lytic metastases. In addition, prostate cancer, which has predominantly sclerotic bone metastases, is one of the few tumours where FDG-PET identifies metastases less well than 99mTc MDP bone scintigraphy (SANZ et al. 1999; SHREVE et al. 1996; YEH et al. 1996). The reason for less uptake of FDG in sclerotic metastases is unclear but it may reflect a lower glycolytic rate and smaller absolute tumour volume. The F 18-fluoride ion has been used in imaging bones for over 40 years (BLAU et al. 1962) and with the recent expansion and availability of PET scanning is being re-evaluated for defining metastatic disease. It shows a high contrast between normal and abnormal bone and has high uptake in both lytic and sclerotic metastases (SCHIRRMEISTER et al. 1999).

5.4.5
Arthritides

In arthritides, bone scintigraphy may be useful to define active joint disease by showing increased uptake in the joint margins. This is due to osteoblastic reaction at the joint and in the case of osteoarthritis reflects new bone formation. Inflammatory arthropathy can occur even in osteoarthritis and in this case the three phase bone scan will be positive in all phases. In arthritides of the hip and pelvis a useful role is in the assessment of sacroiliitis of any cause including ankylosing spondylitis. Acute sacroiliitis produces a positive bone scintigraph even when X-ray is negative (LENTLE et al. 1977; NAMEY et al. 1977). Some difficulties do arise though as in normal studies the uptake in the sacroiliacs can be increased compared to the surrounding pelvis and sacrum due to altered mechanical stresses and particularly so in younger people who are more likely to have sacroiliitis. Quantitative techniques have been developed and help to overcome these interpretation difficulties. An uptake ratio is measured comparing the uptake of tracer in each sacroiliac joint to the other, to the normal sacrum or surrounding bone (RUSSELL et al. 1975; DAVIES et al. 1984) (Fig. 5.10). In acute or early disease the ratio will be increased. In end stage ankylosing spondylitis the ratio will have returned to normal as fusion of the joints occurs. SPECT imaging is also both sensitive and specific for detection of established sacroiliitis and is more specific than MR for this condition (HANLY et al. 1994).

5.4.6
Sporting Injuries

The pelvis can be affected in some sporting injuries and a knowledge of the relevant anatomy can lead to accurate diagnosis on bone scintigraphy. Increased uptake on the bone scintigraph due to abnormal osteoblastic activity at tendon and ligament insertion indicates tendon/ligamentous injury/tear/rupture with accuracy. Due to the excretion of tracer through the bladder part of the pelvis can be obscured on the standard image and often, extra views, such as the subpubic or obliques, are required. With this extra imaging, conditions such as osteitis pubis, muscle avulsion from the inferior pubic ramus or apophyseal avulsion from the ischial spines (an important site of injury in adolescent athletes) (KUJALA et al. 1997) will not be missed. Nowadays many of these conditions could be diagnosed with MR imaging but the long waiting lists for the procedure, particularly in the some countries, e.g. UK, mean that the bone scintigraph remains a valuable and quickly obtainable alternative.

Multiple injuries in sports people and others are also possible in the hip. These can be easily diagnosed on bone scintigraphy. In particular, further imaging with pinhole collimators has been useful in identifying Perthes disease, slipped capital femoral epiphysis in children and fractures in the neck of femur in athletes (typically at the inferior aspect of the femoral neck).

5.4.7
Metabolic Bone Disease

In metabolic bone disease the main use of the bone scintigraph in the hip and bony pelvis will be for the assessment of Paget's disease. Paget's is a process of osteoblastic activation and deposition of bone in an abnormal pattern leading to bone formation and increase in size of affected bones. The bone scan appearance of Paget's is classically one of intense high uptake of tracers in the affected bone. The bone scan allows rapid assessment of the whole skeleton and is more sensitive for detecting sites of disease than conventional radiology (FOGELMAN and CARR 1980) (Fig. 5.11). In addition the level of uptake reflects the degree of disease activity (SHIRAZI et al. 1974) and can be used to monitor response to therapy such as bisphosphonates (RYAN et al. 1992).

5.5
Conclusion

In imaging of the hip and bony pelvis the nuclear medicine bone scintigraph can be of enormous value. It is a highly sensitive technique for determining abnormal bone. When normal patterns of physiological uptake and symmetry are taken into account it is a powerful tool for identifying altered skeletal metabolism in a wide range of disorders. Many conditions also have a well-known pattern of uptake which, if seen, aid in diagnosis. Other tests such as for infection can be used alone or together

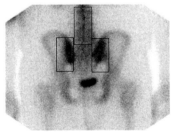

```
                    Percentages compared to Spine.
                         Raw            Norm.
               Left   : 86.2  %        98.2  %
               Right  : 98.8  %       112.5  %

POST PELVIS    L/R Ratio : 0.87        0.87
```

Fig. 5.10. Quantitative SI study in a patient with possible sacroiliitis. The posterior view of the pelvis from the bone scan (*left*) shows normal uptake in the sacroiliacs. The count profile confirms normal ratios between the two sides and compared to the spine

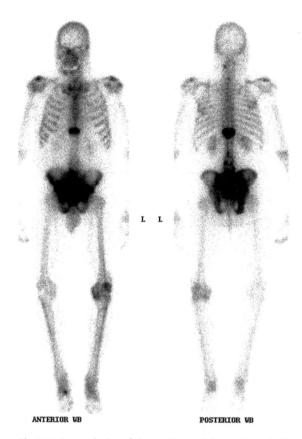

ANTERIOR WB   POSTERIOR WB

Fig. 5.11. Bone scintigraph in a patient with known Paget's disease in the pelvis. The scan identifies uptake at T12 identifying a further undiagnosed site of Paget's. Note also the large bladder obscuring accurate viewing of the pelvis

with bone scintigraphy to define with high sensitivity and specificity infection in soft tissue, bone and joint replacements. PET scanning is a relatively new technique which in the hip and pelvis can define metastatic disease and shows enormous potential in imaging infection.

References

Blau M, Nagler W, Bender MA (1962) A new isotope for bone scanning. J Nucl Med 3:332-334

Brown CV, Miller JH (1994) Extraskeletal extravasation of MDP in soft tissue seconadry to methotrexate infiltration. Clin Nucl Med 19:357-358

Cawley KA, Dvorak AD, Wilmot AD (1983) Normal anatomical variant: scintigraphy of the ischiopubic synchondrosis. J Nucl Med 24:14-16

Cheran SK, Herndon JE, Patz EF Jr (2004) Comparison of whole body FDG-PET to bone scan for bone metastases in patients with a new diagnosis of lung cancer. Lung Cancer 44:317-325

Chew FS, Hudson TM, Enneking WF (1981) Radionuclide imaging of soft tissue neoplasms. Semin Nucl Med 11:277-288

Citrin DL, Bessent RG, Greig WR (1977) A comparison of the sensitivity and accuracy of the 99m-Tc-phosphate bone scan and skeletal radiography in the diagnosis of bone metastases. Clin Radiol 28:107-117

Collier BD, Carrera GF, Johnson RP et al (1985) Detection of femoral head avascular necrosis in adults by SPECT. J Nucl Med 26:979-987

Constable AR, Cranage RW (1981) Recognition of the superscan in prostatic bone scintigraphy. Br J Radiol 54:122-125

Cook GJ, Houston S, Reubens R et al (1998) Detection of bone metastases in breast cancer by 18FDG-PET: differing metabolic activity in osteoblastic and osteolytic lesions. J Clin Oncol 16:3375-3379

Davis MC, Turner DA, Charters JR et al (1984) Quantitative sacroiliac scintigraphy: the effect of method of selection of the region of interest. Clin Nucl Med 9:334-340

Deutsch AI, Mink JH, Waxman AD (1989) Occult fractures of the proximal femur: MR imaging. Radiology 170:113-116

Fogelman I (1980) Skeletal uptake of diphosphomate: a review. Eur J Nucl Med 3:224-225

Fogelman I, Carr DA (1980) A comparison of bone scanning and radiology in the assessment of patients with symptomatic Paget's disease. Eur J Nucl Med 5:417-421

Hain SF, Cooper RA, Aroney RS et al (1999) Soft-tissue uptake of colonic metastases Clin Nucl Med 24:358-359

Handmaker H, Leonard R (1976) The bone scan in inflammatory osseous disease. Semin Nucl Med 6:95

Hanly JG, Mitchell MJ, Barnes DC et al (1994) Early recognition of sacroilitis by magnetic resonance imaging and single photon emission computed tomography. J Rheumatol 21:2088-2095

Harris WH, Barrack RL (1993) Contemporary algorithms for the evaluation of the painful total hip prosthesis. Orthopaed Rev 22:531-539

Janssen S, Piers DA, Rijswick MH et al (1990) Soft tissue uptake of 99m Tc-disphonate and Tc-99m pyrophosphate in amyloidosis. Eur J Nucl Med 16:663-670

Kujala UM, Orava S, Karpakka J et al (1997) Ischial tuberosity apophysitis and avulsion among athletes. Int J Sports Med 18:149-155

Lentle BC, Russell As, Percy JS et al (1977) The scintigraphic investigation of sacroiliac disease. J Nucl Med 18:529-533

Martin P (1979) The appearance of bone scans following fractures, including immediate and long-term studies. J Nucl Med 20:1227-1231

Miles KA, Harper WH, Finlay DBL et al (1992) Scintigraphic abnormalities in patients woth painful hip replacements treated conservatively. Br J Radiol 65:491-494

Namey TC, McIntyre J, buse M et al (1977) Nucleographic studies of axial spondarthritides. I. Quantitative sacroiliac scintigraphy in early HLA-B27-associated sacroilitis. Arthritis Rheum 20:1058

Orzel JA, Rudd TG, Nelp WB (1984) Heterotopic bone formation(myositis ossificans) and lower extremity swelling mimicking deep vein thrombosis. J Nucl Med 25:1105-1107

Oswald SG, van Nostrand D, Savory CG et al (1989) Three phase bone and indium white cell scintigraphy following porous coated hip arthroplasty: a prospective study of the prosthetic hip. J Nucl Med 30:1321-1331

Pistenma DA, McDougall IR, Kriss JP (1975) Screening for bone metastases: are only scans necessary? JAMA 231:46-50

Rossleigh MA, Lovergrove FTA, Reynolds PM et al (1982) Serial bone scans in the assessment of response to therapy in advanced breast carcinoma. Clin Nucl Med 7:397-402

Rossleigh MA, Lovergrove FTA, Reynolds PM et al (1984) The assessment of response to therapy of bone metastases in breast carcinoma. Aust NZ J Med 14:19-22

Russell AS, Lentle BD, Percy JS (1975) Investigations of sacroiliac joints: comparative evaluation of radiological and radionuclide techniques. J Rheumatol 2:45-51

Ryan PJ, Gibson T, Fogelman I (1992) Bone scintigraphy following pamidronate therapy for Paget's disease. J Nucl Med 33:1589-1593

Sanz G, Robles JE, Gimenez M et al (1999) Positron emission tomography with 18fluorine-labelled deoxyglucose: utility in localised and advanced prostate cancer. BJU Int 84:1028-1031

Seabold JE, Nepola JV, Marsh JL et al (1991) Post-operative bone marrow alterations: potential pitfalls in the diagnosis of osteomyelitis with In 111 labelled leucocyte scintigraphy. Radiology 180:741-747

Schirrmeister H, Guhlmann A, Kotzerke J et al (1999) Early detection and accurate description of extent of metastatic disease in breast cancer with flouride ion and positron emission tomography. J Clin Oncol 17:2381-2389

Shirazi PH, Ryan WG, Fordham EW (1974) Bone scanning in evaluation of Paget's disease of the bone. CRC Crit Rev Clin Radiol Nucl Med 5:523-528

Shreve PD, Grossman HB, Gross MD et al (1996) Metastatic prostate cancer: initial findings with 2-deoxy-2-[f-18]fluoro-D-glucose. Radiology 199:751-756

Tofe AJ, Francis MA, Harvey WJ (1975) Correlation of neoplasms and incidence and localisation of skeletal metastases: an analysis of 1355 diphosphonate bone scans. J Nucl Med 16:986

Truit CL, Hartshorne MF, Peters VJ (1998) Subcutaneous ossification of the legs examined with SPECT. Clin Nucl Med 13:423-425

Utz G, Lull RJ, Galvin EG (1986) Asymptomatic total hip prosthesis: natural history determined using tc-99m MDP bone scans. Radiology 16:509-512

Yeh SD, Imbriaco M, Larson SM et al (1996) Detection of bony metastases of androgen dependent prostate cancer by FDG-PET. Nucl Med Biol 23:693-697

Zhuang H, Duarte PS, Pourdehand M et al (2001) The promising role of 18F-FDG PET in detecting infected lower limb prosthesis implants. J Nucl Med 42:44-48

Zuckier LS, Patle KA, Wexler JP et al (1990) The hot clot sign: a new finding in deep venous thrombosis on bone scintigraphy. Clin Nucl Med 15:790-793

6 Interventional Procedures

Afshin Gangi, Antonio Basille, Houman Alizadeh, Xavier Buy, Juan Cupelli, and Guillaume Bierry

CONTENTS

6.1
Introduction

Percutaneous musculoskeletal procedures are widely accepted as low invasive, effective and safe techniques in a vast amount of pathologies of the bone either in diagnostic or in therapeutic management. These procedures are usually performed with a single imaging technique: ultrasound, fluoroscopy, CT, or MR.

A. Gangi, MD, PhD; A. Basille, MD; H. Alizadeh, MD;
X. Buy, MD; J. Cupelli, MD; G. Bierry, MD
Department of Radiology B, University Hospital of Strasbourg,
Pavillion Clovis Vincent, BP 426, 67091 Strasbourg, France

Fluoroscopy and CT are the most frequently used guidance techniques. Fluoroscopy offers multiple planes and direct imaging with the disadvantages of poor soft-tissue contrast and non-negligible radiation exposure for both patient and operator. CT is well suited for precise interventional needle guidance because it provides good visualization of bone and surrounding soft tissues. It also avoids damage to adjacent vascular, neurological, and visceral structures. FluoroCT technique is rarely necessary. FluoroCT with six to eight images per second are helpful if the region of interest moves during the procedure (breathing).

6.2
Bone Biopsy

6.2.1
Introduction

Histopathological and bacteriological analyses are often required in musculoskeletal lesions of the pelvic bone and hip to establish a definitive diagnosis. In such cases imaging-guided percutaneous biopsy (IGPB) is a routine, safe and cost effective technique. Percutaneous biopsies of musculoskeletal lesions allow fast diagnosis of disease with an accuracy up to 98% (Jelinek et al. 2002), and have a major impact on the decision of appropriate treatment (Fraser-Hill et al. 1992; Bickels et al. 1999).

6.2.2
Indications

Percutaneous biopsy is performed whenever pathologic, bacteriologic or biological examination is required for definitive diagnosis or treatment. The following are the major indications of percutaneous biopsy. The most common situation is a lytic or blastic bone lesion, less often a soft tissue mass, in a patient with history of neoplasia. The metastatic origin is frequently obvious; however, before beginning a specific treatment, e.g. radiotherapy, hormone therapy, confirmation is necessary. In some cases, the metastatic lesion is discovered many years after the diagnosis of cancer. In this situation, the problem is to decide whether the metastasis is that of the original tumor or of a new neoplasm. Other situations with blastic or lytic lesions occur without a history of cancer. To establish whether the lesion is primary or metastatic, a biopsy is necessary. Benign lesions may be confused with malignancies (granuloma, intraosseous ganglion, eosinophilic granuloma, and infection). In septic clinical history, percutaneous biopsies frequently enable discovery of the organism in question or exclusion of the diagnosis of infection. More generally, soft tissue or bone masses, in the absence of any clinical and biological diagnosis may require a biopsy. A musculoskeletal lesion discovered by CT, MRI, or radiography without a precise diagnosis may require percutaneous biopsy (GHELMAN 1998).

6.2.3
Contraindications

The expected results of biopsy should outweigh the risks of the procedure. Careful review of imaging findings and of previous studies should assist the radiologist in avoiding unnecessary biopsies (benign bone islands, subchondral sclerosis, etc.). A thorough knowledge of the anatomy of the pelvis is always mandatory in order to obviate inappropriate maneuvers that can result in complications; in cases where the biopsy should be performed before surgical resection, the pathway should be chosen with the surgeon in order to obviate alteration of surgical treatment (ANDERSON et al. 1999). The risk of tumor seeding should be considered, particularly with sarcomas. Well-known contraindications are the following: bleeding diatheses (INR > 1.5, prothrombin time > 1.5 times control, platelets < 50,000/mm^3) and soft tissue infection with high risk of contamination of bone.

6.2.4
Technique

The choice between fluoroscopy and CT guidance is determined by the characteristic of the bone lesions, i.e. large lesions can be considered for fluoroscopic biopsy, while small lesions are commonly approached by using CT scan imaging. In the latter cases the CT scan localizes the lesion precisely, the entry point and the pathway, avoiding neural, vascular and visceral structures. For the pelvic girdle a posterior approach is used to avoid sacral canal and nerves. For hip bone biopsy, the shortest way should be chosen in order to minimize tissue lesions during passage. The approach must avoid tendons as well as neural, vascular, visceral, and, articular structures.

Bone biopsy is usually performed under local anesthesia. Neuroleptanalgesia may be necessary for painful lesions. General anesthesia is used for children. The procedure is carried out under strict sterility. The skin's subcutaneous layers, muscles and the periosteum are infiltrated by local anesthesia (1% lidocaine) with a 22-gauge needle. For bone puncture the biopsy needle is advanced safely under CT guidance. The choice of the needles also depends to the consistence of the lesion. As well described by JELINEK et al. (2002), bone lesions can be divided in three subtypes: (I) sclerotic lesions; (II) solid non-sclerotic lesions; (III) cystic lesions.

For sclerotic lesions, defined as lesions with more than 50% bone component, large needles (7–14 Gauge) are used. In solid non-sclerotic lesions (mild ossification or with a thin cortex surrounding the lesion) a 14-gauge Ostycut (Angiomed/Bard, Karlsruhe, Germany) bone biopsy needle is used and penetration is performed with a surgical hammer. In cases of mild condensation, and for primary tumors or lymphoma we use an 8-gauge trephine needle (Laredo type). In blastic lesions, or lesions with thick cortex, drilling is necessary. In these cases a 2 mm diameter hand drill or a 14-gauge Bonopty Penetration set (Radi Medical Systems Uppsala, Sweden) are used. (Figs. 6.1, 6.2)

A 16- to 14-gauge biopsy gun can be used in solid non-sclerotic lesions, with a soft tissue component of greater than 50% per cent, and for subperiosteal lesions without ossification. For cases in which normal biopsy needles are used either core or cytological samples can be obtained coaxially. For cystic lesions, fluid aspiration is frequently insufficient and a soft tissue component biopsy is mandatory (JELINEK et al. 2002; AYALA et al. 1995).

For pathological examination the specimen is fixed in 10% formalin. Material is sent for histology. If bacteriological analysis is necessary the specimens are not fixed and are sent for culture. Single use needles are preferred for biopsies. The presence

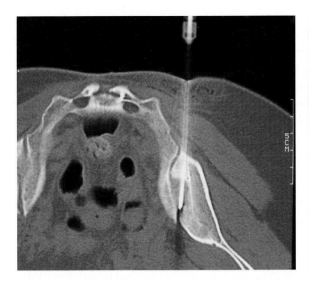

Fig. 6.1. CT-guided sacroiliac biopsy of a lytic lesion. After local anesthesia a 14-gauge biopsy needle is introduced into the lesion. The needle is advanced into the lesion to obtain a core tissue sample

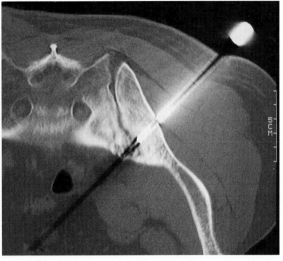

Fig. 6.2. Percutaneous biopsy of a sclerotic sacroiliac lesion. The biopsy is performed with a coaxial system using an 8-gauge trephine needle

of a pathologist in the intervention room can be very helpful.

6.2.4
Results

Complications of IGPB are very rare. A major complication is infection, thus strict sterility is mandatory. Hematoma, reflex sympathetic dystrophies, and neural or vascular injuries are other reported complications.

At our institution, 440 percutaneous musculoskeletal biopsies were reviewed retrospectively. There were 63% female and 37% male patients ranging in age from 4 to 87 years (mean 58 years). Biopsy was performed in 55% of the cases for lytic lesions, in 24% of the cases for condensing or mixed lesions, in 18% of the cases for vertebral compression fractures. In 17% of the cases the biopsies were performed for pelvic girdle. Specificity and sensitivity were, 100% and 93.9%, respectively, while positive predictive value and negative predictive values were 100% and 87.5%, respectively. Only three complications were observed among 440 IGPB: two paravertebral hematomas, spontaneously resolved, and a needle tip breakage in cortical bone. This low complication rate seems to be related to the systematic use of CT or dual guidance providing excellent monitoring.

MURPHY et al. (1981), in a large review of 9500 percutaneous skeletal biopsies, identified 22 complica-

tions (0.2%). They reported nine pneumothoraces, three cases of meningitis, and five spinal cord injuries. Serious neurological injury occurred in 0.08% of procedures. Death occurred in 0.02%. The authors concluded that the historical accuracy of the procedure is approximately 80%, but this figure is probably an underestimation because true-negative cases may not have been well documented or tabulated. In more recent series the accuracy rate ranges between 74% and 98% (WARD and KILPATRICK 2000; YAO et al. 1999; JELINEK et al. 2002), and the best results were obtained in series in which a cytopathologist assisted the procedure, with the aim to immediately determine the adequacy of the specimen and the need for further biopsies.

6.3
Sacroiliac Intraarticular Injection

6.3.1
Introduction

The sacroiliac (SI) joint is responsible for low back pain at a rate ranging between 3% and 22% of cases (BERNARD and CASSIDY 1991). SI joint injection is useful in both diagnosis and treatment management of low back pain. The diagnostic tests consist either of pain provocation or pain relief after intraarticular injection. In the former case, if the injection of hypertonic saline or of contrast medium into the SI joint and the subsequent distension of the joint causes pain within the distribution previously described by the patient the test is positive, and SI joint syndrome can be considered (FORTIN et al. 1994). If the intraarticular injection of local anesthetics into the SI joint produces 80% or more post-injection pain relief, the presumed diagnosis can be supported (INTERNATIONAL SPINAL INJECTION SOCIETY, ISIS, 1997).

6.3.2
Indications

SI joint injection is indicated in the diagnosis and treatment of low back pain. An SI Joint injection can establish the component of pain related to the SI joint. SI injection is very useful to treat inflammatory and degenerative SI joint pain.

6.3.3
Contraindications

Imaging guidance is essential for accurate intra-articular needle placement and reduction of complication. Usual contraindications are the following: bleeding diatheses (INR > 1.5, prothrombin time > 1.5 times control, platelets < 50,000/mm^3) and soft tissue infection with a high risk of bone contamination. Specific contraindications of steroid administration should be considered.

6.3.4
Technique

SI joint injection is a simple and safe procedure that can be performed under CT or fluoroscopic control. The SI joint has a curved complex configuration that can be difficult to show even with medial or lateral obliquity of the fluoroscopic tube. The fluoroscopic technique is fast and cost effective. The patient is in prone position and the tube is perpendicular to the table and the C-arm is angled 20°–30° caudad. The needle is inserted in the inferior margin of the SI joint. The intra-articular position of the needle is confirmed with injection of 0.5 ml of contrast medium.

For CT guidance, the patient is placed in a prone position. The SI joint is evaluated with 3 to 5 mm axial images obtained from its mid-portion through the inferior margin. CT scan of the affected level is used to determine the needle pathway and the entry point. The needle should be placed in the lower third of the joint. Once the skin's subcutaneous layers, muscles and the periosteum have been infiltrated by local anesthesia (1% lidocaine) a 22-gauge needle is advanced into the joint and the ideal needle tip position is about 1 cm above the inferior aspect of the joint. After arthrography confirming the correct needle position, in the case of provocative test, 0.2–0.5 ml of 5% saline or contrast medium is injected smoothly. In the case of the pain relief test, 2 ml of lignocaine 2% is injected. For therapeutic injections, a solution of cortivazol and lignocaine 2% is injected into the joint. Cortivazol is provided in 1.5 ml solution (3.75 mg of long acting steroid) and with the addition of 1.5 ml of lignocaine 2%, a 3 ml solution is obtained. Usually the injection is performed bilaterally and 1.5 ml of this solution is injected into each side. The global dose of 3.75 mg of cortivazol per session should not be exceeded (Fig. 6.3).

6.3.5
Results

In the literature, immediate pain relief after SI steroid injections varies between 50% and 80% with good pain relief for up to 17 months (DUSSAULT et al. 2000; SLIPMAN et al. 2001). A reduction in success of < 50% has been noted in patients undergoing surgical interventions in the spine (PULISETTI and EBRAHEIM 1999).

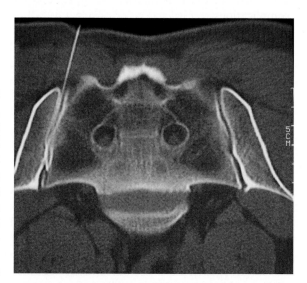

Fig. 6.3. Sacroiliac joint injection. Axial CT image. The needle is inserted parallel to the joint. The injection is easier in the lower part of the articulation

The complications of SI joint injection with precise needle positioning are rare. Severe allergic reactions to local anesthetics are uncommon. Steroid injections can produce local reactions, which generally occur immediately after the injection. These reactions last 24–48 h, and they can be relieved by the application of ice. The greatest complication is septic arthritis and can be avoided by an appropriate aseptic technique. Other complications are transitory lower extremity weakness and paresthesia.

6.4
Hip Intraarticular Injection

6.4.1
Introduction

Osteoarthritis is the most common form of arthritis, and can be a major source of disability. Intraarticular corticosteroids have been widely used for the symptomatic treatment of osteoarthritis (CRAWFORD et al. 1998; JAMES and LITTLE 1976). Corticosteroid and lidocaine have been demonstrated as effective in the treatment of osteoarthritis of the hip as long ago as 1956 (LEVEAUX and QUIN 1956), and are still used in different painful pathologies of the hip (PLANT et al. 1997). There are no guidelines for the administration of corticosteroids, and they can be associated with increased risk of tendon rupture and infection. Viscosupplementation has gained popularity in the treatment of osteoarthritis and intraarticular injections of hyaluronic acid have been shown to decrease pain and improve functional outcomes (WEN 2000). By improving the joint's elasticity and viscosity, viscosupplementation provides shock absorption and lubrication to cushion and protect the joint, thus reducing pain and increasing mobility. It aims at supplying replacement hyaluronic acid into the joint space to return the elasticity and viscosity of the synovial fluid to normal.

6.4.2
Indications

The hip infiltrations are used for the symptomatic treatment of osteoarthritis, rheumatoid arthritis, ankylosing spondylitis, and trochanteric bursitis (DIEPPE 1993). Intraarticular injections of hyaluronic acid are used in the treatment of osteoarthritis.

6.4.3
Contraindications

The usual contraindications are the following: bleeding diatheses (INR > 1.5, prothrombin time > 1.5 times control, platelets < 50,000/mm^3) and soft tissue infection with high risk of contamination of articulation. Specific contraindications of steroid administration should be respected. Hyaluronic acid is usually extracted from rooster combs and a contraindication to treatment would be an allergy to eggs or chicken.

6.4.4
Technique

Under fluoroscopic or CT guidance a 22-gauge spinal needle is advanced into the synovial cavity of the affected hip. Fluoroscopic guidance is generally preferred. The patient is placed supine on the table and the 90° direct-anterior approach arthrography technique is used. After confirmation of the intraarticular position by instillation of a few milliliters of contrast medium the diagnostic or therapeutic injection is performed. The injections must be intraarticular. Intrasynovial or extraarticular injections will not work and are much more likely to produce inflammatory reactions. The incidence of local reactions can vary depending on the product injected, but is typically 1%–2%. Occurrence of transient pain at the injection site is the most common reaction (Fig. 6.4).

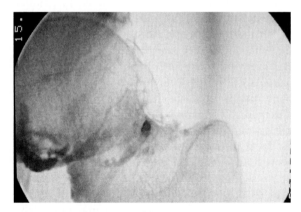

Fig. 6.4. Painful osteoarthritis of the hip. Anterior approach, after the arthrography confirming the intraarticular position of the needle, the synovial liquid is aspirated and one syringe of hyaline G-F 20 (Synvisc; Genzyme, USA) is injected in the articulation

6.4.5
Results

In the literature, effectiveness of the therapeutic injections varies in a range of 69% to 75% of cases (FLANAGAN et al. 1988; SMITH et al. 1994). Severe allergic reactions to local anesthetics or hyaluronic acid are rare. Steroid injections can produce local reactions, which usually occur immediately after the injection. These reactions last 24–48 h, and they can be relieved by applying ice. The greatest complication is septic arthritis and can be avoided by an appropriate aseptic technique. Hyaluronic acid, a polysaccharide, is a natural component of cartilage and plays an essential part in the viscoelastic properties of the synovial fluid. Although there is still insufficient information to draw a conclusion concerning the effect of this treatment on the progression of osteoarthritis in humans, considerable evidence supports the positive effects of hyaluronic acid on joint cellular and immunological function with improvement of patient mobility and reduction of osteoarthritic symptoms.

6.5
Bone Neoplasms Therapeutic Percutaneous Interventions

6.5.1
Introduction

Malignant bone neoplasms of pelvis and hip commonly affect the quality of life of patients causing refractory pain, fractures, and related functional disability (MERCADANTE 1997). Surgical resection is considered the only potentially curative option for primary and secondary malignant bone tumors. However, in secondary bone tumors only few patients are surgical candidates and some benign bone tumors like osteoid osteoma are the perfect indications of percutaneous management. Radiation therapy represents the standard palliative treatment for focal metastatic neoplasms; it prevents tumor growth, achieving effective pain control in 50%–90% of cases (GILBERT et al. 1977; HOSKIN 1991; MITHAL et al. 1994; JANJAN 1997), within 10–14 days.

Several minimally invasive percutaneous techniques for the treatment of primary and secondary bone tumors have been described in the literature, such as cementoplasty, alcoholization (ethanol ablation), and radiofrequency ablation (GANGI et al.

1994, 1996). The stimulation of sensory cortical or periosteal afferent nerves in cases of bone metastases is responsible of pain transmission (MACH et al. 2002); furthermore, certain tumor-derived cytokines and tumor factors are involved in promoting painful osteoclastic activity (WOOLF et al. 1997; GOKIN et al. 2002; HONORE et al. 2000). Cementoplasty such as alcoholization and radiofrequency (RF) ablation, locally destroy, in different methods, sensory nerves and tumor cells, interrupting pain transmission and reducing the humoral cascade involved in both nerve sensitization and osteoclastic activity, thus resulting in pain relief.

We review and debate the aspects of each technique including mechanism of action, equipment, patient selection, treatment technique, and recent patient outcome. For the particular characteristics of the treatment we also describe the percutaneous treatment of osteoid osteoma.

6.5.2
Percutaneous Cementoplasty

6.5.2.1
Introduction

Percutaneous cementoplasty with acrylic glue (polymethylmethacrylate: PMMA) is a procedure aimed at relieving pain and improving quality of life in patients with painful unresectable bone metastasis of pelvis and hip. This technique is well studied in the spine (vertebroplasty) (DERAMOND et al. 1998; GANGI et al. 2003), where it prevents vertebral body crushing and pain in patients with pathological vertebral bodies. There is a growing interest in its use for painful bone lesions outside the spine.

The pain reducing effect of cement can be due to multiple factors. As already reported for spine lesions (WEILL et al. 1996), the bone pain is due to the activation of pain nerves of the periosteum (MACH et al. 2002); it has been hypothesized that internal reinforcement of the trabecular bone, operated by the PMMA, could lead to stabilization of the fragile bone, with subsequent analgesic effects (HIEROLZER et al. 2003). However, the effect of PMMA cannot be explained by the consolidation of the pathological bone alone. In fact, good pain relief is obtained after injection of only 2 ml of methyl methacrylate in metastasis. In these cases the consolidation effect is minimal. The methyl methacrylate is cytotoxic due to its chemical and thermal effect during polymerization. The temperature during polymerization is high enough to produce coagulation of the tumoral cells, and to destroy, as already described, sensory nerve terminal and chemical stimuli inside the tumor (WEILL et al. 1996). Therefore, good pain relief can be obtained with a low volume of glue.

6.5.2.2
Indications

Percutaneous injection of acrylic cement in pelvic and hip regions is proposed in the palliative management of patients with painful pelvic metastasis, recurrence, no relief after radiotherapy (COTTEN et al. 1999), or even before radiation (MURRAY et al. 1974; WEILL et al. 1998), and to prevent bone crushing. Percutaneous injection of methylmethacrylate for malignant acetabular osteolyses is a palliative procedure that should be offered only to patients who are unable to tolerate surgery. The best indications are painful osteolytic tumors with risk of pathological fractures.

6.5.2.3
Contraindications

General contraindications are bleeding diatheses (INR > 1.5, prothrombin time > 1.5 times control, platelets < 50,000/mm^3) and soft tissue infection with high risk of contamination of bone. For acetabular lesions, COTTEN et al. (1999) suggested cementoplasty only if bone destruction is not too extensive and the cement may be expected to produce a mechanical effect. However, new studies have not reported clinically relevant complications in patients treated with larger bone destruction (HIERHOLZER et al. 2003).

6.5.2.4
Technique

Radiography and CT including contiguous thin-section acquisition must be performed prior to therapeutic percutaneous injection to assess location and extent of the lytic process, presence of cortical destruction or fracture, and presence of soft tissue involvement. The procedure is performed with the patient under sedation (COTTEN et al. 1999). A 10-gauge needle is advanced into the tumor via a posterior or posterolateral access route with the bevel ori-

ented to spread the cement in the desired direction (COTTEN et al. 1999; GANGI et al. 1996). For a metastasis of the S1 vertebral body a transiliac approach was also proposed (DEHDASHTI et al. 2000). When the needle is in the optimal position, the mandrill is extracted and a screw syringe is filled with PMMA and connected at the hub of the needle to facilitate the injection of this viscous cement under continuous fluoroscopic control (Fig. 6.5).

The acrylic cement (OsteopalV, Biomet Merck, Darmstadt, Germany; Vertebroplastic, DePuy, Acro Med, England) is prepared by mixing the powder and the fluid monomer.

During the first 30–50 s after mixing, the glue is thin but then becomes pasty. The acrylic cement has to be injected during its pasty polymerization phase to prevent distal venous migration. A total of 0–8 ml of acrylic glue are injected using a screw syringe (Cemento RE, Optimed, Karlsruhe, Germany) to facilitate the injection of this viscous mixture and to allow better control of the injection. At this stage, the intervention has to be performed quickly because the glue begins to thicken after 3–5 min (depending on the temperature of the operating room) and any further injections become impossible (Fig. 6.6).

The injection of the cement is monitored under strict anteroposterior and lateral fluoroscopic guidance and is stopped if leakage of bone cement into the joint space or soft tissue is detected. After tumor filling, the mandrill of the needle is replaced under fluoroscopic control and the needle is removed care-

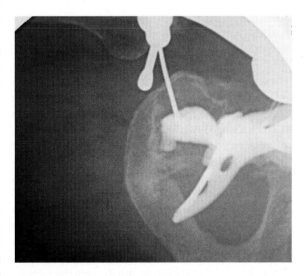

Fig. 6.5. Thyroid cancer with painful lytic metastases of the ischial tuberosity. A percutaneous cementoplasty is performed with a 15-gauge needle to consolidate and treat pain. Excellent clinical response

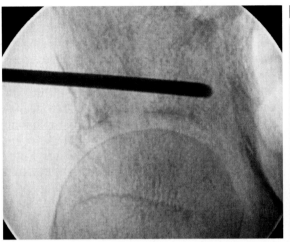
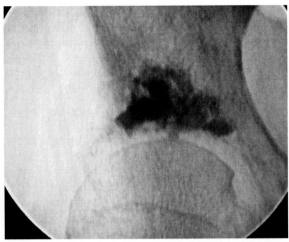

a

b

Fig. 6.6a,b. Percutaneous cementoplasty of acetabulum in painful metastasis. The cementoplasty is performed under fluoroscopic control. **a** The 10-gauge cementoplasty needle is inserted in the lytic lesion. **b** A total of 5 ml of cement is injected in the acetabulum. Excellent pain reduction

fully before the cement begins to set. At approximately 6–7 min after mixing, the methyl methacrylate begins to harden. During this hardening time, the methyl methacrylate becomes hot (+/-90°C). The patient should be under sedation to control pain. Monitoring arterial pressure is necessary during the procedure because methyl methacrylate injections can induce brief drops in arterial pressure. It is highly recommended that a CT, which allows assessment of lesion filling as well as detection of PMMA leakage, be performed in the hours following the procedure (COTTEN et al. 1999).

6.5.2.5
Results

Cementoplasty presents a reported effectiveness on pain relief in patients with pelvic and hip bone metastases in a range of 81.8%–100% of cases (COTTEN et al. 1995; MARCY et al. 2000; WEILL et al. 1998; HIERHOLZER et al. 2003). Fever and transitory worsening of pain may occur secondary to inflammatory reaction in the hours following injection, usually resolving with the administration of non-steroidal anti-inflammatory drugs within 1–3 days (COTTEN et al. 1995; GANGI et al. 1996). The most common complication is cement leak, occurring in a range of 0%–50% of patients (HIERHOLZER et al. 2003; WEILL et al. 1998); in most cases the cement leaks are without clinical significance. However, a case of chondrolysis after intraarticular leak has been reported (LECLAIR et al. 2000). Other possible

delayed complications include vascular injury, nerve injury, infection, and thrombophlebitis of the lower limbs (COTTEN et al. 1995; WEILL et al. 1998). The risk of allergic accidents and hypertension is limited in these procedures, because the quantities of acrylic glue injected in percutaneous cementoplasty are far less than those used in orthopedic surgery.

6.5.3
Alcoholization

Mainly used in the past for the management of liver tumors, ethanol ablation has shown good results also in the treatment of bone malignancies in poorly controlled pain in cancer patients. Within cells, ethanol causes dehydration of the cytoplasm and subsequent coagulation necrosis, followed by fibrous reaction.

6.5.3.1
Indication

The size and shape of the induced necrosis with ethanol is not always reproducible. It varies with the degree of vascularization, necrosis and tissue consistency. Therefore, ethanol is mainly used in palliative management of painful osteolytic bone metastases instead of tumor management. Percutaneous alcoholization of bone metastasis is well suited in patients with painful severe osteolytic bone metastases, in whom conventional anti-cancer therapy is ineffective and high doses of opiates are necessary to control pain; another possible indication is the need for rapid pain relief (radiation or chemotherapy usually requires a 2 to 4 week delay) (GANGI et al. 1994). When osteolysis does not involve the weight-bearing part of the acetabulum or when extensive osteolysis or soft-tissue involvement is present, we prefer to perform ethanol injections because pain relief is the sole object of the procedure. Percutaneous injection may result in reduction in tumor volume, especially with repeat ethanol injections. Ethanol and methylmethacrylate injections may be performed together if both weight-bearing and non-weight-bearing parts of the acetabulum are involved or extensive soft-tissue involvement is present. Furthermore, these injections could be performed prior to radiation therapy, which complements their action due to similar effects on pain, or also after radiation therapy that has failed to relieve pain, or in cases of local recurrence (COTTEN et al. 1999).

Ethanol injection in neoplasms has recently been used prior to RF ablation of highly vascularized metastases (thyroid, renal cell carcinoma) because of its immediate vasoconstrictive effect, to increase the thermal effect of RF.

6.5.3.2
Contraindications

The contraindications of alcoholization treatment of bone neoplasms perfectly match the ones already described for the other percutaneous procedures. However, the use of 22-gauge spinal needles necessary for the injections makes the procedure even less risky. The major contraindication of alcoholization is the risk of leakage of ethanol. Nevertheless, radiologists must be aware of the risk of such diffusion into vital structures (GANGI et al. 1996), such as nerves and vascular structures adjacent to the tumor (GANGI et al. 1994).

6.5.3.3
Technique

The procedure is performed under neuroleptanalgesia or general anesthesia to palliate the painful alcohol injection with the patient in positions already described for pelvic or hip bone biopsies. After delineation of tumor location and size on contiguous CT scans, the optimal puncture site and angle are defined. Contrast-enhanced CT is performed to determine the necrotic part of the tumor. Alcoholization equipment consists of a syringe, sterile 95% ethanol, and a 22-gauge spinal needle, connecting tube, contrast media, and lidocaine.

Following local anesthesia (lidocaine 1%) a 22-gauge needle is placed in the tumor. Initially, contrast medium (non-ionic) 25% diluted with lidocaine is injected into the lesion. Intratumoral instillation of lidocaine is performed to reduce the pain caused by the injection of alcohol. The distribution of contrast media within the tumor is imaged by CT and predicts the diffusion of ethanol in the lesion. In cases in which diffusion of the contrast medium extends beyond the tumor boundaries, particularly when reaching contiguous neurologic structures, or in the case of vascular leak, the procedure is discontinued. Depending on tumor size, 3–30 ml of 96% ethanol is instilled into the tumor. In large tumors, alcohol is selectively instilled into regions considered to be responsible for pain, usually the periphery of the metastases and osteolytic areas. After injection of 2–3 ml of alcohol, the distribution in the tumor is again evaluated by CT. The ethanol is visualized by the dilution of contrast media and by hypodense areas. If the ethanol was accidentally injected in contact with neural structures or other vital structures, the alcohol must be immediately diluted with the injection of an isotonic solution. If the distribution of alcohol is uneven within the tumor (particularly in large metastases), the needle is repositioned in regions of poor diffusion and the injection is repeated (Fig. 6.7).

6.5.3.4
Results

Alcoholization is successful in pain reduction in 74% of cases (GANGI et al. 1994, 1996). In 26% of cases a reduction in tumor size is observed. Liquefactive necrosis is found in 76% of metastases after the first ethanol instillation. The best results are obtained with small metastases (diameters ranging from 3–6 cm). One of the major advantages of the injection of alcohol into bone metastasis is the rapid relief of pain occurring within 24–48 h. Duration of pain relief ranges from 2–9 months. In 4% of cases, alcoholization could not be performed due to rich vascular communication and/or leakage of contrast media (GANGI et al. 1994).

Ethanol injection usually does not lead to serious complications. Possible complications are neurolysis and massive tumor necrosis with fever and hyper-

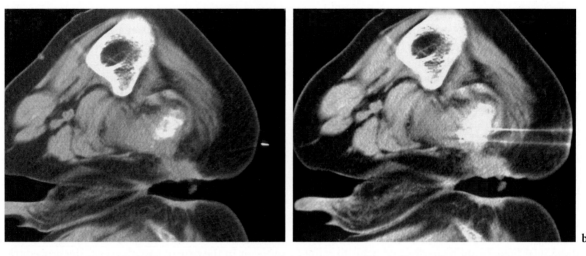

a   b

Fig. 6.7a,b. Percutaneous alcoholization under sedation. **a** Painful metastases of the ischium with soft tissue extension. **b** The spinal needles are inserted under CT guidance in the lytic part of the metastases and after contrast media injection, 3 ml of 95% ethanol is injected

uricemia (GANGI et al. 1994, 1996). Transitory worsening in pain may occur secondary to inflammatory reaction in the hours following injection; these side effects resolve spontaneously within 1–3 days after the procedure. No intraarticular leaks of ethanol have been reported (COTTEN et al. 1999).

6.5.4
Radiofrequency Ablation

6.5.4.1
Introduction

Alternating electric current operated in the range of RF can produce a focal thermal injury in living tissue. Shielded needle electrodes are used to concentrate the energy in selected tissue. The tip of the electrode conducts the current, which causes local ionic agitation and subsequent frictional heat, which leads to localized coagulation necrosis. Basically, the term radiofrequency refers not to the emitted wave but rather to the alternating electric current that oscillates in the range of high frequency (200–1200 kHz). Schematically, a closed-loop circuit is created by placing a generator, a large dispersive electrode (ground pad), a patient, and a needle electrode in series.

For irreversible cellular damage, and immediate protein coagulation, the temperature should reach 60–100°C (GOLDBERG et al. 2000). Tissue carbonization and vaporization happen with temperature above 100°C. Effective ablation needs optimized

heat production and minimized heat loss. For effective tumor destruction, the entire volume of the lesion should be exposed to cytotoxic heat. As the cytotoxic volume around the needle electrode is limited, some modified technique should be used to increase the diameter of coagulation necrosis. These are: (a) the use of multiprobe, hooked, and bipolar needle arrays; (b) intraparenchymal injection of saline during RF ablation; (c) internally cooled RF electrodes; (d) algorithms for RF current application that maximize energy deposition but avoid tissue boiling, charring, or cavitations (GAZELLE et al. 2000).

Percutaneous RF ablation has been studied mainly for the treatment of liver neoplasms (MCGAHAN and DODD 2001). Recent studies have advocated RF ablation of bone metastases in the same indications as alcoholization or cementoplasty (DUPUY et al. 2001; CALLSTROM et al. 2002; GOETZ et al. 2004). RF ablation, such as PMMA cementoplasty and alcoholization, locally destroys sensory nerves and tumor cells, interrupting pain transmission and reducing the humoral cascade involved in both nerve sensitization and osteoclastic activity.

6.5.4.2
Indications

RF is actually reserved for tumor management and/or pain relief if alcoholization is contraindicated or too risky. Palliative RF ablation is used for malignant tumors after other conventional tumor therapy failed to control pain or to slow progression. For a complete ablation, the tumor size should be less than 4 cm in diameter. RF is more suitable in sensitive regions because of the predictable size and well shaped lesion produced by this technique. Thermocoagulation is contraindicated if the lesion is close to neurological structures and in bone tumors consolidated with osteosynthesis.

6.5.4.3
Contraindications

The contraindications of RF treatment for bone neoplasms are bleeding diatheses (INR > 1.5, prothrombin time > 1.5 times control, platelets < 50,000/mm^3) and soft tissue infection with high risk of bone contamination. Specific contraindications are: risk of thermal damage to adjacent structures such as visceral organs, neurologic or vascular structures adjacent to the tumor. These contraindications could be relative if precise cooling techniques such as continuous water infusion are used.

6.5.4.4
Technique

Before the procedure, CT and MR imaging should be performed to assess the location and extent of the lytic process, the presence of cortical destruction or fracture, the presence of soft tissue involvement, and the relationship to visceral pelvic organs. The procedure is performed under general anesthesia. The RF probe is advanced into the tumor via a posterior or posterolateral access route. For lesions requiring cortical perforation, a 14-gauge bone biopsy needle (Ostycut) may be used. For tumors surrounded by dense cortical bone, a 14-gauge Bonopty penetration set (RADI Medical Systems, Uppsala, Sweden) may be needed.

Different RF probes are now available, with different shapes (straight or umbrella shaped), and different modalities (dry, cooled tip, with saline infusion, multipolar). In our department, we are using an electrode with continuous saline infusion to increase the coagulation size (Berchtold, Tuttlingen, Germany). The continuous infusion of saline at the tip of the needle allows increasing heat and electrical conductivity. Increased impedance can be detected by the generator, which can then reduce the current output and increase the saline flow. Injection of NaCl solution during RF ablation can increase energy

deposition, tissue heating, and induced coagulation (GERALD et al. 2000; RHIM et al. 2001).

The infused electrode of 18–16 gauges is inserted inside the tumor and a power of 40–60 Watts is used for 10–15 min. For large lesions (4 cm) the procedure should be repeated after modification of the position of the needle electrode. In our institution, we also use the bipolar technique with insertion of two needle electrodes, allowing the alternative current transmission between two needles. Ablation strategies must vary with the size of each lesion. On the basis of a 3 cm thermal injury, tumors less than 2 cm in diameter can be treated with one or two ablations, tumors 2–3 cm require at least six overlapping ablations, and tumors greater than 3 cm require at least 12 overlapping ablations. The length of a single procedure depends on the number of ablations performed. The guidance system is chosen largely on the basis of operator preference and local experience. We routinely use CT guidance for liver and bone tumor ablations; however, MRI can be used for needle insertion and thermal monitoring during ablation.

The minimum coagulation diameter inside bone with a single electrode is about 35 mm in diameter. At 2 weeks after ablation, MR imaging is performed. The procedure is repeated if the ablation is not complete or if symptoms persist. Large bone metastases require multiple applications. For lesions larger than 4 cm, two to three sessions could be necessary. The procedure can be repeated every 2 weeks.

During the first hours after the procedure, major pain killers should be used. The septic risk is reduced by strict sterility. Neurological complications are avoided by a precise anatomical knowledge, precise CT control, bipolar ablation, and cooling technique (Figs. 6.8, 6.9).

6.5.4.5
Results

In the literature a range of 80%–95% of patients who undergo RF ablation of bone metastases experience a clinically significant decrease in pain, and the complication rate varies from 0% to 6.9% (CALLSTROM et al. 2002; GOETZ et al. 2004). In our institution we treated 68 patients with painful osteolytic bone metastases using RF ablation. Nine well differentiated thyroid cancer patients with metastatic bone lesions were treated by the combination of RF ablation and radioisotope therapy (iodine–131). All treated lesions were osteolytic. The mean diameter of the tumors was 4.6 cm (2.4–10 cm). If no previous

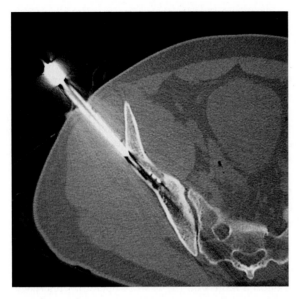

Fig. 6.8. Percutaneous RF ablation of symptomatic eosino-philic granuloma. Coaxial insertion of the RF electrode in the lesion with ablation for 10 min (40 watts)

histological or cytological proof of the patient's malig-nancy had been obtained, a percutaneous biopsy was performed prior to treatment. Before the ablation, all patients underwent physical examination and a CT and MR imaging (maximum 2 weeks before the procedure). The best ablations were obtained in large metastases of differentiated thyroid cancer. As a matter of fact, the treatment was performed in two steps. Initially, RF ablation was performed with destruction of more than 90% of the lesion followed

by iodine-131 therapy to complete the ablation of residual tumor. Complete necrosis was observed in 85% of these cases. Besides the classic potential side effects due to the approach, such as vascular injury, nerve injury, and infection described earlier, cases of skin burn at the grounding pad site, transient bowel and bladder incontinence and fractures of the acetabulum have also been reported following RF ablation of pelvic and hip bone neoplasms (GOETZ et al. 2004). No major complications in patients treated in our department have been reported. In one case, along with the necrosis of the metastasis, there was also a muscular necrosis with major pain for 1 week. RF ablation appears to be an efficient means of pal-liative management of painful primary bone tumors and metastases (GANGI et al. 2002).

6.5.5
Combination of RF and Cementoplasty

6.5.5.1
Introduction

Recently, some authors have advocated the combi-nation of both RF ablation and cementoplasty in the management of bone metastases (SCHAEFER et al. 2002, 2003; GRONEMEYER et al. 2002; NAKATSUKA et al. 2004). The combination of both techniques allows the addition of the antitumoral effect of RF ablation to the stabilizing action of cementoplasty to prevent subsequent fractures.

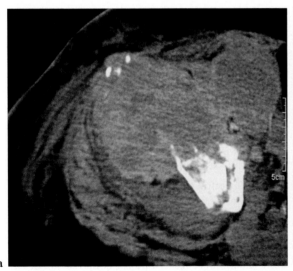
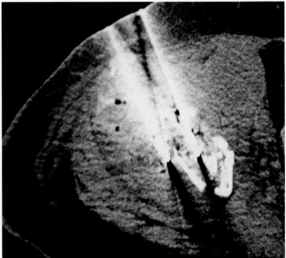

a   b

Fig. 6.9a,b. Bipolar RF ablation of large thyroid metastases of iliac bone. **a** Axial CT scan of the lesion with soft tissue exten-sion. **b** Two parallel electrodes are inserted in the tumor. Ablation was performed for 40 min with 60 W of power. The needle's position was modified during the procedure to allow complete ablation

6.5.5.2
Indications and Contraindications

The indications and contraindications of this technique are the same as those already mentioned for each technique. RF ablation and methylmethacrylate injections may be performed together if both weight-bearing and non-weight-bearing bone is involved or extensive soft-tissue involvement is present. This combination is used specially in large iliac bone tumors with extension to the acetabulum. The treatment is indeed complex in these cases. The RF ablation is used to reduce and treat the tumor and its extension to the soft tissue and the cementoplasty is performed for consolidation of the acetabulum.

6.5.4.3
Technique

The technique is very similar to cementoplasty. The 10-gauge needle can be used as a cannula for coaxial insertion of the needle electrode and after RF ablation the procedure is ended by injection of cement. The treatment has been used widely in bone metastases of the spine, and only six cases of pelvic bone metastases have been reported in the larger published series (NAKATSUKA et al. 2004).

6.5.4.4
Results

High technical and clinical success of up to 100% is reported with no major complications, although there is a rate of up to 24% of neurological complications in patients with spinal metastases (SCHAEFER et al. 2002, 2003; GRONEMEYER et al. 2002; NAKATSUKA et al. 2004) (Fig. 6.10).

6.5.6
Percutaneous Management of Osteoid Osteoma

6.5.6.1
Introduction

Osteoid osteoma is a benign neoplasm of bone that occurs more often in men ranging in age from 2 to 50 years, with 90% of cases before the age of 25 and with a common localization at the femur. Osteoid osteoma produces local pain that is worse at night and improves dramatically with aspirin. The char-

acteristic findings of this tumor in clinical and radiological examinations can lead to a high level of diagnostic confidence in many instances. The treatment of this tumor is achieved with complete removal of the nidus. The conventional treatment is surgical or percutaneous excision. Some alternative percutaneous techniques have been proposed to treat osteoid osteoma, including surgical excision, percutaneous extraction, alcoholization, RF ablation and interstitial laser photocoagulation (ILP).

6.5.6.2
Indications

Patient selection is crucial for treatment effectiveness. The indication is osteoid osteomas confirmed by CT scan, MR imaging, and scintigram with positive and consistent clinical findings.

6.5.6.3
Contraindications

The contraindications are: hemorrhagic diathesis (INR > 1.5, prothrombin time > 1.5 times control, platelets < 50,000/mm^3), soft tissue infection with high risk of contamination of bone, and lesions near neurological structures (distance < 5 mm). No safe access to the tumor.

6.5.6.4
Technique

The technique consists of percutaneous insertion of optical fibers into the tumor. The tumor is coagulated and destroyed by direct heating. With a low power laser technique, a well-defined coagulation of predictable size and shape can be obtained in bone tissue. Experimental works have shown that a reproducible area of coagulative necrosis is obtained around the fibers, with good correlation between energy delivered and the lesion size, and with conservation of the biomechanical properties of the bone tissue in the treated area. The size of osteoid osteomas falls within the range that can effectively be coagulated by one or two fibers (GANGI et al. 1997).

The procedure is performed under CT guidance. CT is used to measure the diameter of the nidus. The largest diameter of the nidus determines the energy that will be necessary to coagulate the tumor. For

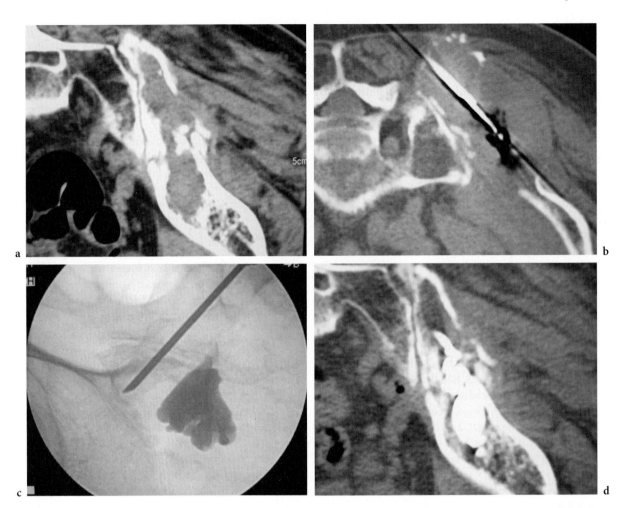

Fig. 6.10a–d. Combination of RF ablation and cementoplasty in large metastases of iliac bone with painful pathological fracture. **a** Lytic lesion with pathological fracture. **b** Percutaneous RF ablation is performed to treat the soft tissue mass especially in the upper portion of the tumor. The RF electrode is inserted coaxially trough a vertebroplasty needle. The RF electrode position is modified inside the tumor during the procedure to produce a larger ablation. **c** After the RF ablation is performed the vertebroplasty needle is used to inject cement to consolidate the fragile tumor. This part of the procedure is performed under fluoroscopic control. A second vertebroplasty needle is positioned through the fracture and the cement is injected inside the gap. **d** CT control after the procedure visualizing the cement filling the pathological fracture. Excellent pain reduction

diameters larger than 10 mm we usually use two fibers to ensure tumor destruction. The entry point and the pathway are determined by CT, avoiding nervous vascular and visceral structures. The penetration of the needle into the nidus is always extremely painful; therefore ILP is performed under general anesthesia or blocks. The procedure is performed under strict sterility.

Subperiostal nidi or cortical nidi without major ossification are directly punctured with an 18-gauge spinal needle (Becton Dickinson, Rutherford, NJ). In cases with mild ossification or small cortex surrounding the lesion, a 14-gauge bone biopsy needle is more adequate (Ostycut).

In cases of dense ossification, or of dense cortical bone surrounding the lesion, drilling is necessary. In these cases we use a 2 mm diameter hand drill or a 14-gauge Bonopty penetration set (Radi Medical Systems Uppsala, Sweden) to allow insertion of the 18-gauge needle. The 18-gauge needle tip is inserted into the centre of the nidus. Before the optical fiber is placed, it is inserted in an 18-gauge needle mounted by a side-arm fitting to measure the appropriate length of the fibers. The 400 µm fiber is then inserted through the needle; the needle is withdrawn about 5 mm so that the tip of the bare fibers lies within the centre of the tumor (Fig. 6.11).

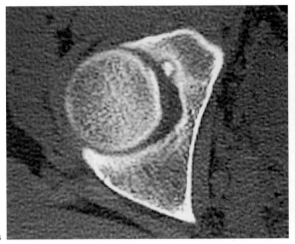
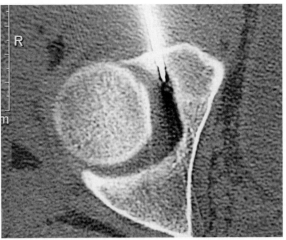

a   b

Fig. 6.11a,b. Osteoid osteoma of the acetabular cup. Percutaneous photocoagulation of the nidus. **a** CT scan of the nidus. **b** After injection of 15 ml of saline inside the hip joint to avoid thermal lesion of the femoral head, a 14-gauge needle is inserted in the nidus under CT guidance. A total of 1200 joules of energy was delivered. No complications arose. The patient was able to walk the day after the procedure

The diode laser (Diomed 805 nm; Diomed Ltd., London, UK) is turned on in continuous wave mode, at a power of 2 watts for 200–600 s depending on the nidus size (energy delivered 400–1200 joules) (nidus size in mm×100 Joules) + 200 Joules. If a maximum energy of 1200 Joules is necessary to coagulate the tumor, a minimum distance of 8 mm must be present between the fibers tip and the neurological structure. If this minimum distance could not be obtained, a cooling solution should be given to the surrounding region as used in one of the sacrally located nidi in our series, to prevent thermal neural damage. Due to the limitation in coagulation size that can be produced in bone by precharred fibers (maximum thermal lesion of 16 mm), two or rarely three 18-gauge spinal needles are placed to ensure adequate tumor coagulation. In these cases, the fibers are fired simultaneously with a 1×4-fiber splitter and a total energy of 2000–3000 Joules (1000 Joules delivered through each fiber) is delivered to the nidus.

In patients with a nidus located in the subarticular region like the acetabular roof, or femoral head of the hip joint, about 10 ml of normal saline is infused into the joint space prior to delivery of laser energy into the nidus to reduce thermal injury to the cartilage. At the end of the procedure 5–10 ml of Naropin 2% is injected subperiosteally to ease post-procedural local pain.

In the case of RF ablation, electrode placement should be such that no portion of the tumor is more that 5 mm from the exposed tip. The technique of RF ablation is similar to RF neurolysis with thermal technique. The RF electrode is inserted in the nidus and the power is increased progressively to reach 90°C. The nidus is exposed to this temperature for a maximum of 6–10 min (ROSENTHAL et al. 2003). To avoid large necrosis of bone, the cooling system or infusion should not be used in osteoid osteoma.

CT control scans are performed during the procedure to detect vaporization gas.

After a period of 6–12 months sclerosis of the nidus is observed on CT controls. Return to normal activities is usually prompt; most patients were able to return to work or school within 1 week.

6.5.6.5
Results

In the literature pain, relief after RF ablation is reported in recent series in between 79% and 86% of cases (ROSENTHAL et al. 2003; CIONI et al. 2004) with a complication rate ranging from 0% to 2% (WORTLER et al. 2001; CIONI et al. 2004). Ethanol injection into the nidus seems promising in case reports; however, further evaluation is required (CANTWELL et al. 2004). The ILM series have a clinical success rate ranging from 91% to 100% of cases (WITT et al. 2000; GANGI et al. 1998) with a minor complication rate in a range of 4%–33% (WITT et al. 2000; GANGI et al. 1998).

At our institution, updating the data already present in the literature, 114 patients with suspected osteoid osteoma based on clinical and typical imaging findings were treated by ILP on an out-patient basis or 24 h hospitalization. Among these patients, 30 had nidi in a pelvic region (femoral head=21, acetabular roof=5, ilium=2, sacrum=2). ILP was successful in 113/114 patients. Pain relief was observed to occur rapidly: 88% of the patients were completely pain-free within 24 h of the procedure, 6% were pain-free within 48–72 h, one patient was pain-free only after 2 months due to a reflex sympathetic dystrophy syndrome. Although we had six recurrences in our series (5.2%) with an average follow-up of 58.4 months (range 3–120 months) these recurrences were successfully treated with a second ILP. Complications of ILP were very rare. Only one complication was observed among our 114 patients. This consisted of a mild reflex sympathetic dystrophy of the wrist. Symptoms were entirely relieved after 2 months of treatment. Other possible complications are infection and hematoma.

6.6
Conclusion

With the advent of new imaging technologies and new minimally invasive techniques, it appears that minimally invasive interventions have a bright and exciting future. The interventional radiologist is part of a multidisciplinary team where he/she contributes actively in the management of musculoskeletal lesions and should play an active role in therapeutic approaches. However, precise patient selection is essential to the success of each of these techniques. The decision to perform one of these procedures should be made by a multidisciplinary team because the choice between these options and alternative methods of treatment depends on several factors including location of the lesion, local and general extent of the disease, pain and functional disability experienced by the patient, and the patient's state of health and life expectancy.

References

Anderson MW, Temple HT, Dussault RG et al (1999) Compartmental anatomy: relevance to staging and biopsy of musculoskeletal tumors. AJR Am J Roentgenol 173:1663–1671

Ayala AG, Ro JY, Fanning CV et al (1995) Core needle biopsy and fine needle aspiration in the diagnosis of bone and soft tissue lesions. Hematol Oncol Clin North Am 9:633–651

Bernard TN, Cassidy JO (1991) The sacroiliac joint syndrome. In: Frymoyer JW (ed) The adult spine: principles and practice. Raven, New York

Bickels J, Jelinek JS, Shmookler BM et al (1999) Biopsy of musculoskeletal tumors: current concepts. Clin Orthop 368:212–219

Callstrom MR, Charboneau JW, Goetz MP et al (2002) Painful metastases involving bone: feasibility of percutaneous CT- and US-guided radio-frequency ablation. Radiology 224:87–97

Cantwell CP, Obyrne J, Eustace S (2004) Current trends in treatment of osteoid osteoma with an emphasis on radiofrequency ablation. Eur Radiol 14:607–617

Cioni R, Armillotta N, Bargellini I et al (2004) CT-guided radiofrequency ablation of osteoid osteoma: long-term results. Eur Radiol 14:1203–1208

Cotten A, Deprex X, Migaud H et al (1995) Malignant acetabular osteolyses: percutaneous injection of acrylic bone cement. Radiology 197:307–310

Cotten A, Demondion X, Boutry N et al (1999) Therapeutic percutaneous injections in the treatment of malignant acetabular osteolyses. Radiographics 19:647–653

Crawford RW, Gie GA, Ling RSM et al (1998) Diagnostic value of intra-articular anaesthetic in primary osteoarthritis of the hip. J Bone Joint Surg 80B:279–281

Deramond H, Depriester C, Galibert P et al (1998) Percutaneous vertebroplasty with PMMA. Radiol Clin North Am 36:533–546

Dehdashti AR, Martin JB, Jean B et al (2000) PMMA cementoplasty in symptomatic metastatic lesions of the S1 vertebral Body. Cardiovasc Interv Radiol 23:235–241

Dieppe PA (1993) Management of osteoarthritis of the hip and knee joints. Curr Opin Rheumatol 5:487–493

Dussault RG, Kaplan PA, Anderson MW (2000) Fluoroscopy guided sacro-iliac joint injection. Radiology 214:273–277

Dupuy D, Ahmed M, Rodrigues B et al (2001) Percutaneous radiofrequency ablation of painful osseous metastases: a phase II trial. Proc Am Soc Clin Oncol 20:385a, abstract 1537

Flanagan J, Thomas TL, Casale FF et al (1988) Intraarticular injection for pain relief in patients awaiting hip replacement. Ann R Coll Surg Engl 70:156–157

Fortin JD, Aprill CN, Ponthieux B et al (1994) Sacroiliac joint: pain referral maps upon applying a new injection/arthrography technique. II. Clinical Evaluation. Spine 19:1483–1490

Fraser-Hill MA, Renfrew DL, Hilsenrath PE (1992) Percutaneous needle biopsy of musculoskeletal lesions. Effective accuracy and diagnostic utility. Am J Roentgenol 158:809–812

Gangi A, Kastler B, Klinkert A et al (1994) Injection of alcohol into bone metastases under CT guidance. J Comput Assist Tomogr 18:932–995

Gangi A, Dietemann JL, Schultz A et al (1996) Interventional radiologic procedures with CT guidance in cancer pain management. Radiographics 16:1289–1304

Gangi A, Dietemann JL, Gasser B et al (1997) Interstitial laser photocoagulation of osteoid osteomas with use of CT guidance. Radiology 203:843–848

Gangi A, Dietemann JL, Guth S et al (1998) Percutaneous laser photocoagulation of spinal osteoid osteoma under CT guidance. Am J Neuroradiol 19:1955–1958

Gangi A, Guth S, Imbert JP, Marin H, Wong LLS (2002) Percutaneous bone tumor management. Semin Intervent Radiol 19:279–286

Gangi A, Guth S, Imbert JP et al (2003) Percutaneous vertebroplasty: indications, technique, and results. Radiographics 23:e10

Gazelle GS, Goldberg SN, Solbiati L et al (2000) Tumor ablation with radio-frequency energy. Radiology 217:633–646

Gerald D. Dodd GD, Soulen MC et al (2000) Minimally invasive treatment of malignant hepatic tumors: at the threshold of a major breakthrough. Radiographics 20:9–27

Ghelman B (1998) Biopsies of the musculoskeletal system. Radiol Clin North Am 36:3:567–580

Gilbert HA, Kagan AR, Nussbaum H et al (1977) Evaluation of radiation therapy for bone metastasis: pain relief and quality of life. AJR Am J Roentgenol 129:1095–1096

Goetz MP, Callstrom MR, Charboneau JW et al (2004) Percutaneous image-guided radiofrequency ablation of painful metastases involving bone: a multicenter study. J Clin Oncol 22:300–306

Gokin AP, Fareed MU, Pan HL et al (2002) Local injection of endothelin-1 produces pain-like behaviour and excitation of nociceptors in rats. J Neurosci 21:5358–5366

Goldberg SN, Gazelle, GS, Mueller PR (2000) Thermal ablation therapy for focal malignancy: a unified approach to underlying principles, techniques, and diagnostic imaging guidance. AJR Am J Roentgenol 174:323

Gronemeyer DH, Schirp S, Gevargez A (2002) Image-guided radiofrequency ablation of spinal tumors: preliminary experience with an expandable array electrode. Cancer J 8:33–39

Hierolzer J, Anselmetti G, Fuchs H et al (2003) Percutaneous osteoplasty as a treatment for painful malignant bone lesions of the pelvis and femur. J Vasc Interv Radiol 14:773–777

Honore P, Luger NM, Sabino MA et al (2000) Osteoprotegerin blocks bone cancer-induced skeletal destruction, skeletal pain and pain-related neurochemical reorganization of the spinal cord. Nat Med 6:521–528

Hoskin PJ (1991) Palliation of bone metastases. Eur J Cancer 27:950–951

International Spinal Injection Society (ISIS) (1997) Guidelines for the performance of spinal injection procedures. Clin J Pain 32:285–302

James CDT, Little TF (1976) Regional hip blockade. Anesthesia 31:1060–1067

Janjan NA (1997) Radiation for bone metastases: conventional techniques and the role of systemic radiopharmaceuticals. Cancer 80 [Suppl 8]:1628–1645

Jelinek JS, Murphey MD, Welker JA et al (2002) Diagnosis of primary bone tumors with image-guided percutaneous biopsy: experience with 110 tumors. Radiology 223:731–737

Leclair A, Gangi A, Lacaze F et al (2000) Rapid chondrolysis after an intra-articular leak of bone cement in treatment of a benign acetabular subchondral cyst: an unusual complication of percutaneous injection of acrylic cement. Skeletal Radiol 29:275–278

Leveaux VM, Quin CE (1956) Local injection of hydrocortisone and procaine in osteoarthritis of the hip. Ann Rheum Dis 15:33

McGahan JP, Dodd GD (2001) Radiofrequency ablation of the liver: current status. AJR Am J Roentgenol 176:3–16

Mach DB, Rogers SD, Sabino MC et al (2002) Origin of skeletal pain: sensory and sympathetic innervations of the mouse femur. Neuroscience 133:155–166

Marcy PY, Palussiere J, Magne N et al (2000) Percutaneous cementoplasty for pelvic bone metastasis. Support Care Cancer 8:500–503

Mercadante S (1997) Malignant bone pain: pathophysiology and treatment. Pain 69:1–18

Mithal NP, Needham PR, Hoskin PJ (1994) Re-treatment with radiotherapy for painful bone metastases. Int J Radiat Oncol Biol Phys 29:1011–1014

Murphy WA, Destoutet JM, Gilula LA (1981) Percutaneous skeletal biopsy: a procedure for radiologists. Radiology 139:545–549

Murray JA, Bruels MC, Lindberg R (1974) Irradiation of polymethylmethacrylate. J Bone Joint Surg 56A:311–312

Nakatsuka A, Yamakado K, Maeda M et al (2004) Radiofrequency ablation combined with bone cement injection for the treatment of bone malignancies. J Vasc Interv Radiol 15:707–712

Plant MJ, Borg AA, Dziedzic K et al (1997) Radiographic pattern and response to corticosteroid hip injection. Ann Rheum Dis 56:476–480

Pulisetti D, Ebraheim NA (1999) CT-guided sacroiliac joint injections. J Spinal Disord 12:310–312

Rhim H, Goldberg SN, Dodd GD III et al (2001) Essential techniques for successful radio-frequency thermal ablation of malignant hepatic tumors. RadioGraphics 21:17S–35S

Rosenthal, DI Hornicek FJ, Torriani M (2003) Osteoid osteoma: percutaneous treatment with radiofrequency energy. Radiology 229:171–175

Schaefer O, Lohrmann C, Herling M et al (2002) Combined radiofrequency thermal ablation and percutaneous cementoplasty treatment of a pathologic fracture. J Vasc Interv Radiol 13:1047–1050

Schaefer O, Lohrmann C, Markmiller M et al (2003) Combined treatment of a spinal metastasis with radiofrequency heat ablation and vertebroplasty. AJR Am J Roentgenol 180:1075–1077

Slipman CW, Lipetz JS, Plastaras CT et al (2001) Fluoroscopically guided therapeutic sacroiliac joint injections for sacroiliac joint syndrome. Am J Phys Med Rehabil 80:425–432

Smith RW, Cook PL, Cawley MID (1994) A survey of arthrography and intra-articular corticosteroid injection of the hip joint. Br J Rheumatol 33:76

Ward WG Sr, Kilpatrick S (2000) Fine needle aspiration biopsy of primary bone tumors. Clin Orthop 373:80–87

Weill A, Chiras J, Simon JM et al (1996) Spinal metastases: indications for and results of percutaneous injection of acrylic surgical cement. Radiology 199:241–247

Weill A, Kobaiter H, Chiras J (1998) Acetabulum malignancies: technique and impact on pain of percutaneous injection of acrylic surgical cement. Eur Radiol 8:123–129

Wen DY (2000) Intra-articular hyaluronic acid injections for knee osteoarthritis. Am Fam Physician 62:565–570

Woolf CJ, Allchorne A, Safieh-Garabedian B et al (1997) Cytokines, nerve growth factor and inflammatory hyperalgesia: the contribution of tumor necrosis factor alpha. Br J Pharmacol 121:417–424

Witt JD, Hall-Graggs A, Ripley P et al (2000) Interstitial photocoagulation for the treatment of osteoid osteoma. J Bone Joint Surg Br 82B:1125–1128

Wortler K, Vestring T, Boettner F et al (2001) Osteoma osteoid: CT-guided percutaneous radiofrequency ablation and follow-up in 47 patients. J Vasc Interv Radiol 12:717–722

Yao L, Nelson SD, Seeger LL, Eckardt JJ, Eilber FR (1999) Primary musculoskeletal neoplasms: effectiveness of core-needle biopsy. Radiology 212:682–686

Clinical Problems

7 Congenital and Developmental Abnormalities

Karl J. Johnson and A. Mark Davies

CONTENTS

7.1
Embryology and Development

The lower limb bud develops as an outgrowth from the ventral surface of the embryonic mass at approximately 4 weeks' gestational age. The club-shaped femoral pre-cursors along with the iliac, ischial and pubic pre-modal centres develop at around 6 weeks. Between 6 and 11 weeks the femoral head can be identified as a mass of cells interposed between the distal femur and the pelvis, at the same time the primitive femoral neck and greater trochanter

K. J. JOHNSON, MD
Department of Radiology, Princess of Wales Birmingham Children's Hospital, Steelhouse Lane, Birmingham, B4 6NH, UK
A. M. DAVIES, MD
The MRI Centre, Royal Orthopaedic Hospital, Birmingham, B31 2AP, UK

form. Cavitation occurs between this cell mass and the femur creating the joint space. Any incongruity present at birth is therefore secondary to abnormal development from 11 weeks onwards. After 11 weeks vascular invasion, cartilage formation and ligament development become apparent. The hip joint is completely developed by 5 months of gestational age (FRANCIS 1951).

Ossification is initially seen in the centre of the femur and appears at the level of the lesser trochanter at 4 months of gestational age. Primary ossification centres appear in the ilium, ischium and pubis at 2, 3 and 4 months respectively. The sacrum is formed from five segments each of which constitutes a vertebral body and paired neural arches. Ossification occurs in a craniocaudal direction beginning at about 14 weeks' gestational age. The vertebral bodies are the first to ossify, followed by the neural arches and lateral masses (CAFFEY and MADELL 1956; OSBORNE et al. 1980).

Following birth ossification of the proximal femoral epiphysis is generally seen in girls between 2 and 6 months of age and in boys between 3 and 7 months. Femoral head ossification is seen in 50% of children by 4 months and in 90% by 7 months of age (PETTERSSON and THEANDER 1979; STEWART et al. 1986).

Secondary ossification centres appear in the iliac crest, ischial tuberosity the pubic symphysis, the superior acetabulum and the anterior superior and inferior iliac spines around puberty and are usually fused by early adulthood. Fusion of the posterior spinal elements of the sacrum fuse in a craniocaudal direction and is complete by around 17 years of age (EICH et al. 1992).

7.2
Normal Variants

The multiple centres of ossification and the variation in their appearance and timing need to be con-

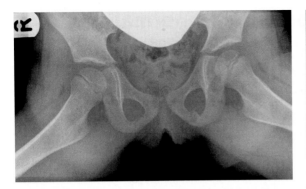

Fig. 7.1. AP radiograph of the pelvis in a 5-year-old boy. There is asymmetry in the appearances of the ischiopubic synchondrosis. The left side is larger and more prominent than the right

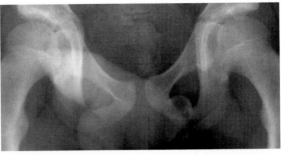

Fig. 7.2. AP radiograph of the pubic bones in a 13-year-old boy. The left ischium pubic synchondrosis is large and prominent. The right is almost absent

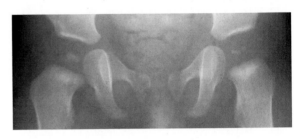

Fig. 7.3. AP radiograph showing two separate ossification centres in the left proximal femoral epiphysis. This is a normal variant

sidered when evaluating radiographs of the pelvis. These normal variants are very well illustrated in *Atlas of Normal Roentgen Variants* (KEATS and ANDERSON 2001).

At birth the pelvis is more rounded with the bony outline of the acetabulum appearing shallower. Minor irregularities in the outline of the acetabulum, iliac crest and pubic bones can be seen from 3 years of age until early adulthood.

Fusion of the ischiopubic synchondrosis has a very variable appearance and times of closure. It can appear as early as 3 years of age, with complete fusion seen in the majority of children by 12 years of age. Closure may be preceded by increase in size of the cartilaginous component giving a swollen or bubbly appearance which may last up to 3 years (Figs. 7.1 and 7.2) (CAFFEY and ROSS 1956). This expansion can be unilateral and it may also show unequal uptake on bone scintigraphy. The uptake in the synchondrosis should not be greater than that seen around the triradiate cartilage (KLOIBER et al. 1988).

Vertical clefts and multiple ossific centres can be seen in the superior pubic ramus and the superior margin of the acetabulum may be irregular with beaking of its intra-pelvic portion (PONSETI 1978).

A wide variety of appearances and times of ossification of the proximal femoral epiphysis can occur, asymmetry of 2 mm in height being recognised in any individual (LEMPERG et al. 1973).

During infancy the ossification centres can have a crenated, or stippled outline with vertical clefts within them. There may also be central defect in the epiphysis due to the ligamentous teres attachment (OZONOFF and ZITER 1987) (Fig. 7.3).

In the sacrum transitional vertebrae are commonly seen to involve the sacrococcygeal and lumbosacral junctions. The L5 vertebrae can be incorporated into the sacrum (sacralized) or the S1 vertebrae can be incorporated into the lumbar spine (lumbarized). These transitional vertebrae retain partial features of the segments involved above and below so the total number of vertebra remains constant. Transitional vertebrae are usually an incidental asymptomatic finding on pelvic and abdominal radiographs. Enlarged transverse processes have been described to cause soft tissue irritation (EICH et al. 1992).

7.3
Femoral Neck-Shaft Angulation

At birth the femoral neck to shaft angle, as measured in the coronal plane, is 150° which decreases to 120°–130° in the adult. Coxa vara is a smaller and coxa valga is a larger than normal angle (PAVLOV et al. 1980; LINCOLN and SUEN 2003; STAHELI et al. 1985).

The alteration in neck angle shaft during childhood is as a result of different growth rates of the greater trochanter and femoral neck. This is a consequence of the gravitational forces that act on the proximal femur that occur as the child starts to walk upright.

7.3.1
Coxa Vara

A Coxa vara deformity is the result of either congenital or acquired conditions, which may be a localised abnormality or associated with a more generalised skeletal disorder. Once coxa vara is identified it is important to find a causative deformity to determine prognosis, any likely associations and plan management.

Localised acquired conditions include treated congenital hip dislocations with or without subsequent avascular necrosis, Gaucher's disease, Perthes' disease, slipped capital femoral epiphysis, trauma and sepsis (Fig. 7.4).

Generalised acquired conditions are usually associated with reduced bone density including osteomalacia, renal osteodystrophy and rickets. In these children there is remodelling of the femoral necks, metaphyseal widening, irregularity, slipped capital femoral epiphysis and bowed femurs. The coxa vara can be progressive.

Coxa vara that is present at birth (congenital coxa vara) can be isolated or associated with other anomalies. When associated with proximal focal femoral deficiency, congenital short femur or congenitally bowed femur, there is usually minimal progression (Fig. 7.5).

A list of the disorders associated with coxa vara is given in Table 7.1.

7.3.2
Infantile Coxa Vara

Infantile or developmental coxa vara is a localised abnormality that is usually not detected until the child begins to walk at around 2 years of age, radiographs being normal at birth (BLOCKEY 1969; AMSTUTZ 1970). It is of unknown aetiology but may be the result of a defect in cartilaginous development, with an abnormal transition from resting to proliferating cartilage cells; in the medial portion of the growth plate being described (Bos et al. 1989). There is no sex predilection but familial cases have been reported. Bilateral involvement is seen in 30%–50% of cases (CALHOUN and PIERRET 1972).

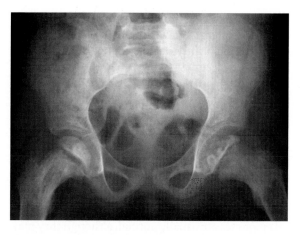

Fig. 7.4. AP radiograph of a child with Gaucher's disease. The bone density is abnormal. There is fragmentation and irregularity of the left femoral epiphysis as a result of avascular necrosis. There is bilateral coxa vara

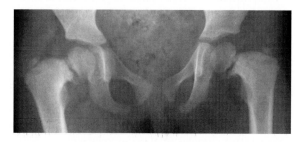

Fig. 7.5. Congenital coxa vara. The physis is almost vertical. There is fragmentation around the distal metaphysis, with a small ossification fragment on the inferior aspect

Table 7.1. Causes of Coxa vara (unilateral or bilateral)

Idiopathic coxa vara of childhood
Legg-Perthes' disease, old
Neuromuscular disorders
Malunited fracture
Developmental dysplasia of the hip
Fibrous dysplasia
Paget's disease
Rheumatoid arthritis
Rickets; osteomalacia
Proximal focal femoral deficiency
Diastrophic dwarfism
Enchondromatosis (Ollier's disease)
Fibrous dysplasia
Hyperparathyroidism, secondary
Hyperphosphatasia
Hypothyroidism
Kniest's disease
Metaphyseal chondrodysplasia
Multiple epiphyseal dysplasia
Osteogenesis imperfecta
    Osteopetrosis
    Slipped capital femoral epiphysis
Spondyloepiphyseal dysplasia

Children often complain of fatigue, thigh pain and an abnormal gait between 1–6 years of age. A unilateral deformity results in a Trendelenburg limp, while a waddle and prominent lumbar lordosis is seen with bilateral disease. The gait abnormality is related to the short femoral neck and the abnormal insertion of the abductor muscles.

Radiographically the neck shaft angle is decreased and the physis is widened and vertically orientated, being more than 30° to the horizontal pelvic baseline. Angles between 30–45° usually resolve spontaneously, while angles greater than 60° worsen (WEINSTEIN et al. 1984) (Fig. 7.6). The capital femoral epiphyses are usually normal, although they may be slightly osteopaenic and rounder than usual, with some metaphyseal irregularity. There is no femoral bowing or shortening greater than 5.0 cm, with a normal fibula, to differentiate it from proximal focal femoral deficiency (PAVLOV et al. 1980).

In children under 9 years of age there is a characteristic separate triangular osseous fragment medial and inferior to the physis. These fragments fuse with the shaft in adolescence. Remodelling and thickening of the medial cortex of the femoral neck and upper shaft, with abnormal orientation of the acetabulum, occurs due to abnormal loading stresses. Secondary degenerative changes may occur relatively early in adulthood. Treatment in childhood is surgical with valgus osteotomies (PAVLOV et al. 1980).

7.3.3
Coxa Valga

An increased neck-shaft angle is usually seen where there is abnormal muscular and gravitational forces acting upon the upper femur. It occurs in neuromuscular disorders such as cerebral palsy and poliomyelitis.

Those disorders associated with coxa valga are given in Table 7.2.

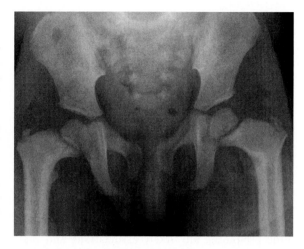

Fig. 7.6. Congenital coxa vara. AP radiograph of a 3-year-old boy. There is marked coxa vara. The proximal femoral epiphysis is vertically orientated. There is a tiny ossification fragment on the inferior aspect of the proximal femoral metaphysis

Table 7.2. Causes of Coxa valga

Paralytic disorder (e.g. meningomyelocele, cerebral palsy, muscular dystrophy, poliomyelitis)

Abductor muscle weakness

Juvenile idiopathic arthritis

Chronic leg injury

Cleidocranial dysplasia

Dysplasia epiphysealis hemimelica (Trevor's disease)

Turners syndrome

Hypoplasia of sacrum

Mucopolysaccharidosis (e.g. Hurler, Hunter, Morquio); mucolipidosis

Myositis (fibrodysplasia) ossificans progressiva

Osteodysplasia (Melnick-Needles)

Osteopetrosis

Prader-Willi syndrome

Progeria

Femoral neck fractures

Diastrophic dwarfism

Multiple enchondromatosis

7.4
Femoral Anteversion

Femoral anteversion (femoral torsion) is the projected angle between a line through the femoral neck and dicondylar coronal plane of the distal femur. At birth the femoral neck is normally anteverted by 32° or greater. This gradually decreases through childhood to a mean value of 16° at 16 years of age. This

reduction is the result of the development of the hip extensors and tightening of the anterior capsule of the hip joint (FABRY et al. 1973; GELBERMAN et al. 1987; GUENTHER et al. 1995).

The imaging techniques for measuring the degree of femoral anteversion are described in Chap. 2.

Persistence or increased anteversion (antetorsion or lateral femoral torsion) results in a decreased range of lateral rotation in hip extension. When the child walks they internally rotate their femurs and adduct their feet. This may cause compensatory torsion of the tibias resulting in foot eversion and valgus deformity with medially displaced patellae.

An increase in the angle of anteversion is associated with developmental hip dysplasia, cerebral palsy and Perthes' disease. In cerebral palsy the angles are normal at birth but do not decrease in the normal way from 2–3 years of age and the femoral necks become elongated. The degree of paraplegia does not affect the degree of anteversion. It may also be seen in otherwise normal children; when it occurs it is usually bilateral and is more common in girls (BOBROFF et al. 1999; REIKERAS and BJERKREIM 1982).

7.5
Sacral Agenesis
(Caudal Regression Syndrome)

This is a rare condition that occurs in less than 0.01% of the population, its incidence is higher in the children of diabetic mothers. Up to 20% of children with sacral agenesis have diabetic mothers (Fig. 7.7).

There is a spectrum of sacral agenesis and it has been classified into four types. With type 1 there is partial unilateral agenesis localised to the sacrum or coccyx. In type 2 there are bilateral partial defects in the sacrum. The distal sacrum and coccyx fail to develop with the iliac bones articulating with S1 and in type 3 there is total sacral agenesis with the iliac bones articulating with the lowest available lumbar vertebra. In type 4 there is complete absence of the sacrum with fusion of the iliac bone posteriorly (Fig. 7.7).

MR imaging is important to exclude an underlying spinal abnormality which include a club shaped conus, syrinx, lipoma and lipomyelomeningocele (DIEL et al. 2001).

7.6
Acetabular Protrusion (Protrusio Acetabuli)

Acetabular protrusion is medial displacement of the inner wall of the acetabulum. It may be primary with no recognisable cause or secondary to causes which include metabolic (Paget's disease and osteomalacia), infective (gonococcal, tuberculosis and acute pyogenic), traumatic, inflammatory (rheumatoid arthritis and ankylosing spondylitis), chronic steroid use and sickle cell anaemia. It also a feature of Marfan's syndrome, occurring in 45% of cases, of which 50% are unilateral and 90% have associated scoliosis (STEEL 1996).

Primary acetabular protrusion (protrusio acetabuli) is an isolated condition in which the other aetiological factors have been excluded. It is usually bilateral and is commoner in females. It may present in adolescence, while often it is not detected until adulthood, when there are concerns regarding obstetric delivery or secondary osteoarthritis (FRANCIS 1959; MACDONALD 1971).

On anterior-posterior radiographs the appearances of the acetabulum gradually progress from a normal configuration to obvious medial protrusion. The division between normal and abnormal appear-

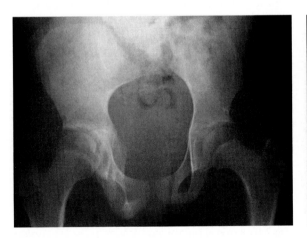

Fig. 7.7. There is complete sacral agenesis. This a child of a diabetic mother

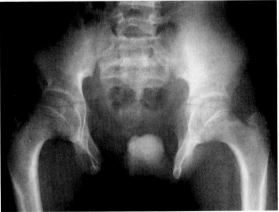

Fig. 7.8. There is ectopia vesicae. There is wide spacing of pubic symphysis

ances of the acetabulum is slightly arbitrary but is based on recognised radiographic signs (HOOPER and JONES 1971) (Fig. 7.9).

On the AP radiograph there is a tear (or pear) drop sign. This is formed by the acetabular floor laterally and the pelvic wall medially. If this pattern is disrupted, particularly if the medial wall of the acetabulum is located medially to the lateral wall of the pelvis it indicates protrusio acetabuli. The femoral head will become intrapelvic and the acetabulum will bulge inward (BOWERMAN et al. 1982).

A more objective method of assessment is from an abnormal C/E angle of Wiberg. This is the angle between a perpendicular line through the midpoint of the femoral head and a line along the upper outer margin of the acetabulum. An angle of 20°–40° is normal (McBRIDGE et al. 2001).

The disorder can be associated with local symptoms and reduced joint mobility. The more severe the protrusion the more likely the individual will be predisposed to develop early osteoarthritis. Treatment is usually supportive with physiotherapy.

7.7
Proximal Focal Femoral Deficiency

Proximal focal femoral deficiency (PFFD) describes a spectrum of disorders that ranges from mild shortening of the femur but with varus deformity of the femoral neck to nearly complete absence with small rudimentary femoral stub (ANTON et al. 1999; EPPS 1983; GILSANZ 1983). There are significant abnormalities of the iliofemoral articulation with rotational deformities. PFFD excludes mild shortening of the femur with normal hip articulation and complete absence of the femur.

The incidence is less than 1 in 50,000, with the majority of cases being sporadic, while some familial patterns are described. Approximately 15% of abnormalities are bilateral and up to 60% of patients have ipsilateral fibular hemimelia. Deformity of the feet and absence of the cruciate ligaments have been described. Clinically children present in early infancy with short bulky thighs, leg length discrepancy or fixed flexion deformity of the hip and knee joints (KALAMCHI et al. 1985).

Radiographs show a short femur displaced superiorly and posteriorly, the distal end of the femur is usually normal. A wide variety of classification systems have been described based on the radiographic findings and the osseous integrity of the proximal

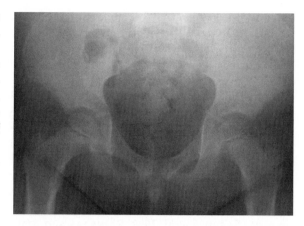

Fig. 7.9. Protrusio acetabuli. AP radiograph of the pelvis. There is medial displacement of the inner wall of the acetabulum bilaterally. The medial wall of the acetabulum is more medial than the lateral or the pelvis

femur and acetabulum. They are used mainly to try and predict prognosis and function (COURT and CARLIOZ 1997; FIXEN 1995; GILLESPIE and TORODE 1983; GILSANZ 1983; GODDARD et al. 1995; HILLMANN et al. 1987; LANGE et al. 1978; LEVINSON et al. 1997; PANTING and WILLIAMS 1978; SANPERA and SPARKS 1994).

The most widely used classification is that described by Aitken in which there are four types, type A represents the least severe form with a short femur but a femoral head and adequate acetabulum while D is the most severe form where there is complete absence of the femoral head and acetabulum (Figs. 7.10 and 7.11). A classification by Pappas gives a broader description of congenital femoral abnormalities that range from agenesis of the femur (class 1) to femoral hypoplasia or mild shortening (class 9). Patients may move into different categories and sub-classifications depending on how the cartilaginous structures develop (PAPPAS 1983).

Even in the milder forms of the disease a pseudoarthrosis may develop in the proximal femur. This

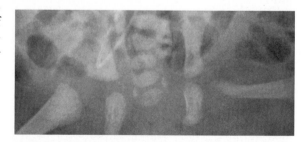

Fig. 7.10. Proximal femoral focal deficiency. The left proximal femur is absent. Small rudimentary femoral head. This is an Atkins Grade IV

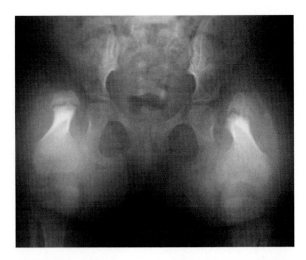

Fig. 7.11. Bilateral focal femoral deficiency. Both acetabulae are poorly developed and the femoral heads are dislocated

can occur in two places: either subtrochanteric, just below the level of the lesser trochanter or between the proximal femur and femoral head.

Imaging is important to estimate the degree of functionality of the hip, the size of the joint space and to try and predict if any pseudoarthrosis will fuse. The initial radiograph at birth is of limited value, particularly as the presence or absence of the femoral head is important in the classification system. The radiography taken in early infancy is poor in predicting what areas will develop at skeletal maturity. The secondary ossification centres being delayed in PFFD, that of the femoral head may be delayed up to 2 years. Radiographs performed between 12 months and 2 years are of better prognostic significance.

Ultrasound and MRI are increasingly being used to evaluate the extra-osseous structures, which govern treatment of prognosis in these children.

MR imaging provides earlier definition of both cartilaginous and soft tissue structure. MR imaging has shown that the muscles around the affected hip are less well developed but with enlargement of the sartorius, which may account for the flexion deformities (PIRANI et al. 1991).

Ultrasound (GRISSOM and HARKE 1999) is able to identify the femoral heads and improve the classification of the PFFD; however, it is technically challenging, as the normal imaging planes are disrupted.

Treatment is individualised and is aimed at improving function and reducing disability; reducing any limb length disparity will maximise the potential for ambulation.

7.8
Skeletal Dysplasias

Skeletal dysplasias may effect any part of the bony pelvis and proximal femur. An exact diagnosis will depend on a detailed radiological, clinical, genetic and biochemical evaluation. It is important that the full extent of the disorder is documented along with any phenotypic or systemic abnormalities. A full skeletal survey is needed to assess the distribution both within an individual bone and also the areas of skeleton involved.

Within each of the disorders there is considerable heterogeneity, which can also make the diagnosis difficult. It may be necessary that numerous repeat radiographs are performed over time, particularly as a child grows and the skeleton ossifies, to fully detail and monitor the disorder.

Irregularity and fragmentation of the proximal femoral epiphysis is a common manifestation of a skeletal dysplasia (Fig. 7.12), but it is a radiological feature with a wide differential diagnosis that is shown in Table 7.3.

7.8.1
Meyer's Dysplasia
(Dysplasia Epiphysealis Capitis Femoris)

This is a localised dysplasia of the femoral head, which is bilateral in up to 50% of cases. There is a small or delayed ossification centre of the proximal femoral epiphysis; the delay may between 18 months to 3 years. Bilateral involvement may cause a waddling gait, while more often the defect is picked up

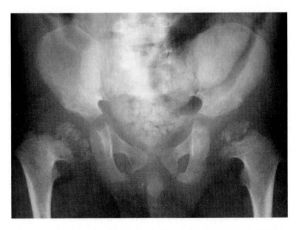

Fig. 7.12. There is bilateral coxa vara and bilateral epiphyseal irregularity. The epiphyses have a stippled appearance. This is the result of congenital hypothyroidism

Table 7.3. Fragmented or irregular femoral head

Common
Normal Variant
Avascular necrosis
Congenital dislocation of the hip
Legg-Perthes' disease
Uncommon
Chondrodysplasia punctata (congenital stippled epiphyses, Conradi-Hunerman)
Cretinism, congenital hypothyroidism
Haemophilia
Hereditary arthro-ophthalmopathy (Stickler syndrome)
Infection
Leukaemia
Mucopolysaccharidosis (e.g. Hurler, Hunter, Morquio, Maroteaux-Lamy)
Multiple epiphyseal dysplasia and Meyer dysplasia
Osteochondromuscular dystrophy (Schwartz syndrome)
Renal osteodystrophy
Rickets, all types
Slipped capital femoral epiphysis (late)
Trisomy 18 and 21
Prenatal infections
Warfarin embryopathy
Cerebrohepatorenal syndrome (Zellweger syndrome)
Fetal alcohol syndrome

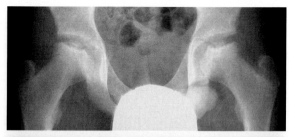

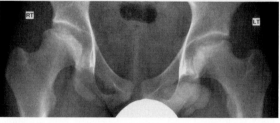

Fig. 7.13a,b. Meyer's dysplasia in a child and subsequent adult. There is irregularity and a granular appearance to the femoral heads. Over time the femoral heads have remained flattened and irregular

as an asymptomatic finding (KHERMOSH and WIEN-TROUB 1991).

On radiographs the ossification centre can be granular or multiple, with up to six separate centres. Fusion of these centres starts to occur by around 5–6 years of age, which may give the femoral head an irregular outline. The most confusing differential diagnosis is that of Perthes' disease (HESSE and KOHLER 2003). Typically in Perthes' disease bilateral lesions (when present) are asymmetric, and the superolateral weight bearing area is most commonly involved (see Chap. 11). In Meyers dysplasia the appearances are symmetrical and they gradually improve over time unlike in Perthes' where there is often further sclerosis and flattening of the femoral head with abnormality of the acetabulum. Bone scintigraphy is normal in Meyer's dysplasia with no evidence of ischaemia and MR imaging has shown a normal appearance of the unossified epiphysis. There appears to be a spontaneous resolution of the dysplasia, which may leave no residual trace apart from some slight femoral flattening (Fig. 7.13).

7.8.2
Multiple Epiphyseal Dysplasia

Multiple epiphyseal dysplasia (MED) is a heterogeneous group of abnormalities that commonly affect the hip and pelvis causing epiphyseal irregularity and deformity, the bone density and texture are normal. If there is significant spinal involvement, then they are described as spondyloepiphyseal (SED). The primary defect in MED is believed to be within the chondrocytes of the unossified skeleton (HAGA et al. 1998; LACHMAN et al. 1973).

The modern definition and classification of the MED is now based upon genetic studies and chromosomal linkage (UNGER et al. 2001). Phenotypically two classical forms have been described a milder form (Ribbing type) and the severe variety (Fairbank type). The condition is however heterogeneous with some patients exhibiting features of the mild form of the disease in certain bones but more severe changes elsewhere in the skeleton. It is most commonly autosomal dominantly inherited with variable penetrance, but there dose appear to be some consistency in the distribution of affected epiphyses between families (AMIR et al. 1985).

The hips, knees and ankles are the most commonly involved joints and children present with reduced mobility, difficult on walking and altered gait. Severe involvement of the limb long bones will cause them to be short and 'stubby'. Often patients have reduced stature, and a thoracic kyphosis. The milder forms of MED are difficult to diagnose in a neonate and they can be an incidental diagnosis in the older child. Generalised joint and back pain are common symptoms, with mild cases not presenting until adulthood.

The radiographic abnormalities are visible between the second and third years of life. There is abnormal ossification of 2 or more pairs of epiphyses. The proximal femoral epiphysis is commonly involved and it is fragmented, small and misshapen with an abnormal pattern of ossification. Multiple centres of ossification have been described as 'mulberry like', alternatively the central ossification centre may be surrounded by specks of calcification. The multiple ossification centres coalesce at maturity, with the adult the femoral head being flattened and irregular. There may be a coxa valga deformity with metaphyseal widening, with the acetabulum becoming become shallow and dysplastic. The more severe dysplasias result in poor acetabular and joint development joint that results in earlier osteoarthritis. Ossification of the epiphysis of the hands and feet is delayed while there is distal shortening of the short and long bones (TREBLE et al. 1990) (Figs. 7.14 and 7.15).

Vertebral end plates irregularity, especially at the thoracolumbar junction, Schmorl's nodes and vertebral wedging is a feature of MED. While more severe spinal changes are in keeping with spondyloepiphyseal dysplasia.

MED may be confused with Perthes' disease, but with the latter there are no other affected epiphyses and the appearances are usually asymmetrical. In MED the ossific nucleus gradually enlarges with ossification becoming more uniform, without the sequential changes usually seen in Perthes'. The differential diagnosis includes juvenile idiopathic arthritis, progressive pseudo-rheumatoid dysplasia, congenital hypothyroidism and the mucopolysaccharidosis (MANDELL et al. 1989).

7.8.3
Spondyloepiphyseal Dysplasia

There are a variety of forms of SED that are distinguished by clinical, genetic and radiological defects. In the long bone, particularly around the hips the appearances are similar to MED, depending on the severity of the disorder (LANGER et al. 1990). In the SED the spinal abnormalities are more pronounced and include platyspondylia, with short pear shaped or more flattened vertebral bodies, with widening of

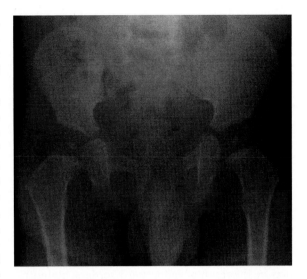

Fig. 7.14. Multiple epiphyseal dysplasia. Symmetrical abnormality of both femoral heads. Both femoral epiphyses are small and irregular. There is metaphyseal irregularity

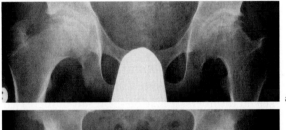
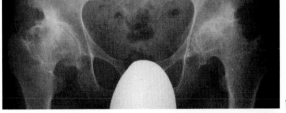

Fig. 7.15a,b. Progression of the femoral heads changes in multiple epiphyseal dysplasia. The epiphyses are initially small and irregular. The epiphyses become widened and flattened with evidence of bone remodelling and loss of joint space

the disc spaces. Children may develop a kyphosis. The spinal changes in SED may be confused with Morquio's disease but they are usually none of the digital hand abnormalities and the bone texture is normal.

7.8.4
Accelerated Ossification

Accelerated ossification is an important marker for a small number of skeletal dysplasias and metabolic disorders. These disorders have accelerated skeletal maturation defects elsewhere within the body, particularly the hands and skull, with metaphyseal irregularity and abnormal phalanges (STELLING 1973).

Advanced pelvic ossification is seen in the femoral heads either at birth or shortly after in asphyxiating thoracic dysplasia and chondroectodermal dysplasia. In the pelvis it is seen in Marshall-Smith syndrome, chondroectodermal dysplasia, congenital adrenal hyperplasia, Weaver syndrome and Beckwith-Wiedemann syndrome.

7.8.5
Delayed Ossification

Delayed ossification is a non-specific finding and may be the result of endocrine disorders, malnutrition, chronic disease or a skeletal dysplasia. It is most often seen in the pubis, ischium and femoral epiphysis, but may affect any part of the skeleton (STELLING 1973).

7.8.6
Increased Bone Density

Increased bone density is seen in a wide range of skeletal disorders. It may be the result of increased calcium deposition, diminished resorption, exces-

sive new bone formation or be the result of a sclerosing bone dysplasia. The pattern may be diffuse or focal. The more common sclerosing dysplasias include Camurati-Engelmann disease, metaphyseal dysplasia (Pyle disease), dysosteosclerosis, endosteal hyperostosis (Worth and van Buchem), osteopetrosis, melorheostosis, pyknodysostosis and osteopoikilosis (Figs. 7.16 and 7.17).

7.8.7
Decreased Bone Density

Decreased bone density is a non-specific finding that may be part of a bone dysplasia, e.g. osteogenesis imperfecta, metabolic disorder, chronic illness, malignancy, chronic steroid use and hyperparathyroidism. Reduced bone density can lead to coax valga and acetabular remodelling. If severe there may be an increase risk of fracturing, bone remodelling and pseudoarthrosis (Fig. 7.18).

7.8.8
Abnormal Shape and Appearance of Pelvis

The relative size of the ilium should always be considered with respect to the gestational age of the child (EICH et al. 1992). A small ilium is associated with dysplasias that are detectable at birth, some of which are lethal, which includes asphyxiating thoracic dysplasia, chondroectodermal dysplasia, Kniest dysplasia and the short rib polydactyly dysplasias (OESTREICH and PRENGER 1992). The small ilium may be squared or flared and is usually associated with a horizontal acetabular roof. The pubis

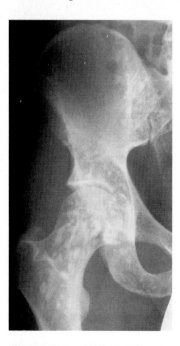

Fig. 7.16. Osteopoikilosis. There are multiple oval densities around the hip joint. They are parallel to the long axis of the femur

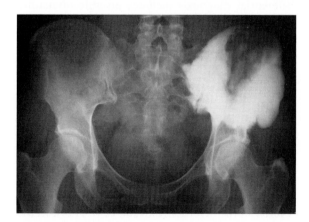

Fig. 7.17. Melorheostosis. There is increased sclerosis around the left iliac wing and cortical hyperostosis with a wavy outline

and ischium may also be small. In some dysplasias a small sciatic notch may be present such as in achondroplasia (Fig. 7.19).

Small iliac wings are an isolated finding in some syndromes that includes scapuloiliac dysplasia and thoracic-pelvic dysostosis. Narrowing of the ilium at the base , with flaring of the wings is a feature of lysosomal storage disorders. Flared iliac wings are a feature of Downs syndrome, as are decreased acetabular and iliac angles. Iliac horns are a marker for osteo-onycho-dysostosis (nail patellar syndrome) where the pelvis may be small.

Hypoplasia of the ischium and pelvis is seen in disorders that cause delayed or deficient ossification and also camptomelic dysplasia, cleidocranial dysplasia and spondyloepiphyseal dysplasias.

A steep or slanted acetabular roof is often an isolated finding that can be attributed to a congenital dysplasia or dislocation of the hip. It is also seen in neuromuscular disorders. It is a feature of some bone dysplasias in particular the storage disorders (Eich et al. 1992).

A flat or horizontal acetabular roof is a feature of those dysplasias associated with a small ilium, in

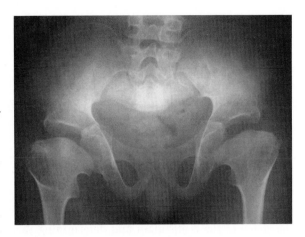

Fig. 7.19. Achondroplasia. There is squaring of the iliac wings, and a short narrow sacrosciatic notch. The sacrum is horizontal and articulates low on the ileum. The acetabulum are shallow. There is marked remodelling and deformity of both femoral heads

particular the neonatal lethal dysplasias, but also pseudoachondroplasia, trisomy-21 and Rubinstein-Taybi syndrome.

Diastasis of the pubic symphysis is associated with some dysplasia , most commonly cleidocranial dysostosis. It is also a feature of bladder exstrophy, due to incomplete formation and rotation of the pelvic girdle due to abnormal bladder development (Fig. 7.8). There are often other associated renal tract anomalies.

7.9
Arthrogryposis Multiplex Congenita

Arthrogryposis multiplex congenita is characterised by joint contractures, muscle fibrosis and a significant reduction in function. It is often recognised at birth due to limited movement of the joints.

Radiographically there is decreased muscle mass, and incongruity around joints. Dislocation of the hip is a feature. Fractures and scoliosis can occur.

A classical appearance is the diamond deformity with the hips adducted, flexed and internally rotated with flexed knees.

7.10
Neuromuscular Hip Dysplasia

Children with cerebral palsy who do not walk before the age of 5 years have increased incidence of hip dysplasia. The more severe the neurological dis-

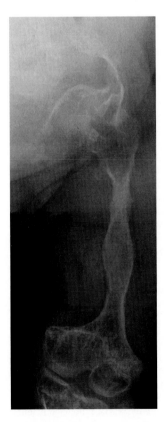

Fig. 7.18. Osteogenesis imperfecta. There is marked reduction in bone density, numerous healing fractures, acetabuli protrusio and remodelling around the acetabulum

order the greater the incidence and degree of the dysplasia, and the more likely that it will be bilateral. Lack of muscle balance and function results in coxa valga deformity, abnormal anteversion of the femoral neck (AKTAS et al. 2000). The proximal epiphysis is often poorly developed and may be flattened or notched. The acetabulum is often shallow, with lateral uncovering of the femoral head with an increased incidence of hip subluxation or dislocation (MORRELL et al. 2002).

Serial radiographs are useful for assessing hip development, acetabular remodelling and femoral head coverage over time. CT is useful in evaluating the shape of the acetabulum and determining the degree of femoral anteversion (DAVIDS et al. 2003).

Surgical treatment may involve soft tissue releases to improve muscle balance. Osteotomies are used to improve the coverage of the femoral head and help hip development. Correction of any inversion abnormality is important in improving surgical outcome.

References

Aktas S, Aiona MD, Orendurff M (2000) Evaluation of rotational gait abnormality in the patients cerebral palsy. J Pediatr Orthop 20:217–220

Amir D, Mogle P, Weinberg H (1985) Multiple epiphyseal dysplasia in one family: a further review of seven generations. J Bone Joint Surg 67B:809–813

Amstutz HC (1970) Developmental (infantile) coxa vara – a distinct entity: report of two patients with previously normal roentgenograms. Clin Orthop 72:242–247

Anton CG, Applegate KE, Kuivila TE, Wilkes DC (1999) Proximal Femoral Focal Deficiency (PFFD): more than an abnormal hip. Semin Musculoskelet Radiol 3:215–226

Blockey NJ (1969) Observations on infantile coxa vara. J Bone Joint Surg 51B:106 –111

Bobroff ED, Chambers HG, Sartoris DJ, Wyatt MP, Sutherland DH (1999) Femoral anteversion and neck-shaft angle in children with cerebral palsy. Clin Orthop 364:194–204

Bos CF, Sakkers RJ, Bloem JL, vd Stadt RJ, vd Kamp JJ (1989) Histological, biochemical, and MRI studies of the growth plate in congenital coxa vara. J Pediatr Orthop 9:660–665

Bowerman JW, Sean JM, Chang R (1982) The teardrop shadow of the pelvis: anatomy and clinical significance. Radiology 143:659–662

Calhoun JD, Pierret G (1972) Infantile coxa vara. AJR 115:561–568

Caffey J, Madell SH (1956) Ossification of the pubic bones at birth. Radiology 67:346–350

Caffey J, Ross SE (1956) The ischiopubic synchondrosis in healthy children: some normal roentgenologic findings. AJR 76:488–494

Court C, Carlioz H (1997) Radiological study of severe proximal femoral focal deficiency. J Pediatr Orthop 17:520–524

Davids JR, Marshall AD, Blocker ER, Frick SL, Blackhurst DW,

Skewes E (2003) Femoral anteversion in children with cerebral palsy. Assessment with two and three-dimensional computed tomography scans. J Bone Joint Surg 85(A):481–488

Diel J, Ortiz o, Losada RA, Price DB, Hayt MW, Katz DS (2001) The sacrum: pathologic spectrum, multimodality imaging, and subspecialty approach. Radiographics 21:83–104

Eich GF, Babyn P, Giedion A (1992) Paediatric pelvis: radiographic appearance in various congenital disorders. Radiographics 12:467–484

Epps CH (1983) Proximal femoral focal deficiency. J Bone Joint Surg 65A:867–870

Fabry G, MacEwen GD, Shands AR (1973) Torsion of the femur. A follow-up study in normal and abnormal conditions. J Bone Joint Surg 55(A):1726–1738

Fixen JA (1995) Major congenital shortening of the lower limb and congential pseudarthrosis of the Tibia. J Ped Orthop 49B:142–144

Francis CC (1951) Appearance of centres of ossification in the human pelvis before birth. AJR 65:778–783

Francis HH (1959) The etiology, development, and the effect upon pregnancy of protusio acetabuli (otto pelvis). Surg Gynecol Ostet 103:295–308

Gelberman RH, Cohen MS, Desai SS, Griffin PP, Salamon PB, O'Brien TM (1987) Femoral anteversion. A clinical assessment of idiopathic in toeing gait in children. J Bone Joint Surg 69(B):75–79

Gillespie R, Torode IP (1983) Classification and management of congenital abnormalities of the femur. J Bone Joint Surg 65 (B):557–568

Gilsanz V (1983) Distal focal femoral deficiency. Radiology 147:105–107

Goddard NJ, Hashemi-Nejad A, Fixsen JA (1995) Natural history and treatment of instability of the hip in proximal femoral focal deficiency. J Pediatr Orthop 4(B):145–149

Grissom LE, Harke HT (1999) Developmental dysplasia of the pediatric hip with emphasis on sonographic evaluation. Semin Musculoskelet Radiol 3:359–370

Guenther KP, Tomczak R, Kessler S, Pfeiffer T, Puhl W (1995) Measurement of femoral anteversion by magnetic resonance imaging – evaluation of a new technique in children and adolescents. Eur J Radiol 21:47–52

Haga N, Nakamura K, Takikawa K, Manabe N, Ikegawa S, Kimizuka M (1998) Stature and severity in multiple epiphyseal dysplasia. J Pediatr Orthop 18(B):394–397

Hesse B, Kohler G (2003) Does it always have to be Perthes' disease? What is epiphyseal dysplasia? Clin Orthop 414:219–227

Hillmann JS, Mesgarzadeh M, Revesz G Bonakdarpour A, Clancy M, Betz RR (1987) Proximal femoral focal deficiency: radiologic analysis of 49 cases. 165:769–773

Hooper JC, Jones EW (1971) Primary protrusion of the acetabulum; J Bone Joint Surg 53(B):23–29

Kalamchi A, Cowell HR, Kim KI (1985) Congenital deficiency of the femur. J Pediatr Orthop 5:129–134

Keats T, Anderson M (2001) Atlas of normal roentgen variants, 4th edn. Mosby, Chicago

Khermosh O, Wientroub S (1991) Dysplasia epiphysealis capitis femoris. Meyer's dysplasia. J Bone Joint Surg 73(B):621–625

Kloiber R, Udjus K, McIntyre W, Jarvis J (1988) The scintigraphic and radiographic appearance of the ischiopubic synchondroses in normal children and in osteomyelitis. Pediatr Radiol 18:57–61

Lachman RS, Rimoin DL, Hollister DW (1973) Athropathy of the hip: a clue to the pathogenesis of the epiphyseal dysplasias. Radiology 108:317–322

Lange DR, Schoenecker PL, Baker CL (1978) Proximal femoral focal deficiency: treatment and classification in forty-two cases. Clin Orthop 135:15–25

Langer LO, Brill BW, Ozonoff MB et al (1990) Spondylo-metaphyseal dysplasia, corner fracture type: a heritable condition associated with coxa vara. Radiology 175:761–766

Lemperg R, Liliequist B, Mattson S (1973) Asymmetry of the epiphyseal nucleus in the femoral head is stable and unstable hip joints. Pediatr Radiol 1:191–195

Levinson ED, Ozonoff MB, Royen PM (1997) Proximal femoral focal deficiency (PFFD). Radiology 125:197–203

Lincoln TL, Suen PW (2003) Common rotational variations in children. J Am Acad Orthop Surg 11:312–320

Macdonald D (1971) Primary protrusio acetabuli. Report of an affected family. J Bone Joint Surg 53(B):30–36

Mandell GA, MacKenzie WG, Scott CI Jr, Harcke HT, Wills JS, Bassett GS (1989) Identification of avascular necrosis in the dysplastic proximal femoral epiphysis. Skeletal Radiol 18:273–281

McBridge MT, Muldoon MP, Santore RF, Trousdale RT, Wenger DR (2001) Protrusio acetabuli: diagnosis and treatment. J Am Acad Orthop Surg 9:79–88

Morrell DS, Pearson JM, Sauser DD (2002) Progressive bone and joint abnormalities of the spine and lower extremities in cerebral palsy. Radiographics 22:257–268

Oestreich AE, Prenger EC (1992) MR demonstrates cartilaginous megaepiphyses of the hips in Kniest dysplasia of the young child. Pediatr Radiol 22:302–303

Osborne D, Effmann E, Broda K, Harrelson J (1980) The development of the upper end of the femur, with special reference to its internal architecture. Radiology 137:71–76

Ozonoff MB, Ziter FMH Jr (1987) The femoral head notch. Skeletal Radiol 16:19–22

Panting AL, Williams PF (1978) Proximal femoral focal deficiency. J Bone Joint Surg 60B:46–52

Pappas AM (1983) Congenital abnormalities of the femur and related lower extremity malformations: classification and treatment. J Pediatr Orthop 3:45–60

Pavlov H, Goldman AB, Freiberger RH (1980) Infantile coxa vara. Radiology 135:631–639

Pettersson H, Theander G (1979) Ossification of femoral head in infancy. I. Normal standards. Acta Radiol [Diagn] 20:170–179

Pirani S, Beauchamp RD, Li D, Sawatzky B (1991) Soft tissue anatomy of proximal femoral focal deficiency. J Pediatr Orthop 11:563–570

Ponseti IV (1978) Growth and development of the acetabulum in the normal child. J Bone Joint Surg 60(A):575–585

Reikeras O, Bjerkreim I (1982) Idiopathic increased anteversion of the femoral neck. Radiological and clinical study in non-operated and operated patients. Acta Orthop Scand 53:839–845

Sanpera I Jr, Sparks LT (1994) Proximal femoral focal deficiency: does a radiologic classification exist? J Pediat Orthop 14:34–38

Staheli LT, Corbett M, Wyss C, King H (1985) Lower-extremity rotational problems in children. Normal values to guide management. J Bone Joint Surg 67(A):39–47

Steel HH (1996) Protrusio acetabuli: its occurrence in the completely expressed Marfan syndrome and its musculoskeletal component and a procedure to arrest the course of protrusion in the growing pelvis. J Pediatr Orthop 16:704–718

Stelling FH (1973) The hip in heritable conditions of connective tissue. Clin Orthop 90:33–49

Stewart RJ, Patterson CC, Mollan RAB (1986) Ossification of the normal femoral capital epiphysis. J Bone Joint Surg 68(B):653

Treble NJ, Jensen FO, Bankier A, Rogers JG, Cole WG (1990) Development of the hip in multiple epiphyseal dysplasia. Natural history and susceptibility to premature osteoarthritis. J Bone Joint Surg 72(B):1061–1064

Unger SL, Briggs MD, Holden P, Zabel B, Ala–Kokko L, Paassiltra P, Lohiniva J, Rimoin DL, Lachman RS, Cohn DH (2001) Multiple epiphyseal dysplasia: radiographic abnormalities correlated with genotype. Pediatr Radiol 31:10–18

Weinstein NJ, Kuo KN, Millar EA (1984) Congenital coxa vara. A retrospective review. J Pediatr Orthop 4:70–77

8 Developmental Dysplasia of the Hip 1: Child

Helen Williams and Karl J. Johnson

CONTENTS

8.1 Introduction

Normal growth and development of the hip joint depends on congruent stability of the femoral head within the acetabulum. This allows balanced growth between the acetabular and triradiate cartilages and a well-located femoral head. Developmental dysplasia of the hip (DDH) is a disorder with a spectrum of abnormalities involving the growing acetabulum, proximal femur and surrounding soft tissues. It may be defined as abnormal formation of the hip joint occurring between organogenesis and maturity, as a result of instability. Formerly congenital dysplasia or congenital dislocation of the hip (CDH), the more

H. Williams, MD; K. J. Johnson, MD
Department of Radiology, Princess of Wales, Birmingham Children's Hospital, Steelhouse Lane, Birmingham, B4 6NH, UK

recent term developmental dysplasia of the hip is preferable because the process is not restricted to congenital abnormalities of the hip, and includes some hips that were normal at birth and subsequently became abnormal.

In 98% of cases, DDH results from an alteration in development of a previously normal hip during the last 4 weeks of pregnancy or in the postnatal period. The remaining 2% of cases result from an earlier in-utero alteration. During gestation the hip is at risk of dislocation during the 12th week when the lower limb rotates medially, and during the 18th week as the hip muscles develop. Dislocations during these developmental stages are termed teratologic and are the result of congenital abnormal neuromuscular development. Strictly, DDH applies to idiopathic hip dysplasia, but hip dysplasia can occur secondary to neurological conditions (e.g. myelomeningocele, cerebral palsy), connective tissue diseases (e.g. Ehlers-Danlos syndrome), and myopathic disorders (e.g. arthrogryposis multiplex congenita).

Early diagnosis and treatment of DDH is important because the longer the condition is unrecognised, the higher the incidence of treatment failure. Furthermore, the treatment of DDH can differ significantly depending upon the age at diagnosis. In the long term, DDH is an important cause of gait disturbance, restricted joint mobility and degenerative joint disease in adolescence and adulthood.

8.2 Epidemiology and Aetiology of DDH

The incidence of DDH varies with race and gender. The true incidence is not known because statistics vary due to differences in methods used for diagnosis and there is no agreed 'gold standard' for the diagnosis of DDH. The prevalence of DDH varies between 1 per 100 births in clinically screened populations to 80 per 1000 in sonographically screened populations (Dwek et al. 2002). There is a four to eight fold increased incidence of DDH in female infants. This is attributed to potentiation (by endogenous oestrogens produced by the female infant) of the transiently increased ligamentous laxity in the perinatal period caused by high levels of circulating maternal hormones. Firstborn children are affected more frequently than subsequent siblings, which may be related to the confining effects of an unstretched primigravid uterus and abdominal wall, with subsequent effects on fetal limb position and hip joint development. DDH occurs three times more frequently on the left side, probably because the most common position in non-breech babies is head down with the fetal spine on the mothers left side. In this position the left hip lies posteriorly against the mother's spine and abduction is limited. Postural deformities, oligohydramnios, foot abnormalities such as metatarsus varus and talipes equinovarus are all associated with DDH. Congenital torticollis is also associated with DDH (WALSH and MORRISSY 1998). Breech presentation independent of method of delivery is associated with a higher incidence of hip dysplasia, particularly the extended breech position. Breech position is also commoner in females, and in first-born infants (GUILLE et al. 2000).

Both genetic and environmental factors are important in the aetiology of DDH. An increased probability of having a child with DDH has been estimated to be 6% if there is one prior affected child but both parents have normal hips. It is 12% if one parent is affected but no prior affected child, and 36% if there is one affected parent and one affected child (WYNNE-DAVIS 1970; LINGG et al. 1981). Monozygotic twins are more likely to have DDH than dizygotic twins. DDH is also affected by cultural and racial factors. It is commonest in white neonates and there is a very low incidence in black African and Chinese populations (WEINSTEIN 1987). An increased incidence in Laplanders and native American Indians is thought to be associated with the cultural tradition of strapping infants to a cradleboard or swaddling them with the hips together in extension. In adduction, the femoral head is directed posteriorly and away from the joint. If the acetabulum is shallow or there is ligamentous laxity, swaddling can accentuate instability and contribute to the incidence of hip subluxation or dislocation. An anti-swaddling campaign in Japan decreased the incidence of DDH from 3.5% to 0.2% (YAMAMURO and ISHIDA 1984). Traditionally African and Chinese mothers hold their infants against the waist with the infants hips in flexion and abduction, this position is more conducive to acetabular-femoral development.

The history obtained on first presentation of an infant with suspected DDH should include pertinent risk factors such as family history of hip dysplasia, maternal obstetric history, presentation and delivery. Infants with known associations and certain risk factors such as breech presentation are offered ultrasound screening in many centres in addition to clinical screening tests. A low threshold for hip ultrasound in the neonatal period should theoretically reduce the incidence of late diagnosis.

DDH is clearly a multifactorial condition although several theories have been proposed to account for the disease process (NOVACHECK 1996). These place increased importance on: (1) mechanical factors such as restricted uterine space and breech positioning, (2) ligamentous laxity and (3) the concept of 'primary acetabular dysplasia' as a basis for the development of hip dysplasia. Genetic predisposition may significantly contribute to the latter two aetiological theories.

8.3
Hip Embryology, Anatomy and Pathological Changes in DDH

Embryologically all components of the hip joint arises from a single block of mesenchymal tissue. During the 7th week of gestation a cleft appears in the pre-cartilaginous cells and by the 11th week this cleft separates the acetabulum and femoral head. Acetabular and femoral head development continues throughout intrauterine life but the femoral head grows disproportionately faster so that at birth, relative coverage of the femoral head by the acetabulum is at its least. Within a few weeks of birth however, labral growth accelerates resulting in increased coverage of the femoral head. It is during the perinatal period and for several months after birth that the femoral head has the least structural support from the acetabulum and hip capsule, and is at the highest risk of subluxation or dislocation (DONALDSON and FEINSTEIN 1997). In most cases if a dislocation is found in the newborn period it can be easily reduced. However if subluxation or dislocation is allowed to persist, adaptive changes occur within the hip structures making concentric reduction of the femoral head more difficult.

The acetabular cartilage comprises a cup shaped structure forming the outer two-thirds of the joint cavity and the triradiate cartilage located deep in the joint. The lateral aspect of the acetabular cartilage has three epiphyses or secondary ossification centres; the acetabular epiphysis is adjacent to the ilium, the os acetabuli is next to the pubis and there is a small posterior epiphysis next to the ischium. Most acetabular development occurs by eight years of age, but at puberty these epiphyses develop and enhance the depth of the acetabulum. The fibrocartilaginous labrum rims the anterior, superior and posterior aspects of the acetabular cartilage, inferiorly it is known as the transverse acetabular ligament. The labrum contributes to hip stability by deepening the hip capsule and constricting its orifice.

In infancy the femoral head, neck, greater and lesser trochanters, intertrochanteric zone and a portion of the proximal femur are composed entirely of cartilage. The ossification centre for the femoral head appears between 2 and 7 months of age. Growth occurs mostly at the physis, growth plate of the greater trochanter and the cartilage of the femoral neck isthmus situated between these two structures. The balance of growth between these three structures, and the effect of muscle pull and weight-bearing forces on the proximal femur determines the eventual shape and congruency of the femoral head. Disruption of blood supply to the proximal femoral physis results in femoral shortening and varus deformity because of unbalanced growth of the femoral neck isthmus and greater trochanteric growth plate.

In a dysplastic hip the acetabulum loses its cup-like shape. As the femoral head migrates superiorly, the labrum becomes everted and flattened. Growth of the acetabulum is altered in the absence of a normally located femoral head. The acetabulum becomes shallow and the slope of the roof becomes steeper. If the femoral head dislocates, the inferior capsular fibres and the transverse acetabular ligament are pulled up over the empty socket. Capsular constriction and shortening of the iliopsoas tendon can prevent hip reduction. The ligamentum teres thickens, and the socket becomes filled with fibro-fatty tissue known as the pulvinar. Interposition of capsular tissue or inverted labral tissue may present mechanical blocks to reduction of the femoral head. Fibrous tissue develops and merges with hyaline cartilage at the rim of the acetabulum. This fibrous tissue is a pathological structure known as the limbus, and may also contribute to failure of concentric hip reduction.

Growth of the femoral head is affected when it is no longer correctly seated within the acetabulum. It loses its spherical shape, and may become smaller or develop areas of flattening. In untreated hip dis-

location a neoacetabulum can form in the iliac bone above the native joint (Fig. 8.1). Acetabular growth is affected most in complete hip dislocations when there is no contact with the femoral head. In these cases both anterior and posterior columns of the acetabulum are stunted due to lack of pressure stimulation. When the hip is subluxed or the acetabulum is shallow, weight-bearing forces are altered and there is increased pressure at the edge of the steep, shallow acetabulum (Fig. 8.2).

Generally the longer the femoral head remains out of the acetabulum or persistently subluxed, the greater the severity of acetabular dysplasia and distortion of the femoral head. Closed reduction of the femoral head within the acetabulum results in spon-

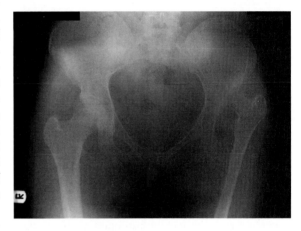

Fig. 8.1. A 16-year-old female patient with longstanding "missed" left DDH. The left femoral head articulates with a neo-acetabulum in the iliac bone. The left femoral shaft is reduced in diameter and there is wasting of the thigh muscles

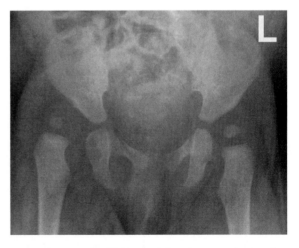

Fig. 8.2. A 5-month-old female with right DDH. The acetabulum is dysplastic and the right femoral head is subluxed superolaterally. Shenton's line is disrupted on the right

taneous resolution of the pulvinar. Open reduction of a fixed dislocated hip involves resection of the ligamentum teres and the pulvinar to ensure congruent reduction. Incision of the transverse acetabular ligament is also essential for complete reduction.

8.4
Clinical Detection of DDH – Definitions

- Dysplasia – abnormal formation of tissues including the femur, acetabulum, or soft tissues.
- Subluxation – the protrusion of the femoral head beyond the acetabulum, with contact still maintained.
- Dislocation – loss of contact of the femoral head with the acetabulum. A dislocated hip may be reducible or irreducible.
- Instability refers to subluxatable or dislocatable hips.
- A dislocatable hip is one in which the femoral head is located within the acetabulum but can be completely displaced from it by the application of posteriorly directed forces to the hip positioned in adduction. In most cases the dislocated proximal femur lies postero-superior to the acetabulum. A subluxatable hip is one in which the femoral head slides in the acetabulum into a position of partial contact with the acetabulum upon application of similar forces.

8.4.1
Clinical Detection of DDH – Birth to 6 Months

A full inspection of the lower limbs is a vital part of the clinical examination for DDH. Asymmetric inguinal or thigh skin folds (with extra folds on the affected side) may be an indicator of hip abnormality but asymmetry is also seen in infants with normal hips. There may be lower limb shortening due to superior displacement of the affected femur. A positive Galeazzi or Allis sign indicates femoral shortening and is elicited by lower position of the knee on the affected side with flexion of the hips and knees. Femoral shortening may be congenital or due to unilateral hip dislocation. Limited abduction of an affected hip may not be present for several months, resulting from contraction and shortening of associated muscles, the hip joint capsule and other soft tissues. When there is bilateral hip abnormality, asymmetry may not be a feature.

The Ortolani and Barlow manoeuvres are the mainstay of clinical diagnosis in the first months of life. Both are performed with the infant supine, and each hip is examined individually with the opposite hip held in maximum abduction to stabilise the pelvis. The Ortolani test checks for reduction of a dislocated hip. It is performed with the baby's hip and knee in flexion. The examiner holds the baby's thigh with their middle finger behind the greater trochanter and their thumb in front on the upper inner thigh. Gentle but sustained abduction whilst pressing forwards on the greater trochanter (lifting away from the examination couch) results in reduction of the femoral head into the acetabulum. A 'clunk' or jerk during this procedure is felt when the femoral head passes over the posterior labrum (ORTOLANI 1937, 1976).

Barlow's manoeuvre attempts to produce subluxation or dislocation of a normally located femoral head. It is performed with the knee flexed to 90° and the hip adducted and partially flexed to 45°–60°. The knee is gently pushed posteriorly (towards the examination couch) and superiorly. In a normal child no movement occurs. In a child with a dislocatable hip a palpable 'clunk' is felt as the head of the femur slips out over the posterior labrum, returning immediately pressure on the upper femur is released (BARLOW 1962). Audible 'clicks' during this procedure generally have no pathological significance and result from stretching of the joint capsule and tendons (GUILLE et al. 1999). Even in the best hands physical examination can fail to detect DDH, and after 3 months of age the Ortolani and Barlow tests become negative due to progressive soft tissue contractures.

8.4.2
Clinical Detection of DDH – the Older Child

It is inevitable that despite clinical screening and early ultrasound examination of patients with known risk factors for the development of DDH, some children will have a delayed presentation or late diagnosis of DDH. In these children timing is important because the treatment of children presenting at 6 months of age or later is different to those presenting under the age of 6 months. Also included in this group of patients are those who were identified early but in whom Pavlik harness treatment has failed, or the changes of DDH have developed late as a result of maturation even though no physical abnormality was identified in the neonatal period.

Physical examination is still the main method for detection of DDH up to walking age. After several months of age the Ortolani and Barlow manoeuvres are no longer useful as soft tissues around the hip joint tighten and contract. Abduction becomes more limited which is particularly noticeable when there is unilateral disease. Femoral shortening (positive Galeazzi test) may be apparent but this can be difficult to appreciate with bilateral disease. Ambulatory children will have a Trendelenburg gait in addition to limited hip abduction (VITALE 2001).

8.5
Natural History of DDH

The natural history of DDH in the newborn is variable. Many unstable newborn hips will stabilise shortly after birth. Neonates with a dysplastic acetabulum but without instability may go on to develop normal hips without treatment. Those with instability or frank dislocation often develop progressive radiographic changes, followed by loss of motion and pain (YAMAMURO and ISHIDA 1984; COLEMAN 1995). Over the age of 6 months spontaneous resolution of dysplasia is unlikely and usually more aggressive treatment is required compared with younger children. Older children tend to have more advanced changes in the soft tissues and bony structures. Ossification of the acetabulum is delayed and this is often abnormally shallow, anteverted, and deficient anterolaterally. Delayed ossification of the femoral head also occurs and there is exaggerated femoral anteversion.

Persistence of hip dysplasia into adolescence and adulthood can lead to an abnormal gait, restricted abduction, reduced strength and an increased rate of degenerative joint disease. In general the outcome of untreated unilateral DDH is less favourable compared with bilateral disease, due to the associated problems with limb length discrepancy, asymmetrical movement, strength, and knee disorders. Degenerative joint disease tends to present earlier in subluxated hips than in dysplastic hips without subluxation (COOPERMAN et al. 1980). The most severely affected patients with subluxation develop symptoms in their second decade, but the mean age at which symptoms appear is 36.6 years in women and 54 years in men. Severe radiographic changes then develop over the next 10 years (MURRAY and CRIM 2001). Symptom-

atic disease in patients with acetabular dysplasia without subluxation is more difficult to predict. It remains clinically silent until secondary degenerative changes develop.

The natural history of untreated complete hip dislocations is also variable. There may be little functional disability but this depends on whether there is a well-developed neoacetabulum and if the dislocation is bilateral. Bilateral hip dislocations without a false acetabulum normally have a good prognosis, although hyperlordosis of the lumbar spine can lead to pain. The development of well-formed acetabulum is more likely to result in early degenerative disease and pain whether unilateral or bilateral (WEINSTEIN 1998).

8.6
The Role of Imaging in DDH

Imaging is fundamental in the screening, diagnosis, treatment and follow-up of patients with DDH. The choice of imaging method for evaluation of hip dysplasia will depend upon the age of the child and the indication for imaging. In the newborn period the hip is cartilaginous and although radiographs can confirm DDH or congenital abnormalities of the hip, a normal radiograph does not exclude the presence of instability. Radiographs are only useful after ossification of the acetabulum and femoral head has occurred and are generally used in the follow-up of treated DDH. The femoral head ossifies between 2 and 6 months in girls and between 3 and 7 months in boys. By 4 months of age ossification of the proximal femoral epiphysis is seen in only 50% of normal infants (OZONOFF 1992). Caution should be taken in the interpretation of radiographs before adequate ossification has occurred as they may provide false negative information. Ultrasound is the technique of choice in the first few months of life. Generally beyond 6 months of age ossification prevents adequate evaluation with ultrasound. CT is useful in the post-operative evaluation of infants when the use of radiographs and ultrasound is limited due to the presence of a plaster cast, and in the evaluation of treated and untreated DDH. Magnetic resonance imaging has a role in DDH and can be used to evaluate both ossified and unossified components of the hip but is still infrequently used. This may be related to limited availability, cost and issues such as requirement for sedation.

8.6.1
Interpretation of Radiographs

Radiographs of infants should be obtained with the pelvis in neutral position in relation to the examination table, the lower limbs held in neutral rotation and slight flexion. If the lower limbs are held down the pelvis rotates anteriorly, distorting acetabular anatomy. Pelvic rotation to one side results in spurious deficiency of acetabular coverage of one hip and normal coverage of the opposite hip. In older children who are walking, a weight bearing AP radiograph with the hips in neutral position (patellae facing directly forward) is the optimum view.

Several reference lines and angles are useful in the interpretation of anteroposterior radiographs of the pelvis for DDH (Fig. 8.3 and 8.4). Many of these lines were devised to help localise the unossified cartilaginous femoral head in infancy prior to the use of ultrasound. Values obtained by these methods are not absolute and should be considered in conjunction with clinical information provided by history and examination. Furthermore, abnormal pelvic positioning adversely affects the diagnostic value of these reference lines and this must be considered in their interpretation.

1. Hilgenreiner's line is a horizontal line drawn through the tops of both triradiate cartilages.
2. Perkins' line is drawn perpendicular to Hilgenreiner's line at the lateral edge of the acetabulum, which can be difficult to identify in the dysplastic hip. These two lines divide the hip area into four quadrants. The femoral head should lie within the inner lower quadrant. In a dislocated hip it lies in the upper outer quadrant.
3. Shenton's line is a continuous arc drawn along the medial border of the femoral neck, and superior border of the obturator foramen. Displacement of the femoral head or severe external rotation of the hip results in discontinuity of Shenton's line. Imperfect positioning can result in spurious disruption of this line.
4. The acetabular index or angle is a measure of the apparent slope of the acetabular roof. It is calculated by drawing an oblique line through the outer (superolateral) edge of the acetabulum and superolateral edge of the triradiate cartilage, tangential to Hilgenreiner's line. If there is an acetabular notch this should be included to its superolateral edge but the presence of the notch can increase the margin of error in measurement. At birth the normal acetabular angle is $26°\pm5°$ in males, and $30°\pm4°$ in females. This gradually decreases to $18°\pm4°$ in boys and $20°\pm3°$ in girls by 12 months of age (DWEK et al. 2002). Acetabular angle measurements greater than this strongly suggest acetabular dysplasia.
5. Proximal migration of the femur is determined by shortening of the vertical distance from the femoral ossific nucleus or the femoral metaphysis to Hilgenreiner's line.

When the proximal femoral ossific nucleus is present the centre edge (CE) angle of Wiberg may be calculated. First a horizontal line is drawn linking the centres of the two femoral heads. A second line

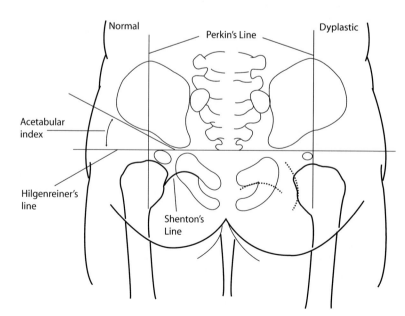

Fig. 8.3. Diagram showing the lines and angles used to assess the developing hip. *Hilgenreiner's line* is a horizontal line drawn through the tops of both triradiate cartilages. *Perkins' line* is drawn perpendicular to Hilgenreiner's line at the lateral edge of the acetabulum. *Shenton's line* is a continuous arc drawn along the medial border of the femoral neck, and superior border of the obturator foramen. The *acetabular index* or angle is calculated by drawing an oblique line through the outer (superolateral) edge of the acetabulum and superolateral edge of the triradiate cartilage, tangential to Hilgenreiner's line. Proximal migration of the femur is determined by shortening of the vertical distance from the femoral ossific nucleus or the femoral metaphysis to Hilgenreiner's line

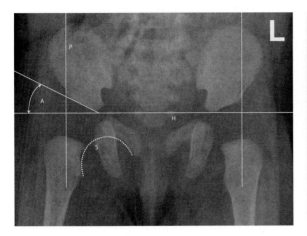

Fig. 8.4. AP pelvic radiograph of a normal 11-week-old infant showing position of lines used to localise the unossified femoral head on pelvic radiographs prior to the use of ultrasound. *H*, Hilgenreiner's line; *P*, Perkins' line; *A*, acetabular index; *S*, Shenton's line

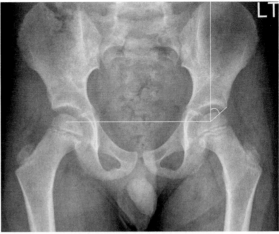

Fig. 8.5. AP pelvic radiograph of a normal 5-year-old boy. Calculation of the centre edge (CE) angle of Wiberg

is then drawn vertically through the centre of the femoral head, perpendicular to the first line. A third line connects the centre of the femoral head to the most lateral point of the acetabulum. The CE angle is determined by the intersection of the last two lines (Fig. 8.5). Angles greater than 25° are normal, angles of 20°–25° borderline, and angles less than 20° are abnormal (WIBERG 1939). The CE angle is difficult to measure in children less than 3 years of age due to incomplete or irregular ossification of the femoral head and ideally this measurement should be reserved for children over 5 years of age (WEINTROUB et al. 1979).

With growth, the adaptive changes of untreated or unsuccessfully treated DDH become more evident on radiographs of the pelvis. The characteristic findings include superior and lateral migration of the proximal femur with a shallow dysplastic acetabulum that lacks the normal slight central depression and well-defined lateral edge. There may also be abnormal sclerosis at the superolateral edge of the acetabulum. Delayed ossification of the proximal femoral epiphysis which remains relatively small is a characteristic finding and the acetabular teardrop may not develop normally (Fig. 8.6). Delay in appearance of the ossification centre for the femoral head occurs when there is persistent instability, but can result from a vascular insult following intervention. If ossification of the femoral head has not occurred by one year of age, avascular necrosis is believed to be present (OZONOF 1992). The teardrop is produced by the acetabular fossa laterally and the pelvic wall medially. It is absent at birth but develops

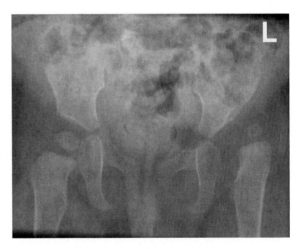

Fig. 8.6. AP pelvic radiograph of an 8-month-old female with left DDH. The left acetabulum is shallow and the hip is dislocated. The left proximal femoral ossification centre is small compared with the normal right side. The normal right acetabulum has a central depression and well-defined lateral edge. The acetabular teardrop is developing on the right but not on the dysplastic left side

in response to the articulating femoral head. Abnormal hip articulation such as persistent subluxation of the femoral head or hip instability may result in either delayed appearance of the teardrop or persistent widening, absence of the acetabular line or an abnormal V-shaped configuration (COLEMAN 1983; KAHLE and COLEMAN 1992). Widening of the teardrop in the older child may signify occult low-grade instability (GUILLE et al. 1999). With appropriate treatment the radiographic signs of DDH regress although disparity in size of the ossified femoral head can persist for 6–12 months. Appearance of the acetabular teardrop is a reliable sign of successful concentric reduction (SMITH et al. 1997).

8.6.2
Ultrasound

Ultrasound is capable of visualising the cartilaginous anatomy of the hip in the first few months of life prior to ossification. Over the past 20 years development of the technique has advanced the evaluation and understanding of DDH. The obvious advantages of ultrasound are that it does not use ionising radiation, is non-invasive, can be performed without the use of sedation and is inexpensive largely because the equipment is widespread. However, accurate use of hip ultrasound does require training and experience.

8.6.2.1
Ultrasound Technique

The two techniques commonly used for evaluating DDH are static or morphological evaluation, and dynamic evaluation which assesses the stability of the femoral head in the acetabulum as well as morphology of the joint. Both methods require a high frequency linear transducer of 7.5 MHz or more from birth to 3 months. After 3 months a 5 MHz transducer is usually adequate. Static or morphological evaluation developed by GRAF (1980, 1984) is widely used in Europe. This technique uses measurements taken in a standard plane to describe acetabular depth and shape. The standard plane is a coronal view representing the centre of the deepest point of the acetabulum (Fig. 8.7 and 8.8). This is best obtained with the infant scanned in a decubitus position with knees slightly flexed. The hip can be placed in neutral position (extended and in slight internal rotation) as originally described by GRAF, or flexed to 90°. The ultrasound approach is slightly posterolateral. The ultrasound beam first penetrates the gluteal muscle lateral to the hip and beneath this the joint capsule, which follows the contour of the femoral head. The femoral head is seen as a stippled, low echogenicity sphere normally centred over the hypoechoic triradiate cartilage. The triradiate cartilage is an important landmark because it represents the centre and deepest part of the acetabulum. From the upper part of the acetabulum the ilium extends superiorly to form the iliac wing. The junction of the

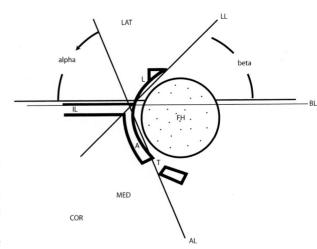

Fig. 8.7. Diagram showing hip anatomy on standard coronal ultrasound plane and lines used to evaluate hip dysplasia using the Graf method. The femoral head (*FH*) is centred over the hypoechoic triradiate cartilage (*T*). The promontory is at the junction of the iliac wing (*IL*) and the bony acetabular roof (*A*). *L*, labrum. The alpha angle reflects the depth of the bony acetabular roof and is formed by the intersection of the baseline (*BL*) and acetabular roof line (*AL*). In a normal mature hip the alpha angle is greater than 60°. The beta angle reflects cartilaginous coverage and is formed by the intersection of the baseline with the labral line (*LL*). A normal beta angle is less than 55°

iliac wing and the acetabular roof is called the promontory or transition point where the acetabulum deviates medially. The shape of the promontory is important because the sharper it appears, the more mature the hip. With an immature hip the promontory appears rounded and flattened (Fig. 8.9). The correct ultrasound view is obtained when the sonographer identifies the mid-coronal scan showing the greatest depth of the acetabular cup, and the greatest diameter of the femoral head. The bony interface of the iliac wing must be horizontal, parallel to the transducer. The bony acetabular promontory and cartilaginous acetabular roof with echogenic tip at the point of the labrum are sharply defined. Rotation of the transducer out of the mid-coronal plane can underestimate acetabular depth. The iliac wing flares laterally when the scan plane is too anterior, and a concave appearance of the ilium is seen when scans are obtained too posteriorly so visualising the concave gluteal fossa of the ilium (GERSCOVICH 1997b). Graf described two angles taken from the standard coronal plane and formed by the intersection of three lines (Fig. 8.8). The baseline (iliac line) is drawn running along the iliac wing perpendicular to the iliac crest. A second line is drawn from the

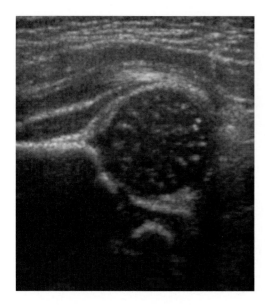

Fig. 8.8. Standard coronal ultrasound of the normal infant hip joint. The promontory is sharply defined and the bony acetabular roof is steep. The ossification centre for the femoral head has not yet developed

promontory to the lower edge of the acetabulum along the medially oriented osseous acetabular roof (acetabular roof line). The intersection of these lines forms the alpha (á) angle. The alpha angle reflects the depth of the bony acetabular roof and coverage of the femoral head. In a normal mature hip the alpha angle is 60° or more. A smaller alpha angle indicates a shallow bony acetabulum. The smaller the alpha angle the shallower the bony acetabulum with a correspondingly increased degree of dysplasia. The beta (à) angle is less important than the alpha angle and is used to assess the cartilaginous acetabular roof. It is formed by the intersection of the baseline with a third line drawn from the promontory to the middle of the acetabular labrum, known as the labral line. In a normal infant the beta

angle is less than 55°. The smaller the beta angle the less the cartilaginous coverage which is a manifestation of better bony containment. An increased beta angle reflects superior displacement of the femoral head. It is mainly used to subclassify dysplastic hips (GRAF 1987).

The Graf classification of hip types is based on calculation of the alpha and beta angles (Table 8.1). Although an alpha angle of less than 60° is abnormal, many infants will demonstrate an alpha angle of between 50° and 59° in the first 3 months of life due to immaturity (Graf type IIA). These require follow up and should normalise. The same measurements in a child over 3 months of age are abnormal. An angle below 50° is abnormal at any age. In the Graf technique there are four basic hip types. Type 1 is normal and requires no treatment. Type 2 needs to be closely observed clinically. Types 3 and 4 require immediate treatment.

The Graf technique is widely used to evaluate the morphology of the acetabulum but an important consideration is that it does not take into account the position of the femoral head, although the two are interdependent. In a normal hip at least half of the femoral head should lie within the acetabulum. This is evaluated sonographically by assessing the percentage of femoral head that lies below the iliac line or baseline. A continuation of the iliac line should bisect the cartilaginous femoral head. With increasing subluxation the percentage of femoral head coverage decreases (Figs. 8.10–8.12) (DWEK et al. 2002). An increased thickness of acetabular cartilage has been described in patents with DDH (SOBOLESKI and BABYN 1993). Cartilage thickness is measured from the baseline at the promontory to the upper aspect of the femoral head. Abnormal values are above 3.5 mm.

Dynamic ultrasound examination of the infant hip was originally described by HARCKE et al. (1984). The technique allows similar morphologic

Table 8.1. Sonographic classification of hip dysplasia (GRAF 1987)

Type	Alpha angle	Beta angle	Comment
I	> 60	-	Normal
IIA	50–59	-	Physiological immaturity (< 3 months old)
IIB	50–59	-	Delayed ossification (> 3 months old)
IIC	43–49	< 77	Critical zone; labrum not everted
IID	43–49	> 77	Subluxed; labrum everted
III	< 43	> 77	Dislocated
IV	< 43 or not measurable	> 77	Dislocated with labrum interposed between femoral head and acetabulum

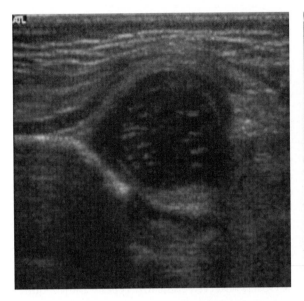

Fig. 8.9. Coronal ultrasound of an immature hip with a rounded flattened promontory indicating a shallow acetabulum. Continuation of the baseline here does bisect the femoral head and in this position (adduction) the femoral head is not significantly subluxed

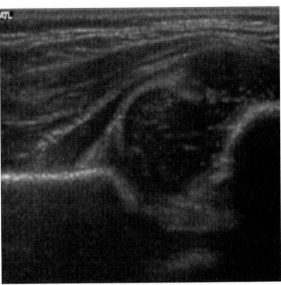

Fig. 8.10. Coronal ultrasound of an immature, subluxed hip. The promontory is slightly rounded and approximately 25% of the femoral head is within the bony acetabulum. The left femoral head is decentred

examination of the hip joint to the Graf technique using static images but emphasises hip instability as the primary abnormality for monitoring. The ultrasound examination incorporates the clinical manoeuvres for provoking subluxation or dislocation of an unstable hip (Barlow test), and reducing a dislocated hip (Ortolani test). The hip is scanned in coronal and transverse planes with the patient supine. In the coronal plane, femoral head coverage, acetabular and labral morphology are evaluated from static views. Stability is assessed while pistoning the hip anteroposteriorly with the knee flexed (Barlow test). The sonographer looks for posterior movement of the femoral head with respect to the triradiate cartilage. This may be achieved by obtaining a slightly posterior view compared with the standard plane. In this view the greatest diameter of the femoral head is not transected and therefore the femoral head appears slightly smaller. If there is subluxation of the femoral head during stress a greater diameter of the femoral head is visualised.

In the transverse plane with the hip flexed ultrasound images are analogous to axial computed tomography (CT) scans of the hip. The femoral head is viewed between two echogenic limbs created by the proximal femoral physis anteriorly and the ischium at the posterior lip of the acetabulum (Fig. 8.13). These form a V shape with the hip in adduction and

a U shape in abduction, with the hypoechoic triradiate cartilage at the base of the acetabular cup. Instability can be assessed in a relaxed infant by performing adduction with gentle stress or pistoning (Barlow test), and reduction of a dislocated hip can be assessed by abduction (Ortolani test). A positive examination is identified if the femoral head subluxes posteriorly over the ischium. In both coronal and transverse planes up to 6 mm posterior displacement can be seen up to 2 weeks of age and is considered to be physiological laxity (KELLER et al. 1988). After this age there should be minimal displacement of no more than 1 mm (HARCKE and GRISSOM 1990; BELLAH 2001). Using the dynamic ultrasound technique hips are classified as either normal, lax with stress, subluxated, or dislocated-dislocatable. Both static and dynamic techniques are subject to significant inter-observer variability, however most studies have shown that this does not have a significant effect on outcome (BAR-ON et al. 1998; JOMHA et al. 1995; ROSENDAHL et al. 1995; DIAS et al. 1993).

Ultrasound is important in follow-up of patients, particularly those undergoing Pavlik harness treatment. Patents may be scanned in the harness (without stressing the joint) to assess the position of the femoral head during its use, and to monitor resolution of dysplasia. With progressive maturity a vascular nidus appears at the centre of the femoral head, followed by the ossification centre beginning as a

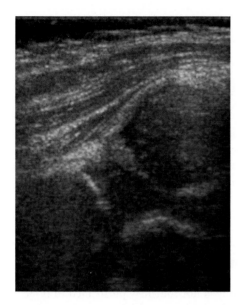

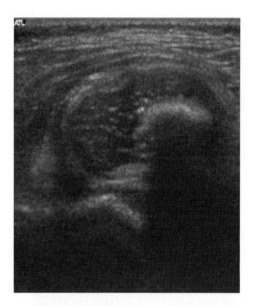

Fig. 8.11. Decentred femoral head on coronal ultrasound. Less than 25% acetabular coverage. The femoral head is significantly displaced from the bony acetabular roof with echogenic material interposed. Appearances suggest labral inversion

Fig. 8.12. Dislocated hip on coronal ultrasound. The femoral head is not aligned with the acetabulum and is seen posterolaterally, beneath the gluteal muscles

small echogenic focus. This is seen on ultrasound earlier than on radiographs (Fig. 8.14). Increased ossification eventually obscures the sonographic landmarks and by 7 to 12 months of age ultrasound can no longer be used to evaluate the hip joint.

8.6.2.2
Use of Ultrasound in Screening for DDH

Screening for DDH is a controversial issue and many studies have evaluated the value of screening programmes. Practice varies in different countries and between centres in the same country. Some European centres screen all newborns whereas the American approach is to offer ultrasound screening to newborns with known risk factors such as family history, breech presentation or abnormality found on physical examination (LEHMANN et al. 2000; AAP GUIDELINE 2000). Clinical screening alone is used in Canada (PATEL 2001). An effective screening programme detects a disease whilst it is asymptomatic, enabling early treatment that aims to prevent or reduce later morbidity. The ideal screening programme is also cost effective. Clinical screening decreases the incidence of late presenting or 'missed' DDH by 50% (TREDWELL and DAVIES 1989). Although the specificity of clinical examination is high, the sensitivity is low with false positive

results leading to over treatment and false negative results leading to late presentation. Sensitivity is improved with increased training and experience of the examiners (EASTWOOD 2003).

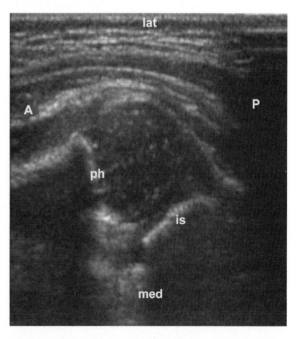

Fig. 8.13. Axial ultrasound demonstrating anatomical landmarks. This image was taken with the hip in adduction. *A*, assecion; *P*, possecion; *lat*, lsteral; *ph*, physis; *is*, ischium; *med*, medial

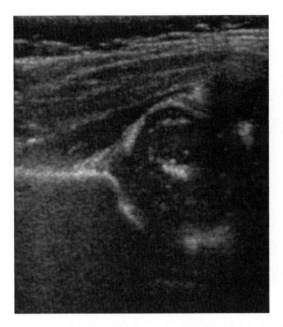

Fig. 8.14. Normal mature hip with ossification centre for the femoral head present

Ultrasound is a very sensitive test for acetabular dysplasia and subluxation and ultrasound detects one third more abnormalities than with clinical examination alone (BOEREE and CLARKE 1994). However the routine use of ultrasound does increase the treatment rate. This inevitably leads to over treatment of some infants whose hips would have become normal without intervention; these are mostly infants with mild acetabular dysplasia or immaturity (MARKS et al. 1994; ROSENDAHL et al. 1996). Treatment with harnessing or splints generally has a low complication rate but there are cost implications for these patients in terms of clinical and imaging follow up. A large-scale study has

shown that selective ultrasound screening of infants with known risk factors did not alter the incidence of surgery in patients with DDH (DEZATEAUX and GODWARD 1996; GODWARD and DEZATEAUX 1998). Policy decisions concerning the use of ultrasound in conjunction with clinical screening will vary depending on the available information regarding the effectiveness of alternative policies, relative disadvantages and cost. The question of whether ultrasound screening for DDH is effective and justified is sure to remain a subject of much debate and further research.

8.6.3
Arthrography

Arthrography is not routinely performed in typical cases of DDH but has an important role in determining whether open or closed reduction is to be performed in infants and toddlers. The procedure is particularly helpful if a dislocation is discovered late, or if sequential radiographs do not demonstrate a satisfactory response to treatment. Arthrography is either performed before surgery or intraoperatively. The goal of arthrography in DDH is to demonstrate the position of the femoral head with respect to other joint structures both at rest and during reduction or stress manoeuvres (Fig. 8.15). It also outlines any deformities or obstructions to concentric reduction, such as inverted limbus, capsular constriction, pulvinar or a hypertrophied ligamentum teres (ALIABADI et al. 1998). Furthermore, arthrography is a dynamic test to evaluate stability and quality of reduction. Most arthrography is performed under general anaesthetic in theatre so that muscle relaxation is maximal and the hip

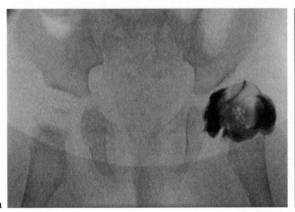
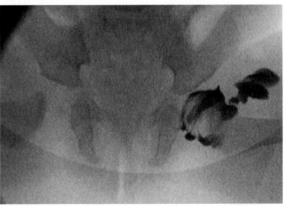

a   b

Fig. 8.15a,b. Images taken during arthrography in a child with left DDH. In neutral position (**a**) the femoral head is dislocated but the hip reduces fully in abduction (**b**)

joint can be fully manipulated. Spot films are taken with the hip in some or all of the following positions: (1) extension-external rotation, (2) extension-neutral position, (3) extension-internal rotation, (4) abduction-neutral position, (5) abduction-internal rotation, (6) abduction-flexion, (7) adduction, (8) adduction-push and (9) adduction-pull (Dwek et al. 2002). Arthrography overcomes the potential for a false impression of concentric reduction being achieved on radiographs because of compression of structures such as an infolded labrum and capsule.

8.6.4
Computed Tomography

There are two main indications for computed tomography (CT) in patients with DDH. CT is used to document hip reduction post-operatively if a child is placed in a spica cast, and also to assist in pre-operative planning for children with severely dysplastic hips that require corrective procedures. For children in a spica cast radiographs provide insufficient information (Fig. 8.16) and there is not usually a large enough ultrasound window to adequately assess the hip, and so a low dose limited CT examination is performed to confirm position of the femoral head with respect to the acetabulum (Eggli et al. 1994). This usually consists of a small number of slices through the hip joint, using low tube current and without the use of sedation or intravenous contrast. CT cannot reliably differentiate between unossified cartilage and other soft tissues and therefore is of most use when the femoral heads are at least partly ossified. When the femoral head is unos-

sified, its position can only be inferred based on the alignment of the metaphysis with the acetabulum (Figs. 8.17 and 8.18). With the hips in abduction, the femoral head should be seated in the acetabulum, slightly posterior to the triradiate cartilage. The axis of the femoral neck should be oriented toward the triradiate cartilage at the centre of the acetabulum.

Acetabular depth and morphology is more accurately assessed with CT compared with radiographs particularly with the use of multiplanar and three-dimensional reconstructions. This is particularly usefully in determining which part of the acetabulum is most deficient in order to plan acetabuloplasty. CT evaluation for femoral anteversion can be helpful in planning derotational osteotomies in children with DDH and hip dysplasia secondary to neuromuscular disease (Hernandez et al. 1981).

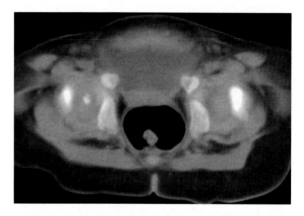

Fig. 8.17. Axial CT scan following left hip reduction. The left hip is dysplastic and the proximal femoral ossification centre is not yet present. Both femoral heads are aligned with the acetabulum, confirming successful hip reduction

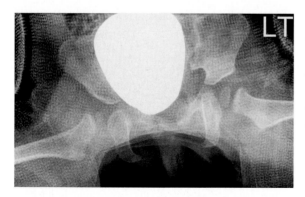

Fig. 8.16. AP radiograph of an 8-month-old child in a spica cast. The right hip is dysplastic with a shallow acetabulum and small left proximal femoral epiphysis. The left femoral head is aligned with the acetabulum but anterior or posterior displacement cannot be assessed from this view alone

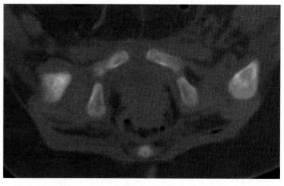

Fig. 8.18. Axial CT scan following open reduction of the left hip. The left femoral metaphysis is not aligned with the acetabulum and the femoral head is displaced posteriorly. The spica cast was removed and patient underwent further manipulation under anaesthesia to achieve successful reduction

8.6.5
Magnetic Resonance Imaging

Magnetic resonance (MR) imaging offers distinct advantages over both CT scanning and arthrography in pre-operative imaging in patients with DDH. Most importantly, MR imaging has the ability to differentiate between different types of soft tissue which enables visualisation of unossified cartilage, ligaments, fat, muscle and fluid including those soft tissues that present an obstruction to concentric reduction such as pulvinar, the labrum and joint capsule. A further advantage is the lack of ionising radiation, although MR imaging is more time-consuming than CT or arthrography. In newborns and infants sedation may be required, except if patents are in a spica cast since this limits movement. The main disadvantages of MR imaging is increased cost and limited availability. MR imaging is still infrequently used in the evaluation of patients with DDH.

MR imaging scan sequences are tailored to the individual clinical problem. In order to confirm hip reduction post-operatively, identify obstructions to concentric reduction or avascular necrosis acutely, axial T1- and T2-weighted spin echo sequences are adequate. Use of gradient echo sequences may reduce the imaging time (GERSCOVICH 1997a). T1-weighted sequences are used to evaluate the bony anatomy because they provide the highest spatial resolution. Fast spin echo T2-weighted sequences with fat saturation (FSET2W-FS) or fast inversion recovery (FSEIR) sequences optimally demonstrate cartilage and marrow oedema (MURRAY and CRIM 2001). Coronal images provide excellent detail of the acetabular roof and labrum (Fig. 8.19), and parasagittal images show the extent of anterior and posterior coverage. The axial images are generally the least useful for evaluating the joint except when confirming post-operative hip reduction and for measuring femoral anteversion. MR arthrography is useful in the evaluation of articular cartilage and the acetabular labrum which is at risk of tearing or detachment in the dysplastic hip because of altered loading forces (MURRAY and CRIM 2001).

Abducted positioning of hips in a spica cast following reduction of DDH may cause avascular necrosis and femoral head perfusion can be assessed using T1-weighted spin echo or three-dimensional spoiled gradient recalled sequences (SPGR) following bolus infusion of gadolinium-chelate (JARAMILLO et al. 1998). Alternatively subtraction images can be obtained using T1-weighted sequences before and after administration of intravenous gadolinium-chelate (SEBAG et al. 1997). This allows detection of decreased femoral head perfusion in the early post-operative period when it is still reversible.

8.7
Treatment of DHH

A full and detailed account of treatment for DDH is outside the scope of this book but it is important for radiologists to be aware of general principles regarding the treatment of DDH in order to direct appropriate imaging, interpret the findings and relate them to the clinical question when treatment options are being considered. Initial treatment may be conservative or operative and will depend upon the age at presentation, pathological and adaptive changes that have taken place within the hip joint

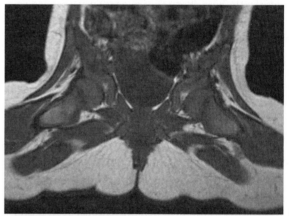

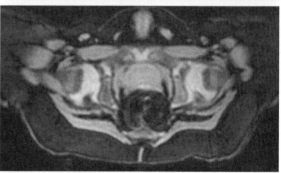

Fig. 8.19. a Coronal T1-weighted MR imaging scan of the pelvis following left hip reduction. The left hip is satisfactorily reduced but there is increased fatty tissue within the hip joint. **b** Axial proton density fast spin echo fat-saturated MR imaging scan of the pelvis (same patient) following left hip reduction. This sequence demonstrates the cartilaginous anatomy well. The femoral heads, triradiate cartilages and the pubic symphysis have high signal. Both hips are in joint

and previous treatment failure. It should be borne in mind that practice will vary between different centres dependent upon current treatment concepts and to an extent upon personal experience of the clinician. Treatment will also depend upon considerations related to the individual patient. Therefore the following information is a general guide only.

At all ages the goal of treatment is to obtain and maintain a concentrically reduced hip joint at the earliest stage possible while minimising complications. Ideally this should result in restoration of normal biomechanical forces about the joint so that remodelling will occur and prevent the development of early degeneration. The longer the hip remains non-congruent the greater the chance of residual dysplasia. Remodelling of the acetabulum is generally considered to be most predictable up to the age of 4 years (ZIONTS and MACEWEN 1986; VITALE and SKAGGS 2001) but the earlier a successful reduction can be achieved, ideally before 18 months of age, the better the outcome.

Subluxation of the hip diagnosed at birth often corrects spontaneously and may be observed for several weeks without treatment. Application of double or triple nappies has previously been used to prevent hip adduction but is not proven to be of any benefit compared with no treatment in the first weeks of life (GUILLE et al. 1999). This practice also encourages hip extension which is an unfavourable position for hip development. When there is actual hip dislocation at birth, or clinical or ultrasound evidence of dysplasia or instability beyond 3–6 weeks of age treatment is indicated. The Pavlik harness or similar abduction devices are used to treat infants presenting with DDH under 6 months of age, with the exception of infants with irreducible hip dislocation which requires an operation. The Pavlik harness is a dynamic positioning device that allows a certain amount of movement whilst maintaining the hips in flexion and abduction, and preventing adduction. The hips are held in 100°–110° of flexion, and abduction is maintained in the so-called safe zone (usually between 30° to 40°), which is between the position of re-dislocation and forced uncomfortable abduction. The harness must be worn at all times and patients in Pavlik harness require close clinical follow-up to monitor treatment and allow harness adjustment during this rapid period of growth. Therefore cooperation of the parents or carers during Pavlik harness treatment is mandatory. Length of treatment is variable but not usually less than 6 weeks, and the incidence of complications with this method of treatment is very low. Avascular necrosis can occur

as a result of excessive hip abduction, and inferior or obturator dislocation occurs rarely secondary to excessive hip flexion. In most cases Pavlik harness treatment is successful but if not, closed or open hip reduction with application of a spica cast is usually necessary. The Pavlik harness is not suitable for older children who are stronger, more active and able to overcome the positioning.

Over the age of 6 months most dislocated hips are not manually reducible. Traction may be used to stretch the contracted soft tissues, prior to attempted closed or open reduction and application of a spica cast (NOVACHECK 1996). Manipulation under anaesthesia with or without operative intervention is also required in order to achieve congruency in persistently subluxed or unstable hips, after which the child is placed in a spica cast. Children over the age of 6 months spend a longer period of time in a spica cast compared with Pavlik harness treatment (typically a minimum of 3 months) to allow the acetabulum to develop. The increased length of time reflects the relatively advanced dysplastic changes seen over the age of 6 months. Spica casts are changed during this period to allow for growth. After 18 months of age secondary changes are usually too severe to respond to non-operative intervention. Traction and closed reduction are rarely successful, and open surgical reduction is required. Patients are at risk of post-operative avascular necrosis, and operative procedures to produce femoral shortening and release the soft tissues are helpful to reduce pressure on the femoral head after reduction. Care must also be taken to avoid excessive abduction in the spica cast as this can also lead to avascular necrosis.

Residual or long standing acetabular dysplasia is more likely to require a redirective or salvage procedure. Femoral varus derotational osteotomy is performed to correct excessive anteversion of the femoral neck, and valgus deformity. It involves varus angulation of the proximal femur, with or without rotation in order to redirect the femoral head into the acetabulum. Iliac osteotomies address the problem of deficient acetabular containment of the femoral head, and aim to increase acetabular coverage, achieve better congruence, decrease pressure loading of the femoral head and improve efficiency of the hip musculature. There are various methods but the most commonly used is the innominate (Salter) osteotomy which reorientates the acetabulum without changing its size or shape. This is indicated for patients with persistent subluxation and mild to moderate acetabular dysplasia. The circumacetabular (Pemberton) osteotomy is a means of reducing acetabular size and increasing articular congruence in moderate to severe DDH. Both Salter and Pemberton osteotomies increase pressure on the femoral head and may lead to avascular necrosis (Fig. 8.20). A median displacement (Chiari) osteotomy medialises the femoral head and provides greater femoral head coverage by enlarging the acetabulum. Success of acetabular osteotomies is dependent on there being sufficient bone to achieve coverage, therefore these procedures are generally not performed before 18 months of age. A combina-

tion of innominate bone and femoral osteotomies is sometimes recommended in older children. After surgery patients are placed in a spica cast for several months. Some patients may require secondary procedures particularly if radiographic appearances begin to deteriorate following a period of resolution of the changes of DDH. A full account of the various operative procedures and surgical techniques can be found in standard paediatric orthopaedic textbooks and in the surgical literature (GILLINGHAM et al. 1999; WENGER and BOMAR 2003).

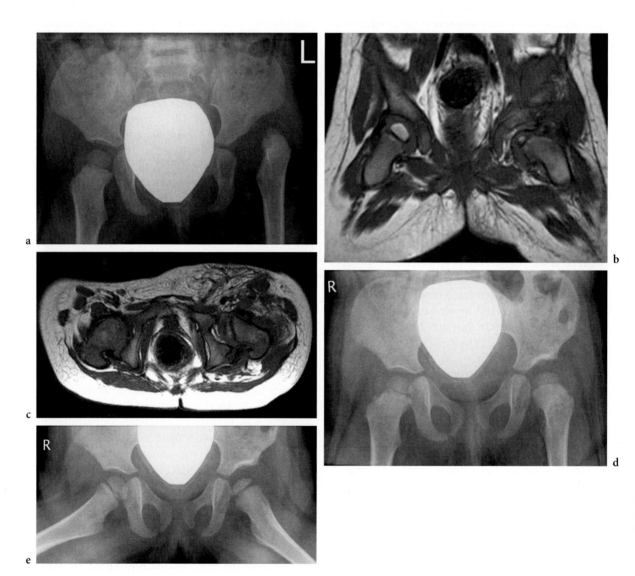

Fig. 8.20. a AP pelvic radiograph. A 2-year-old female with dislocated left hip and markedly dysplastic acetabulum. Small left proximal femoral epiphysis. This child underwent open reduction and Salter osteotomy. **b** Coronal T1-weighted MR imaging scan of the pelvis in the same child following open reduction and Salter osteotomy. **c** T2-weighted axial MR imaging scan of the pelvis demonstrating satisfactory alignment of the left femoral head and acetabulum post-reduction. Post-operative changes in the soft tissues. **d,e** AP and frog-lateral radiographs of the pelvis taken 1 year after surgery. The left proximal femoral epiphysis is small, irregular and fragmented consistent with avascular necrosis. The pelvic osteotomy has healed well and there is good acetabular coverage.

8.8
Conclusions

DDH is a multifactorial condition with a spectrum of abnormalities that can very from mild changes that spontaneously resolve to severe changes that are incapacitating later in life. It may present at birth or become apparent months or years later. Imaging has an important role in both diagnosis and follow up of patients undergoing treatment. Goals of treatment are to achieve congruency of the femoral head and acetabulum and normalise the distribution of biomechanical forces about the joint. The ultimate aim of treatment is to reduce the incidence of symptoms and secondary degeneration later in life.

References

Aliabadi P, Baker ND, Jaramillo D (1998) Hip arthrography, aspiration, block and bursography. Radiol Clin North Am 36:673–690

American Academy of Pediatrics (2000) Clinical practice guideline: early detection of developmental dysplasia of the hip. Pediatrics 105:896–905

Barlow TG (1962) Early diagnosis and treatment of congenital dislocation of the hip. J Bone Joint Surg Br 44:292–301

Bar-On E, Meyer S, Harari G et al (1998) Ultrasonography of the hip in developmental hip dysplasia. J Bone Joint Surg Br 80:321–324

Bellah R (2001) Ultrasound in pediatric musculoskeletal disease. Radiol Clin North Am 39:597–618

Boeree NR, Clarke NM (1994) Ultrasound imaging and secondary screening for congenital dislocation of the hip. J Bone Joint Surg Br 76:525–533

Coleman SS (1983) Reconstructive procedures in congenital dislocation of the hip. In: McKibbin B (ed) Recent advances in orthopedics. Churchill Livingstone, Edinburgh, pp 23–44

Coleman SS (1995) The subluxating or wandering femoral head in developmental dysplasia of the hip. J Pediatr Orthop 15:785–788

Cooperman DR, Wallensten R, Stulberg SD (1980) Post-reduction avascular necrosis in congenital dislocation of the hip. J Bone Joint Surg Am 62:247–258

Desateaux C, Godward S (1996) A national survey of screening for congenital dislocation of the hip. Arch Dis Child 74:445–448

Dias JJ, Thomas IH, Lamont AC et al (1993) The reliability of ultrasonographic assessment of neonatal hips. J Bone Joint Surg Br 75:479–482

Donaldson JS, Feinstein KA (1997). Imaging of developmental dysplasia of the hip. Pediatr Clin North Am 44:591–614

Dwek JR, Chung CB, Sartoris DJ (2002) Developmental dysplasia of the hip. In: Resnick D (ed) Diagnosis of bone and joint disorders, 4th edn. Saunders, Philadelphia, pp 4355–4381

Eastwood DM (2003) Neonatal hip screening. Lancet 361: 595–97

Eggli KD, King SH, Boal DKB et al (1994) Low-dose CT of developmental dysplasia of the hip after reduction: diagnostic accuracy and dosimetry. Am J Roentgenol 163:1441–1443

Gerscovich EO (1997a) A radiologist's guide to the imaging in the diagnosis and treatment of developmental dysplasia of the hip I. General considerations, physical examination as applied to real time sonography and radiography. Skeletal Radiol 26:386–397

Gerscovich EO (1997b) A radiologist's guide to the imaging in the diagnosis and treatment of developmental dysplasia of the hip II. Ultrasonography: anatomy, technique, acetabular angle measurements, acetabular coverage of femoral head, acetabular cartilage thickness, three-dimensional technique, screening of newborns, study of older children. Skeletal Radiol 26:447–456

Gillingham BL, Sanchez AA, Wenger DR (1999) Pelvic osteotomies for the treatment of hip dysplasia in children and young adults. J Am Acad Orthop Surg 7:325–337

Godward S, Desateaux C (1998) On behalf of the MRC Working Party on congenital dislocation of the hip. Surgery for congenital dislocation of the hip in the UK as a measure of outcome of screening. Lancet 351:1149–1152

Graf R (1980) The diagnosis of congenital hip-joint dislocation by the ultrasonic Combound treatment. Arch Orthop Trauma Surg 97:117–133

Graf R (1984) Classification of hip joint dysplasia by means of sonography. Arch Orthop Trauma Surg 102:248–255

Graf R (1987) Guide to sonography of the infant hip. Thieme Medical, New York

Guille JT, Pizzutillo PD, MacEwen GD (2000) Developmental dysplasia of the hip from birth to six month. J Am Acad Orthop Surg 8:232–242

Harcke HT, Grissom LE (1990) Performing dynamic sonography of the infant hip. Am J Roentgenol 155:837–844

Harcke HT, Clarke NM, Lee MS et al (1984) Examination of the infant hip with real-time ultrasonography. J Ultrasound Med 3:131–137

Hernandez RJ, Tachdijian MO, Poznanski AK et al (1981) CT determination of femoral torsion. Am J Roentgenol 137:97–101

Jaramillo D, Villegas-Medina O, Laor T et al (1998) Gadolinium enhanced MR imaging of pediatric patients after reduction of dysplastic hips: assessment of femoral head position, factors impeding reduction and femoral head ischemia. Am J Roentgenol 170:1633–1637

Jomha NM, McIvor J, Sterling G (1995) Ultrasonography in developmental hip dysplasia. J Pediatr Orthop 15:101–104

Kahle K, Coleman SS (1992) The value of the acetabular teardrop figure in assessing pediatric hip disorders. J Pediatr Orthop 12:586–591

Keller MS, Weltin GG, Rattner Z et al (1988) Normal instability of the hip in the neonate: US standards. Radiology 169:733–736

Lehmann HP, Hinton R, Morello P et al (2000) In conjunction with the Committee on Quality Improvement, Subcommittee on Developmental Dysplasia of the Hip. American Academy of Pediatrics. Developmental dysplasia of the hip practice guideline: technical report. Pediatrics 105:1–25

Lingg G, von Torklus D, Nebel G (1981) Hip dysplasia and congenital hip dislocation: a roentgenometric study in 110 families. Radiologe 21:538–541

Marks DS, Clegg J, al-Chalabi AN (1994) Routine ultrasound screening for neonatal hip instability: can it abolish late-presenting congenital dislocation of the hip? J Bone Joint Surg Br 76:534–538

Murray KA, Crim JR (2001) Radiographic imaging for treatment and follow-up of developmental dysplasia of the hip. Semin Ultrasound CT MRI 22:306–340

Novacheck (1996) Development dysplasia of the hip. Pediatr Clin North Am 43:829–905

Ortolani M (1937) Un segno poco noto e sua importanza per la diagnosi precoce de prelussazione congenita dell'anca. Pediatr Med Chir 45:129

Ortolani M (1976) The classic: congenital hip dysplasia in the light of early and very early diagnosis. Clin Orthop 119:6–10

Ozonoff MB (1992) The hip. In: Pediatric orthopaedic radiology, 2nd edn. Saunders, Philadelphia, pp 164–303

Patel H (2001) Preventive health care, 2001 update: screening and management of developmental dysplasia of the hip in newborns. Can Med Assoc J 164:1669–1677

Rosendahl K, Aslaken A, Lie RT et al (1995) Reliability of ultrasound in the early diagnosis of developmental dysplasia of the hip. Pediatr Radiol 25:219–224

Rosendahl K, Markestad T, Lie RT (1996) Developmental dysplasia of the hip: a population based comparison of ultrasound and clinical findings. Acta Pediatr 85:64–69

Sebag G, Docou Le Pointe H, Klein I et al (1997) Dynamic gadolinium enhanced subtraction MR imaging – a simple technique for the diagnosis of Legg-Calvé-Perthes disease: preliminary results. Pediatr Radiol 27:216–220

Smith JT, Matan A, Coleman SS et al (1997) The predictive value of the development of the acetabular teardrop figure

in developmental dysplasia of the hip. J Pediatr Orthop 17:165–169

Soboleski DA, Babyn P (1993) Sonographic diagnosis of developmental dysplasia of the hip: importance of increased thickness of acetabular cartilage. Am J Roentgenol 161:839–842

Tredwell SJ, Davies L (1989) A prospective study of congenital dislocation of the hip. J Pediatr Orthop 9:386–390

Vitale MG, Skaggs DL (2001) Developmental dysplasia of the hip from six months to four years of age. J Am Acad Orthop Surg 9:401–411

Walsh JJ, Morrissy RT (1998) Torticollis and hip dislocation. J Pediatr Orthop 18:219–221

Weinstein SL (1987) Natural history of congenital hip dislocation (CDH) and hip dysplasia. Clin Orthop 255:62–76

Weinstein SL (1998) Natural history and treatment outcomes of childhood hip disorders. Clin Orthop 344:227–242

Weintroub S, Green I, Terdiman R, Weissman SL (1979) Growth and development of congenitally dislocated hips reduced in early infancy. J Bone Joint Surg Am 61:125–130

Wenger DR, Bomar JD (2003) Human hip dysplasia: evolution of current treatment concepts. J Orthop Sci 8:264–271

Wiberg G (1939) Studies on dysplastic acetabula and congenital subluxation of the hip joint. Acta Chir Scand 58:5

Wynne-Davis R (1970) Acetabular Dysplasia and familial joint laxity: two aetiological factors in CDH. J Bone Joint Surg Br 52:704–716

Yamamuro T, Ishida K (1984). Recent advances in the prevention, early diagnosis and treatment of congenital dislocation of the hip in Japan. Clin Orthop 184:34–40

Zionts LE, MacEwen GD (1986) Treatment of congenital dislocation of the hip in children between the ages of one and three years. J Bone Joint Surg Am 68:829

9 Developmental Dysplasia of the Hip 2: Adult

Kaj Tallroth

CONTENTS

9.1 Introduction

Developmental dysplasia of the hip, abbreviated to DDH, is a complex entity. The second 'D' originally referred to 'dislocation' but the word 'dysplasia' is more accurate since this term nowadays comprises all variations and stages of congenital hip dysplasia, subluxation and dislocation. DDH has thus replaced congenital dysplasia of the hip (CDH) as we have become aware of its later form, the residual dysplasia in which a hip that has been clinically normal at birth is later found to be dysplastic or subluxated. So today DDH is considered to be a developmental condition with a variance in shape, size and orientation of the acetabulum, frequently exhibiting a deficient coverage of the femoral head. In addition it may be associated with an abnormal orientation of the femoral neck and changes in size and shape of the femoral head (SIEBENROCK et al. 1999). This chapter deals with the patho-aetiology, diagnostic presentation and sequelae of DDH in adults, as well as radiological evaluation in preparation for the current periacetabular osteotomy named after professor Reinhold Ganz, who developed the method and performed the first operations at the University of Bern in 1984.

9.2 Aetiology

The aetiology of DDH is multifactorial involving both genetic and intrauterine environmental factors (WEINSTEIN et al. 2004). In a study published by WYNNE-DAVIES (1970) the results demonstrated that first degree relatives of children with DDH had lax joint ligaments and undoubtedly also a shallower acetabulum than the normal population. Ethnic factors also contribute to development of DDH as the incidence is 2.5%–5% in Lapps and North American Indians whereas it is extremely low in Chinese and black Africans (WENGER 1993). Furthermore, risk factors for pure hip dysplasia with a shallow acetabulum include e.g. breech delivery, female gender and first-born, as well as positive family history.

9.3 Development

The majority of the abnormalities in dysplastic hips are on the acetabular side. The concave shape of the acetabulum is determined by the presence of a spherical femoral head and later during adolescence by several secondary ossification centres which deepen the joint cavity. Acetabular growth and development are affected by the primary disease such as abnormal acetabular cartilage, pressure changes from the femur or disturbances from treatment (WEINSTEIN et al. 2004).

K. TALLROTH, MD
Associate Professor, Orton Orthopedic Hospital, Tenalavagen 10, 00280 Helsinki, Finland

9.4
Anatomy

An obliquely orientated hip joint socket with deficient lateral coverage of the femoral head characterises the pathoanatomy of the acetabular dysplasia. Computed tomography (CT) analysis of dysplastic hips has revealed that the hip is not concentrically reduced, nor is the acetabular anteversion statistically different from normal (MILLIS and MURPHY 1992). Rather than a hemisphere, the dysplastic acetabulum is typically only one third of a sphere. There are varying degrees of deficiency and individual patients may have, alone or in combination, different degrees of insufficiency of the roof, and of the anterior or posterior wall (TRUMBLE et al. 1999). Furthermore, another classic pattern, present to a greater or lesser extent depending on the severity of dysplasia, is the typically shallow, anteverted and lateralized acetabulum deficient anteriorly and superiorly. On the femoral side, the femoral head may be deformed, the femoral neck may be short, have a excessive anteversion or the neck-shaft angle may be increased (SANCHEZ-SOTELO et al. 2002).

9.5
Natural History

If the diagnosis of DDH or dislocation is missed at birth the joint can still become normal later, it can go on to complete dislocation or subluxation, or the acetabulum can retain dysplastic features and lead to what is called residual dysplasia. This is a condition with anatomic abnormalities, which in some subjects can eventually lead to premature degenerative joint disease, usually in the third or fourth decade. The real incidence of degenerative joint disease in residual dysplastic hips is difficult to assess since it is only discovered in subjects with symptoms or as an incidental finding in radiological examinations.

9.6
Clinical Presentation

Most often the adult DDH patients are females who presented no clinical symptoms in the hips throughout childhood and adolescence. Mild DDH is frequently symptom free and is often unrecognised unless there are symptoms from the contralateral side. Usually symptoms commence at the age of 30–40 years with pain in the region of the groin that radiates to the medial side of the thigh, combined with a sensation of weakness in the leg. These symptoms are thought to be caused by a slight subluxation of the femoral head and the pain can be provoked with hyperextension and external rotation of the hip. Later the pain increases with physical activity, it can be associated with catching episodes and eventually it may lead to a limp at normal walking. Characteristically the pain occurs with the first few steps after a period of rest and it rarely awakens the patient from sleep. In physical examinations the pain can by reproduced with hyperextension and external rotation. Furthermore, there is quite often a limitation of the range of motion in the hip joint. Feeling of giving-way, catching, snapping and locking are symptoms that may indicate a labral pathology. A provocation test with forced internal rotation in flexion has been used as a sign of possible labral lesion anterior-superiorly (SIEBENROCK et al. 1999). Unfortunately, standard screening radiographs of the hips are often taken supine and not in a standing position, which reveals mild subluxations more clearly.

9.7
Pathogenesis of Osteoarthrosis

Osteoarthrosis (OA) may be considered as an idiopathic primary or secondary degenerative process. In the hip the latter is most often due to a pre-existing anatomic deformation (ARONSON 1986). The anatomic abnormalities of DDH lead to increased contact pressure on a decreased contact area which may predispose to the development of OA (SANCHEZ-SOTELO et al. 2002; TRUMBLE et al. 1999). Lateralization of the acetabulum and hip rotation also increase the body-weight lever arm. MURPHY et al. (1995) have demonstrated that the probability of development of OA is relative to the severity of the DDH. Other factors influencing the evolution and progression of OA are abnormal hip biomechanics, mild hip instability or labral pathology (MCCARTHY et al. 2001). Labral alterations may progress and explain premature OA with subchondral bony cyst formation and paralabral cysts.

In a large analysis of five series consisting of 474 patients with OA, ARONSON (1986) found that 76% had an underlying deformity which predisposed the hip to mechanical failure. The underlying deformity was caused by dysplasia of the hip in 43%. An increased femoral anteversion can even be the only manifestation of DDH (ALVIK 1962). TERJESEN et al. (1982) demonstrated in a series of 50 primary OA patients that their median femoral anteversion was significantly increased in relation to a control group. They concluded that an increased femoral anteversion is a predisposing factor for OA. WIBERG (1939) in his classic monograph *Studies on Dysplastic Acetabula and Congenital Subluxation of the Hip Joint* presents findings that showed that all patients with a pathologic lateral coverage developed OA. To determine the natural history of acetabular dysplasia COOPERMAN et al. (1983) followed up 32 hips for an average of 22 years; of these, 30 developed OA. Furthermore, it has been reported that up to one half of patients with untreated hip dysplasia are known to suffer from OA already at the age of 50 years (PAJARINEN and HIRVENSALO 2003).

9.8
Indications for Surgical Interventions

Patients with DDH that do not present symptoms should be treated conservatively. They should however be urged to look out for symptoms of commencing OA. If clinical symptoms of residual DDH appear during late childhood surgical treatment is preferable rather than waiting to see if the symptoms become severe. Nowadays, there are several options of surgical interventions. The main goal of these procedures is to offer pain relief and restore hip function. Several factors should be considered: the main ones include the age of the patient, the severity of the dysplasia and the presence of OA. Available alternatives are, at least theoretically, arthroscopic surgery, osteotomy of the femur, osteotomy of the pelvis either alone or complemented with a femoral osteotomy, arthroplasty and arthrodesis. Some surgeons prefer to inspect the joint and acetabular labrum at the osteotomy, whereas other do not perform arthrotomy. An outpatient arthroscopy procedure allows not only joint observation but also an opportunity to excise labral tears and remove loose bodies which may accelerate joint wear and promote premature OA. In young patients a total hip arthroplasty does not represent a sound alternative because it would imply bony reconstruction of the socket and subsequent increasingly complex surgery in an active young population (SIEBENROCK et al. 1999).

9.9
Reconstructive Surgery

The goals of reconstructive osteotomies in the treatment of DDH in adults are to restore nearly normal hip anatomy, improve symptoms and diminish the risk of degenerative joint changes. This is done by reorienting the acetabulum so pressures are better distributed over cartilage joint surface, and reorienting the acetabulum to contain the femur and stabilise it (HIPP et al. 1999). An improvement in the biomechanics of the hip decreases the pathological load on the articular cartilage and dysplastic bony joint surfaces. It is widely accepted that properly selected patients benefit from properly performed acetabular positioning and the progression of secondary OA may slow down or even reverse by better distributing forces applied through the hip joint.

Many different reconstructive osteotomies have been described. The choice depends on the age of the patients, but also on the experience and preferences of the surgeons. There is Salter's single innominate osteotomy for children but it is often insufficient for adults. Chiari's osteotomy is a salvage procedure for dysplastic and incongruent hips of children. Double and triple osteotomies, for example Sutherland's, Le Coeur's and Steels's procedures, can lead to notable asymmetry and deformity of the pelvis. Tönnis juxta-articular triple osteotomy allows increased correction with less pelvic obliquity but a larger extent of correction can result in a defect between the ischium and the osteotomized acetabulum. Periacetabular osteotomies described by Eppright, Wagner and Ninomiya and Tagawa provide good lateral coverage, but the amount of anterior coverage and the ability to medialise the hip joint are often limited (SANCHEZ-SOTELO et al. 2002).

9.10
Bernese Periacetabular Osteotomy

Since this chapter deals mainly with the diagnosis of residual DDH in adults and preoperative radiological evaluation used for planning of the Bernese periacetabular osteotomy it is appropriate to describe this osteotomy technique. Nowadays the advantages of the periacetabular osteotomy are well recognised and the procedure is widely used. It is preferred by many surgeons in skeletally mature adolescents once the triradiate cartilage has closed. The current main challenge is to choose patients for surgery who have dysplasia predisposing for OA but not yet developed severe degenerative changes. In hips with severe degenerative changes and irreversible deformity no realigning osteotomy is likely to improve the mechanics enough to give relief or arrest the progression of OA.

The Bernese periacetabular osteotomy has many advantages compared to other osteotomies. The operation is usually done through one incision, it is performed with straight reproducible extra-articular cuts and a controlled fracture to separate the acetabular cup from the rest of the pelvis. The cup is realigned and fixed to the pelvis to improve the femoral head coverage and contact pressure distribution in the hip joint (Fig. 9.1). The posterior column remains intact which allows early mobilisation after surgery. The vascularity of the acetabular fragment is preserved and the vascular supply from the inferior gluteal artery remains intact. It is possible to examine the acetabular labrum through capsulotomy when there is clinical suspicion of a torn labrum without the risk of osteonecrosis of the osteotomy fragment (TROUSDALE et al. 1995; MILLIS et al. 1996). A well-performed osteotomy does not compromise the pertinent pelvic dimensions in young women allowing them to have normal vaginal child delivery (TROUSDALE et al. 2002). One of the disadvantages of periacetabular osteotomy is that it is a technically demanding procedure requiring an expertise in anatomic knowledge.

In follow up studies of operated patients reported results have been good. MATTA and co-workers (1999) studied 66 hips of 58 patients that had undergone periacetabular osteotomy on average 4 years after surgery and the final clinical results were graded as 17% excellent, 59 % good, 12% fair and 12% poor. None of their patients who met the ideal indications for surgery had poor results. Similarly TROUSDALE and co-workers (1995) followed up 42 patients with DDH after an average duration of 4 years. Of 33 patients with an established preoperative grade 1 or 2 OA 32 had an excellent or good results. MURPHY and DESHMUKH (2002) performed a prospective study of 95 consecutive hips in 87 patients. They concluded that excellent prognosis after periacetabular osteotomy can be anticipated for spherical hips with grades 0–2 OA and a good prognosis with hips with grade 3 OA provided that the joint shows an improved cartilage space interval on preoperative functional radiographs. Aspherical hips represent high risk cases that need to be considered individually.

The reversal of degenerative joint destruction evident by decrease in subchondral sclerosis, resolution of cysts and even increase of joint space, has also been reported. TRUMBLE et al. (1999) noticed on radiographic examinations at an average follow up of 4.3 years in patients undergoing periacetabular osteotomy some degree of bone regeneration in more than 80% (82 of 100) of the hips with degenerative preoperative changes in periarticular bone.

9.11
Femoral Osteotomy

Proximal femoral osteotomy can be performed when the periacetabular osteotomy alone does not produce

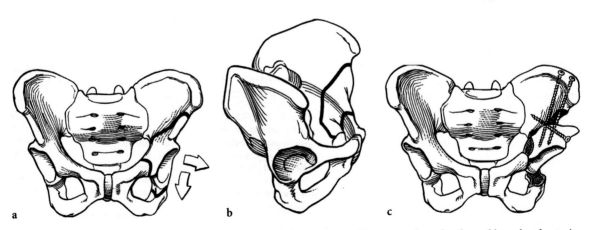

Fig. 9.1. a Frontal diagram showing location of the periacetabular osteotomy. The *arrows* show the planned lateral and anterior correction. **b** Oblique view of hip showing location of cuts with the posterior column intact. **c** Diagram showing osteotomized fragment that has been medialised, tilted laterally and anteriorly. The fragment is fixed with three screws. [Reprinted with permission from CROCKARELL et al. (1999)]

satisfactory coverage and congruity or when femur is the primary site of deformity. It is not uncommon for patients with acetabular dysplasia to have an associated proximal femoral anatomy, as for example increased valgus or anteversion (MATTA et al. 1999). Since PAUWELS in the 1960s (1968) described his biomechanical theory on intertrochanteric osteotomy for hip dysplasia many surgeons have applied this procedure for OA due to DDH. In a follow up study by IWASE et al. (1996) of more than 15 years of intertrochanteric osteotomy in patients with prearthrosis or early degenerative stage of OA good clinical results were obtained when coverage postoperatively was significantly improved.

In DDH the femur is usually slightly anteverted compared to the normal 10°–20°. Increased anteversion can also be the only manifestation of a DDH (ALVIK 1962). In some reported series femoral rotational osteotomy has been performed in conjunction with periacetabular osteotomy in up 27% of cases (SANCHEZ-SOTELO et al. 2002). However, it is important to realise that no degree of correction provided by varus osteotomy will compensate for the anatomic instability created by a dysplastic acetabulum.

9.12
Imaging Features: Preoperative

Today, in many centres, the preoperative evaluation of DDH for joint-preserving reconstructive surgery involves both conventional radiology and computed tomography (CT), sometimes complemented with MR. Conventional radiographs allow a two-dimensional interpretation of the hip but the information depends on multiple projections and on inconclusive assessments of landmarks. CT imaging and three-dimensional reconstruction offers reliable magnifications and measurements without undesirable and disturbing superimposition of bony structures. Additionally, evaluations provide clinicians information to choose suitable candidates for operation and to avoid, i.e. patients with severe OA. Preoperatively it is of paramount importance to determine the varying types and degrees of deficiency to be able to define the goals of surgery and to plan the appropriate adjustments. Just as the preoperative examinations are important for characterisation of DDH and planning of surgery, the postoperative examinations are important to assess the results of surgery (Fig. 9.2).

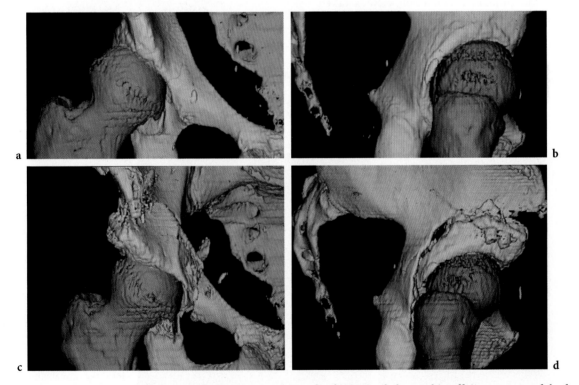

Fig. 9.2. a,b In the upper row preoperative 3D images show a dysplastic acetabulum and insufficient coverage of the femoral head. **c,d** In the lower row after periacetabular osteotomy there is a marked improvement in the coverage of the femoral head

Numerous terms are used to describe the radio-logical changes occurring in DDH. These include anteversion of the acetabulum and femur, inclina-tion, abduction, subluxation, cover and coverage, containment, tilt, opening. Unfortunately defini-tions and terms are used differently in anatomical, radiographic and operative assessments of orienta-tion (Murray 1993). The increasing use of preoper-ative CT evaluation have even manifold conception and measurement methods.

9.12.1
Conventional Radiography

The initial routine radiographic evaluation of DDH includes a functional AP radiograph of the pelvis and a frog-leg view of the symptomatic hip. The AP radiographs should be taken weight-bearing and centred on the pubis symphysis to show the bio-mechanical aspects of the pelvis and hip (Fig. 9.3). The recumbent frog-leg view is to look for changes in the morphology of the femoral head and neck (Fig. 9.4). In many centres these radiographs are completed with views in abduction and adduction to inspect the full range of motion and the coverage of the femoral head under the dysplastic acetabulum (Fig. 9.5). The functional abduction view is taken to simulate the appearance of the hip after periac-etabular osteotomy.

Earlier a frequently used radiograph was the faux-profile, false-profile view (Lequesne and de Sèze 1961) which is a true lateral radiograph of the acetabulum. The patient stands at an angle of 65° oblique to the X-ray beam, with the foot on the

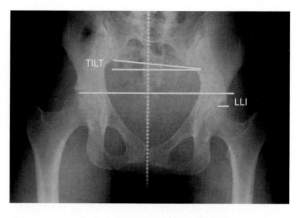

Fig. 9.3. A weight-bearing anteroposterior radiograph show-ing leg-length disparity, pelvic tilt and a dysplastic left hip

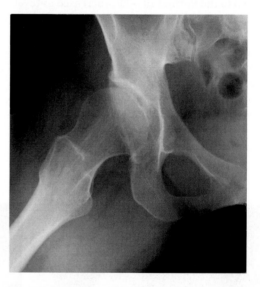

Fig. 9.4. A recumbent frog-leg view shows well the morphol-ogy of the femoral head and neck

a

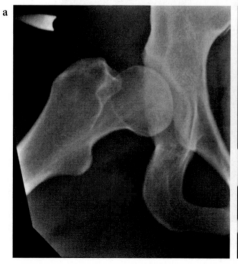

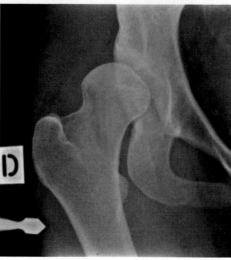

b

Fig. 9.5a,b. Abduction (a) and adduction (b) films show the range of motion in the hip as well as how the femoral head will fit into the acetabulum after reorientation osteotomy

a 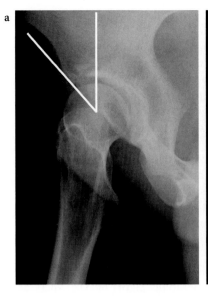 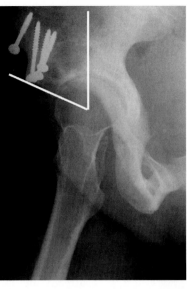 b

Fig. 9.6. a Preoperative false-profile view showing the superior-anterior coverage of the femoral head (ACE angle). b Postoperative false-profile radiograph showing an increased anterior coverage

affected side parallel to the X-ray cassette. The view shows the superior-anterior coverage of the femoral head. This anterior centre-edge angle (ACE) is composed of a vertical line through the centre of the femoral head and a second line through the centre of the hip and the foremost aspect of the acetabulum (Fig. 9.6). Angles of less than 20° are considered abnormal (CROCKARELL et al. 2000).

A false profile-view of hip in flexion simulates the anterior coverage after osteotomy. Abduction view and false profile view in flexion often show proper reduction of a subluxated joint and improvement of the cartilage space interval and thus suggest that the hip will respond well to acetabular redirection (MURPHY and DESHMUKH 2002).

The main preoperative radiographic assessments consist of several observations and measurements done from weight-bearing frontal radiograph of the pelvis.

- Pelvic tilt. Deviation in pelvic tilt is measured as the angle between the horizon plane and a plane through the tear-drops, a plane through the caudal contours of the lower ramus or a plane through the lower margin of the SI joint (Fig. 9.3).
- Leg length discrepancy. Estimation of leg-length discrepancy is commonly measured from the weight-bearing joint surfaces of the femoral heads (Fig. 9.3).
- The lateral centre-edge angle of Wiberg (CE angle) is perhaps the most used indicator of the lateral coverage of the femoral head (WIBERG 1939). The angle is formed between a line connecting the femoral head centre and the most lateral edge of the acetabulum, and a line drawn

through the femoral head centre perpendicular to the pelvic horizon (Fig. 9.7). WIBERG on the basis of his study deduced that CE angles of greater than 25° were normal, angles 24°–20° borderline normal, and angles less than 20° were pathologic. A large CE angle correlates with a deep acetabulum (TÖNNIS 1987)

- The acetabular index angle of the weight-bearing zone of the acetabulum (TÖNNIS 1987), (the lateral tilt of the opening of acetabulum, AA angle, also called AC angle, i.e. acetabular cartilage angle) (normal 10°±2°) The angle is formed between a line parallel to the weight-bearing dome (*sourcil*) and a line parallel to the horizontal plane of the pelvis (Fig. 9.8).

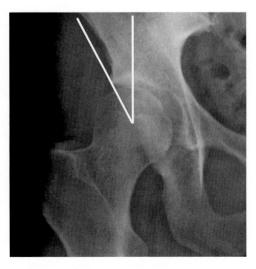

Fig. 9.7. The lateral centre-edge angle of Wiberg (CE angle) shows the lateral coverage of the femoral head

- Cranial subluxation of the femoral head is best appreciated as a broken Shenton's line (Fig. 9.9).
- Lateral subluxation of the femoral head can be measured as the shortest distance between the medial aspect of the femoral head and the ilioischial line (Fig. 9.10) (SIEBENROCK et al. 1999) or from the lateral side of the tear-drop to the medial edge of the femoral head (Fig. 9.10b) (TROUSDALE et al. 1995).
- A caudal stress examination (Fig. 9.11) shows whether the femoral head can be pulled downwards permitting a reorientation of the acetabulum.
- For the joint congruity and containment the femoral neck and head are as important as the acetabulum. Before correction of malposition of the head radiographs in abduction and adduction are taken to see whether the re-orientated head fits into the acetabulum (Fig. 9.5).
- Femoral neck-shaft angle. An easy way to judge the neck-shaft angle is to draw a line through the tip of the greater trochanter perpendicular to the long axis of the femur (Fig. 9.12). Normally, this line runs through the centre of the femoral head but in coxa vara the line runs above it and in coxa valga below the centre (DIHLMAN 1985). This relationship between the trochanter and the centre of the femoral head is independent of the rotation of the leg. In normal subjects the neck-shaft angle is between 130° and 140°.

At the time of clinical presentation there might already be radiographic signs of OA such as increased subchondral sclerosis in the joint surfaces of the weight-bearing areas, joint space narrowing, degenerative cysts and osteophytes (Fig. 9.13). Sometimes a subchondral acetabular cyst located anterior-superiorly (Egger's cyst) may be the first conspicuous sign of OA. Presence of OA is often graded according to the criteria of Tönnis: Grade 0 no joint space narrowing, Grade 1 slight joint space narrowing, Grade 2 moderate joint space narrowing, and Grade 3 joint space narrowing (TÖNNIS 1987; TRUMBLE et al. 1999). Another commonly used grading system is the one introduced by KELLGREN and LAWRENCE (1957). A dysplastic hip can falsely show a narrow joint space on the AP radiograph if the femoral head is subluxated anteriorly and superimposed on the roof of the acetabulum.

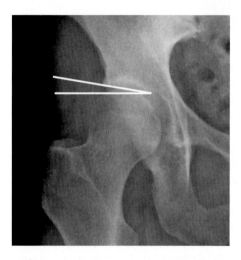

Fig. 9.8. The lateral slope of the acetabulum, the acetabular index angle (AA angle), is measured as shown on the anteroposterior radiograph

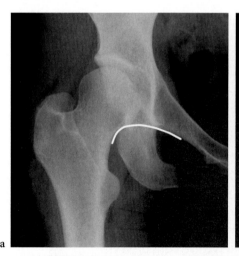
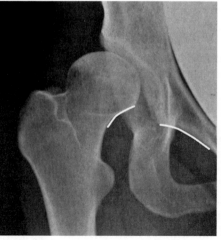

a   b

Fig. 9.9. a A normal Shenton's line is an even, continuous line between the medial border of the neck of the femur and the superior border of obturator foramen. **b** A broken and interrupted Shenton's line is a sign of a superior displacement of the femoral head

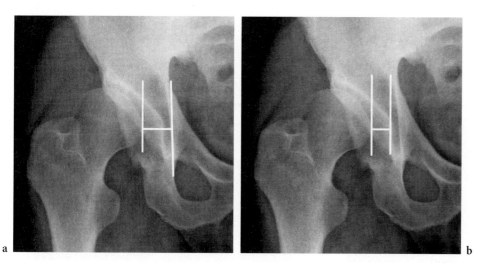

Fig. 9.10. a Lateralization of the femoral head is measured as the distance from the medial aspect of the femoral head to the ilioischial line. **b** Lateralization can also be measured as the distance from the medial portion of the femoral head to the lateral edge of the tear drop.

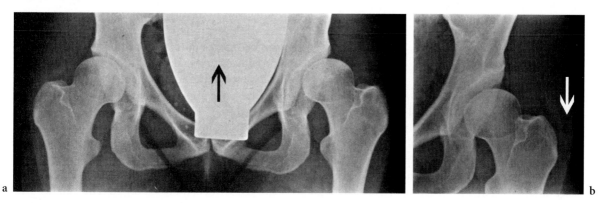

Fig. 9.11a,b. The mobility of the displaced femoral head on a weight-bearing radiograph (**a**) can be examined with a preoperative inferior stress view (**b**)

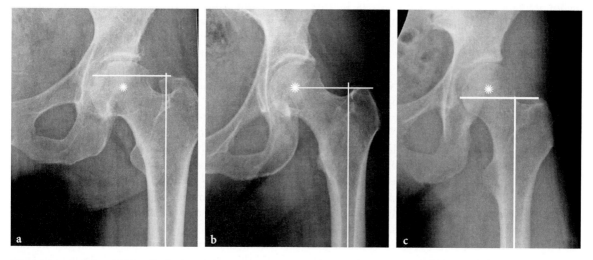

Fig. 9.12a–c. In a decreased neck-shaft angle, a coxa vara, a perpendicular line to the long axis of femur drawn as a tangent to the greater trochanter runs above the centre of the femoral head (**a**), in a normal hip approximately level with the centre (**b**) and in coxa valga below this reference point (**c**)

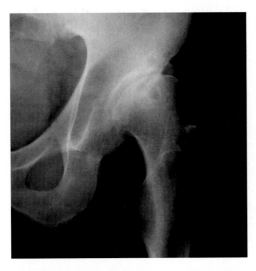

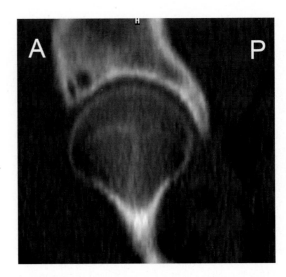

Fig. 9.13. Typical degenerative OA changes in a dysplastic hip: joint space narrowing, sclerotic bone formation and cysts in the femoral head as well as in the acetabulum

Fig. 9.14. Early signs of degenerative OA of a dysplastic hip are shown on a sagittal CT reformat as an anterior-superior acetabular cyst (Egger's cyst) and slight narrowing of the anterior joint space

9.12.2
Computed Tomography

Many of these above-mentioned measurement methods based on conventional radiography have been replaced by CT which has proven to be more accurate for the planning and simulation of pelvic and femoral osteotomies. CT helps clarify anatomic deformity and is particularly helpful in complex cases of DDH (KLAUE et al. 1988), to evaluate femoral anteversion and to detect early OA (Fig. 9.14). The CT angular measurements are as a rule convenient and fast for routine diagnostic work as well as for demanding preoperative analysis in three dimensions (HADDAD et al. 2000). CT scanning has become an irreplaceable imaging tool in most centres in which multiplanar re-orientation of the acetabula are performed.

Volume scanning, regardless of which technique is used, in association with contemporary software programs enables reformats in various planes and rendering of three-dimensional (3D) images. The scanning technique must be simple and reproducible. We scan the patient supine with the pelvis horizon perpendicular to the central axis of the scanning table. The feet are stabilised in a neutral position, and care is taken to ensure that there is no pelvic tilt or flexion of the hips or knees. Slice thickness of 4 mm is sufficient and obtained through both hip joints and femoral condyles. At most diagnostic workstations it is possible to simultaneously view the transaxial scans, and sagittal and coronal refor-

mats. The centre point of the femoral head is identified and used as a reference for the measurements of the coverage of the acetabulum.

- Centre-edge angle (CE angle, lateral coverage of the femoral head, normal 33°±10° (JANZEN et al. 1998) is measured from a coronal reformat through the centre of the femoral head (Fig. 9.15). It is the angle between the vertical axis of the pelvis and a line through the centre point and the lateral acetabular margin. The smaller this angle is the smaller the weight-bearing surface above the femoral head.
- Acetabular index angle (AA angle, lateral tilt or loading zone of the acetabulum) is calculated from a coronal reformat through the centre of the femoral head (Fig. 9.15c). It is the angle between the pelvic horizon and a line through the lateral rim of the acetabulum and the superior edge of the fovea, that is approximately a line along the *sourcil*.
- The superior-anterior coverage of the acetabulum (or anterior centre-edge angle, ACE angle) is measured from a sagittal reformat through the centre point of the femoral head (Fig. 9.16). The angle is bound by the horizon and a line through the most cranial point of the acetabular joint surface and the anterior rim of the acetabulum.
- Acetabular anteversion (AcetAV angle, normal 20°±7° (MURPHY et al. 1990) is measured from a transverse reformat through the centres of the femoral heads (Fig. 9.17). The acetabular antever-

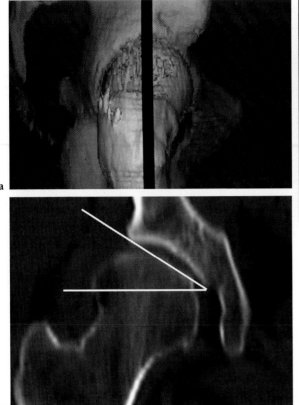

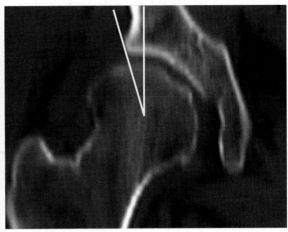

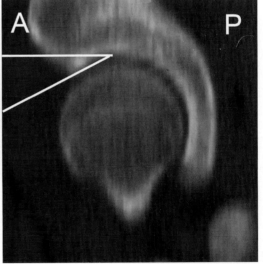

Fig. 9.15a–c. A lateral 3D image of a hip (**a**) showing the plane of 2D reformats for measurement of the lateral centre-edge angle of Wiberg (CE angle) (**b**), and acetabular index angle (AA angle) (**c**)

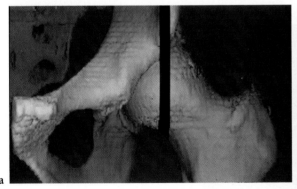

Fig. 9.16a,b. A frontal 3D hip image (**a**) showing the plane of a 2D reformat for measurement of the superior-anterior angle (ACE angle) (**b**)

sion is the angulation between a line combining the anterior and posterior margins of the acetabulum and a line perpendicular to the intercapital centreline (Fig. 9.17b) (ANDA et al. 1991a,b).

- Anterior and posterior coverage (anterior acetabular sector angle, AASA, normal 63°±6° and posterior acetabular sector angle, PASA, normal 105°±8°) (Fig. 9.17a) in the transverse plane are measured as the angles of the intercapital centreline and lines from the centre point of the heads to the anterior and posterior rims of the acetabulum (Fig. 9.17b) (ANDA et al. 1986, 1991a,b).
- Femoral anteversion. Femoral neck and condyles are scanned for the assessment of the femoral neck

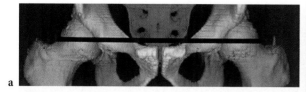

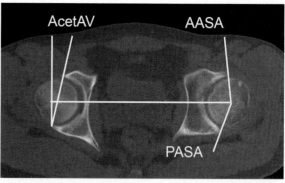

Fig. 9.17a,b. A frontal 3D image (**a**) showing the plane for the 2D reformat through the centres of the femoral heads from which the acetabular anteversion (*AcetAV*), anterior acetabular sector angle (*AASA*) and posterior acetabular sector angle (*PASA*) are measured (**b**)

anteversion. Looking at the volume of the knee from the feet, the femoral condyles are rotated so that the posterior aspects are horizontal. When the neck is are rotated to the same degree it is possible to measure the anteversion as the angle between the horizon and a line combining the centre point of the femoral head and the midpoint of the neck (Fig. 9.18). Normal femoral anteversion in adults is 10°–20°. This technique with the measurements presented below is fast: a hip and the femoral anteversion can be scanned and analysed in approximately 10 min. It is easily reproducible with small interobserver variability.

At the calculations of the magnitude of acetabular corrections in different planes one has to remember that position of the pelvis on the scanner table is not the same as in standing position. The vertical tilt of the pelvis due to imaging position, i.e. lumbosacral lordosis or kyphosis, is assessed by comparing the pelvic tilt on an erect lateral pelvic radiograph and on a supine lateral CT scout view.

CT data can also be presented in 3D mode which usually is visual and perspicuous for the orthopaedic surgeon when planning an optimal re-orientation of the acetabulum. 3D images show well the relationship between the acetabular containment, femoral

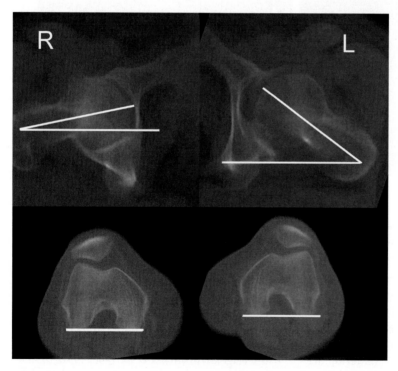

Fig. 9.18. The anteversion of the femoral neck is the angle between the axis of the neck and the horizon when the femur is rotated so that the posterior borders of the femoral condyles are horizontal. The anteversion of the left femur is increased

head and neck. Most radiologists, however, prefer to make their exact measurements from 2D reformats in different planes.

9.12.3
Magnetic Resonance Imaging (MR)

MR has also been used to measure various spatial relations between the acetabulum, femoral head and labrum (Horii et al. 2003). According to these authors measurements of the different coverage angles are easily performed on radial MR images. It is even possible to evaluate the coverage labrum provides the femoral head. The better ability of MR to show intraarticular damage is an advantage compared to conventional radiography. In recent years MR has become more common in the evaluation of DDH patients with clinical signs of labral or rim disease (Figs. 9.19 and 9.20). These lesions are depicted on MR arthrography (Siebenrock et al. 1999) as labral pathology shows abnormal signal intensity (Horii et al. 2003). Recent studies with diluted gadolinium combined with off axis tangent reconstruction views have increased the sensitivity for detecting labral tears (McCarthy and Lee 2002). The same authors have presented a study of 170 arthroscopically treated hips with DDH in mature adults. In all, 72% of the hips had labral tears, and 93% of these lesions occurred anteriorly. Additionally, of 113 patients with dysplasia with a labral tear, 78 (69%) had an ante-rior acetabular chondral lesion. They concluded that even in mild dysplasia labral and chondral injuries occur, and they occur most frequently in the ante-rior region of the acetabulum. Similarly, Hasagewa et al. (1996) have reached the same conclusion that MR demonstrates well degeneration and thinning of adjacent cartilage next to labral lesion. Degenerative acetabular OA cysts show up as high signal spots on T2-weighted images. Thus, MR may be useful in alerting the surgeon to the location and nature of intraarticular disorders that can be addressed at the time of surgery (Siebenrock et al. 1999).

9.13
Imaging Features: Postoperative

After reconstructive surgery the same radiological examinations and measurements as preoperatively are performed to evaluate to what extent the plan-ning and performance of surgery have been suc-cessful. On plain weight-bearing radiographs of the pelvis leg length parity as well as horizontal bal-ance of the pelvis are seen. The centre-edge angle (CE angle), the acetabular index angle (AA angle) (Fig. 9.21), and superior-anterior angle (ACE angle) (Figs. 9.6b), reveal to what extent surgery has cor-rected the faulty containment. Healing of the supra-acetabular part of the periacetabular osteotomy, as well as the upper ramus osteotomy, are easily

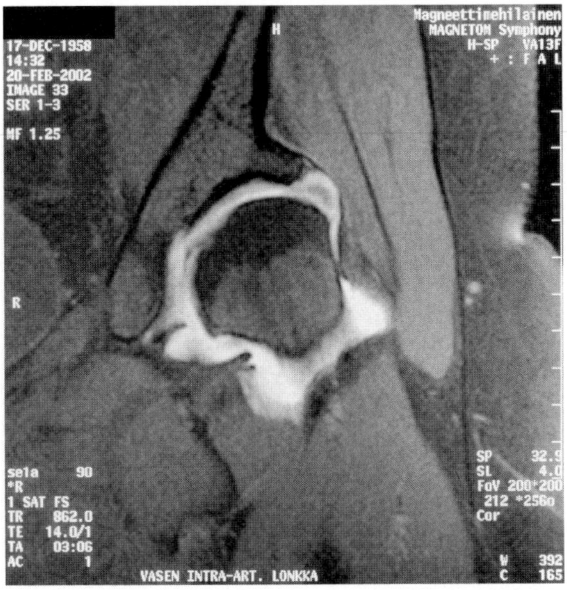

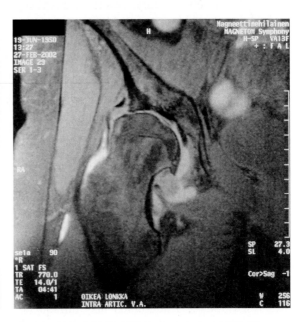

Fig. 9.19. Coronal MRI with intra-articular gadolinium con-trast demonstrating a fissure of the labrum

Fig. 9.20. Coronal MRI with intra-articular gadolinium con-trast demonstrating a torn and superiorly displaced labrum

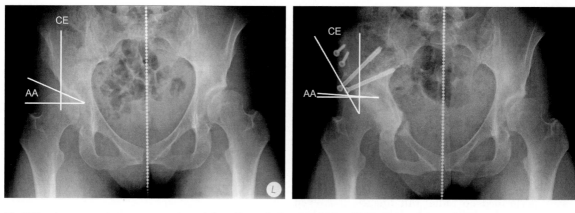

a   b

Fig. 9.21. a A preoperative anteroposterior pelvic radiograph showing the insufficient AA and CE angles. **b** Radiograph obtained 4 months after periacetabular osteotomy showing the corrections of the AA and CE angles

appreciated whereas the union of the posterior part is frequently not detectable due to unfavourable projections or superimposition of other bone structures. There is no need for additional oblique radiographs if CT is performed since the union of the entire osteotomy is well demonstrated with 2D curved reformats (Fig. 9.22 and 9.23). The CE, AC and ACE angles are measured in sagittal and coronal CT reformats through the centre of the femoral head and compared to the preoperative values.

The effect of the Bernese periacetabular osteotomy has been successfully studied with biomechanical analysis using computer-aided simulation of joint contact pressure on conventional AP radiographs (LEPISTÖ et al., in press).

Correlation between clinical results and radiological findings have been reported by several groups. TROUSDALE et al. (1995) reported a series of patients with dysplasia and degenerative changes treated with the Bernese periacetabular osteotomy. Radiologically the average correction of the lateral coverage was 28% and of the anterior 26%. The clinical Harris hip scores (HARRIS 1969) improved significantly from 62 to 86 points.

Failed corrections of femoroacetabular congruency, either because of an overly extensive correction or an inadequate one, can be concluded from plain and CT films. An intraoperative fracture of the base of the lower ramus just under the acetabular joint is not uncommon. However, this usually heals in 4–6 months. A lasting non-union of the upper ramus osteotomy is more frequent. This non-union does not cause pain or discomfort for the patients according to postoperative clinical evaluations of patients. However, a non-union may infrequently become associated with a stress fracture of the medial part of the lower ramus (Fig. 9.24).

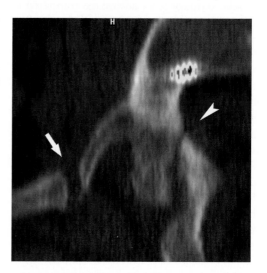

Fig. 9.22. Postoperative curved CT reformat of the hip shows the osteotomy of the upper ramus (*arrow*) and a perioperative posterior fracture of the acetabulum (*arrowhead*)

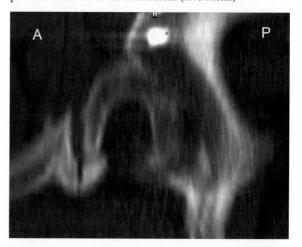

Fig. 9.23. At 4 months after a periacetabular osteotomy the upper ramus osteotomy is still unfused whereas the posterior osteotomy cut is well fused

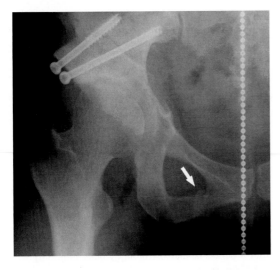

Fig. 9.24. An anteroposterior hip radiograph demonstrates a stress fracture in the medial part of the lower ramus (*arrow*). This type of fracture may appear as a complication to a delayed healing of the osteotomy

9.14
Summary

The most characteristic feature of DDH is a decreased acetabular lateral coverage of the femoral head. Many patients are symptom-free but it has been shown that moderate and severe dysplasia lead to premature OA. Surgery is to be considered when the patients have persistent symptoms which restrict everyday activities. Today the Bernese periacetabular rotational osteotomy is a common procedure to recreate relatively normal anatomy. To establish the diagnosis of DDH plain radiographs and measurements of the CE and AA angles are sufficient. However, to choose the right patients for surgical correction more sophisticated radiographic and CT measurements are needed in order to obtain a thorough visualisation and knowledge of the underlying abnormalities, as well as the magnitude of malpositions and malalignments so that reconstruction of a deficient acetabular roof and malrotated femur can be planned and performed appropriately. A radiological follow up after surgery makes it possible to determine performed coverage corrections, possible complications and a possible progression of degenerative joint disease.

References

Alvik I (1962) Increased anteversion of the femur as the only manifestation of dysplasia of the hip. Clin Orthop 22:16–20

Anda S, Svenningsen S, Dale LG, Benum P (1986) The acetabular sector angle of the adult hip determined by computed tomography. Acta Radiol Diagn 27:443–447

Anda S, Terjesen T, Kvistad KA, Svenningsen S (1991a) Acetabular angles and femoral anteversion in dysplastic hips in adults. CT investigation. J Comput Assist Tomogr 15:115–120

Anda S, Terjesen T, Kvistad KA (1991b) Computed tomography measurements of the acetabulum in adult dysplastic hips: which level is appropriate? Skeletal Radiol 20:267–271

Aronson J (1986) Osteoarthritis of the young adult hip: etiology and treatment. Instr Course Lect 35:119–128

Cooperman DR, Wallensten R, Stulberg SD (1983) Acetabular dysplasia in the adult. Clin Orthop 175:79–85

Crockarell J Jr, Trousdale RT, Cabanela ME, Berry DJ (1999) Early experience and results with the periacetabular osteotomy. The Mayo Clinic experience. Clin Orthop 363:45–53

Crockarell JR Jr, Trousdale RT, Guyton JL (2000) The anterior centre-edge angle. A cadaver study. J Bone Joint Surg Br 82:532–534

Dihlman W (1985) Joints and vertebral connections. Thieme, Stuttgart, p 232

Haddad FS, Garbuz DS, Duncan CP, Janzen DL, Munk PL (2000) CT evaluation of periacetabular osteotomies. J Bone Joint Surg Br 82:526–531

Harris WH. (1969) Traumatic arthritis of the hip after dislocation and acetabular fractures: treatment by mold arthroplasty. An end-result study using a new method of result evaluation. J Bone Joint Surg 5:737–755

Hasegawa Y, Fukatsu H, Matsuda T, Iwase T, Iwata H (1996) Magnetic resonance imaging in osteoarthrosis of the dysplastic hip. Arch Orthop Trauma Surg 115:243–248

Hipp JA, Sugano N, Millis MB, Murphy SB (1999) Planning acetabular redirection osteotomies based on joint contact pressures. Clin Orthop 364:134–143

Horii M, Kubo T, Inoue S, Kim WC (2003) Coverage of the femoral head by the acetabular labrum in dysplastic hips: quantitative analysis with radial MR imaging. Acta Orthop Scand 74:287–292

Iwase T, Hasegawa Y, Kawamoto K, Iwasada S, Yamada K, Iwata H (1996) Twenty years' followup of intertrochanteric osteotomy for treatment of the dysplastic hip. Clin Orthop 331:245–255

Janzen DL, Aippersbach SE, Munk PL, Sallomi DF, Garbuz D, Werier J, Duncan CP (1998) Three-dimensional CT measurement of adult acetabular dysplasia: technique, preliminary results in normal subjects, and potential applications. Skeletal Radiol 27:352–358

Kellgren JH, Lawrence JS (1957) Radiological assessment of osteo-arthrosis. Ann Rheum Dis 16:494–502

Klaue K, Wallin A, Ganz R (1988) CT evaluation of coverage and congruency of the hip prior to osteotomy. Clin Orthop 232:15–25

Lepistö J, Armand M, Tallroth K, Elias J, Chao E Outcomes of periacetabular osteotomy – joint contact pressure calculation using standing AP radiographs: 12 patients followed up for average 2 years. Acta Orthop Scand (in press)

Lequesne M, de Sèze S (1961) Le faux profile du bassin: nouvelle incidence radiographique pour l'etude de la hance. Son utilite dans les dysplasies et les differentes coxopathies. Rev Rhum Mal Osteoartic 28:643–652

Matta JM, Stover MD, Siebenrock K (1999) Periacetabular osteotomy through the Smith–Petersen approach. Clin Orthop 363:21–32

McCarthy JC, Lee JA (2002) Acetabular dysplasia: a paradigm of arthroscopic examination of chondral injuries. Clin Orthop 405:122–128

McCarthy JC, Noble PC, Schuck MR, Wright J, Lee J (2001) The Otto E. Aufranc Award: the role of labral lesions to development of early degenerative hip disease. Clin Orthop 393:25–37

Millis MB, Murphy SB (1992) Use of computed tomographic reconstruction in planning osteotomies of the hip. Clin Orthop 274:154–159

Millis MB, Murphy SB, Poss R (1996) Osteotomies about the hip for the prevention and treatment of osteoarthrosis. Instr Course Lect 45:209–226

Murphy S, Deshmukh R (2002) Periacetabular osteotomy: preoperative radiographic predictors of outcome. Clin Orthop 405:168–174

Murphy S, Kijewski PK, Millis MB, Harless A (1990) Acetabular dysplasia in the adolescent and young adult. Clin Orthop 261:214–223

Murphy S, Ganz R, Muller ME (1995) The prognosis in untreated dysplasia of the hip. A study of radiographic factors that predict the outcome. J Bone Joint Surg Am 77:985–989

Murray DW (1993) The definition and measurement of acetabular orientation. J Bone Joint Surg Br 752:228–232

Pajarinen J, Hirvensalo E (2003) Two-incision technique for rotational acetabular osteotomy: good outcome in 35 hips. Acta Orthop Scand 74:133–139

Pauwels F (1968) The place of osteotomy in the operative management of osteoarthritis of the hip. Triangle 8:196–210

Sanchez-Sotelo J, Berry DJ, Trousdale RT, Cabanela ME (2002) Surgical treatment of developmental dysplasia of the hip in adults. II. Arthroplasty options. J Am Acad Orthop Surg 10:334–344

Siebenrock KA, Scholl E, Lottenbach M, Ganz R (1999) Bernese periacetabular osteotomy. Clin Orthop 363:9–20

Terjesen T, Benum P, Anda S, Svenningsen S (1982) Increased femoral anteversion and osteoarthritis of the hip joint. Acta Orthop Scand 53:571–575

Tönnis D (1987) Congenital dysplasia and dislocation of the hip in children and adults. Springer, Berlin Heidelberg New York

Trousdale RT, Ekkernkamp A, Ganz R, Wallrichs SL (1995) Periacetabular and intertrochanteric osteotomy for the treatment of osteoarthrosis in dysplastic hips. J Bone Joint Surg Am 77:73–85

Trousdale RT, Cabanela ME, Berry DJ, Wenger DE (2002) Magnetic resonance imaging pelvimetry before and after a periacetabular osteotomy. J Bone Joint Surg Am 84A:552–556

Trumble SJ, Mayo KA, Mast JW (1999) The periacetabular osteotomy. Minimum 2 year followup in more than 100 hips. Clin Orthop 363:54–63

Wenger DR (1993) Developmental dysplasia of the hip. In: Wenger DR, Rang M (eds) The art and practice of children's orthopaedics. Raven, New York, pp 256–296

Weinstein SL, Mubarak SJ, Wenger DR (2004) Developmental hip dysplasia and dislocation, part I. Instr Course Lect 53:523–530

Wiberg G (1939) Studies on dysplastic acetabula and congenital subluxation of the hip joint: With special reference to the complication of osteo-arthritis. Acta Chir Scand 83 [Suppl 58]:1–135

Wynne-Davies R (1970) Acetabular dysplasia and familial joint laxity: two etiological factors in congenital dislocation of the hip. A review of 589 patients and their families. J Bone Joint Surg Br 52:704–716

10 Imaging of the Irritable Hip and Hip Infection

James Teh and David Wilson

10.1
The Irritable Hip

Irritability or pain around the hip, with limping or refusal to weight bear, is a common reason for acute presentation of children in accident and emergency, orthopaedic and paediatric units. The assessment of hip pain in children can be extremely difficult and an organised approach is therefore essential. The vast majority of patients have a benign self-limiting condition, transient synovitis, but this may be clinically indistinguishable from more serious conditions, particularly septic arthritis, Perthes disease and slipped upper femoral epiphysis (SUFE) (see Table 10.1).

10.1.1
Management

Investigation of the irritable hip in the child should always include a thorough history and clinical exam-

J. Teh, MD
Department of Radiology, Nuffield Orthopaedic Centre, Windmill Road, Headington, Oxford, OX3 7LD, UK
D. Wilson, MD
Department of Radiology, Nuffield Orthopaedic Centre, NHS Trust, Windmill Road, Headington, Oxford, OX3 7LD, UK

ination. Blood tests should be routinely obtained, including a full blood count, erythrocyte sedimentation rate (ESR) and/or C-reactive protein and blood cultures. Imaging should begin with a plain AP radiograph of the pelvis, with frog leg views in children at risk of SUFE, followed by an ultrasound examination. The plain radiograph is obtained to exclude conditions such as Perthes disease, SUFE and tumours, whilst the ultrasound is performed for detecting joint effusions. The management of the patient with an effusion is controversial; many institutions opt to aspirate all hip effusions demonstrated, whereas others take a minimally invasive approach, with aspiration only undertaken when certain features or clinical prediction algorithms indicate a moderate to high risk of sepsis.

- With the minimally invasive approach, children with irritable hips are often admitted to hospital for observation and pain relief (Vidigal and da Silva 1981; Taylor and Clarke 1994). As no single factor or blood test is diagnostic, several variables have to be taken into consideration for assessing risk of sepsis (Taylor and Clarke 1994; Eich et al. 1999; Kocher et al. 1999; Luhmann et al. 2004). Kocher et al. (1999) identified four main diagnostic variables associated with septic arthritis of the hip: a history of fever, non-weight bearing, ESR of greater than 40 mm/h and a white cell count of greater than 12000/mm^3.

Table 10.1. Differential diagnosis for the irritable hip in children

Transient synovitis
Sepsis including septic arthritis, osteomyelitis and pyomyositis
Perthes disease
Primary bone tumours
Leukaemia
Haemarthrosis due to trauma or coagulation disorder
Fracture, including non-accidental injury
Inflammatory arthropathy
Idiopathic chondrolysis
In children around the age of puberty, slipped upper femoral epiphysis

They formulated a clinical prediction algorithm which showed that if all of these variables were present a child had a 99.6% chance of having septic arthritis of the hip. TAYLOR and CLARKE (1994) used the slightly different criteria of spasm, tenderness, pyrexia >38° and ESR of > 20 mm/h and found that a combination of any two of these produced a sensitivity for sepsis of 95%.

There is however disagreement regarding the effectiveness of clinical prediction algorithms, as there is significant overlap between these various factors for septic arthritis and transient synovitis (LUHMANN et al. 2004; DEL BECCARO et al. 1992; FINK et al. 1995; BENNETT and NAMNYAK 1992). LUHMANN et al. (2004) evaluated the clinical prediction algorithm proposed by KOCHER et al. (1999), and found that if all four variables were present, the predictive probability of hip sepsis was only 59% in their cohort of patients. It has therefore been proposed that a more proactive approach for excluding sepsis should be used, with aspiration of all hip effusions shown on ultrasound (EICH et al. 1999; LUHMANN et al. 2004; FINK et al. 1995; BERMANN et al. 1995; FISCHER and BEATTIE 1999). This has the following advantages:

- The diagnosis of septic arthritis is made at the earliest opportunity. Septic arthritis of the hip is considered a surgical emergency usually requiring arthrotomy in addition to antibiotic treatment (SHETTY and GEDALIA 1998; DONATTO 1998). Delayed diagnosis may have disastrous consequences including femoral head destruction, degenerative arthritis and growth disturbance. Immediate aspiration prevents a delay in the diagnosis and subsequent therapy.
- Avoidance of admission to hospital. Hospital admission consumes considerable resources, and is both upsetting for the child and disruptive to the family. In cases of transient synovitis, hospital admission can usually be avoided (TAYLOR and CLARKE 1994; FINK et al. 1995). The most reliable way of ensuring that patients with septic arthritis are not inadvertently sent home is to obtain a sample of joint fluid for analysis.
- Relief of joint tamponade. Although controversial, it has been argued that the presence of a hip effusion may lead to an increase in intra-articular pressure which may compromise the blood supply to the capital femoral epiphysis causing Perthes disease (VEGTER 1987; KALLIO and RYOPPY 1985; WINGSTRAND et al. 1985; KEMP 1981). Hip aspiration with relief of joint tamponade may therefore decrease the incidence of Perthes disease.

- Pain relief. Transient synovitis may be extremely painful. Aspiration of the joint has been shown to significantly alleviate symptoms and decrease the requirement for analgesia (FINK et al. 1995; HILL et al. 1990; WINGSTRAND 1986). This simple diagnostic and therapeutic measure often removes the need for analgesia, bed rest, traction therapy and hospital admission.

The protocol outlined below is the authors' approach to the management of the irritable hip in children.

10.2
Transient Synovitis

Several synonymous terms are used to describe this condition including irritable hip, observation hip and toxic synovitis. The diagnosis can only be made by exclusion of other causes of hip pain. Transient synovitis is the most common cause of acute hip pain in children aged 3–10 years. It has however been described in an infant of 3 months and also in adults (DZIOBA and BARRINGTON 1977; LAROCHE et al. 2000). Epidemiological studies have shown an average annual incidence of two per thousand, with an accumulated risk of 3%. Boys are affected twice as often as girls (FISCHER and BEATTIE 1999; LANDIN et al. 1987).

The onset of symptoms may be relatively sudden or insidious, developing over several days. Unilateral hip pain with reluctance to weight bear is the most common presentation but some patients may complain of thigh or knee pain. Most patients are afebrile but sometimes a mild pyrexia is present.

The condition is of unknown cause. Infection, usually of the upper respiratory tract is said to be common in the preceding 2–3 weeks but children of this age commonly have such symptoms and no seasonal variation has been demonstrated. Studies have shown an increase in viral antibody titres suggesting an infective cause (LEIBOWITZ et al. 1985; TOLAT et al. 1993). Trauma, recent vaccination and an allergic disposition have also been linked to transient synovitis (SAINSBURY et al. 1986; DENMAN et al. 1983). On histological examination the affected synovium reveals non-specific inflammation and hypertrophy of the synovial membrane. The synovial fluid contains increased proteoglycans which are released from the articular cartilage as a result of degradation by chondrocytes (LOHMANDER et al. 1988).

Transient synovitis usually follows an entirely benign course (SHARWOOD 1981; MUKAMEL et al.

1985). A possible long term consequence of the condition is asymptomatic overgrowth of the femoral head, coxa magna, which is of no clinical significance (KALLIO 1988). Controversy exists regarding a possible relationship between transient synovitis and Perthes disease (ERKEN and KATZ 1990; GERSHUNI et al. 1983; KALLIO et al. 1986). It has been argued that an effusion may lead to joint tamponade which can compromise the blood supply to the capital femoral epiphysis causing Perthes disease (VEGTER 1987; KALLIO and RYOPPY 1985; WINGSTRAND et al. 1985; KEMP 1981). In patients diagnosed with transient synovitis there is an incidence of Perthes disease of around 1%–3.4% (LANDIN et al. 1987; SHARWOOD 1981).

10.2.1
Imaging Findings in Transient Synovitis

The main roles for imaging in transient synovitis are to exclude other more serious conditions and to allow early discharge.

10.2.1.1
Plain Radiographs

Plain radiographs have an important role in excluding bony abnormalities such as Perthes disease, osteomyelitis, tumours and fractures, and are normally obtained as part of the initial investigation of patients with an irritable hip.

A possible exception is in children below the age of 8 years when SUFE would be very unlikely, when there is a joint effusion that has been proven by ultrasound and aspirated to show a clear, uninfected and non-haemorrhagic effusion. In these circumstances, septic arthritis, haemorrhage and fracture are ruled out. If the child recovers within 24 h then Perthes disease, juvenile arthritis and osteomyelitis are effectively excluded. Therefore plain films might be avoided.

In patients with a large effusion, radiographs may demonstrate widening of the medial joint space (Waldenstrom's sign) which is measured from the ossified part of the femoral head to the acetabulum (lateral margin of Kohler's teardrop). This measurement includes the unossified portion of the femoral head, the articular cartilage and any joint fluid, and is therefore only a poor estimate of joint effusion. Compared to the other side, this distance should be the same or within 2 mm (Fig. 10.1). Most children with joint effusions will not demonstrate this sign.

Indeed it is more likely that this abnormality is the result of cartilage oedema which invariably is associated with an effusion. It is a rare but useful early sign in Perthes disease (KEMP and BOLDERO 1966).

Displacement of fat pads around the hip has also been used for the assessment of joint effusions (JUNG et al. 2003) but several studies have shown that these are unreliable, as the fat pads are often simply displaced due to the abduction posture adopted by an irritable hip (BROWN 1975; EGUND et al. 1987) (Fig. 10.2). The capsular fat pad is formed by the fatty layer that lies just adjacent to the joint capsule. The medial iliopsoas fat pad lies between the joint capsule and the iliopsoas muscle. The intergluteal fat pad lies between the gluteus minimus and gluteus medius muscles.

10.2.1.2
Ultrasound

Ultrasound is an extremely sensitive technique for the detection of hip joint effusion (WILSON et al. 1984; WILSON 2004) and is an invaluable aid joint aspiration.

A high resolution linear probe is optimum but other configurations may be effective. The child should be examined supine with the legs extended and held in neutral, and the transducer orientated longitudinally along the femoral neck. With the probe centred on the epiphysis, the image should include part of the acetabulum, the epiphysis, the articular cartilage, the growth plate and the femoral neck. The ossified rim of the acetabulum should be clearly distinguished from the partly ossified femoral epiphysis. This image is obtained by rotat-

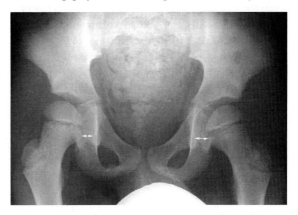

Fig. 10.1. Plain radiograph of the pelvis in a child with transient synovitis of the left hip. There is widening of the medial joint space of the left hip (arrows) indicating a positive Waldenstrom's sign

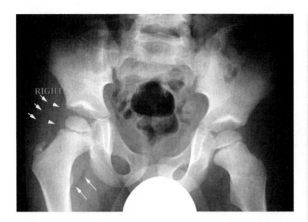

Fig. 10.2. Plain radiograph of the pelvis in a child demonstrating asymmetric widening of the left medial joint space (Waldenstrom's sign) in a patient with transient synovitis who had a joint effusion shown on ultrasound. The normal fat pads around the right hip are illustrated: the *short arrows* delineate the intergluteal fat pad, the *arrowheads* delineate the capsular fat pad and the *long arrows* delineate the iliopsoas fat pad

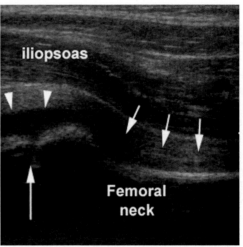

Fig. 10.3. Normal US anatomy of the hip joint. The low echogenicity articular cartilage of the femoral head is marked by *arrowheads*, whilst the echogenic iliofemoral ligament is marked by the *arrows*. The low echogenicity cleft marked by the *long arrow* in the femoral head represents the growth plate

ing the alignment of the probe to the plane of the femoral neck. The growth plate is seen as a low echogenicity cleft separating the epiphysis from the metaphysis. The joint capsule appears as an echogenic band extending from the acetabulum to the inter-trochanteric line. In the normal hip the synovium cannot normally be distinguished from the bone and overlying capsule. The normal capsule to bone distance should measure no more than 3 mm and the difference between sides should be less than 2 mm (WILSON et al. 1984) (Fig. 10.3).

An effusion is usually seen as an area of low echogenicity anterior to the femoral neck with convex anterior bulging of the echogenic joint capsule (Fig. 10.4). Synovial thickening may be evident both anterior to the fluid and in the synovial reflection along the femoral neck. An echo-free effusion does not exclude infection or haemorrhage (MATHIE et al. 1991; MARCHAL et al. 1987). Furthermore the absence of flow on power Doppler sonography does not allow exclusion of septic arthritis (STROUSE et al. 1998). As ultrasound cannot differentiate transient synovitis from infection, aspiration of all effusions has been advocated (EICH et al. 1999; FINK et al. 1995; BERMAN et al. 1995; FISCHER and BEATTIE 1999).

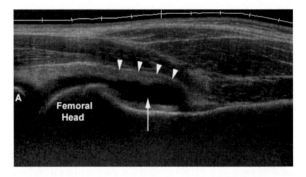

Fig. 10.4. Extended field of view ultrasound scan demonstrating a hip joint effusion (*arrow*) and bulging iliofemoral ligament (*arrowheads*) in a patient with transient synovitis. The acetabulum (*A*) is seen adjacent to the femoral head

10.2.1.3
Technique for Aspiration

A technique for ultrasound guided aspiration has been described by BERMAN et al. (1995). Aspiration should be performed under strict aseptic conditions. At least 1 h prior to the ultrasound scan local anaesthetic cream is applied over the hip. Informed consent is obtained from the parent or guardian, explaining the risks of pain, infection and bruising. Using ultrasound guidance the skin is marked directly over the centre of the effusion, avoiding the femoral vessels. The child is shielded from observing the procedure by an assistant leaning over their chest and gently immobilising the arms. The skin is then cleaned and punctured using a 19-gauge needle which is advanced in a true vertical direction until the femoral neck is reached. It is rarely necessary to use the ultrasound machine to image the needle. Suction is then applied using a 10-ml syringe. Normal joint fluid should be clear or straw coloured, highly viscous and non turbid. Infection results in purulent grey, yellow or green synovial fluid (HERNDON et al. 1986). Sometimes however non-infected synovial fluid may have a cloudy appearance (FINK et al. 1995). Once obtained, the sample is sent for immediate Gram stain and culture. This procedure will relieve pain and allow immediate discharge of most patients.

10.2.1.4
Bone scintigraphy

The use of bone scintigraphy varies widely according to local practice and availability of MRI. Bone scintigraphy is normally reserved for those patients in whom the symptoms have failed to settle and the diagnosis remains uncertain after plain radiography and ultrasound. Its value lies in excluding other more serious conditions rather than confirming transient synovitis as it is one of the most effective techniques for detecting musculoskeletal inflammatory processes, particularly osteomyelitis and septic arthritis. The examination is performed using technetium 99-m labelled mono diphosphonate (Tc 99^m MDP). The examination typically involves three phases of acquisition: the initial flow phase, the blood pool phase (5–10 min after injection) and the equilibrium/delayed phase (3–6 h after the injection). A fourth phase (24 h after injection) can be useful in patients who have equivocal findings after the three phase examination (GREENSPAN and TEHRANZADEH 2001).

On a three phase bone scintigram the findings in transient synovitis are non-specific (CONNOLLY and CONNOLLY 2003). In the blood pool phase there may be mild diffuse increased joint activity reflecting hyperaemia. On the delayed images the activity in the joint may be normal, increased or decreased. Decreased uptake, or the "cold hip" sign is thought to be due to an effusion resulting in tamponade and thus impaired perfusion of the joint (UREN and HOWMAN-GILES 1991).

10.2.1.5
Magnetic Resonance Imaging (MR Imaging)

In many institutions the use of scintigraphy for investigating the irritable hip has been supplanted

by MR imaging which provides much more anatomical detail. As with bone scintigraphy, MR imaging tends to be reserved for those patients in whom the symptoms do not settle, and when conditions other than transient synovitis are suspected.

The typical MR imaging findings in transient synovitis are of a simple effusion without specific changes in bone marrow (TOBY et al. 1985; LEE et al. 1999) (Fig. 10.5). There may be minor signal intensity alterations in the soft tissue around the hip joint, indicating reactive soft-tissue oedema. The use of intravenous Gadolinium allows the distinction between an enhancing rim of inflamed synovial membrane and hypointense joint effusion, but this finding may be seen in transient synovitis as well as septic arthritis (LEE et al. 1999).

LEE et al. (1999) have shown that MR imaging can help differentiate between transient synovitis and septic arthritis on the basis of peri-articular marrow changes. In this study 14 patients diagnosed with transient synovitis had normal bone marrow signal, whilst eight out of nine patients with proven septic arthritis had marrow signal changes (i.e. low signal intensity on T1-weighted images and high signal intensity on fat-suppressed T2-weighted images). There were mild peri-articular marrow signal changes in six patients without osteomyelitis, and extensive changes in the femoral head and neck in two patients with coexistent osteomyelitis. In septic arthritis, mild signal intensity alterations in bone marrow may be caused by reactive oedema. When there is coexistent osteomyelitis, the marrow changes tend to be more diffuse, particularly on T1 weighted images (KARCHEVSKY et al. 2004).

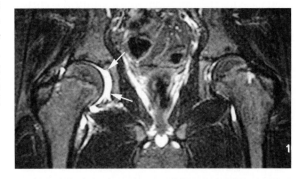

Fig. 10.5. Transient synovitis of the right hip. Coronal STIR image of both hips demonstrating a unilateral right hip joint effusion (*arrows*). The peri-articular bone marrow signal is normal

10.3
Hip Infection

Infection around the hip may be caused by haematogenous seeding, local spread from contiguous infection or inoculation, including trauma and surgery (WALD 1985) (Table 10.2). The infecting organism differs according to the patient's age and immune status, and the presence of a prosthetic joint.

10.3.1
Osteomyelitis

Osteomyelitis may be classified according to the chronicity of symptoms, the route of infection or the causative organism. The normal developmental changes that affect the bone, growth plate and cartilage have a strong influence on the manifestations of osteomyelitis (OGDEN and LISTER 1975; BOUTIN et al. 1998). In neonates and infants, infection can spread across the growth plate, along transphyseal vessels, to penetrate the epiphysis, resulting in an increased incidence of joint infections (OGDEN and LISTER 1975). Between 6–18 months of age the diaphyseal vessels terminate in slow-flowing metaphyseal vascular sinusoids, with involution of the transphyseal vessels. The growth plate therefore comes to act as a natural barrier for the spread of infection. As a consequence, the metaphysis is the usual site for childhood osteomyelitis. When the growth plate fuses, the vascular connection between the metaphysis and epiphysis is restored and the joint is once again subject to contiguous spread of infection.

Acute osteomyelitis results in bone marrow oedema, cellular infiltration and vascular engorgement. As the pressure builds within the intramedullary cavity the infection spreads into the cortex and subperiosteal space, and eventually into the surrounding soft tissue (WILLIS and ROZENCWAIG 1996). The hip joint is particularly susceptible to infection as a result of the synovial membrane inserting distal to epiphysis, allowing bacteria to spread directly from the metaphysis to the joint (DORMANS and DRUMMOND 1994). Apart from septic arthritis, complications of osteomyelitis around the hip include pathological fractures, slipped capital femoral epiphysis, bone modelling deformity (coxa magna), premature growth plate closure and chronic infection (BETZ et al. 1990).

In infants and children, acute osteomyelitis is usually caused by haematogenous spread. The most

Table 10.2. Risk factors for septic arthritis

Increased risk off haematogenous seeding
- Simultaneous bacterial infection particularly ear and respiratory infections in children and gonorrhoea in adults
- Immuno-compromise including HIV disease and patients on chemotherapy
- Diabetes
- Sickle cell disease
- Intravenous drug abuse

Increased risk of local infection
- Prosthetic joint
- Indwelling vascular catheter
- Adjacent soft tissue infection
- Rheumatoid arthritis

Inoculation
- Trauma
- Arthroscopy or recent surgery

common infective agents are bacterial. *Staphylococcus aureus* is the commonest organism, followed by Beta-haemolytic *Streptococcus*, *Streptococcus pneumoniae* and *E. Coli* (NELSON 1991). Until recently *Haemophilus influenzae b* (HIB) was a commonly cultured organism but the introduction of HIB vaccination has led to a marked decline in cases (BOWERMAN et al. 1997; LIPTAK et al. 1997). Patients with sickle cell anaemia are particularly prone to *Salmonella* osteomyelitis due to micro-infarctions of the bowel wall allowing the organism to enter the blood stream from the gastrointestinal tract (EBONG 1987; ADEYOKUNNU and HENDRICKSE 1980) although they are also commonly affected by the organisms seen in children without the haemoglobinopathy.

10.3.2
Septic Arthritis

Septic arthritis is also referred to as bacterial, suppurative, purulent or infective arthritis. It causes inflammation of the synovial membrane with purulent effusion into the joint capsule. In the hip the onset of the symptoms is usually rapid with joint irritability, intense pain, limp, non-weight-bearing and fever.

Septic arthritis may occur at any age. In children, it often affects those less than 3 years old, particularly infants, when the diagnosis can be very difficult as there may initially be no obvious localising signs (SHETTY and GEDALIA 1998). Concomitant osteomyelitis occurs in approximately 50% of neonates with septic arthritis, but only 20% of infants with septic arthritis.

In neonates and infants, *Staphylococcus aureus* and gram-negative anaerobes are the main organisms involved in septic arthritis (FINK and NELSON 1986). As with osteomyelitis, the incidence of *Haemophilus influenzae* has dramatically decreased due to widespread use of the HIB vaccine (BOWERMANN et al. 1997). In children aged over the age of 1 year, *Staphylococcus aureus* is the major cause of infection (WELKON et al. 1986). As sexual activity begins, *Neisseria gonorrhoeae* becomes a common pathogen. Women are three times more likely to develop Gonococcal arthritis than men (CUCURULL and ESPINOZA 1998).

Septic arthritis may have severe consequences, resulting in avascular necrosis and femoral head destruction, modelling deformity, ankylosis and premature osteoarthritis (BETZ et al. 1990; DORMANS and DRUMMOND 1994).

10.3.3
Imaging of Osteomyelitis and Septic Arthritis

The early diagnosis and treatment of osteomyelitis and/or septic arthritis is essential to prevent long-term morbidity. The various imaging methods have individual strengths and benefits.

10.3.3.1
Plain Radiographs

For patients with suspected osteomyelitis or septic arthritis, plain radiographs should be obtained as valuable information regarding joint morphology, soft tissue gas, calcifications and prostheses may be provided. It is however recognised that the plain radiographic findings of osteomyelitis may not manifest for 10–14 days after the onset of symptoms (DALINKA et al. 1975; ABERNETHY and CARTY 1997; WRIGHT et al. 1995; GASH et al. 1994; LORD and CARTY 1993; JONES et al. 1990; CARTY and OWEN 1985).

In patients with acute osteomyelitis, soft tissue swelling with blurring or loss of the normal fat planes may be the only sign of infection, indicating the presence of cellulitis. After several days, local hyperaemia and cellular infiltration of the bone marrow results in osteolysis. Between 30%–50% of bone mineral may need to be lost before the plain radiograph becomes positive (JARAMILLO et al. 1995). As infection extends into the cortex cortical destruction and periostitis can be seen. The sensitiv-

ity of plain radiographs for osteomyelitis is quoted as ranging from 43%–75%, with a specificity of 75%–83% (BOUTIN et al. 1998; SANTIAGO RESTREPO et al. 2003).

Chronic osteomyelitis is present when symptoms have been present for more than 1 month, or when existing osteomyelitis has been inadequately treated (WILLIS and ROZENCWAIG 1996). Plain radiographs show mottled areas of lucency due to areas of trabecular resorption and cortical thickening due to established periostitis. A draining sinus may be demonstrated as a focal cortical defect. Dense necrotic bone or sequestrum may also be identified on radiography. This can persist as a focus for infection, resorbed or discharged through a sinus tract. Involucrum is seen as new bone formed beneath elevated periosteum that surrounds sequestrum (Fig. 10.6).

With acute septic arthritis plain radiographs may be completely normal or may demonstrate widening of the joint space with soft tissue swelling and blurring of adjacent fat planes (MITCHELL et al. 1988) – findings which may be indistinguishable from transient synovitis in children. In a study involving 19 children with aspiration-proven septic arthritis of the hip, the radiograph was abnormal in all neonates, showing widening of the joint space, but normal in eight out of 10 over the age of 1 year

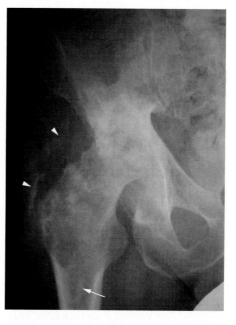

Fig. 10.6. Plain radiograph of the right hip demonstrating chronic osteomyelitis of the proximal femur with chronic septic arthritis of the hip. There is cortical destruction and bony fragmentation (*arrowheads*) in addition to sequestrum in the femoral shaft (*arrow*). The femoral head has been destroyed and the hip is subluxed

(VOLBERG et al. 1984). With certain organisms, particularly *Escherichia coli*, *Enterobacter* and *Clostridium perfringens* gas formation may be seen in the joint and soft tissues. Joint dislocation may occur (Fig. 10.7). If there is associated osteomyelitis, osteolysis and periostitis may be evident (JARAMILLO et al. 1995; CURTISS 1973).

In more advanced stages of infection there may be peri-articular osteoporosis and marginal or central erosions. Subsequently the subchondral bone may be destroyed and the joint may become subluxed or eventually ankylosed (GREENSPAN and TEHRANZADEH 2001) (Figs. 10.6, 10.8). WELKON et al showed that complications following acute septic arthritis were significantly associated with infection at age less than 6 months, a delay in treatment of 4 or more days, infection due to *Staphylococcus aureus* and the concomitant presence of osteomyelitis (WELKON et al. 1986).

10.3.3.2
Bone Scintigraphy

The three phase bone scintigraphy has a very high sensitivity for detecting osteomyelitis and excluding infection if the plain radiograph is normal, but it does have a relatively low specificity (CRIM and SEEGER 1994; ISRAEL et al. 1987; HOWIE et al. 1983). Other conditions such as Perthes disease, trauma and tumour can also produce a "hot" bone scan (BOWER et al. 1985) (Fig. 10.9a,b). In osteomyelitis there is usually increased uptake during all phases. Increased vascularity at the site of infection allows early concentration of isotope whilst the bone repair process explains the increased uptake on delayed imaging. There is, however, a wide spectrum of findings as both "cold" and "hot" abnormalities may be present (GALPERINE et al. 2004; HANDMAKER 1980). A "cold" spot occurs as a result of medullary thrombosis and compression of arteries by intra-osseous pus (ALLWRIGHT et al. 1991).

With septic arthritis the typical finding is of increased peri-articular uptake during all phases of imaging (Fig. 10.10). Unfortunately the findings are non-specific and may be seen in a variety of conditions including inflammatory arthropathy and transient synovitis. The "cold hip" sign on bone scan is due to fluid in the hip joint under pressure causing impaired perfusion of the structures within the joint capsule. In a retrospective review, 22% of patients with this sign were found to have septic arthritis at surgery (UREN and HOWMAN-GILES 1991).

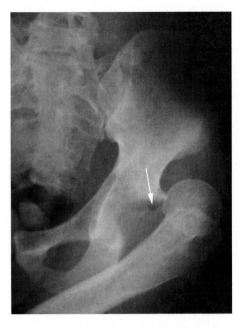

Fig. 10.7. Plain radiograph of the pelvis demonstrating dislocation of the left hip joint in an IV drug user with acute septic arthritis. Note the presence of gas in the joint (*arrow*)

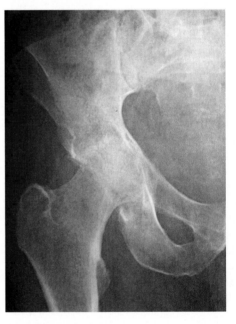

Fig. 10.8. Plain radiograph of the right hip demonstrating early ankylosis following chronic septic arthritis

10.3.3.3
Other Scintigraphic Techniques

In uncomplicated situations the three phase bone scintigram usually suffices for detection of osteomyelitis. In certain situations, particularly when

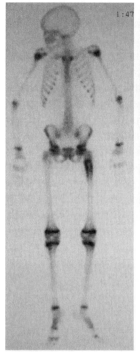

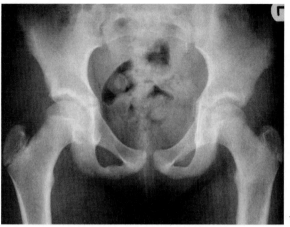

Fig. 10.9. a Equilibrium phase technetium 99ᵐ MDP bone scintigram demonstrating non-specific increased uptake in the proximal left femur in a 12-year-old girl with a Ewing's sarcoma. b Same patient as (a). Plain radiograph of the pelvis demonstrating a lytic intramedullary lesion in the proximal femur

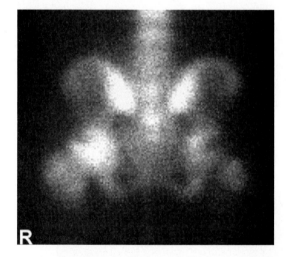

Fig. 10.10. Equilibrium phase technetium 99ᵐ MDP bone scintigram demonstrating increased periarticular uptake in a patient with septic arthritis of the right hip

orthopaedic hardware is present, complementary scintigraphic techniques may be useful (WELLMAN et al. 1988).

Labelled leucocyte (with Indium 111 or hexamethylpropyleneamine, HMPAO) imaging is a technique capable of detecting infections at various anatomical sites. However, the in vitro labelling process is labour intensive, not always available, and involves direct handling of blood products. For musculoskeletal infection, the need to frequently perform comple-mentary marrow or bone imaging adds complexity and expense to the procedure (LOVE and PALESTRO 2004). The accuracy of combined bone scintigraphy and labelled leucocyte imaging for osteomyelitis varies with the chronicity and location of the lesion (SCHAUWECKER et al. 1984). Acute osteomyelitis in the peripheral skeleton is accurately detected, whilst chronic lesions in the axial skeleton are poorly demonstrated.

Gallium 67 citrate imaging improves the accuracy for detection of osteomyelitis by granulocyte and bacterial uptake at the site of infection. It is however not specific for infection with increased uptake seen in inflammatory arthropathies and trauma (LEWIN et al. 1986). A combination of bone scintigraphy and gallium scanning improves the accuracy for osteomyelitis: if the gallium activity is greater than the bone scintigraphy activity osteomyelitis is considered likely.

With the increased availability of MR these additional techniques are less often appropriate.

10.3.3.4
Ultrasound

As ultrasound is unable to penetrate the cortex of bone its use in the detection of osteomyelitis is limited. Nevertheless, the diagnosis of osteomyelitis can be made by ultrasound demonstration of subperiosteal or juxta-cortical fluid collections (HOWARD et al. 1993; ABIRI et al. 1989). HOWARD et al. (1993) showed three main abnormalities in children who were shown to have osteomyelitis on ultrasound: These were thickening of the periosteum, elevation of the periosteum by more than 2 mm, and swelling of overlying muscle or subcutaneous tissue. However, the absence of these signs on ultrasound examination does not exclude osteomyelitis.

Ultrasound is an excellent means of detecting early joint effusions and synovial thickening and is therefore the ideal means of excluding acute septic arthritis. If an effusion is detected, aspiration is required for diagnosis of infection as the findings are non-specific (WILSON et al. 1984; WILSON 2004) (Fig. 10.11). It has been shown that osteomyelitis associated with hip septic arthritis is not reliably demonstrated by ultrasound (ZAWIN et al. 1993).

10.3.3.5
Computed Tomography (CT)

Computed tomography allows excellent delineation of the osseous structures and is very well suited to guiding drainage or biopsy. In patients with osteomyelitis CT can be a useful method to detect early osseous erosion and to document the presence of sequestrum, foreign body, or gas formation (SANTIAGO RESTREPO et al. 2003; GOLD et al. 1991; RAM et al. 1981). The presence of intra-osseous gas is virtually diagnostic for osteomyelitis (RAM et al. 1981) (Fig. 10.12). Contrast enhanced studies are necessary to assess soft tissue abnormalities and collections but do not help to identify bony changes. Increased density may be seen in the intramedullary canal following intravenous contrast administration but this finding is non-specific and may also be seen with tumours, haemorrhage, irradiation and fractures,

as well as with infection (ALIABADI and NIKPOOR 1994). CT has an important role in characterising osseous lesions; in particular it can be diagnostic for osteoid osteoma, which may mimic osteomyelitis clinically and radiographically (Fig. 10.13).

Using CT a variety of features can be seen in septic arthritis including effusions and abscesses. Bone changes range from minor erosion of articular surfaces to gross destruction of the proximal femur and acetabulum (RESNIK et al. 1987). Sinus tracts may be demonstrated. Intravenous contrast agents improve soft tissue contrast and may show rim enhancement around abscesses. The presence of gas within the hip joint is highly suggestive of septic arthritis unless the patient has recently undergone

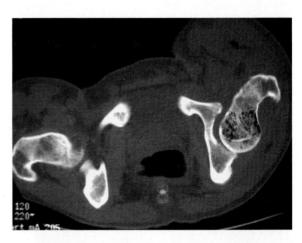

Fig. 10.12. CT scan of the hips demonstrating multiple foci of intra-osseous gas in the femoral head in an adult with osteomyelitis

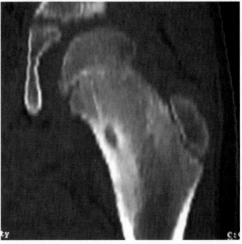

Fig. 10.13. CT scan of the left hip with a coronal reformat demonstrating the lucent nidus of an osteoid osteoma. The cortical thickening alone might suggest infection

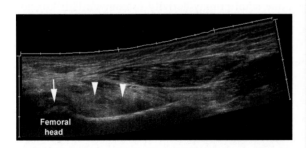

Fig. 10.11. Extended field of view ultrasound scan demonstrating a joint effusion (*arrow*) and increased echogenicity in the iliopsoas muscle (*arrowheads*) in a 3-year-old child with septic arthritis and pyomyositis

surgery, joint puncture or traumatic dislocation of the hip (Fairbairn et al. 1995) (Fig. 10.14).

A limitation of conventional CT used to be in the assessment of regions with metallic implants or prostheses, due to beam hardening artefact (Santiago Restrepo et al. 2003). However, with advances in multislice CT and the ability to perform 3D volume rendered reformats, a significant amount of this artefact can be eliminated allowing the relationship between the hardware and adjacent bones to be clearly shown (Pretorius and Fishman 1999). CT therefore has an increasingly important role to play in the assessment of suspected prosthetic joint infections (Fig. 10.15).

10.3.3.6
MR Imaging

MR imaging is an extremely valuable technique for evaluating musculoskeletal infections around the hip and has a very important role in the early diagnosis and staging of infections. Numerous studies have shown the utility of MRI for detecting osteomyelitis in various anatomical locations (Table 10.3).

MR imaging allows exquisite characterisation and delineation of infection of the bones and soft tissues in multiple planes. With osteomyelitis the bone marrow is infiltrated with oedema, pus and inflammatory cells, leading to a loss of the normal fatty marrow signal on T1 weighted sequence, with ill-defined low signal intensity and high signal intensity on T2 weighted sequences. Fat suppressed and short tau inversion recovery (STIR) sequences have extended the dynamic range of tissue contrast by decreasing the interfering signal of fat on both

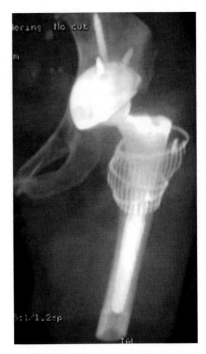

Fig. 10.15. Three-dimensional volume rendered CT scan of a left total hip replacement showing a good position and normal prosthesis bone interface in a patient with a painful hip. Note the lack of artefact from the metal prosthesis

Table 10.3. Utility of MRI for detecting osteomyelitis in various anatomical locations

Reference	Sensitivity %	Specificity %	Anatomic location
Unger et al. (1988)	92	96	various
Erdman et al. (1991)	98	75	various
Mazur et al. (1995)	97	92	various
Huang et al. (1998)	98	89	pelvis/hip

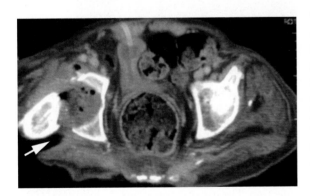

Fig. 10.14. CT scan of the hips demonstrating gas bubbles and an effusion within the right hip joint in a paraplegic patient with septic arthritis and subluxation of the femoral head. The *arrow* indicates the site of a deep sinus in the buttock which communicates with the hip

T1 and T2 weighted sequences, leading to increased conspicuity of lesions with high water content (Huang et al. 1998; Morrison et al. 1993). In children the signal intensity of normal haemopoietic marrow must be recognised to avoid over-diagnosis of marrow signal change. Usually osteomyelitis is of higher signal intensity on T2 and STIR sequences than normal haemopoietic marrow (Abernethy and Carty 1997; Jaramillo et al. 1995; Erdman et al. 1991).

The surrounding soft tissues are usually abnormal in the acute phase of osteomyelitis, with oedema, loss of the normal fat planes and collections. The cortical bone can be disrupted and may return increased signal intensity on T2 weighted and STIR sequences (Santiago Restrepo et al. 2003) (Fig. 10.16a,b).

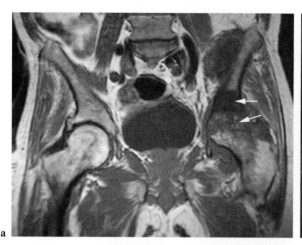
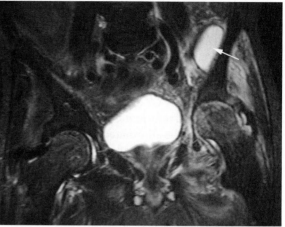

a   b

Fig. 10.16. a Coronal T1 weighted image demonstrating joint space loss and loss of the normal fatty marrow signal in a peri-articular distribution (*arrows*) in a patient with acute septic arthritis, osteomyelitis and pyomyositis. Although symptoms had only been present for 3 weeks there is flattening of the femoral head and marked joint space loss. **b** Same patient as in (**a**). Coronal FSTIR image demonstrating a collection in the iliopsoas muscle (*arrow*) and extensive oedema in the muscles surrounding the hip

Subacute osteomyelitis occurs when acute osteo-myelitis progresses to intra-osseous abscess formation, otherwise known as a Brodie's abscess. There is usually reactive bone marrow oedema surrounding a Brodie's abscess reflecting hyperaemia. The internal wall of the abscess is lined by a layer of vascularised granulation tissue that results in a rim of increased signal hyperintensity relative to the main abscess contents on T1 weighted sequences, described as the "penumbra sign" (GREY et al. 1998; TEHRANZADEH et al. 1992). In around 50% of cases the findings in subacute osteomyelitis may be confused with a tumour. The differential diagnosis often includes Langerhans cell histiocytosis, Ewing's sarcoma and osteoid osteoma (Fig. 10.17).

MR imaging combined with plain films can help differentiate between acute and chronic osteomyelitis (ERDMAN et al. 1991; DANGMAN et al. 1992). In acute osteomyelitis there is no cortical thickening and the interface between normal and abnormal marrow is difficult to define clearly. In contrast there is usually cortical thickening and relatively clear definition between normal and abnormal marrow in chronic osteomyelitis. A peripheral area of low signal intensity ('rim sign') may be seen on all sequences, corresponding to fibrous change in chronic osteo-myelitis (ERDMAN et al. 1991). There may be areas of fibrotic scarring in the marrow leading to low signal intensity on both T1 and T2 weighted sequences (Fig. 10.18a,b). Eventually there may be extensive bony sclerosis with reduction of the marrow cavity. Sinus tracts are often present when there is chronic

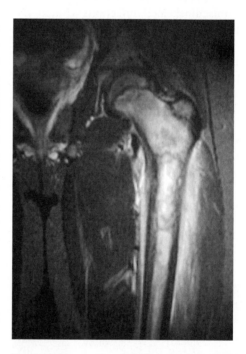

Fig. 10.17. Same patient as in Fig. 10.9a,b. Coronal FSTIR image demonstrates extensive marrow signal abnormality with marked oedema in the surrounding soft tissues in a patient with Ewing's sarcoma. The findings may mimic infection but the diaphyseal location would be unusual for osteomyelitis

infection. The use of intravenous Gadolinium DTPA may yield further information as areas of devascularised sequestration do not enhance. Furthermore the presence of collections can be confirmed by the presence of rim enhancement (Fig. 10.19).

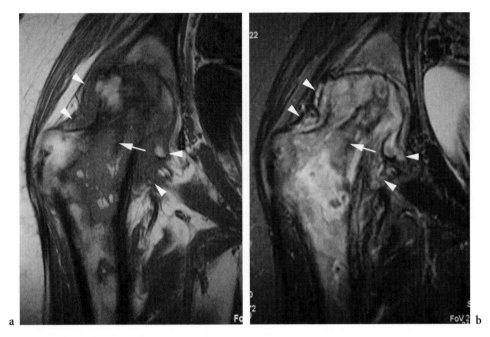

a   b

Fig. 10.18a,b. Coronal T1 weighted (**a**) and FSTIR (**b**) images demonstrating chronic osteomyelitis of the right proximal femur with marked heterogeneity in marrow signal and extensive replacement of fatty marrow. Areas of very low signal are present on both sequences indicating scarring and fibrosis (*arrows*). Associated septic arthritis has resulted in marked loss of joint space and synovial thickening (*arrowheads*)

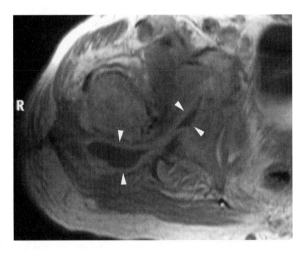

Fig. 10.19. Axial T1 weighted image demonstrating the presence of a rim-enhancing collection in the hip (*arrowheads*) in a patient following a Girdlestone procedure for a primary hip infection

MR imaging is extremely sensitive for the detection of septic arthritis with a much greater specificity than either plain films or CT (UNGER et al. 1988; RANNER et al. 1989). In the early stages of infection, T2 weighted and STIR sequences may reveal a high signal joint effusion or synovial thickening without any marrow signal change (LEE et al. 1999). On T2 weighted sequences, the infected joint effusion coupled with haemorrhage may lead to an inhomogeneous appearance. Patchy abnormal signal intensity in the peri-articular marrow can be seen on T1-weighted and short tau inversion-recovery images indicating reactive marrow oedema (LEE et al. 1999; ERDMAN et al. 1991). This feature may be helpful in differentiating transient synovitis, where there are no marrow changes, from septic arthritis (LEE et al. 1999) although it would be unwise to depend on this sign in alone.

In more advanced stages there may be peri-articular soft tissue inflammation and cellulitis and articular cartilage destruction with narrowing of the joint space (Fig. 10.18a,b). Synovial enhancement, peri-synovial oedema and joint effusions have been shown to have the highest correlation with the clinical diagnosis of a septic joint (KARCHEVSKY et al. 2004).

There are certain conditions that may mimic septic arthritis of the hip on MR and other imaging methods, including rapidly destructive osteoarthritis, rheumatoid and seronegative arthritis, avascular necrosis with secondary osteoarthritis and neuropathic osteoarthropathy (BOUTRY et al. 2002; ROSENBERG et al. 1992). Ultimately biopsy or aspiration is necessary for a definitive diagnosis (Fig. 10.20).

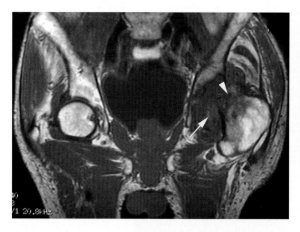

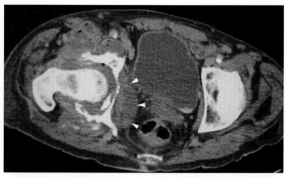

Fig. 10.21. Contrast enhanced CT scan of the hips demonstrating septic arthritis of the right hip with extensive pyomyositis in the surrounding muscles, including obturator internus (*arrowheads*). Note the presence of mild rim enhancement of the intramuscular abscesses and the presence of intra-articular gas

Fig. 10.20. Rapidly destructive osteoarthritis of the hip. Coronal T1 weighted image demonstrating severe erosion of the femoral head (*arrow*) with marked synovial thickening in an elderly man with a rapidly progressive arthropathy. Biopsy of the joint revealed no infection or crystals

10.3.4
Pyomyositis

Pyomyositis is an infectious disease of the skeletal muscle with a wide range of symptoms including pain, fever and swelling. As muscle is normally relatively resistant to infection it is a condition more often encountered in the Tropics, and in immunocompromised patients and those with diabetes (SPIEGEL et al. 1999; TRUSEN et al. 2003). When it involves the muscles around the hip it may mimic a number of conditions including septic arthritis, osteomyelitis and Perthes disease (WONG et al. 2004). Pyomyositis may spread from the muscle to involve the adjacent hip joint, resulting in septic arthritis and osteomyelitis (FREEDMAN et al. 1999; JOU et al. 2000).

On plain radiographs soft tissue swelling with blurring of the deep fat planes may be observed, but the diagnosis usually requires cross-sectional imaging (TRUSEN et al. 2003). Ultrasound demonstrates swelling of the involved muscle with altered echogenicity, with either increased or inhomogeneous echotexture (Fig. 10.11). Low echogenicity areas may be seen at sites of fluid collection or abscess formation.

With CT focal muscle swelling with well-defined area fluid collections may be seen, the latter demonstrating rim enhancement following intravenous contrast (Fig. 10.21). CT may not fully delineate the extent of abnormality unlike MR imaging which is the investigation of choice.

Using MR imaging the involved muscles are hyperintense on T2 weighted and STIR images,

with focal areas of homogeneous signal representing fluid collections (Fig. 10.16a,b). On T1 weighted images the affected muscle may be slightly higher signal than uninvolved muscle due to haemorrhage. Rim enhancement of fluid collections may be seen following intravenous Gadolinium DTPA (TRUSEN et al. 2003). There is usually inflammatory change in the fascial planes with reticulation of the subcutaneous tissue indicating cellulitis. Similar findings may be encountered in trauma, post-viral or auto-immune myositis and diabetic myonecrosis (Fig. 10.22). The latter typically presents with sudden onset of extreme pain but the patients are often afebrile and blood tests do not indicate sepsis (STRUK et al. 2001).

10.3.5
Necrotising fasciitis

Necrotising fasciitis is a rare, rapidly progressive, often fatal infection which causes extensive necrosis of the subcutaneous tissues, fascial planes and muscle. The patients are often immunocompromised and present very rapidly with severe pain, limb swelling and septic shock. Prompt surgical debridement is essential, in addition to intravenous antibiotics (SIMONART 2004). The condition may initially be mistaken for simple cellulitis.

Plain radiographs may show loss of the deep fat planes. Ultrasound usually demonstrates cellulitis with additional finding of fluid in the deep fascial planes. On CT there is thickening of the deep fascia with loss of the fat planes. Muscle swelling small

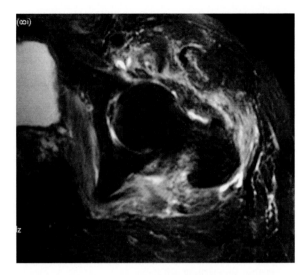

Fig. 10.22. Axial T2 fat-saturated image demonstrating extensive high signal within the muscles surrounding the left hip in a patient with a non-infective inflammatory myositis following a viral infection

gas bubbles and deep collections may also be seen (WALSHAW and DEANS 1996). On MR imaging T2 weighted and STIR images show increased signal intensity in the subcutaneous tissues, deep fascia and muscles (STRUK et al. 2001) (Fig. 10.23). If imaging cannot be performed expeditiously, treatment should not be delayed as the condition may progress quickly and is associated with a high mortality rate.

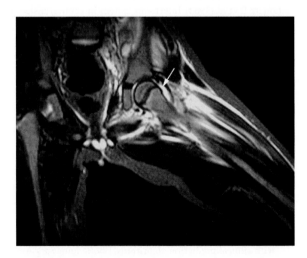

Fig. 10.23. Coronal STIR image of the left hip in a child with septic arthritis and necrotising fasciitis. There is a joint effusion (*arrow*) and high signal within the deep fascial planes of the right thigh indicating extensive oedema and fluid

References

Abernethy LJ, Carty H (1997) Modern approach to the diagnosis of osteomyelitis in children. Br J Hosp Med 58:464-468

Abiri MM, Kirpekar M, Ablow RC (1989) Osteomyelitis: detection with US. Radiology 172:509-511

Adeyokunnu AA, Hendrickse RG (1980) Salmonella osteomyelitis in childhood. A report of 63 cases seen in Nigerian children of whom 57 had sickle cell anaemia. Arch Dis Child 55:175-184

Aliabadi P, Nikpoor N (1994) Imaging osteomyelitis. Arthritis Rheum 37:617-622

Allwright SJ, Miller JH, Gilsanz V (1991) Subperiosteal abscess in children: scintigraphic appearance. Radiology 179:725-729

Bennett OM, Namnyak SS (1992) Acute septic arthritis of the hip joint in infancy and childhood. Clin Orthop 281:123-132

Berman L et al (1995) Technical note: identifying and aspirating hip effusions. Br J Radiol 68:306-310

Betz RR et al (1990) Late sequelae of septic arthritis of the hip in infancy and childhood. J Pediatr Orthop 10:365-372

Boutin RD et al (1998) Update on imaging of orthopedic infections. Orthop Clin North Am 29:41-66

Boutry N et al (2002) Rapidly destructive osteoarthritis of the hip: MR imaging findings. AJR Am J Roentgenol 179:657-663

Bower GD et al (1985) Isotope bone scans in the assessment of children with hip pain or limp. Pediatr Radiol 15:319-323

Bowerman SG, Green NE, Mencio GA (1997) Decline of bone and joint infections attributable to haemophilus influenzae type b. Clin Orthop 341:128-133

Brown I (1975) A study of the "capsular" shadow in disorders of the hip in children. J Bone Joint Surg Br 57:175-179

Carty H, Owen R (1985) Role of radionuclide studies in paediatric orthopaedic practice: a review. J R Soc Med 78:478-484

Connolly LP, Connolly SA (2003) Skeletal scintigraphy in the multimodality assessment of young children with acute skeletal symptoms. Clin Nucl Med 28:746-754

Crim JR, Seeger LL (1994) Imaging evaluation of osteomyelitis. Crit Rev Diagn Imaging 35:201-256

Cucurull E, Espinoza LR (1998) Gonococcal arthritis. Rheum Dis Clin North Am 24:305-322

Curtiss PH Jr (1973) Some uncommon forms of osteomyelitis. Clin Orthop 96:84-87

Dalinka MK et al (1975) The radiology of osseous and articular infection. CRC Crit Rev Clin Radiol Nucl Med 7:1-64

Dangman BC et al (1992) Osteomyelitis in children: gadolinium-enhanced MR imaging. Radiology 182:743-747

Del Beccaro MA et al (1992) Septic arthritis versus transient synovitis of the hip: the value of screening laboratory tests. Ann Emerg Med 21:1418-1422

Denman AM, Mitchell B, Ansell BM (1983) Joint complaints and food allergic disorders. Ann Allergy 51:260-263

Donatto KC (1998) Orthopedic management of septic arthritis. Rheum Dis Clin North Am 24:275-286

Dormans JP, Drummond DS (1994) Pediatric hematogenous osteomyelitis: new trends in presentation, diagnosis, and treatment. J Am Acad Orthop Surg 2:333-341

Dzioba RB, Barrington TW (1977) Transient monoarticular

synovitis of the hip joint in adults. Clin Orthop 126:190-192

Ebong WW (1987) Septic arthritis in patients with sickle-cell disease. Br J Rheumatol 26:99-102

Egund N et al (1987) Conventional radiography in transient synovitis of the hip in children. Acta Radiol 28:193-197

Eich GF et al (1999) The painful hip: evaluation of criteria for clinical decision-making. Eur J Pediatr 158:923-928

Erdman WA et al (1991) Osteomyelitis: characteristics and pitfalls of diagnosis with MR imaging. Radiology 180:533-539

Erken EH, Katz K (1990) Irritable hip and Perthes' disease. J Pediatr Orthop 10:322-326

Fairbairn KJ et al (1995) Gas bubbles in the hip joint on CT: an indication of recent dislocation. AJR Am J Roentgenol 164:931-934

Fink AM et al (1995) The irritable hip: immediate ultrasound guided aspiration and prevention of hospital admission. Arch Dis Child 72:110-113; discussion 113-114

Fink CW, Nelson JD (1986) Septic arthritis and osteomyelitis in children. Clin Rheum Dis 12:423-435

Fischer SU, Beattie TF (1999) The limping child: epidemiology, assessment and outcome. J Bone Joint Surg Br 81:1029-1034

Freedman KB, Hahn GV, Fitzgerald RH Jr (1999) Unusual case of septic arthritis of the hip: spread from adjacent adductor pyomyositis. J Arthroplasty 14:886-891

Galperine T et al (2004) Cold bone defect on granulocytes labelled with technetium-99m-HMPAO scintigraphy: significance and usefulness for diagnosis and follow-up of osteoarticular infections. Scand J Infect Dis 36:209-212

Gash A, Walker CR, Carty H (1994) Case report: complete photopenia of the femoral head on radionuclide bone scanning in septic arthritis of the hip. Br J Radiol 67:816-818

Gershuni DH et al (1983) The questionable significance of hip joint tamponade in producing osteonecrosis in Legg-Calve-Perthes syndrome. J Pediatr Orthop 3:280-286

Gold RH, Hawkins RA, Katz RD (1991) Bacterial osteomyelitis: findings on plain radiography, CT, MR, and scintigraphy. AJR Am J Roentgenol 157:365-370

Greenspan A, Tehranzadeh J (2001) Imaging of infectious arthritis. Radiol Clin North Am 39:267-276

Grey AC et al (1998) The 'penumbra sign' on T1-weighted MR imaging in subacute osteomyelitis: frequency, cause and significance. Clin Radiol 53:587-592

Handmaker H (1980) Acute hematogenous osteomyelitis: has the bone scan betrayed us? Radiology 135:787-789

Herndon WA et al (1986) Management of septic arthritis in children. J Pediatr Orthop 6:576-578

Hill SA, MacLarnon JC, Nag D (1990) Ultrasound-guided aspiration for transient synovitis of the hip. J Bone Joint Surg Br 72:852-853

Howard CB et al (1993) Ultrasound in diagnosis and management of acute haematogenous osteomyelitis in children. J Bone Joint Surg Br 75:79-82

Howie DW et al (1983) The technetium phosphate bone scan in the diagnosis of osteomyelitis in childhood. J Bone Joint Surg Am 65:431-437

Huang AB et al (1998) Osteomyelitis of the pelvis/hips in paralyzed patients: accuracy and clinical utility of MRI. J Comput Assist Tomogr 22:437-443

Israel O et al (1987) Osteomyelitis and soft-tissue infection: differential diagnosis with 24 hour/4 hour ratio of Tc-99m MDP uptake. Radiology 163:725-726

Jaramillo D et al (1995) Osteomyelitis and septic arthritis in children: appropriate use of imaging to guide treatment. AJR Am J Roentgenol 165:399-403

Jones MW et al (1990) Condensing osteitis of the clavicle: does it exist? J Bone Joint Surg Br 72:464-467

Jou IM et al (2000) Synchronous pyomyositis and septic hip arthritis. Clin Rheumatol 19:385-388

Jung ST et al (2003) Significance of laboratory and radiologic findings for differentiating between septic arthritis and transient synovitis of the hip. J Pediatr Orthop 23:368-372

Kallio P, Ryoppy S (1985) Hyperpressure in juvenile hip disease. Acta Orthop Scand 56:211-214

Kallio P, Ryoppy S, Kunnamo I (1986) Transient synovitis and Perthes' disease. Is there an aetiological connection? J Bone Joint Surg Br 68:808-811

Kallio PE (1988) Coxa magna following transient synovitis of the hip. Clin Orthop 228:49-56

Karchevsky M et al (2004) MRI findings of septic arthritis and associated osteomyelitis in adults. AJR Am J Roentgenol 182:119-122

Kemp HB (1981) Perthes' disease: the influence of intracapsular tamponade on the circulation in the hip joint of the dog. Clin Orthop 156:105-114

Kemp HS, Boldero JL (1966) Radiological changes in Perthes' disease. Br J Radiol 39:744-760

Kocher MS, Zurakowski D, Kasser JR (1999) Differentiating between septic arthritis and transient synovitis of the hip in children: an evidence-based clinical prediction algorithm. J Bone Joint Surg Am 81:1662-1670

Landin LA, Danielsson LG, Wattsgard C (1987) Transient synovitis of the hip. Its incidence, epidemiology and relation to Perthes' disease. J Bone Joint Surg Br 69:238-242

Laroche M et al (2000) Do adults develop transient synovitis of the hip? Three case reports. Joint Bone Spine 67:350-352

Lee SK et al (1999) Septic arthritis versus transient synovitis at MR imaging: preliminary assessment with signal intensity alterations in bone marrow. Radiology 211:459-465

Leibowitz E et al (1985) Interferon system in acute transient synovitis. Arch Dis Child 60:959-962

Lewin JS et al (1986) Acute osteomyelitis in children: combined Tc-99m and Ga-67 imaging. Radiology 158:795-804

Liptak GS et al (1997) Decline of pediatric admissions with Haemophilus influenzae type b in New York State, 1982 through 1993: relation to immunizations. J Pediatr 130:923-930

Lohmander LS, Wingstrand H, Heinegard D (1988) Transient synovitis of the hip in the child: increased levels of proteoglycan fragments in joint fluid. J Orthop Res 6:420-424

Lord P, Carty HM (1993) Case report: unexplained symptomatic metaphyseal sclerosis in children: three cases. Br J Radiol 66:737-740

Love C, Palestro CJ (2004) Radionuclide imaging of infection. J Nucl Med Technol 32:47-57; quiz 58-59

Luhmann SJ et al (2004) Differentiation between septic arthritis and transient synovitis of the hip in children with clinical prediction algorithms. J Bone Joint Surg Am 86:956-962

Marchal GJ et al (1987) Transient synovitis of the hip in children: role of US. Radiology 162:825-828

Mathie AG, Benson MK, Wilson DJ (1991) Lessons in the investigation of irritable hip: failure of ultrasound to detect haemarthrosis. J Bone Joint Surg Br 73:518-519

Mazur JM et al (1995) Usefulness of magnetic resonance imaging for the diagnosis of acute musculoskeletal infections in children. J Pediatr Orthop 15:144-147

Mitchell M et al (1988) Septic arthritis. Radiol Clin North Am 26:1295-1313

Morrison WB et al (1993) Diagnosis of osteomyelitis: utility of fat-suppressed contrast-enhanced MR imaging. Radiology 189:251-257

Mukamel M et al (1985) Legg-Calve-Perthes disease following transient synovitis. How often? Clin Pediatr (Phila) 24:629-631

Nelson JD (1991) Skeletal infections in children. Adv Pediatr Infect Dis 6:59-78

Ogden JA, Lister G (1975) The pathology of neonatal osteomyelitis. Pediatrics 55:474-478

Pretorius ES, Fishman EK (1999) Volume-rendered three-dimensional spiral CT: musculoskeletal applications. Radiographics 19:1143-1160

Ram PC et al (1981) CT detection of intraosseous gas: a new sign of osteomyelitis. AJR Am J Roentgenol 137:721-723

Ranner G et al (1989) Magnetic resonance imaging in children with acute hip pain. Pediatr Radiol 20:67-71

Resnik CS, Ammann AM, Walsh JW (1987) Chronic septic arthritis of the adult hip: computed tomographic features. Skeletal Radiol 16:513-516

Rosenberg ZS et al (1992) Rapid destructive osteoarthritis: clinical, radiographic, and pathologic features. Radiology 182:213-216

Sainsbury CP, Newcombe RG, Essex-Cater A (1986) Irritable hips: relationship with trauma. Lancet 1:220

Santiago Restrepo C, Gimenez CR, McCarthy K (2003) Imaging of osteomyelitis and musculoskeletal soft tissue infections: current concepts. Rheum Dis Clin North Am 29:89-109

Schauwecker DS et al (1984) Evaluation of complicating osteomyelitis with Tc-99m MDP, In-111 granulocytes, and Ga-67 citrate. J Nucl Med 25:849-853

Sharwood PF (1981) The irritable hip syndrome in children. A long-term follow-up. Acta Orthop Scand 52:633-638

Shetty AK, Gedalia A (1998) Septic arthritis in children. Rheum Dis Clin North Am 24:287-304

Simonart T (2004) Group a beta-haemolytic streptococcal necrotising fasciitis: early diagnosis and clinical features. Dermatology 208:5-9

Spiegel DA et al (1999) Pyomyositis in children and adolescents: report of 12 cases and review of the literature. J Pediatr Orthop 19:143-150

Strouse PJ, DiPietro MA, Adler RS (1998) Pediatric hip effusions: evaluation with power Doppler sonography. Radiology 206:731-735

Struk DW et al (2001) Imaging of soft tissue infections. Radiol Clin North Am 39:277-303

Taylor GR, Clarke NM (1994) Management of irritable hip: a review of hospital admission policy. Arch Dis Child 71:59-63

Tehranzadeh J, Wang F, Mesgarzadeh M (1992) Magnetic resonance imaging of osteomyelitis. Crit Rev Diagn Imaging 33:495-534

Toby EB, Koman LA, Bechtold RE (1985) Magnetic resonance imaging of pediatric hip disease. J Pediatr Orthop 5:665-671

Tolat V et al (1993) Evidence for a viral aetiology of transient synovitis of the hip. J Bone Joint Surg Br 75:973-974

Trusen A et al (2003) Ultrasound and MRI features of pyomyositis in children. Eur Radiol 13:1050-1055

Unger E et al (1988) Diagnosis of osteomyelitis by MR imaging. AJR Am J Roentgenol 150:605-610

Uren RF, Howman-Giles R (1991) The 'cold hip' sign on bone scan. A retrospective review. Clin Nucl Med 16:553-556

Vegter J (1987) The influence of joint posture on intra-articular pressure. A study of transient synovitis and Perthes' disease. J Bone Joint Surg Br 69:71-74

Vidigal Junior EC, Vidigal EC, Fernandes JL (1997) Avascular necrosis as a complication of septic arthritis of the hip in children. Int Orthop 21:389-392

Vidigal EC, da Silva OL (1981) Observation hip. Acta Orthop Scand 52:191-195

Volberg FM et al (1984) Unreliability of radiographic diagnosis of septic hip in children. Pediatrics 74:118-120

Wald ER (1985) Risk factors for osteomyelitis. Am J Med 78:206-212

Walshaw CF, Deans H (1996) CT findings in necrotising fasciitis—a report of four cases. Clin Radiol 51:429-432

Welkon CJ et al (1986) Pyogenic arthritis in infants and children: a review of 95 cases. Pediatr Infect Dis 5:669-676

Wellman HN, Schauwecker DS, Capello WN (1988) Evaluation of metallic osseous implants with nuclear medicine. Semin Nucl Med 18:126-136

Willis RB, Rozencwaig R (1996) Pediatric osteomyelitis masquerading as skeletal neoplasia. Orthop Clin North Am 27:625-634

Wilson DJ, Green DJ, MacLarnon JC (1984) Arthrosonography of the painful hip. Clin Radiol 35:17-19

Wilson DJ (2004) Soft tissue and joint infection. Eur Radiol 14:E64-71

Wingstrand H et al (1985) Intracapsular pressure in transient synovitis of the hip. Acta Orthop Scand 56:204-210

Wingstrand H (1986) Transient synovitis of the hip in the child. Acta Orthop Scand [Suppl] 219:1-61

Wong-Chung J, Bagali M, Kaneker S (2004) Physical signs in pyomyositis presenting as a painful hip in children: a case report and review of the literature. J Pediatr Orthop B 13:211-213

Wright NB, Abbott GT, Carty HM (1995) Ultrasound in children with osteomyelitis. Clin Radiol 50:623-627

Zawin JK et al (1993) Joint effusion in children with an irritable hip: US diagnosis and aspiration. Radiology 187:459-463

11 Perthes' Disease

NEVILLE B. WRIGHT

CONTENTS

11.1
Historical Background

It is a rather surprising historical fact that the condition now often simply called Perthes' disease was independently described in the same year 1910, by three people: Arthur Thornton Legg (1874–1939), an American surgeon from Boston, Jacques Calve (1875–1954), a French orthopaedic surgeon from Berck, and Georg Clemens Perthes (1869–1927), a German surgeon from Tübingen. Calve described some of the early clinical and radiological features, and Legg is best known for publications on coxa plana. Perthes' disease is therefore more correctly

N. B. WRIGHT, MB, ChB, DMRD, FRCR
Department of Paediatric Radiology, Royal Manchester Children's Hospital, Central Manchester & Manchester Children's University Hospitals NHS Trust, Hospital Road, Pendlebury, M27 4HA, UK

termed Legg-Calve-Perthes syndrome and occurs as a consequence of idiopathic avascular necrosis of the proximal femoral epiphysis.

11.2
Clinical Features

11.2.1
Epidemiology

Perthes' disease mainly affects Caucasian children between 3–12 years of age, primarily 4–8 years, with boys affected about four times more frequently than girls (GUILLE et al. 1998). Bilateral involvement is present in up to 20% of children, but is usually asymmetrical (Fig. 11.1). There is a familial incidence of about 10%. The condition tends to affect children of lower social classes, and there is a strong association with unemployment and low income. There is also a link to low birth-weight and other deprivation measures (MARGETTS et al. 2001). The incidence in the UK is about 7 per 100,000, but in some areas has risen to as high as 25 per 100,000 (HALL et al. 1983).

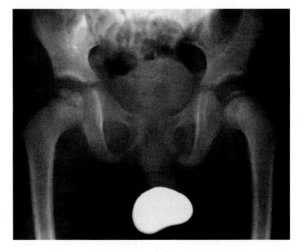

Fig. 11.1. Frontal radiograph of the pelvis showing typical bilateral asymmetrical changes of Perthes' disease

11.2.2
Symptoms and Signs

The clinical features will vary depending on the age of the child, stage of disease and extent of involvement of the femoral head, but usually the child presents with an intermittent limp, which may be painful and made worse with activity. The pain is generally in the hip, groin or inner thigh, but may be referred to the knee via the femoral, sciatic or obturator nerves.

Clinical examination will show an antalgic gait, with reduced and painful hip movement, especially internal rotation. There may be limited abduction (hinge abduction), made worse when the hip is flexed. Passive flexion of the hip may also result in external rotation, a feature known as Catterall's sign (CATTERALL 1971; SCHLESINGER and CRIDER 1988).

Some children will also show signs of delayed skeletal maturation and growth, with small feet being a particular feature (HALL et al. 1988).

11.3
Pathophysiology

11.3.1
Physiology of the Developing Femoral Head

In attempting to understand the pathophysiology of Perthes' disease, it is important to have an understanding of the normal development of the blood supply to the femoral head, since there is certainly evidence to suggest that vascular events have an important role in it's onset.

Initially, in the fetus, the femoral head is supplied by three groups of vessels; metaphyseal vessels, lateral epiphyseal vessels in the retinaculum along the femoral neck and a small supply from the ligamentum teres. With increasing age, the metaphyseal blood supply diminishes and by about the age of 4 is negligible. Conversely the supply via the ligamentum teres increases and becomes significant by about 7 years. For the period between 4–7 years, the ages at which Perthes' disease is commonest, the blood supply may depend entirely on the lateral epiphyseal vessels. This reliance on a single group of vessels makes the femoral head particularly susceptible to vascular events at this time (SALTER 1984).

11.3.2
Aetiology

A number of studies have shown links between abnormal vascular supply to the femoral head and the onset of Perthes' disease. From an arterial perspective, a transient avascular episode has been produced in an immature porcine model resulting in Perthes' like changes, and although angiography is no longer considered a routine imaging modality for the investigation of Perthes' disease, it has shown obstruction of the superior capsular arteries and decreased flow in the medial circumflex femoral and associated arteries in Perthes' affected hips (DE CAMARGO et al. 1984; THERON 1980). Other studies have shown the importance of venous drainage in the development of Perthes' disease. A poorly developed venous drainage can result in increased metaphyseal pressure and is a poor prognostic sign (HEIKINEN et al. 1980). Coagulation abnormalities have also been implicated in the development of Perthes' disease, although this area is still rather contentious. Some authors have suggested familial thrombophilic-hypofibrinolytic disorders have a role (ELDRIDGE et al. 2001) with one study finding 75% of children with abnormalities (GLUECK et al. 1996). Conversely other studies have not found this relationship, although have identified slightly prolonged activated partial thromboplastin time (KEALEY et al. 2000). Reduced levels of manganese in the blood have also been noted in some children with Perthes' disease, although why this is so is unclear (HALL et al. 1989; PERRY et al. 2000).

Hip effusions have long been implicated in the development of Perthes' disease with experimental evidence suggesting they decrease vascular supply (KEMP et al. 1971) and thereby produce ischaemia. In the susceptible hip, this may be sufficient to precipitate avascular necrosis, but it is believed that repeated events are necessary rather than a single episode. With Doppler ultrasound, the resistive index of the anterior ascending cervical arteries of the hip in the presence of an effusion has been shown to be raised, and correlated with the size of the effusion (ROBBEN et al. 2000), although the direct relationship with Perthes' disease was unproven.

11.3.3
Pathological Stages and Natural History

In histopathological terms, Perthes' disease goes through four stages which take between 2 to 4 years to complete:

Stage 1: Ischaemia/necrosis

During the initial stage of ischaemia and necrosis, all or part of the bony femoral head is affected, and the head dies. Although there is no further growth of the affected bony femoral head for the next 6–12 months, the cartilaginous component of the head remains supplied by nutrients via diffusion and continues to grow.

Stage 2: Fragmentation/resorption

During the second stage, which lasts between 12 and 17 months, fractures may appear in the dead bone, especially in the subchondral region. New bone is laid down, the head becomes hyperaemic and revascularised and bone resorption occurs producing some cystic elements.

Stage 3: Reossification/resolution

The bony femoral head begins to reossify, generally at the margins of the epiphysis, so-called paraphyseal ossification, but occasionally this process crosses the physis resulting in a bony bridge and growth arrest. This process combined with remodelling may take between 6 and 24 months.

Stage 4: Remodelling

If revascularisation and repair are prompt, the femoral head may retain its normal shape. However, stresses on weakened areas may lead to further flattening and fragmentation, and if the growth plate is affected this will affect subsequent development, with distortion or arrest. Hypertrophy of the cartilaginous head may also occur, and any alteration in the normal bony architecture may result in early degenerative change in the long term.

11.3.4
Classification

A number of classification systems have been used in Perthes' disease, and these have largely relied on radiographic features. Furthermore new systems continue to be developed and refined (JOSEPH et al. 2003), but the fact that there are a number of systems in use highlights that none is perfect, and that there is considerable inter- and intra-observer variability. A number of studies have looked specifically at this issue, giving conflicting results (AGUS et al. 2004; GIGANTE et al. 2002; LAPPIN et al. 2002; PODESZWA et al. 2000; WIIG et al. 2002). What seems important is that the user of any of the systems is aware of its

limitations and is not too reliant upon any one. In general, the bony femoral head must have begun to fragment and collapse before classification can be performed. Classification systems in common usage are noted below.

11.3.4.1
Catterall Classification

This is the more traditional method of classification devised in 1972, but is subject to a large degree of inter- and intra-observer error. There are four groups described. In group 1, the epiphysis retains it's height, the anteromedial portion of the head is involved, but the metaphysis and epiphyseal plate are spared. In group 2, up to 50% of the head is involved with sclerosis and fragmentation, there may be a central area of collapse, but the uninvolved areas act as buttresses and are able to maintain the femoral head height. There may be localised metaphyseal reaction. In group 3, most of the head is involved and there is insufficient normal bone to support the head, so it collapses. There is more diffuse metaphyseal resorption. In group 4, the worst group, the entire head is involved and collapse occurs early with sclerosis and extensive metaphyseal change. The epiphyseal plate is frequently involved.

11.3.4.2
Herring Classification (HERRING et al. 1992)

This system compares the height of the lateral portion of the epiphysis, the lateral pillar, to the height of the contralateral epiphysis, and is therefore useful in the fragmentation/collapse stage. The femoral head is divided into three parts on the AP radiograph. The appearances are divided into three groups. Group A shows no collapse of the lateral pillar, group B up to 50% loss and group C greater than 50% loss of height (HERRING et al. 1992).

11.3.4.3
Salter-Thompson Classification

A simpler system, dividing the appearances into two groups, stage A in which the lateral portion of the head is present and less than 50% of the head is involved, and stage B in which the lateral portion of the femoral head is absent and more than 50% of the head is affected.

11.3.4.4
Stulberg Classification

This system categorises the appearances after the disease process is complete and attempts to predict likely long-term outcomes with respect to the likelihood of development of osteoarthritis (see Sect. 11.7).

11.4
Imaging Findings

11.4.1
Radiography

The diagnosis of Perthes' disease is often suspected from radiography and the initial examination should include an AP view of the pelvis and frog-lateral view of the hips (Table 11.1). In the early stages when all or part of the femoral head becomes dead, the X-ray is normal. The earliest anatomical abnormality is usually a non-specific effusion of the hip joint, best demonstrated with ultrasound. Plain radiography is not a sensitive method of detecting early effusions, but widening of the medial aspect of the hip joint may be suggestive of fluid. As the bony femoral head stops growing, but the cartilaginous component remains viable, there may also be an increase in the apparent joint space and minor subluxation, Waldenström's sign.

As the disease progresses, a subchondral fracture may occur in the anterolateral aspect of the femoral capital epiphysis, and is an early radiographic feature best seen on the frog-lateral projection. This produces a crescentic radiolucency known as the crescent, Salter's or Caffey's sign (Fig. 11.2). It has been suggested that the extent of this subchondral fracture line is a better predictor of the final outcome of necrosis than MR signal change (Song et al. 1999). As new bone is laid down there is increased sclerosis resulting radiographically as increased bone density (Fig. 11.3). Simultaneously increased blood flow and revascularisation occurs which leads to bone resorption, rarefaction and cyst formation. A focal area of resorption in the superolateral aspect of the femoral head may occur leading to a 'v'-shaped defect known as Gage's sign, which is thought to be an indicator of poor prognosis.

With further progression there is more fragmentation and sclerosis of the epiphysis with collapse of the head (Fig. 11.4). Metaphyseal, ill-defined, focal

Table 11.1. Radiographic features

- Normal appearances
- Widening of the joint space and minor subluxation
- Subchondral crescentic lucency
- Sclerosis
- Fragmentation and focal resorption
- Loss of height
- Metaphyseal cyst formation
- Widening of the femoral neck and head (Coxa Magna)
- Lateral uncovering of the femoral head
- Sagging rope sign
- Acetabular remodelling

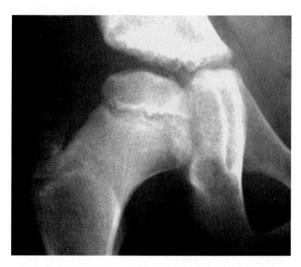

Fig. 11.2. Crescent sign. Frontal view of the right hip shows a subchondral fracture

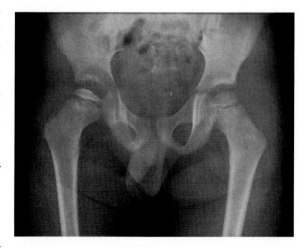

Fig. 11.3. Sclerosis of the epiphysis and widening of joint space in the early stages of Perthes' disease

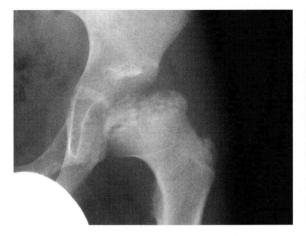

Fig. 11.4. Fragmentation of the femoral capital epiphysis

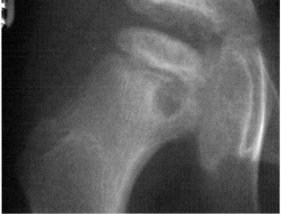

Fig. 11.5. Metaphyseal cyst formation within the femoral neck

radiolucencies may also develop (Fig. 11.5), especially anterolaterally adjacent to the physis and usually described as metaphyseal cysts. Occasionally these are predominant features and they may have an important role in the development of growth disturbance (KIM et al. 2004). As reossification occurs, physeal involvement may produce focal bony bars across the physis itself which result in growth arrest.

In the latter stages, as remodelling occurs, the subsequent shape of the femoral head is determined by the severity and extent of disease. With mild disease and rapid revascularisation, the features may completely resolve and the head retains it's normal shape, but the more severe examples will result in a permanent modelling deformity with a flattened, distorted femoral head and a wide short neck. Clearly focal physeal fusions will distort the head and altered stresses across the growth plate will contribute further to abnormal growth patterns. This, combined with continued growth of overlying epiphyseal cartilage, leads to coxa magna with the epiphysis gradually becoming flatter and wider (Fig. 11.6). Lateral displacement of the cartilaginous head results in uncovering and potential hinge movements of the joint, another important prognostic sign which ultimately may predict premature degenerative change. A common late finding on the anteroposterior radiograph in a mature hip with Perthes' disease is the 'sagging rope sign' (APLEY and WEINTROUB 1981). This a curvilinear sclerotic line running horizontally across the femoral neck which three-dimensional computed tomography studies have confirmed represents the margin of the femoral head (KIM et al. 1995), not a growth arrest line or the distal margin of metaphyseal rarefaction as previously suggested.

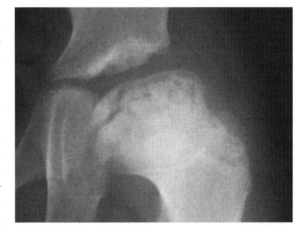

Fig. 11.6. Later stages with widening of the femoral neck, and fragmentation and collapse of the epiphysis

In addition to the changes occurring in the femoral head, secondary acetabular changes also occur including osteopaenia, irregularity of contour and a decrease in depth (MADAN et al. 2003).

11.4.2
Ultrasound

Ultrasound is the most readily available and practical method of demonstrating a hip effusion in Perthes' disease, although the finding is not specific and more commonly due to transient synovitis of the hip (Table 11.2). Typically an echo-free effusion is identified beneath the joint capsule anterior to the femoral neck. It is important that both hips are scanned in the same position to reduce measurement errors. Hip effusions persisting for

Table 11.2. Ultrasound features

- Effusion, especially if persistent
- Synovial thickening
- Cartilaginous thickening
- Atrophy of the ipsilateral quadriceps muscle
- Flattening, fragmentation, irregularity of the femoral head
- New bone formation
- Revascularisation with contrast enhanced power Doppler

more than a couple of weeks should raise the suspicion of Perthes' disease (EGGL et al. 1999). With more chronic presentations there may also be some thickening of the joint capsule itself and also the articular cartilage. Using three criteria combined, widening of the anterior recess, cartilage thickening and atrophy of the ipsilateral quadriceps muscle, considerably improves the specificity and positive predictive value for the diagnosis of Perthes' disease (99% and 95%, respectively; ROBBEN et al. 1998). Irregularity, flattening and fragmentation of the femoral capital epiphysis may also be visible, and in the later healing stages new bone formation can be detected earlier than on radiographs. More recently contrast-enhanced power Doppler ultrasound has been used to evaluate the revascularisation process of the femoral head with some success (DORIA et al. 2002). Whether this technique will be useful in the long term is yet to be confirmed.

11.4.3
Computed Tomography

Computed tomography (CT) assessment of children with Perthes' disease is generally restricted to pre-operative planning in those with severe disease and modelling deformity. Three-dimensional reconstructions enable the surgeon to map out the approach to femoral and innominate bone osteotomy in a similar fashion to that used for hip dysplasia (FRICK et al. 2000; KIM and WENGER 1997; LEE et al. 1991). Assessment of the precise degree of angulation of the femoral neck is useful for the surgeon and can be obtained readily. Additionally, it is recognised that a small number of children with Perthes' disease (between 2%–4%), may develop osteochondritis desiccans, and CT has been shown to be useful in demonstrating the extent, degree, stability and location of free fragments in these children (ROWE et al. 2003). The role of CT includes:

- Pre-operative assessment
- Three dimensional assessment of the modelling deformity
- Assessment of the degree of anteversion of the femoral neck
- Identification of osteochondral fragments

11.4.4
Magnetic Resonance Imaging

There are a number of important additional challenges to be addressed when performing magnetic resonance imaging (MRI) in children compared to adult practise. Firstly is the consideration of the need for sedation, anaesthesia and patient monitoring, which depends on local expertise and practise. Secondly is the understanding of the normal appearances of the developing skeleton, especially the changes in the normal cartilaginous head and bone marrow signal. In the young child, the metaphysis and diaphysis of the femur are composed of red marrow, showing as low signal on T1-weighted sequences. The cartilaginous head is of intermediate signal, but the ossification centre once it develops contains fatty marrow which appears as high signal on T1-weighted sequences, low signal on fat-suppressed and T2-weighted sequences. With time the red marrow signal in the proximal femur is gradually replaced with fatty marrow, but into adolescence, the highest marrow signal on T1-weighted is seen in the normal epiphysis and greater trochanter.

With respect to technique, generally both hips require imaging in Perthes' disease in view of the relative common occurrence of unrecognised bilateral disease. Coronal T1-weighted and transverse T2-weighted spin-echo or fast spin-echo images are generally required as a minimum with the FOV based on patient size. There is some evidence to suggest T1-weighted sequences are as good as T2-weighted in assessing the extent of necrosis (HOCHBERGS et al. 1997). Gradient-echo sequences are useful for fine detail, and T2-weighted fat-suppressed sequences help to define the articular cartilage. Contrast administration may help to define early ischaemic change and the synovium, but on a practical note, if contrast is to be administered, venous access is best sought prior to administering any sedation. MR arthrography is not routinely performed in children, a reflection of the need to minimise invasiveness in paediatric practise.

Both MRI and skeletal scintigraphy are more sensitive than radiographs in the early detection of avascular necrosis. MR imaging has been shown to demonstrate the extent of necrosis better than pinhole scintigraphy (UNO et al. 1995). Clearly MRI has the advantage of providing detail on bone and soft tissue anatomy, but it is important to appreciate the developing hip contains a much greater cartilaginous component and that the marrow signal changes with age (Fig. 11.7) (Bos et al. 1991; HENDERSON et al. 1990; JOHNSON et al. 1989; KANIKLIDES et al. 1995; MITCHELL et al. 1986; PINTO et al. 1989). False-negative scans can occur however, particularly in the very early stages of disease when fat signal may be preserved (ELSIG et al. 1989).

The signal changes seen on MRI reflect the underlying pathological processes and stage of the

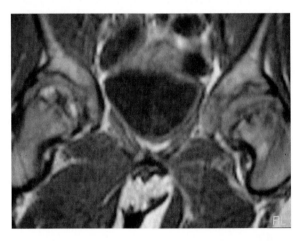

Fig. 11.7. Coronal T1-weighted sequence shows bilateral changes of Perthes' disease, with a central area of infarction in the right femoral capital epiphysis and more advanced changes on the left with generalised loss of height and widening of the femoral neck

disease. In the early stages of infarction, the bright signal of the normal yellow marrow in the femoral capital epiphysis is replaced by lower signal intensity on both T1-weighted and T2-weighted sequences (Fig. 11.8a). This signal change may be patchy or diffuse. Signal change may also involve the metaphyseal region. Once infarction is complete the epiphysis appears very low signal on both sequences. Fluid within the hip joint shows as typical high signal on T2-weighted sequences. Fat-suppressed (STIR) images useful to identify bone oedema (Fig. 11.8b) and contrast enhancement may identify viable bony fragments (MAHNKEN et al. 2002). The state of synovial thickening can be assessed on T2-weighted sequences and has been correlated positively with the severity of disease (HOCHBERGS et al. 1998).

Clearly with time, further structural changes may also develop. As healing progresses, the signal intensity will be restored to normal, although structural changes may persist depending on the severity and extent of the disease. Bone bridges crossing the physis are a strong predictor of abnormal growth and can be detected more readily with MR than radiography (JARAMILLO et al. 1995). Progress can be monitored with MR and the restoration of normal signal intensity may take up to 6 years (HOCHBERGS et al. 1997).

MR imaging is more accurate in defining the extent of involvement of the femoral capital epiphysis than radiography and classification of MR appearances has been attempted and correlates with radiographic extent of disease (HOCHBERGS et al. 1997). Using the proposed system, the femoral head is divided into four zones; two central, two peripheral with one medially and one laterally. The peripheral areas tend to be involved with severe disease and

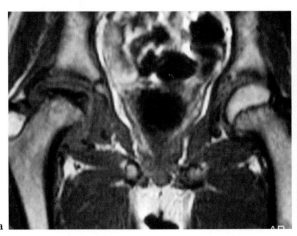
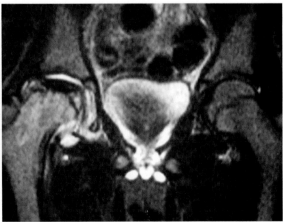

a   b

Fig. 11.8. a Coronal T1-weighted sequence shows complete low of signal from the right femoral capital epiphysis with some loss of height. The left femoral head is normal. **b** Coronal STIR sequence shows low of signal from the central portion of the femoral head, oedema in the femoral neck and medial aspect of the epiphysis and a joint effusion

are also the site of revascularisation. In Catterall group 1 classified disease, the medial zone is never involved, in groups 3 and 4, the entire epiphysis is affected. The closest correlation between the MR appearances, as evidenced by reduced signal intensity on T1-weighted and T2-weighted sequences, and the Catterall classification occurs when imaging is performed 3–8 months after the onset of symptoms (Bos et al. 1991; Lahdes-Vasama et al. 1997).

Dynamic gadolinium-enhanced subtraction MRI has also been shown to improve the detection of epiphyseal ischaemia and analysis of the revascularisation patterns (Lamer et al. 2002; Sebag et al. 1997). The mechanical effect of loss of congruity of the femoral head in the acetabulum has traditionally been assessed with contrast arthrography, often immediately prior to surgery. However dynamic multipositional imaging with an open MR system has been used successfully to assess the potential for hinging of the femoral head and associated congruity using fast spin-echo T2-weighted sequences (Jaramillo et al. 1999). The technique was comparable to contrast arthrography, although it was less successful in assessing deformity. MR has also been shown to be useful in the assessment of sagittal and coronal congruity, and has shown that even if coronal congruity is impaired, sagittal sphericity is preserved (Yazici et al. 2002). The following list summarises changes on MR imaging:

Femoral capital epiphysis
- Reduction in signal on T1- and T2-weighted images
- Central changes initially, peripheral with more severe disease
- Small bony femoral capital epiphysis
- Flattening
- Fragmentation
- Enhancement of revascularising areas
- Congruity of head with acetabulum

Metaphysis
- Bone oedema (STIR)
- Reduction in signal on T1- and T2-weighted images
- Cyst formation

Hip joint
- Synovial thickening
- High signal on T2-weighted sequences reflected joint fluid
- Pooling of fluid medially with incongruous joints

11.4.5
Bone Scintigraphy

Bone scintigraphy is sensitive to Perthes' disease, especially in the early infarction stage when the femoral head shows focal or complete photopenia (Fig. 11.9) (Kaniklides et al. 1996). With recovery and revascularisation, the head may be restored to an isopaenic and even hyperintense appearance. Some prognostic information can be obtained by assessing the pattern of revascularisation of the femoral head with scintigraphy (Conway 1993; Comte et al. 2003). Differentiating recanalisation from neovascularisation has prognostic significance. Recanalisation of existing vessels occurs within weeks to months, whereas neovascularisation may take years and reflects a more severe underlying process requiring the development of new vessels. As scintigraphy relies mainly on perfusion and bone metabolism, the processes of recanalisation and neovascularisation have different and characteristic appearances. Recanalisation is reflected as visualisation of the lateral column and is associated with a good prognosis. Conversely, neovascularisation shows basal filling and mushrooming and is associated with a poor prognosis. SPECT images have also been used to assess the extent of epiphyseal necrosis (Oshima et al. 1992).

11.4.6
Arthrography

The role for arthrography in Perthes' disease lies in three areas; the assessment of congruity of the

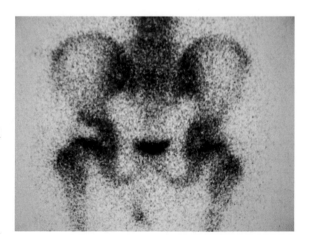

Fig. 11.9. Bone scintigraphy demonstrating complete photopenia in the right femoral capital epiphysis consistent with Perthes' disease. The left hip is normal

femoral head within the acetabulum, the dynamic evaluation of hip mechanics (hinging; Fig. 11.10) and delineation of deformity of the femoral head. Often arthrography is performed immediately prior to surgery, when a dynamic evaluation helps to determine the nature of the subsequent procedure (Fig. 11.11). MR has been shown to be as informative as arthrography and has largely replaced arthrography in static hip assessment, in view of its non-invasive nature, improved anatomical definition and use of non-ionising radiation (EGUND and WINGSTRAND 1991; HOCHBERGS et al. 1994; KANIKLIDES et al. 1995). However, for many orthopaedic surgeons, the dynamic nature of arthrography means that it remains a practical tool for immediate pre-operative assessment of the hip. This may change with the development of MR techniques that allow more dynamic evaluation (JARAMILLO et al. 1999; WEISHAUPT et al. 2000).

During a dynamic study, the presence of contrast pooling confirms loss of congruity and typically occurs medially within the joint, but it may be reduced or effaced with hip abduction. Arthrography has traditionally been used to determine of the degree of corrective abduction required during proximal femoral osteotomy. Hinging occurs when there is failure of movement of the lateral aspect of the femoral head under the acetabulum during internal rotation or abduction. It frequently occurs around an unossified portion of the femoral head, which is difficult to detect on radiographs, but is clearly shown with arthrography (REINKER 1996). Again this information can help the surgeon determine the degree of corrective angulation required with a proximal varus femoral osteotomy and the need for innominate surgery. Lateral subluxation of the hip due to thickening of the ligamentum teres, which has been suggested as an important cause for early subluxation, may also be detected on arthrography (KAMEGAYA et al. 1989).

The technique of arthrography is described elsewhere, but in general terms an anterior approach is usually appropriate, although an inferior approach can be used.

11.5
Differential Diagnosis

The differential diagnosis of avascular necrosis of the hip, one of which is Perthes' disease, is described elsewhere. It is worth noting however that subse-

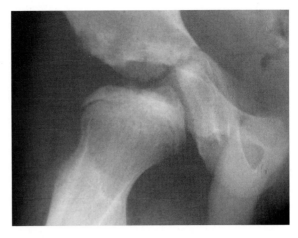

Fig. 11.10. Flattening of the femoral head predisposes the head to 'hinging' during movement

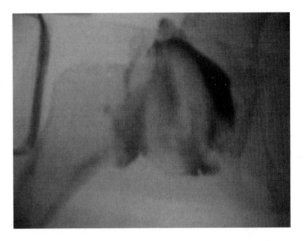

Fig. 11.11. Pre-operative arthrogram showing pooling of contrast medially and confirming loss of congruity

quent investigation should be considered slightly differently if bilateral disease is confirmed, focusing more on metabolic or systemic causes or skeletal dysplasias. Epiphyseal dysplasias particularly can cause confusion, but the key here is that the appearances are generally bilateral and symmetrical, which would be unusual in Perthes' disease (HESSE and KOHLER 2003). In the milder, localised form of multiple epiphyseal dysplasia, Meyer's dysplasia, which is a close mimic of Perthes' disease, there is delay in the appearance of the ossific nuclei of the femoral heads which may appear fragmented, but later development is normal.

The lists below should not be considered exhaustive.

Differential diagnosis of unilateral Perthes' disease:
- Transient synovitis
- Septic arthritis
- Spondyloepiphyseal dysplasia tarda
- Sickle cell disease
- Gaucher's disease
- Eosinophilic granuloma

Differential diagnosis of bilateral Perthes' disease:
- Hypothyroidism
- Multiple epiphyseal dysplasia
- Spondyloepiphyseal dysplasia tarda
- Sickle cell disease

11.6
Treatment

Treatment is based around the relief of symptoms and the maintenance of the normal shape of the femoral head within a normal acetabulum with the long term goal to prevent the development of premature osteoarthritis.

11.6.1
Acute

Acute treatment includes bed rest, skin traction and non-steroidal anti-inflammatory drugs until irritability subsides. This usually takes about 3 weeks.

11.6.2
Long Term

Once the acute symptoms have resolved, the treatment options include 'supervised neglect', where normal activities are resumed supplemented with regular reviews, or 'containment', where the aim is to prevent lateral displacement of the femoral head and maintain its position within the acetabulum. If symptoms or signs return in a 'supervised' patient, containment is commenced.

Containment can be by conservative or surgical means and is thought to improve the sphericity of the hip (GRZEGORZEWSKI et al. 2003). Conservative treatment involves the use of abduction splints, broomstick or brace, but there is some controversy as how useful this is and how long treatment should last (MARTINEZ et al. 1992). Surgical treatment includes the use of pelvic and femoral osteotomy (Fig. 11.12). The femoral osteotomy involves decreasing the varus angulation of the femoral neck with or without a derotation procedure to reduce anteversion and extension. The pelvic osteotomy increases coverage of the femoral head. Pre-operative planning may involve the use of dynamic arthrography and computed tomography, although the role of MR is developing as described above. Using the Catterall Classification, patients in group one require no treatment beyond symptomatic relief. In groups 2 and 3, no treatment is required under 7 years of age, unless there are 'head at risk' signs (see Sect. 11.7). If the child is over 7 years or has 'head at risk' signs, containment is recommended for 6–12 months or until there is recalcification of the femoral head. Children in group 4 require containment. The Herring classification suggests children under 6 years are observed. Between 6 and 8 years, children in group A and group B with a bone age less than 7 years can also be observed. Group B with an older bone age than 7 years and group C children require containment. Most children with changes when older than 8 years are in groups B and C and will require surgery (HERRING 1994).

11.7
Prognosis

Studies on the natural history of Perthes' disease based on the radiological appearance at maturity have suggested that both the sphericity of the femoral head and especially congruity are important predictors of outcome (Fig. 11.13). Three types of

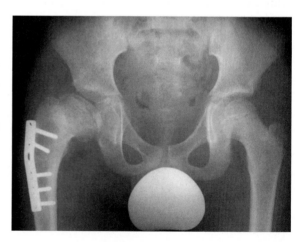

Fig. 11.12. Frontal view of the pelvis following proximal femoral osteotomy for established Perthes' disease. Note the increased varus angulation and the long-standing acetabular changes

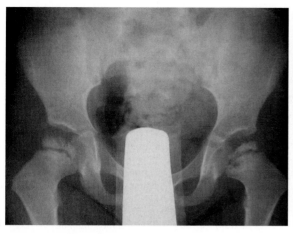
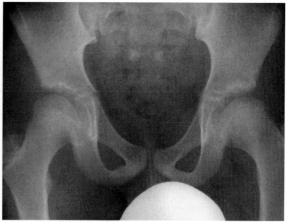

a   b

Fig. 11.13a,b. Bilateral changes of Perthes' disease (**a**) with appearances six years later (**b**). There has been subsequent restoration of femoral head ossification, but with associated modelling changes, more marked on the left

Table 11.3. Stulberg's classification of end result

Congruity group	Class	Appearance	End result[a]			
Spherical congruity	I	Entirely normal	Nil	II	Spherical, coxa magna, short neck	Nil
Aspherical congruity	III	Elliptical head	Mild to moderate OA	IV	Flat femoral head and flat acetabulum	Mild to moderate OA
Aspherical incongruity	V	Flat femoral head and round acetabulum	Severe OA < 50 years			

[a]End result is measured in terms of predisposition to the development of osteoarthritis (OA).

congruity have been described and grouped into a total of five subgroups in association with sphericity (Table 11.4, STULBERG et al. 1981). Those hips showing the greatest loss of sphericity and the most incongruity, not surprisingly, have the worst prognosis, with a tendency to develop severe osteoarthritis before the age of 50 years. The degree of sphericity can be assessed by using rings of increasing diameter (2 mm increments, MOSE et al. 1977). If the head conforms to a single ring in two planes, there is a good prognosis, but if the shape varies from a perfect circle by more than 2 mm in any plane the outcome may be poor. Clearly lesser degrees of asymmetry result in lesser degrees of severity.

A number of other features, termed 'Head at risk' signs (see Table 11.4), have also been identified, both clinical and radiological, which are linked to a poor prognosis.

It is also worth noting that bilateral disease generally undergoes a more severe course than unilateral disease (VAN DEN BOGAERT et al. 1999) and that girls with Perthes' disease have similar outcome to boys (GUILLE et al. 1998). Although young children

Table 11.4. Head at risk signs

Clinical features:

- Progressive loss of movement
- Adduction contractures
- Flexion in abduction
- Heavy child

Radiological features:

- Lateral subluxation of the femoral head (head partially uncovered)
- Entire femoral head involved
- Calcification lateral to the epiphysis
- Metaphyseal cysts
- Gage's sign
- Horizontally orientated physis

(under 5 years) developing Perthes' disease are generally considered to have a good prognosis, this is not always the case (FABRY et al. 2003). Older children (> 8 years) tend to need surgical containment (GRASEMANN et al. 1997).

References

Agus H, Kalenderer O, Eryanlmaz G, Ozcalabi IT (2004) Intraobserver and interobserver reliability of Catterall, Herring, Salter-Thompson and Stulberg classification systems in Perthes disease. J Pediatr Orthop B 13:166–169

Apley AG, Weintroub S (1981) The sagging rope sign in Perthes' disease and allied disorders. J Bone Joint Surg 63B:43–47

Bos CFA, Bloem JL, Bloem RM (1991) Sequential magnetic resonance imaging in Perthes' disease. J Bone Joint Surg Br 73:219–224

Catterall A (1971) The natural history of Perthes' disease. J Bone Joint Surg Br 53:37–53

Comte F, de Rosa V, Zekri H, Eberle MC, Dimeglio A, Rossi M, Mariano-Goulart D (2003) Confirmation of the early prognostic value of bone scanning and pinhole imaging of the hip in Legg-Calve-Perthes disease. J Nucl Med 44:1761–1766

Conway JJ (1993) A scintigraphic classification of Legg-Calve-Perthes disease. Semin Nucl Med 23:274–295

De Camargo FP, de Godoy RM Jr, Tovo R (1984) Angiography in Perthes' disease. Clin Orthop 191:216–220

Doria AS, Guarniero R, Cunha FG, Modena M, de Godoy RM Jr, Luzo C, Neto RB, Molnar LJ, Cerri GG (2002) Contrast-enhanced power Doppler sonography: assessment of revascularization flow in Legg-Calve-Perthes' disease. Ultrasound Med Biol 28:171–182

Eggl H, Drekonja T, Kaiser B, Dorn U (1999) Ultrasonography in the diagnosis of transient synovitis of the hip and Legg-Calve-Perthes disease. J Pediatr Orthop B 8:177–180

Egund N, Wingstrand H (1991) Legg-Calve-Perthes disease: imaging with MR. Radiology 179:89–92

Eldridge J, Dilley A, Austin H, EL-Jamil M, Wolstein L, Doris J, Hooper WC, Meehan PL, Evatt B (2001) The role of protein C, protein S, and resistance to activated protein C in Legg-Perthes disease. Pediatrics 107:1329–1334

Elsig JP, Exner GU, von Schulthess GK, Weitzel M (1989) False-negative magnetic resonance imaging in early stage of Legg-Calve-Perthes disease. J Pediatr Orthop 9:231–235

Fabry K, Fabry G, Moens P (2003) Legg-Calve-Perthes disease in patients under 5 years of age does not always result in a good outcome. Personal experience and meta-analysis of the literature. J Pediatr Orthop B 12:222–227

Frick SL, Kim SS, Wenger DR (2000) Pre- and postoperative three-dimensional computed tomography analysis of triple innominate osteotomy for hip dysplasia. J Pediatr Orthop 20:116–123

Glueck CJ, Crawford A, Roy D, Freiberg R, Glueck H, Stroop D (1996) Association of antithrombotic factor deficiencies and hypofibrinolysis with Legg-Perthes disease. J Bone Joint Surg Am 78:3–13

Gigante C, Frizziero P, Turra S (2002) Prognostic value of Catterall and Herring classification in Legg-Calve-Perthes disease: follow-up to skeletal maturity of 32 patients. J Pediatr Orthop 22:345–349

Grasemann H, Nicolai RD, Patsalis T, Hovel M (1997) The treatment of Legg-Calve-Perthes disease. To contain or not to contain. Arch Orthop Trauma Surg 116:50–54

Grzegorzewski A, Bowen JR, Guille JT, Glutting J (2003) Treatment of the collapsed femoral head by containment in Legg-Calve-Perthes disease. J Pediatr Orthop 23:15–19

Guille JT, Lipton GE, Szoke G, Bowen JR, Harcke HT, Glutting JJ (1998) Legg-Calve-Perthes disease in girls. A comparison of the results with those seen in boys. J Bone Joint Surg Am 80:1256–1263

Hall AJ, Barker DJ, Dangerfield PH, Taylor JF (1983) Perthes' disease of the hip in Liverpool. Br Med J (Clin Res Ed) 287:1757–1759

Hall AJ, Barker DJ, Dangerfield PH, Osmond C, Taylor JF (1988) Small feet and Perthes' disease. A survey in Liverpool . J Bone Joint Surg Br 70:611–613

Hall AJ, Margetts BM, Barker DJ, Walsh HP, Redfern TR, Taylor JF, Dangerfield P, Delves HT, Shuttler IL (1989) Low blood manganese levels in Liverpool children with Perthes' disease. Paediatr Perinat Epidemiol 3:131–135

Heikkinen E, Lanning P, Suramo I, Puranen J (1980) The venous drainage of the femoral neck as a prognostic sign in Perthes' disease. Acta Orthop Scand 51:501–503

Henderson RC, Renner JB, Sturdivant MC, Greene WB (1990) Evaluation of magnetic resonance imaging in Legg-Perthes disease: a prospective, blinded study. J Pediatr Orthop 10:289–297

Herring JA (1994) The treatment of Legg-Calve-Perthes disease. A critical review of the literature. J Bone Joint Surg Am 76:448–458

Herring JA, Neustadt JB, Williams JJ, Early JS, Browne RH (1992) The lateral pillar classification of Legg-Calve-Perthes disease. J Pediatr Orthop 12:143–150

Hesse B, Kohler G (2003) Does it always have to be Perthes' disease? What is epiphyseal dysplasia? Clin Orthop 1:219–227

Hochbergs P, Eckerwall G, Egund N, Jonsson K, Wingstrand H (1994) Femoral head shape in Legg-Calve-Perthes disease. Correlation between conventional radiography, arthrography and MR imaging. Acta Radiol 35:545–548

Hochbergs P, Eckerwall G, Wingstrand H, Egund N, Jonsson K (1997) Epiphyseal bone-marrow abnormalities and restitution in Legg-Calve-Perthes disease. Evaluation by MR imaging in 86 cases. Acta Radiol 38:855–682

Hochbergs P, Eckerwall G, Egund N, Jonsson K, Wingstrand H (1998) Synovitis in Legg-Calve-Perthes disease. Evaluation with MR imaging in 84 hips. Acta Radiol 39:532–537

Jaramillo D, Kasser JR, Villegas-Medina OL, Gaary E, Zurakowski D (1995) Cartilaginous abnormalities and growth disturbances in Legg-Calve-Perthes disease: evaluation with MR imaging. Radiology 197:767–773

Jaramillo D, Galen TA, Winalski CS, DiCanzio J, Zurakowski D, Mulkern RV, McDougall PA, Villegas-Medina OL, Jolesz FA, Kasser JR (1999) Legg-Calve-Perthes disease: MR imaging evaluation during manual positioning of the hip - comparison with conventional arthrography. Radiology 212:519–525

Johnson ND, Wood BP, Noh KS, Jackman KV, Westesson PL, Katzberg RW (1989) MR imaging anatomy of the infant hip. Am J Roentgenol 153:127–133

Joseph B, Varghese G, Mulpuri K, Narasimha Rao KL, Nair NS (2003) Natural evolution of Perthes disease: a study of 610 children under 12 years of age at disease onset. J Pediatr Orthop 23:590–600

Kamegaya M, Moriya H, Tsuchiya K, Akita T, Ogata S, Someya M (1989) Arthrography of early Perthes' disease. Swelling of the ligamentum teres as a cause of subluxation. J Bone Joint Surg Br. 71:413–7.

Kaniklides C, Lonnerholm T, Moberg A, Sahlstedt B (1995) Legg-Calve-Perthes disease. Comparison of conventional radiography, MR imaging, bone scintigraphy and arthrography. Acta Radiol 36:434–439

Kaniklides C, Sahlstedt B, Lonnerholm T, Moberg A (1996) Conventional radiography and bone scintigraphy in the prognostic evaluation of Legg-Calve-Perthes disease. Acta Radiol 37:561–566

Kealey WD, Mayne EE, McDonald W, Murray P, Cosgrove AP (2000) The role of coagulation abnormalities in the development of Perthes' disease. J Bone Joint Surg Br 82:744–746

Kemp HBS, Cholmeley JA, Baijens JK (1971) Recurrent Perthes' disease. Br J Radiol 44:675–681

Kim HT, Wenger DR (1997) "Functional retroversion" of the femoral head in Legg-Calve-Perthes disease and epiphyseal dysplasia: analysis of head-neck deformity and its effect on limb position using three-dimensional computed tomography. J Pediatr Orthop 17:240–246

Kim HT, Eisenhauer E, Wenger DR (1995) The "sagging rope sign" in avascular necrosis in children's hip diseases - confirmation by 3D CT studies. Iowa Orthop J 15:101–111

Kim HK, Skelton DN, Quigley EJ (2004) Pathogenesis of metaphyseal radiolucent changes following ischemic necrosis of the capital femoral epiphysis in immature pigs. A preliminary report. J Bone Joint Surg Am 86:129–135

Lahdes-Vasama T, Lamminen A, Merikanto J, Marttinen E (1997) The value of MRI in early Perthes' disease: an MRI study with a 2-year follow-up. Pediatr Radiol 27:517–522

Lamer S, Dorgeret S, Khairouni A, Mazda K, Brillet PY, Bacheville E, Bloch J, Pennecot GF, Hassan M, Sebag GH (2002) Femoral head vascularisation in Legg-Calve-Perthes disease: comparison of dynamic gadolinium-enhanced subtraction MRI with bone scintigraphy. Pediatr Radiol 32:580–585

Lappin K, Kealey D, Cosgrove A (2002) Herring classification: how useful is the initial radiograph? J Pediatr Orthop 22:479–482

Lee DY, Choi IH, Lee CK, Cho TJ (1991) Assessment of complex hip deformity using three-dimensional CT image. J Pediatr Orthop 11:13–19

Madan S, Fernandes J, Taylor JF (2003) Radiological remodelling of the acetabulum in Perthes' disease. Acta Orthop Belg 69:412–420

Mahnken AH, Staatz G, Ihme N, Gunther RW (2002) MR signal intensity characteristics in Legg-Calve-Perthes disease. Value of fat-suppressed (STIR) images and contrast-enhanced T1-weighted images. Acta Radiol 43:329–335

Margetts BM, Perry CA, Taylor JF, Dangerfield PH (2001) The incidence and distribution of Legg-Calve-Perthes' disease in Liverpool 1982-1995. Arch Dis Child 84:351–354

Martinez AG, Weinstein SL, Dietz FR (1992) The weight-bearing abduction brace for the treatment of Legg-Perthes disease. J Bone Joint Surg Am 74:12–21

Mitchell MD, Kundel HL, Steinberg ME, Kressel HY, Alavi A, Axel L (1986) Avascular necrosis of the hip: comparison of MR, CT, and scintigraphy. Am J Roentgenol 147:67–71

Mose K, Hjorth L, Ulfeldt M, Christensen ER, Jensen A (1977) Legg Calve Perthes disease. The late occurrence of coxarthrosis. Acta Orthop Scand [Suppl] 169:1–39

Oshima M, Yoshihasi Y, Ito K, Asai H, Fukatsu H, Sakuma S (1992) Initial stage of Legg-Calve-Perthes disease: comparison of three-phase bone scintigraphy and SPECT with MR imaging. Eur J Radiol 15:107–112

Perry CA, Taylor JF, Nunn A, Dangerfield PH, Delves H (2000) Perthes' disease and blood manganese levels. Arch Dis Child 82:428

Pinto MR, Peterson HA, Berquist TH (1989) Magnetic resonance imaging in early diagnosis of Legg-Calve-Perthes disease. J Pediatr Orthop 9:19–22

Podeszwa DA, Stanitski CL, Stanitski DF, Woo R, Mendelow MJ (2000) The effect of pediatric orthopaedic experience on interobserver and intraobserver reliability of the herring lateral pillar classification of Perthes disease. J Pediatr Orthop 20:562–565

Reinker KA (1996) Early diagnosis and treatment of hinge abduction in Legg-Perthes disease. J Pediatr Orthop 16:3–9

Robben SG, Meradji M, Diepstraten AF, Hop WC (1998) US of the painful hip in childhood: diagnostic value of cartilage thickening and muscle atrophy in the detection of Perthes disease. Radiology 208:35–42

Robben SG, Lequin MH, Diepstraten AF, Hop WC, Meradji M (2000) Doppler sonography of the anterior ascending cervical arteries of the hip: evaluation of healthy and painful hips in children. Am J Roentgenol 174:1629–1634

Rowe SM, Chung JY, Moon ES, Yoon TR, Jung ST, Lee KB (2003) Computed tomographic findings of osteochondritis dissecans following Legg-Calve-Perthes disease. J Pediatr Orthop 23:356–362

Salter RB (1984) The present status of surgical treatment for Legg-Calve-Perthes disease. J Bone Joint Surg Am 66A:961–966

Schlesinger I, Crider RJ (1988) Gage's sign – revisited! J Pediatr Orthop 8:201–202

Sebag G, Ducou Le Pointe H, Klein I, Maiza D, Mazda K, Bensahel H, Hassan M (1997) Dynamic gadolinium-enhanced subtraction MR imaging–a simple technique for the early diagnosis of Legg-Calve-Perthes disease: preliminary results. Pediatr Radiol 27:216–220

Song HR, Lee SH, Na JB, Cho SH, Jeong ST, Ahn BW, Koo KH (1999) Comparison of MRI with subchondral fracture in the evaluation of extent of epiphyseal necrosis in the early stage of Legg-Calve-Perthes disease. J Pediatr Orthop 19:70–75

Stulberg SD, Cooperman DR, Wallensten R (1981) The natural history of Legg-Calve-Perthes disease. J Bone Joint Surg Am. 63:1095–1108

Theron J (1980) Angiography in Legg-Calve-Perthes' disease. Radiology 135:81–92

Uno A, Hattori T, Noritake K, Suda H (1995) Legg-Calve-Perthes disease in the evolutionary period: comparison of magnetic resonance imaging with bone scintigraphy. J Pediatr Orthop 15:362–367

Van den Bogaert G, de Rosa E, Moens P, Fabry G, Dimeglio A (1999) Bilateral Legg-Calve-Perthes disease: different from unilateral disease? J Pediatr Orthop B 8:165–168

Weishaupt D, Exner GU, Hilfiker PR, Hodler J (2000) Dynamic MR imaging of the hip in Legg-Calve-Perthes disease: comparison with arthrography. Am J Roentgenol 174:1635–1637

Wiig O, Terjesen T, Svenningsen S (2002) Inter-observer reliability of radiographic classifications and measurements in the assessment of Perthes' disease. Acta Orthop Scand 73:523–530

Yazici M, Aydingoz U, Aksoy MC, Akgun RC (2002) Bipositional MR imaging vs arthrography for the evaluation of femoral head sphericity and containment in Legg-Calve-Perthes disease. Clin Imaging. 26:342–346

12 Slipped Upper Femoral Epiphysis

Bernhard J. Tins and Victor N. Cassar-Pullicino

CONTENTS

12.1
Introduction

Slipped upper femoral epiphysis (SUFE) is usually a disease of adolescent teenagers. Diagnostic and treatment options are constantly evolving, partly driven by advances in imaging and therapeutic techniques, partly by a better understanding of its pathology and partly by studies of long-term outcome of treatment methods. This chapter briefly reviews the underlying pathological changes and clinical presentation before describing in more detail the imaging diagnosis, treatment options, complications and their relevance for imaging follow up.

B. J. Tins, MD; V. N. Cassar-Pullicino, MD, FRCR
Department of Diagnostic Radiology, Robert Jones & Agnes Hunt Orthopaedic Hospital, Oswestry, Shropshire, SY10 7AG, UK

12.2
Epidemiology and Pathology

12.2.1
Epidemiology

The incidence of SUFE varies widely between races (Loder 1996a). Absolute numbers therefore need to be interpreted with knowledge of the racial composition of the examined patient population. For white children in the United States an annual incidence of 3.19 per 100000 is quoted based on articles from the early 1970s (Kelsey et al. 1970; Kelsey 1971). In comparison the relative incidence of SUFE is about 4.5 for Polynesian children and only 0.1 for Indo-Mediterranean children (Loder 1996a). In black children in the United States the relative incidence is roughly 2.2 times higher than in white children (Kelsey 1971; Loder 1996a). The relative sex distribution for children with SUFE varies between 90% boys in Indo-Mediterranean children and 50% boys for Native Australian/Pacific Island children. In the United States population as a whole the average sex distribution of children with SUFE is 66% boys and 34% girls (Brown 2004). The average age at onset of SUFE also varies with race and sex. Worldwide the average age at onset is 12 years for girls and 13.5 years for boys (Loder 1996a).

In Germany the incidence of SUFE is about 1:100000, with a boys to girls ratio of 3:1, the average age at diagnosis is 12.5 years for girls and 14.5 years for boys (Harland and Krappel 2002).

There is seasonal variation in the relative incidence of SUFE for children living beyond 40° latitude; the incidence is increased in summer (Loder 1996; Brown 2004) and this effect is more pronounced in white children (Brown 2004).

Increased weight (Loder 1996a) and body mass index (BMI) (Poussa et al. 2003) are risk factors for SUFE. This can potentially cause an increased incidence of SUFE with the growing obesity of children and teenagers in recent years.

Other potential causes for SUFE are manifold. Some authors see a connection between increased mechanical stress (weight and activity/power) and decreased mechanical strength of the cartilage growth plate at the end of puberty. Steroid hormones and STH are thought to be detrimental, but a direct correlation has not been proven. Lack of vitamin C and D, calcium and thyroid hormone are risk factors (Fig. 12.1) as well as increased parathormone levels and renal osteodystrophy (WEINER 1996; MILZ et al. 2002; SCHULTZ et al. 2002; OPPENHEIM et al. 2003). Deeper acetabular depth (LODER et al. 2003) and decreased anteversion of the femoral neck (WEINER 1996; EXNER et al. 2002) have also been identified as risk factors. The occurrence of contralateral SUFE is quoted as being between 20%–80% (ENGELHARDT 2002; HARLAND and KRAPPEL 2002) with a large study quoting 37% (LODER et al. 1993a). Contralateral slips can be clinically asymptomatic is in up to 71% of cases. The longer the time to fusion of the growth plate the larger the risk (SCHULTZ et al. 2002).

12.2.2
Pathology

The pathological changes of SUFE can be discussed as two entities; firstly the primary changes of the physis and adjacent tissues directly involved in or responsible for the development of SUFE and secondly secondary changes resulting from the slip.

Primary pathological changes of SUFE arise in the physis. The cartilage of the growth plate usually fails near the metaphysis since the cartilage is mechanically weakest here. Histologically fibrillar

disintegration can be seen; whether this is cause or effect of the slip is unclear (WEINER 1996; MILZ et al. 2002). Stabilising elements are the perpendicular alignment of the growth plate against the forces acting on it, the additional cupping of the proximal femoral epiphysis around the metaphysis and the formation of grooves in the physis. These grooves are particularly important to counteract rotational forces. The periosteal thickening, the zona orbicularis, around the femoral neck also increases mechanical stability (EXNER et al. 2002; MILZ et al. 2002). After operative internal fixation in patients with SUFE, the residual growth plate can revert to a more normal histological appearance and further growth can take place. This suggests that mechanical factors are probably responsible for the growth plate abnormalities (GUZZANTI et al. 2003).

Secondary pathological changes affect tissues adjacent to the physis. The blood supply to the femoral epiphysis is delivered largely through periosteal vessels. Tears to the periosteum compromise this supply. In slipped upper femoral epiphysis the periosteum does tear opposite to the direction towards which the slip occurs (Fig. 12.2). On the side of the slip the periosteum is usually preserved and initially fairly loose and buckled (Fig. 12.3). With time the sleeve contracts and the metaphysis begins to remodel and form a bony spur in response to the adjacent femoral head. The periosteal sleeve has to stretch over this spur. At about 2 weeks after the slip this process has caused sufficient shortening of the periosteal sleeve to result in a tear at the side of the slip should reduction of the slipped epiphysis occur. This can then result in further compromise of the vascular supply and possible avascular necrosis of

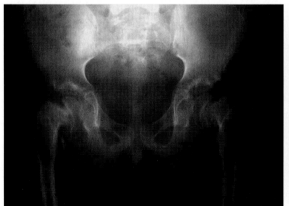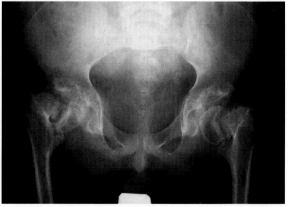

a   b

Fig. 12.1a,b. A boy with severe hypothyroidism. Diagnosed age 13 years. Immature skeleton. **a** Bilateral slipped femoral epiphyses with sclerotic and irregular metaphyses at age 13 years. **b** At 2 years later the slip has worsened, still immature skeleton despite thyroxine therapy. Gross remodelling of the metaphyses, gross femora vara

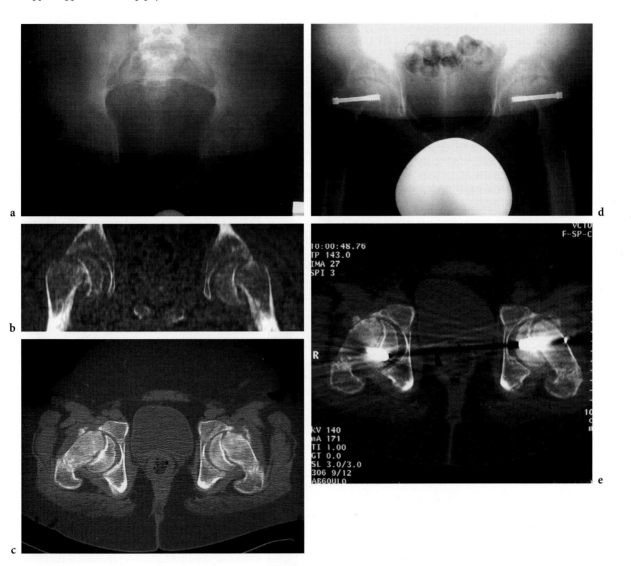

Fig. 12.2a–e. A boy aged 8 years and 7 months. **a** AP view of the hip joints demonstrates bilateral severe slip. Generalised osteopenia. The metaphyses impinge onto the acetabuli. **b** Coronally reconstructed CT confirms the findings. **c** Axial CT demonstrates bilateral severe slip and ossification of the torn periosteal sleeve laterally on both sides. **d** The slips were pinned but the deformity not corrected. **e** CT demonstrates dorsal position of the screw in the right femur, ideally the screw should be central within the femoral epiphysis

the femoral epiphysis (Boyer et al. 1981; Arnold et al. 2002a; Exner et al. 2002; Boero et al. 2003).

12.3
Clinical Presentation and Differential Diagnosis

Clinically patients often present with hip pain but the pain can also be referred to groin, thigh or knee (Harland and Krappel 2002). Referred pain and relatively mild symptoms are responsible for delay in diagnosis and a high index of clinical suspicion in patients with unclear knee, thigh or groin pain is necessary (Ankarath et al. 2002; Kocher et al. 2004). Some authors recommend radiographs of the hips in anterior-posterior (AP) and frog lateral projection for any adolescent with undiagnosed knee or hip pain lasting for 1 week (Ankarath et al. 2002). On examination the internal rotation is often diminished and on flexion of the hip external rotation occurs (Harland and Krappel 2002). The differential diagnosis comprises osteonecrosis, infectious or inflammatory arthritis, tumour and trauma (Lalaji et al. 2002).

Fig. 12.3a–k. A girl aged 11 years and 6 months. Left-sided severe slip, mainly posteriorly, therefore appearances on the AP view (**a**) are deceptive, the true severity is best appreciated on the lateral view (**b**). Coronal STIR (**c**), sagittal (**d**) and axial (**e**) T2-weighted MR images confirm the severe slip. The coronal STIR image shows the elevated peciosteum medially due to the slip (laterally the peciosteum tears). Single screw fixation in malalignment. At 14 months later (**f,g**) deformity of the femoral head due to impingement on the lateral acetabulum. Tc-99m isotope bone scan demonstrates increased activity in the diffusion (**h**) and the bone phase (**i**) indicating activity of the pathological process and raising the possibility on AVN. Normal right-sided hip joint. Further follow up radiograph (**j**) confirms AVN of the cranial part of the femoral head and lateral notch formation. Osteotomy was subsequently performed (**k**)

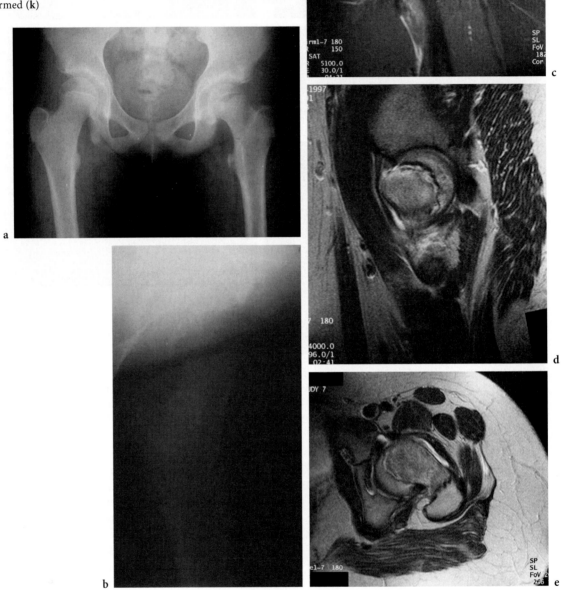

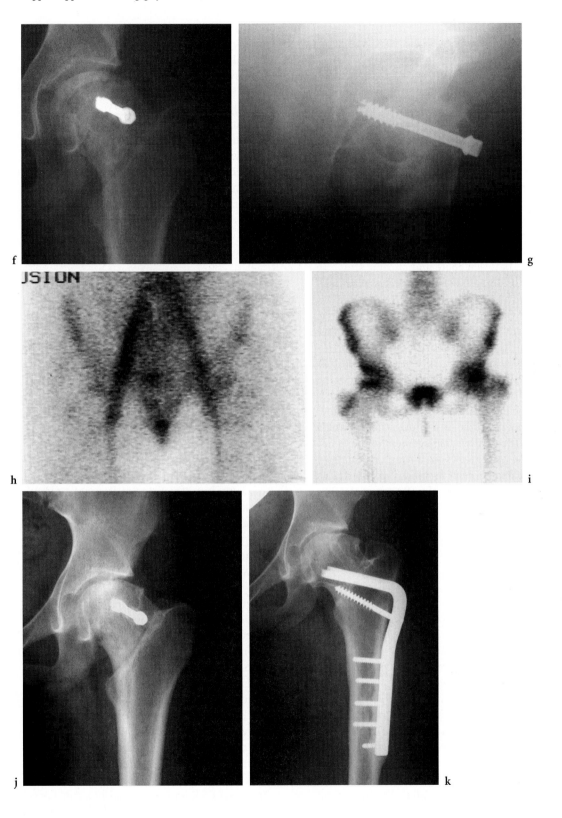

JSION

12.4
Clinical Classifications

Several classification systems exist for the assessment of SUFE. The most commonly used clinical classification differentiates acute, acute-on-chronic and chronic disease. This classification is important because the choice of therapy often depends on it. Acute disease is classed as onset of symptoms less than 3 weeks prior to presentation with acute pain, acute on chronic is defined as presentation with acute pain but onset of some pain more than 3 weeks prior to presentation, chronic disease is defined as symptom onset prior to 3 weeks and presentation without acute symptoms (LODER et al. 1993b). The differentiation between acute and chronic slips can also be based on imaging criteria; this is addressed in detail in Sect. 12.5.

Other classifications define the disease as stable, when the patient is able to weight bear with crutches and as unstable if he is not (LODER et al. 1993b).

The classification of the severity of the slip is based on the slip angle as determined by imaging methods. Slip angles of $< 30°$ are classed as mild, $30°–50°$ as moderate and $> 50°$ as severe (BOYER et al. 1981). If imaging does not allow accurate angle measurement the relative displacement of the femoral head on the neck allows for a rough estimation; $< 1/3$ displacement is seen as mild slip, $1/3–1/2$ as moderate and $> 1/2$ as severe slip (BOYER et al. 1981; KALLIO et al. 1993).

12.5
Imaging of SUFE

The diagnosis of slipped upper femoral epiphysis is made by imaging. Imaging signs of SUFE vary with the stage and severity of disease.

The earliest sign of acute disease may be widening and irregularity of the physeal plate with ill defined metaphysis and epiphysis adjacent to the growth plate and spotty or streaky radiopacities in the growth plate and deossification adjacent to it (Fig. 12.4) (KLEIN et al. 1951; LODER et al. 1993b; GEKELER 2002). Deossification is frequently seen affecting the whole hip joint area (KLEIN et al. 1951). In the most common posteromedial slip the normal lateral overhang of the femoral head over a tangent to the lateral neck of femur disappears with progression of the slip (Fig. 12.3). With further progression the femoral head visibly tilts against the acetabu-

lum and the femoral neck but stays within the acetabulum. Acute slips are often unstable (Fig. 12.5) (KLEIN et al. 1951; GEKELER 2002). Acutely a joint effusion may be seen and this is seen as a sign of instability (HARLAND and KRAPPEL 2002) or acuity of the slip (KALLIO et al. 1991, 1993). Cystic change of the metaphysis may be seen in acute as well as in chronic disease (GEKELER 2002). The main difference between the acute and the chronic stage is the absence of metaphyseal remodelling in the acute stage. Chronic epiphyseolysis usually demonstrates varus deformity of the femoral neck and formation of bone spurs on the medial aspect of the metaphysis. Sloping of the medial metaphysis is also often seen in chronic disease (Fig. 12.6) (GEKELER 2002; LEUNIG et al. 2002).

A systematic approach to radiographs in suspected SUFE is summarized in Tables 12.1 and 12.2.

12.5.1
Radiography

12.5.1.1
Positioning

The most important imaging modality is radiography. Usually AP and specialised lateral views of both hips are taken. Obtaining radiographs of both hips simultaneously allows for comparison between the sides and is also indicated because of the high incidence of bilateral disease. For accurate angle measurements exactly defined patient positioning is a must (ENGELHARDT and ROESLER 1987; GEKELER 2002).

In English speaking countries positioning is usually done according to Southwick's description (SOUTHWICK 1967) which is similar to an earlier description by KLEIN et al. (1951). The AP view is taken with the patients' pelvis flat on the table. The beam is centred exactly in the midline between the hips. The hips are neutral or as near to neutral as possible, i.e. the patellae point straight up. For the frog lateral view the hips are placed in maximal abduction and external rotation. The knees are flexed and the plantar surfaces of the feet face each other. The lateral parts of the feet rest on the table. In cases where frog lateral views are not possible, true lateral radiographs can be used (examined hip extended, opposite hip flexed) (SOUTHWICK 1967).

In German speaking countries positioning is usually done according to Imhäuser. Similar to South-

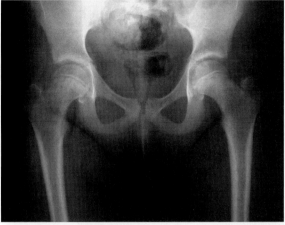
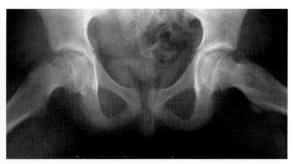

a

b

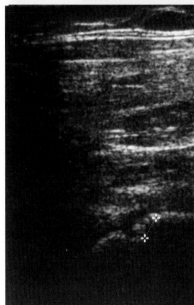
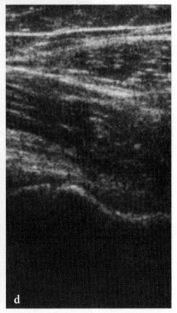

c

d

Fig. 12.4a–d. A female aged 9 years 10 months. Mild slip right hip. On the AP view (a) only irregularity of the growth plate seen. Tangent to the neck of femur still intersecting the femoral head. On the lateral view (b) mild posterior slip. Ultrasound of the right hip (c) demonstrates minor displacement of femoral epiphysis versus the metaphysis by 2.5 mm, ultrasound of the left hip is normal (d)

wick, Imhäuser suggests exact neutral position of the legs for the AP view, the patellae point forward. However, in cases with fixed external rotation in the hip joint he suggests to correct the external rotation by elevating the pelvis. In these cases the hip joints can not be imaged together. For the lateral view Imhäuser suggests to follow Lauenstein's description: the hip joint is flexed by 90° and abducted by 45°. This is easily achieved with a dedicated wedge. The calf has to be parallel to the long axis of the table to avoid rotation (GEKELER 2002).

There is an important caveat for performing lateral views. In high grade slips forced flexion and abduction of the hip joint can cause worsening of the slip. Standard projections should not be forced if painful for the patient (GEKELER 2002).

12.5.1.2
Radiographic Signs of SUFE

Early disease presents with ill defined meta- and epiphyses adjacent to the growth plate and irregular radiopacities in and around the widened growth plate (Fig. 12.4). At this stage there is not always an actual slip seen yet. With an epiphyseal slip an axis perpendicular to the base of the epiphysis is no longer parallel to the femoral neck (Fig. 12.7). Deviation of > 2° is seen as abnormal (FREYSCHMIDT et al. 2001). When the epiphysis begins to slide and tilt, radiographically the growth plate seems to narrow, this is partly a projectional phenomenon and partly true narrowing. In cases of the most common type of slip, the dorsomedial slip, a tangent to the lat-

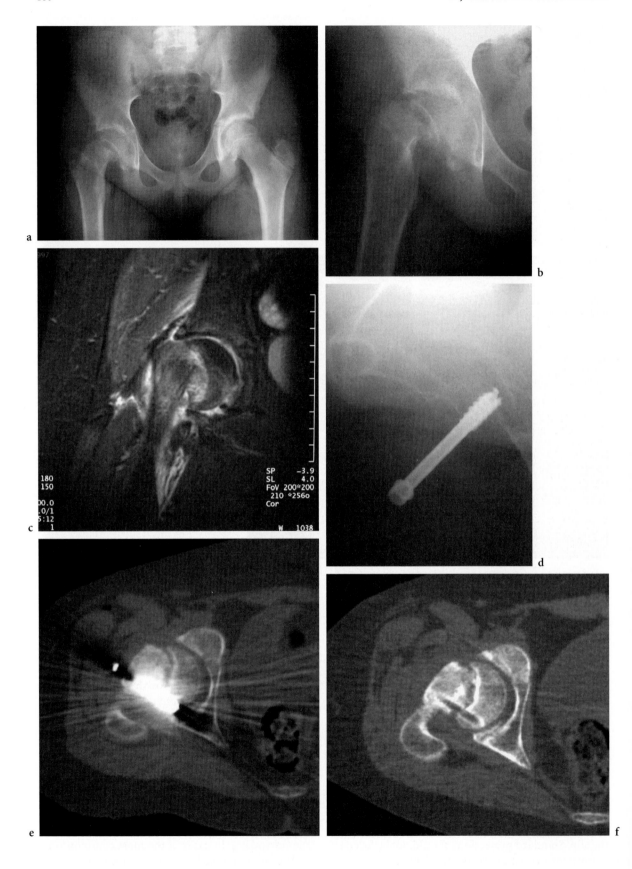

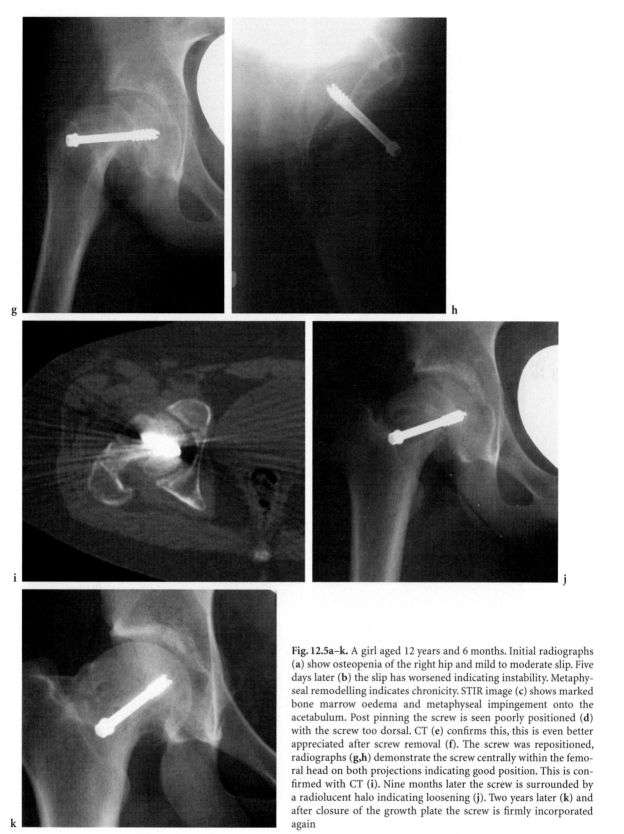

Fig. 12.5a–k. A girl aged 12 years and 6 months. Initial radiographs (**a**) show osteopenia of the right hip and mild to moderate slip. Five days later (**b**) the slip has worsened indicating instability. Metaphyseal remodelling indicates chronicity. STIR image (**c**) shows marked bone marrow oedema and metaphyseal impingement onto the acetabulum. Post pinning the screw is seen poorly positioned (**d**) with the screw too dorsal. CT (**e**) confirms this, this is even better appreciated after screw removal (**f**). The screw was repositioned, radiographs (**g,h**) demonstrate the screw centrally within the femoral head on both projections indicating good position. This is confirmed with CT (**i**). Nine months later the screw is surrounded by a radiolucent halo indicating loosening (**j**). Two years later (**k**) and after closure of the growth plate the screw is firmly incorporated again

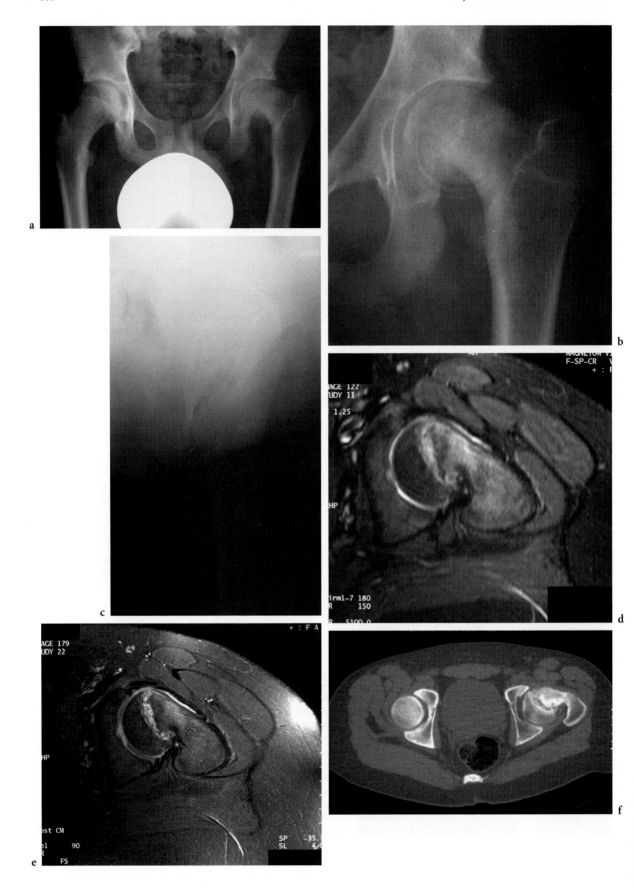

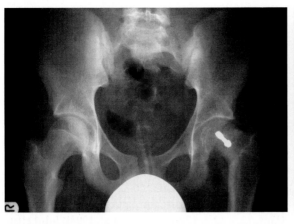
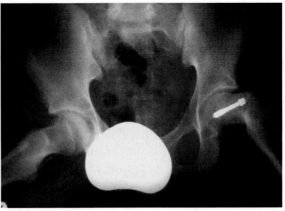

g   c̃   h

Fig. 12.6a–h. A boy aged 16 years and 6 months. AP view of both hips (**a**), coned AP (**b**) and lateral (**c**) view of the left hip show a severe chronic posterior slip with metaphyseal remodelling. Axial STIR (**d**) shows marked oedema in the neck of femur and in the growth plate. Gadolinium contrast enhanced T1-fat saturated (T1-FS) image (**e**) shows contrast uptake in the areas of bone marrow oedema. CT shows beginning ossification of the physis and a cyst in the metaphysis (**f**). AP (**g**) and frog lateral (**h**) views after internal fixation show the persistent marked malalignment of the femoral head with the neck of femur

Table 12.1. Radiographic signs of slipped upper femoral epiphysis

- Growth plate ill defined, possibly widened
- Base of epiphysis no longer perpendicular to the neck of femur (NOF) axis
- In typical dorsomedial slip lateral tangent to NOF no longer intersects with femoral head
- In chronic slip remodelling of metaphysis, possibly with varus (or rarely valgus) deformity of NOF
- Osteopenia

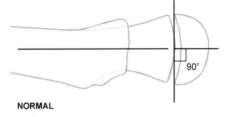

NORMAL

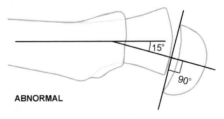

ABNORMAL

Table 12.2. Checklist for reporting of slipped upper femoral epiphysis

- AP and frog lateral views performed and of diagnostic quality?
- Slip present?
- Approximate degree of slip?
- Slip acute, acute on chronic, chronic?
- Secondary complications (chondrolysis, impingement acetabulum/metaphysis)?

Fig. 12.7. Alignment of the upper femoral epiphysis on the lateral view. Normally a line perpendicular to the base line of the epiphysis is parallel to the femoral neck axis. In SUFE the perpendicular to the epiphyseal base line is no longer parallel to the femoral neck axis. In chronic SUFE (not shown) the femoral neck often remodels and the femur shaft axis must then be used as reference line

eral femoral neck no longer intersects the lateral aspect of the femoral head (Fig. 12.3). The lateral view is in most cases more sensitive for the recognition of SUFE (Fig. 12.4) (KLEIN et al. 1951; GEKELER 2002).

In chronic cases signs of metaphyseal remodelling are seen. This comprises formation of a metaphyseal bony spur adjacent to the slip, usually dorsomedially, varus deformity of the femoral neck and possibly signs of secondary joint damage in

higher grade slips due to impingement of the bared metaphysis onto the acetabulum (Figs. 12.3, 12.5, 12.6) (GEKELER 2002; LEUNIG et al. 2002).

In rare cases evidence of loss of cartilage thickness (chondrolysis) is seen on the initial radiographs. Chondrolysis is defined as loss of cartilage thickness of ≥ 2 mm compared to the contralateral normal hip or an absolute cartilage thickness of ≤ 3 mm in cases of bilaterally abnormal hips. Normal hips have a cartilage thickness of 4–5 mm (LODER et al. 1993b).

12.5.1.3
Radiographic Measurements

Angles measured in the AP and lateral projection are not equal to the actual slip angle. For low slip angles, the angles measured in the lateral projection are similar to the real angles (Fig. 12.7), for higher slip angles the real angles can be determined by using conversion tables. Exact positioning is prerequisite for this (GEKELER 2002). In patients with chronic slip and metaphyseal change the angle needs to be measured against the femoral shaft to avoid inaccuracies due to varus, or rarely valgus, deformity of the femoral neck (ENGELHARDT and ROESLER 1987). Despite optimal positioning, angle measurements can have inaccuracies of up to 5° and sometimes even more, especially when the hip joint is in flexion contraction (ENGELHARDT and ROESLER 1987).

In cases where only a single AP view has been acquired there is another method to determine the slip angle. In the AP view the base of the slipped epiphysis appears elliptic. By measuring the long and the short axis of the ellipse and referring to a conversion table the slip angle can be estimated. This method is however inaccurate (GEKELER 2002).

Another classification system for the assessment of poor radiographs, where angle measurement is not possible, uses the relative displacement of the femoral head on the neck for classification. Displacement of < 1/3 is seen as mild, 1/3–1/2 as moderate and > 1/2 as severe slip (BOYER et al. 1981).

12.5.2
MR Imaging

Currently MR imaging for established or suspected cases of SUFE is used as a problem solving tool. It is not usually the primary imaging examination of choice, this is still radiography. MR imaging is useful in equivocal cases and also allows very accurate angle measurements by choosing the most suitable imaging plane, usually the sagittal plane (DASCHNER et al. 1990; HARLAND and KRAPPEL 2002). A few authors see MR imaging as secondary to computed tomography (CT) (ENGELHARDT and ROESLER 1987; ENGELHARDT 2002), but most authors prefer MR imaging to CT in most cases (DASCHNER et al. 1990; HARLAND and KRAPPEL 2002).

The ability of MR imaging to detect cases of SUFE early and even "preslip" is quoted repeatedly in the literature (DASCHNER et al. 1990; STABLER et al. 1992; HARLAND and KRAPPEL 2002; LALAJI et al. 2002). However, it is the opinion of the authors of this chapter that there is no convincing case in the literature proving that MR imaging can diagnose SUFE in the preslip stage. Examples labelled as preslip actually demonstrate evidence of slip on the radiographs illustrated in these articles.

On MR imaging SUFE presents with oedema like signal in the growth plate and adjacent epiphysis and metaphysis, widening and loss of sharpness of the growth plate and slip of the epiphysis (DASCHNER et al. 1990; STABLER et al. 1992; UMANS et al. 1998; HARLAND and KRAPPEL 2002; LALAJI et al. 2002). Metaphyseal sclerosis and spur formation is seen (Figs. 12.3, 12.5, 12.6) (UMANS et al. 1998). Joint effusion is frequently seen, this is however unspecific (ENGELHARDT 2002; HARLAND and KRAPPEL 2002).

In the institution of the authors of this chapter, MR imaging is currently only used as a problem solving tool, particularly for cases of doubtful SUFE, including queried contralateral disease in established cases of SUFE.

The absence of ionising radiation is an advantage of MR imaging but the ease, speed and good sensitivity and specificity of radiographs still favour these as first line examination.

12.5.3
Computed Tomography

Computed tomography attracted early interest, before MR imaging became widely available (ENGELHARDT and ROESLER 1987). Compared to radiography the radiation dose of CT is higher and for routine cases of suspected SUFE CT is not necessary (HARLAND and KRAPPEL 2002). It might have a role for problem solving in patients who can not undergo MR imaging. It is also useful for evaluation whether closure of a growth plate has commenced, this can be important when prophylactic pinning of the asymptomatic side in patients with unilateral SUFE is contemplated (ENGELHARDT 2002).

In SUFE CT demonstrates physeal widening, metaphyseal irregularities with sclerosis and scalloping and in chronic cases metaphyseal beaking (Figs. 12.2, 12.6) (UMANS et al. 1998).

CT, especially with reformatting, can be useful to determine the slip angle in difficult cases, such as in flexion deformity in the hip joint. In these cases it can also depict the joint alignment and possible impingement. It can also be used to determine the position of orthopaedic implants and in particular protrusion of implants into the joint; this can be important in severe slips or when multiple implants are used (Figs. 12.5, 12.8) (FREYSCHMIDT et al. 2001; ENGELHARDT 2002).

12.5.4
Ultrasound

12.5.4.1
Technique and Findings

Ultrasound was proposed as a diagnostic tool for the diagnosis and classification of SUFE in the early 1990s (KALLIO et al. 1991, 1993). There is no ionising radiation and the position of greatest slip can be determined sonographically. This theoretically avoids the problem of projectional error for the slip angle determination. Ultrasound also allows direct assessment of joint effusions (KALLIO et al. 1991, 1993). However ultrasound is operator dependent and the information about bone changes and overall joint appearance is limited. Radiographs are familiar to radiologist and surgeon and ultrasound is not useful for postoperative follow up. Ultrasound has however been proposed for the follow up of asymptomatic contralateral hips after SUFE when a contralateral slip is queried (CASTRIOTA-SCANDERBEG and ORSI 1993). In these cases it provides a sensitive screening test without ionising radiation that is easily complemented by radiography in positive cases.

Generally the use of a 5 MHz probe is advised. The transducer is aligned parallel to the femoral neck and circumferential scanning is performed. This allows to identify the area of maximal displacement of the epiphysis. The displacement of the epiphysis from the metaphysis can then be measured. Similarly the distance of the metaphysis from the acetabulum can be determined.

In acute SUFE an offset between meta- and epiphysis is seen. In typical dorsomedial slips this is easily imaged. Comparison with the contralateral side is also easy (Figs. 12.4, 12.9). In acute cases a joint effusion is usually seen. Joint effusion is diagnosed if there is > 2 mm difference to the normal side or a joint collection of > 6 mm on the symptomatic side. Ultrasound imaging of chronic slips is more difficult, as with time remodelling takes place which causes narrowing of the physeal step. The size of the physeal step is inversely correlated to the duration of symptoms and directly correlated to the degree of displacement (KALLIO et al. 1991). However, small physeal steps can also occur in delayed closure of a physis and Perthes disease (HARLAND and KRAPPEL 2002).

12.5.4.2
Sonographic Measurements

The slip severity is determined indirectly by measuring the epiphyseal displacement either absolute (KALLIO et al. 1991) or relative (KALLIO et al. 1993). Displacement by 7 mm equates roughly to a 30° slip (mild), 11 mm to 50° slip (moderate) and more than 11 mm therefore to more than 50° (severe slip) (KALLIO et al. 1991). Relative displacement relates the amount of displacement to the width of the physis, 33% relative displacement relates to 30°, and 50% displacement to 50° (KALLIO et al. 1993).

12.5.5
Nuclear Medicine

Tc-99m labelled scintigraphy of the hip joints with pin hole collimation technique has been used to assesses the status of femoral head, physis and the hip joint as a whole in patients with SUFE. Bone scintigraphy was (and nowadays rarely is) used for specific management decision during treatment, after the primary diagnosis was made radiographically.

Bone scintigraphy can help diagnose avascular necrosis (AVN) of the femoral head by demonstrating initially absent uptake and later reperfusion and remodelling with increased uptake. It can also assess the status of the growth plate. Radiographically it is often difficult to decide the extent of physeal closure and a Tc isotope bone scan is of help here, increased uptake indicates persistence of the growth plate (Figs. 12.3, 12.10) (SMERGEL et al. 1987).

Bone scintigraphy can also be used for diagnosing chondrolysis after or with SUFE. Generalised increased uptake around the affected joint, premature closure of the femoral capital physis and the apophysis of the greater trochanter with decreased uptake in theses areas are suggestive of chondrolysis (MANDELL et al. 1992; WARNER et al. 1996).

To the authors' knowledge, nuclear medicine is no longer in use for diagnosis or management of SUFE and has been supplanted by CT or MR imaging.

12.6
Treatment Strategies and Problems

There is a large variety of treatment strategies and techniques in orthopaedic textbooks and journals and a number of quite contrasting treatment phi-

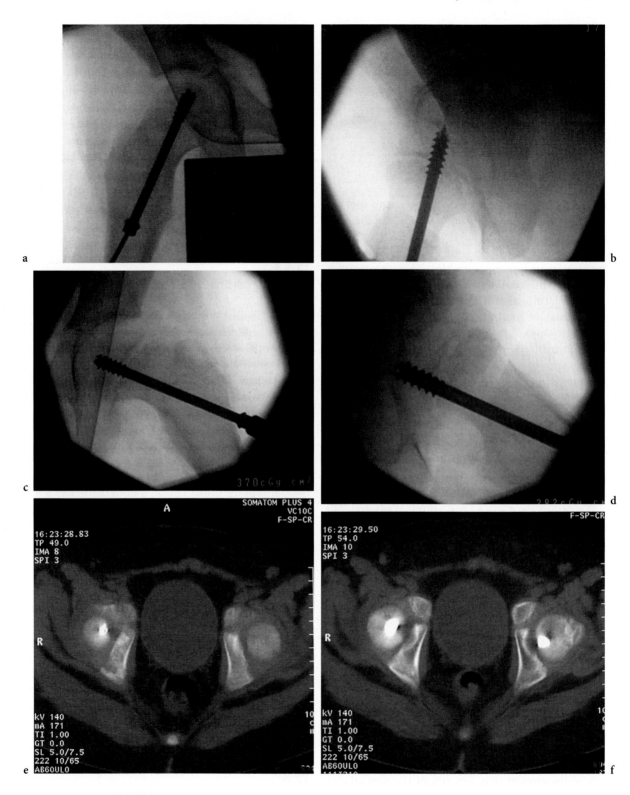

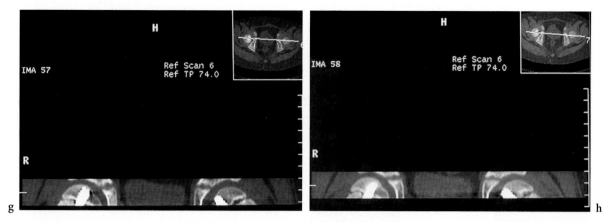

Fig. 12.8a–h. A boy aged 8 years and 1 month; bilateral SUFE. Intraoperatively no obvious cartilage transgression but screw tips near to the cortical bone of the femoral head (**a,b** right; **c,d** left). Axial CT images were equivocal (**e,f**). Coronal reconstructions (**g,h**) demonstrate the right screw contained within the femoral head, the left screw penetrates into the fovea centralis. This case demonstrates the need for thin slices and reconstructions for the assessment of screw position after pinning

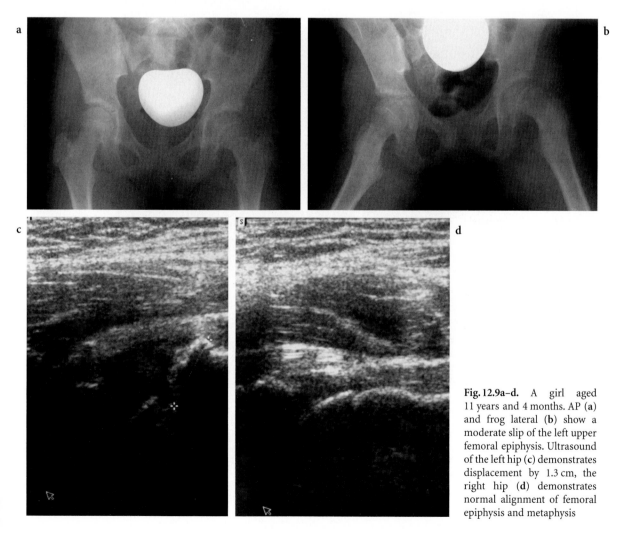

Fig. 12.9a–d. A girl aged 11 years and 4 months. AP (**a**) and frog lateral (**b**) show a moderate slip of the left upper femoral epiphysis. Ultrasound of the left hip (**c**) demonstrates displacement by 1.3 cm, the right hip (**d**) demonstrates normal alignment of femoral epiphysis and metaphysis

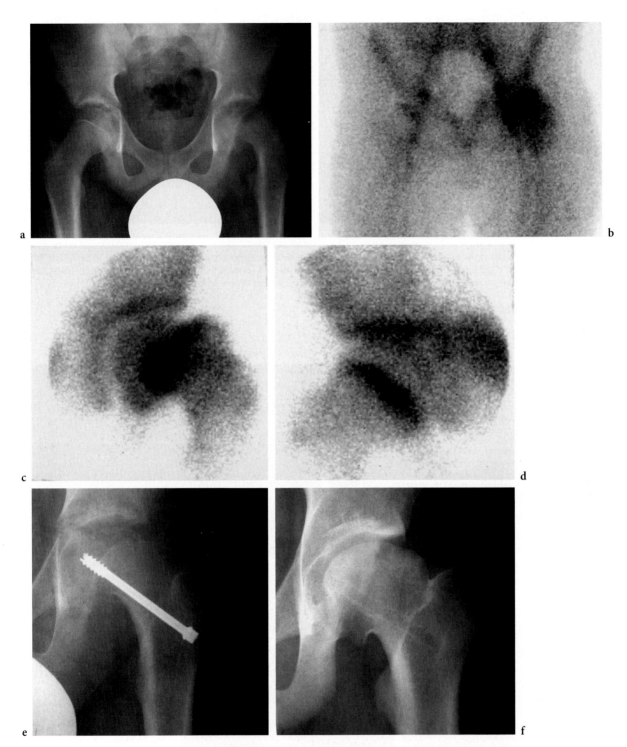

Fig. 12.10a–f. A boy aged 11 years and 4 months. Severe left sided slip (**a**). The diffusion phase of an isotope bone scan (**b**) demonstrates marked increased uptake around the epiphysis of the left proximal femur, no evidence of AVN. The bone phase images demonstrate the slip on the left side (**c**) and normal appearances on the right side (**d**). Single screw fixation in malalignment (**e**) leads to formation of a lateral notch of the femoral head due to impingement (**f**)

losophies exist. This and the following paragraph can by no means be comprehensive but aim to give an overview of the basic principles and problems.

12.6.1
Conservative Treatment

The first decision in the treatment of SUFE patients is whether to treat conservatively or operatively. Conservative treatment means months of immobilisation. The functional outcome is relatively poor and there is an increased incidence of chondrolysis. This treatment approach has largely been abandoned (ARNOLD et al. 2002).

12.6.2
Operative Treatment

All surgical treatment methods for SUFE aim to stabilise the slip. The second goal is to achieve biomechanically sound alignment to prevent or lessen secondary osteo-arthrosis. This can be achieved by reducing the slipped epiphysis or osteotomy (ARNOLD et al. 2002).

The importance of the time span from diagnosis to treatment is subject to debate. There is no clear evidence that immediate intervention in SUFE fares better than urgent (within a few days) intervention, with bed rest until surgery. Treatment should be performed by specialist surgeons (LODER et al. 1993b; ARNOLD et al. 2002; EXNER et al. 2002).

12.6.2.1
Surgical Stabilisation Methods

Surgical stabilisation is achieved by internal fixation of the proximal femur, joining femoral head and neck. Commonly used materials are a single cannulated screw, a dynamic hip screw (DHS) and Kirschner pins (BOYER et al. 1981; ARONSON and CARLSON 1992; ARNOLD et al. 2002; BALLARD and COSGROVE 2002; ENGELHARDT 2002; CARNEY et al. 2003; TOKMAKOVA et al. 2003). Some surgeons still use bone grafts, but this is the exception (ADAMCZYK et al. 2003). Smith Peterson nails, or Steinmann nails are no longer recommended (ENGELHARDT 2002).

The proponents of bone grafts claim a low rate of AVN in its favour (ADAMCZYK et al. 2003). The implantation of two Kirschner pins or small cannulated screws offers the advantage of rotary stability (EXNER et al. 2002), but there is evidence that the complication rate (AVN, chondrolysis) increases with the number of metal implants (Fig. 12.12) (ENGELHARDT 2002; HACKENBROCH et al. 2002; TOKMAKOVA et al. 2003) and many surgeons prefer either a single, larger cannulated screw or a DHS (BOYER et al. 1981; ARONSON and CARLSON 1992; LODER et al. 1993b; ARNOLD et al. 2002a-c; BALLARD and COSGROVE 2002; ENGELHARDT 2002; HACKENBROCH et al. 2002; CARNEY et al. 2003; TOKMAKOVA et al. 2003). A DHS allows for continued growth, thus potentially reducing length discrepancies between the two legs and avoiding shortened femoral necks with elevated trochanters (ARNOLD et al. 2002; EXNER et al. 2002; HACKENBROCH et al. 2002).

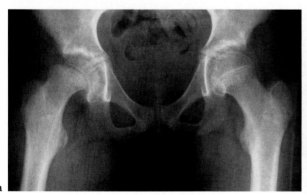

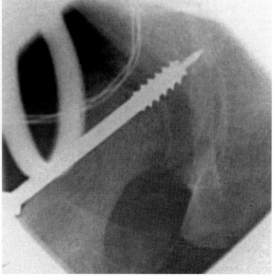

Fig. 12.11a,b. A boy aged 14 years and 8 months. Right-sided moderate to severe slip (a). An intraoperative image shows cartilage injury of the femoral head by the guidewire (b). This should be avoided. Note also the good alignment of femoral head and neck due to spontaneous reduction of the slip

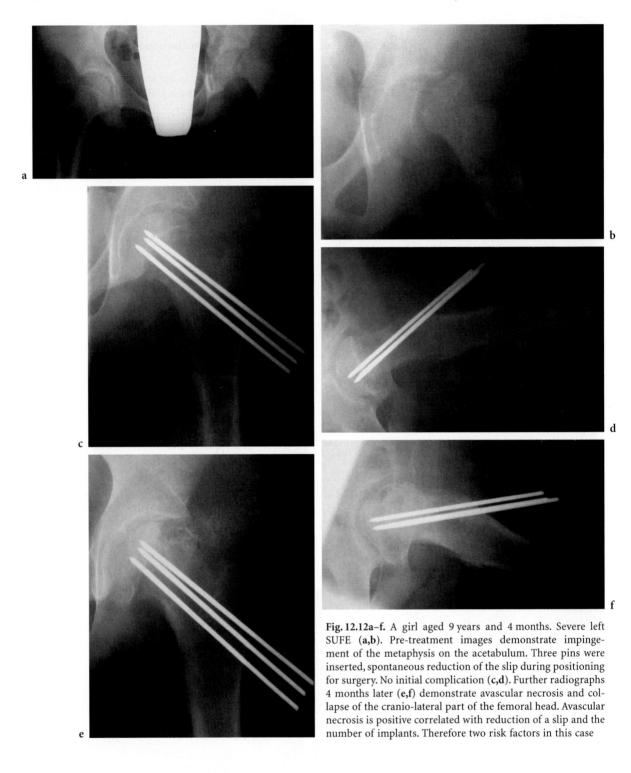

Fig. 12.12a–f. A girl aged 9 years and 4 months. Severe left SUFE (**a,b**). Pre-treatment images demonstrate impingement of the metaphysis on the acetabulum. Three pins were inserted, spontaneous reduction of the slip during positioning for surgery. No initial complication (**c,d**). Further radiographs 4 months later (**e,f**) demonstrate avascular necrosis and collapse of the cranio-lateral part of the femoral head. Avascular necrosis is positive correlated with reduction of a slip and the number of implants. Therefore two risk factors in this case

The injury of joint cartilage by the implants must be avoided because of the increased risk of chondrolysis after cartilage injury (ARNOLD et al. 2002; EXNER et al. 2002; LEUNIG et al. 2002; JOFE et al. 2004). This includes the avoidance of tran-sient cartilage injury by a guidewire during surgery (Fig. 12.11). The use of Kirschner pins is seen criti-cally by some authors as they can work themselves loose with time, resulting in an increased risk of car-tilage damage (ARNOLD et al. 2002).

12.6.2.2
Reduction of SUFE

Reduction can be achieved by open or closed techniques. Open reduction has some proponents (EXNER et al. 2002) but the majority of surgeons do not routinely perform or favour open reduction. Closed reduction can be actively sought by careful flexion, internal rotation and abduction (ARNOLD et al. 2002). Many surgeons however avoid any active reduction for fear of inducing AVN; reduction is however often achieved passively when performing closed fixation (Fig. 12.11, 12.12) (BOYER et al. 1981; BALLARD and COSGROVE 2002).

From a simple biomechanical viewpoint reduction is preferable to in situ fixation without reduction. However active reduction increases the risk of AVN; as the femoral head begins to slip in one direction the periosteal sleeve on the opposite side tears and with it the blood vessels contained in it. A large proportion of the blood supply to the femoral head is then maintained by vessels on the side of the slip. At about 2 weeks after the slip, metaphyseal remodelling with bony spur formation and tightening of the joint capsule has taken place. At 2 weeks and more after the slip, attempts at reduction therefore carry a significant risk of disruption of the surviving capsular blood supply thereby causing femoral head necrosis (BOYER et al. 1981; ARNOLD et al. 2002; EXNER et al. 2002; BOERO et al. 2003). This is the reason why some surgeons suggest open reduction for chronic or even acute SUFE, which makes it possible to resect the bone spur and reduce the slipped head under direct vision, sparing the blood supply. In acute SUFE there should theoretically be no greatly increased risk of AVN from reduction (BOYER et al. 1981; ARNOLD et al. 2002; EXNER et al. 2002).

Some surgeons use the classification of stable (patient can weight bear) and unstable (patient can not weight bear, even with crutches) for the decision whether reduction is safe (yes in unstable, no in stable) (HARLAND and KRAPPEL 2002). However, many surgeons will not try to reduce SUFE at all because of the risk of AVN (HACKENBROCH et al. 2002; CARNEY et al. 2003; TOKMAKOVA et al. 2003) especially in unstable SUFE (BALLARD and COSGROVE 2002).

12.6.2.3
Osteotomy

For corrective osteotomy after SUFE there are four principal techniques. These are subcapital, neck of femur, intertrochanteric and subtrochanteric approaches. The intertrochanteric approach is usually favoured (SOUTHWICK 1967; ARNOLD et al. 2002; EXNER et al. 2002; SCHAI and EXNER 2002) though some surgeons prefer the subtrochanteric approach (BOYER et al. 1981).

The intertrochanteric technique achieves better realignment than the subtrochanteric technique and does not demonstrate the increased risk of AVN that is seen in the subcapital and neck of femur techniques (ARNOLD et al. 2002a,b; EXNER et al. 2002).

12.7
Treatment Philosophies

The previous paragraph outlined common treatments of SUFE, each with its own problems. The treatment choice is partly guided by different philosophies and partly by personal preference.

In the United States most cases of SUFE are treated with in situ surgical fixation only. No attempt of reduction is made (though reduction does often occur with closed fixation) and primary osteotomy is unusual. Most centres opt now for a single cannulated screw for fixation (ARONSON and CARLSON 1992; LODER et al. 1993b; BALLARD and COSGROVE 2002; CARNEY et al. 2003; TOKMAKOVA et al. 2003; JOFE et al. 2004).

In central Europe and in particular in the German speaking countries the treatment of SUFE is more aggressive. There are guidelines from orthopaedic and trauma surgeon organisations advising in situ fixation for slips < 30°, in situ fixation plus subtrochanteric osteotomy for slips between 30° and 50°–60° and for slips of > 50°–60° open reduction and subcapital osteotomy with neck of femur shortening is advised. Some surgeons still try to achieve active reduction before fixation. A single cannulated screw is usually preferred to two Kirschner pins or a DHS (ARNOLD et al. 2002a–c; ENGELHARDT 2002; EXNER et al. 2002; HACKENBROCH et al. 2002; HARLAND and KRAPPEL 2002; LEUNIG et al. 2002; SCHAI and EXNER 2002).

Whether removal of surgical fixation screws is advisable is controversial (ARONSON and CARLSON 1992).

Differences in philosophy can partly explain the difference in treatment approaches. The surgical philosophy favoured in the US aims for minimal trauma at the time of slip to reduce the risk of immediate complication. This results in an increased risk of long term arthrosis. The approach favoured in central Europe is aggressive at the time of slip with a view of reducing long term complications.

Similar differences in approach are seen with regards to prophylactic pinning of the contralateral normal hip joint in patients with unilateral SUFE. While this is not the norm in the US, it is in German speaking countries. A recent extensive review, weighing up the possible advantages and disadvantages now recommends prophylactic pinning also in the US (SCHULTZ et al. 2002).

Whichever general philosophy a surgeon follows, the treatment chosen always has to weigh up the pros and cons for each individual case and guidelines can not be completely prescriptive.

12.8
Imaging Assessment of Surgical Intervention and Complications of SUFE

The most feared immediate complications of SUFE are chondrolysis and AVN. Chondrolysis is diagnosed if there is loss of cartilage thickness of ≥ 2 mm compared to the contralateral normal hip or an absolute cartilage thickness of ≤ 3 mm in cases of bilaterally abnormal hips. Cartilage thickness of normal hip joints is assumed to be 4–5 mm (ARONSON and CARLSON 1992; LODER et al. 1993b; HUGHES et al. 1999). The incidence of chondrolysis after SUFE ranges from 1.1%–11.8% (LUBICKY 1996; TUDISCO et al. 1999). Chondrolysis after SUFE leads to premature closure of the femoral capital growth plate and the apophysis of the greater trochanter. Periarticular osteopenia on radiographs, bone marrow oedema on MR imaging and generalised increased periarticular activity in bone scintigraphy are seen (MANDELL et al. 1992; WARNER et al. 1996). Chondrolysis can be the result of long term immobilisation, direct impingement of the bared metaphysis on the acetabulum or due to surgical intervention with cartilage injury either at the time of surgery or later due to migration of metalwork. An autoimmune mechanism is also controversially discussed, the exact mechanism leading to chondrolysis is not established yet (STERNLICHT et al. 1992; STOVER et al. 1994; LUBICKY 1996; WARNER et al. 1996; ARNOLD et al. 2002a,b; EXNER et al. 2002; HACKENBROCH et al. 2002; LEUNIG et al. 2002; JOFE et al. 2004).

The acute stage of chondrolysis after SUFE lasts about 6 months and presents with joint space narrowing. In the longer term 3 outcomes are seen. There

is joint destruction with painful or painless ankylosis or there can be resolution of the pathological findings with joint space restoration. The latter outcome is seen in 50%–60% of cases (LUBICKY 1996).

AVN presents radiographically with patchy areas of radiolucency and sclerosis and finally epiphyseal collapse (Figs. 12.3, 12.12) (GEKELER 2002). On MR imaging initially oedema like signal is seen within the femoral head. This becomes demarcated by a serpiginous single or less frequently double line, the area enclosed usually demonstrates initially oedema like signal and later fat signal (KAPLAN et al. 2001). The risk is increased in unstable SUFE (LODER et al. 1993b; BALLARD and COSGROVE 2002; TOKMAKOVA et al. 2003) and neck of femur or subcapital osteotomy (ARNOLD et al. 2002). High grade slips are a risk factor for long-term arthrosis but whether they are also a risk factor for AVN is controversial (LODER et al. 1993b; ARNOLD et al. 2002; BALLARD and COSGROVE 2002; TOKMAKOVA et al. 2003). Active closed reduction is thought to be a risk factor for AVN by many (ARONSON and CARLSON 1992; BOERO et al. 2003; TOKMAKOVA et al. 2003) and for chronic slip this is universally accepted (BOYER et al. 1981; ARONSON and CARLSON 1992; ARNOLD et al. 2002; EXNER et al. 2002; BOERO et al. 2003).

Fracture and migration of metal implants, subtrochanteric femur fractures and infection are cited as further complications of surgical treatment (HACKENBROCH et al. 2002). However, no case of infection after closed reduction has been described in the literature (SCHULTZ et al. 2002).

When assessing operative and postoperative images the following features should be checked (Table 12.3).

What is the postoperative slip angle? Has there been reduction?

Has there been an intraoperative or is there a postoperative chondral injury by surgical implants (risk of chondrolysis)?

If a single cannulated screw is used, is it positioned centrally in the femoral head and is it perpendicular to the growth plate (ARONSON and CARLSON 1992)? Are five threads of the screw in the femoral head (the fewer threads the higher the risk of instability and secondary slip; CARNEY et al. 2003)?

Is there possible impingement of the femoral metaphysis onto the acetabulum?

In longer term follow up (Table 12.4), is there implant migration? Is there evidence of instability of a surgically fixed slip? Is there evidence of AVN or chondrolysis? Is there evidence of secondary degenerative change?

Table 12.3. Checklist for reporting immediate postoperative SUFE cases

- Approximate slip angle post op, reduction of slip?
- Intraoperative or postoperative injury to the femoral head cartilage by metal implants?
- Position of metal implants, if single cannulated screw used: five threads beyond the physis? Cartilage injury intraoperative or even persisting postoperative?
- Impingement acetabulum/metaphysis?

Table 12.4. Checklist for long term follow up of SUFE cases

- Impingement?
- Stability of epiphysis?
- Implant migration?
- AVN or chondrolysis?
- Secondary degenerative change?

12.9
Conclusion and Outlook

Slipped upper femoral epiphysis is not a frequent disease but it is potentially well treatable and early diagnosis is important. In undiagnosed hip, groin, thigh or knee pain, AP and frog lateral radiographs (ideally after Imhäuser) can be diagnostic or reassure a normal status.

If SUFE is diagnosed urgent advice and treatment from a specialised centre should be sought. The radiologist's role is to confirm the diagnosis, help with the classification, advise on imaging in more complex cases and to assess pre- and postoperative images for possible complications especially mechanical impingement, AVN and chondrolysis.

With the growing obesity problem in the young population SUFE is unfortunately likely to increase in incidence.

References

Adamczyk MJ, Weiner DS et al (2003) A 50-year experience with bone graft epiphysiodesis in the treatment of slipped capital femoral epiphysis. J Pediatr Orthop 23:578–583

Ankarath S, Ng AB et al (2002) Delay in diagnosis of slipped upper femoral epiphysis. J R Soc Med 95:356–358

Arnold P, Jani L et al (2002a) Results of treating slipped capital femoral epiphysis by pinning in situ. Orthopade 31:880–887

Arnold P, Jani L et al (2002b) Management and treatment results for acute slipped capital femoral epiphysis. Orthopade 31:866–870

Arnold P, Jani L et al (2002c) Significance and results of subcapital osteotomy in severe slipped capital femoral epiphysis. Orthopade 31:908–913

Aronson DD, Carlson WE (1992) Slipped capital femoral epiphysis. A prospective study of fixation with a single screw. J Bone Joint Surg Am 74:810–819

Ballard J, Cosgrove AP (2002) Anterior physeal separation. A sign indicating a high risk for avascular necrosis after slipped capital femoral epiphysis. J Bone Joint Surg Br 84:1176–1179

Boero S, Brunenghi GM et al (2003) Pinning in slipped capital femoral epiphysis: long-term follow-up study. J Pediatr Orthop B 12:372–379

Boyer DW, Mickelson MR et al (1981) Slipped capital femoral epiphysis. Long-term follow-up study of one hundred and twenty-one patients. J Bone Joint Surg Am 63:85–95

Brown D (2004) Seasonal variation of slipped capital femoral epiphysis in the United States. J Pediatr Orthop 24:139–143

Carney BT, Birnbaum P et al (2003) Slip progression after in situ single screw fixation for stable slipped capital femoral epiphysis. J Pediatr Orthop 23:584–589

Castriota-Scanderbeg A, Orsi E (1993) Slipped capital femoral epiphysis: ultrasonographic findings. Skeletal Radiol 22:191–193

Daschner H, Lehner K et al (1990) Imaging of epiphyseolysis of the femur head in the magnetic resonance tomogram. Rofo Fortschr Geb Rontgenstr Neuen Bildgeb Verfahr 152:583–586

Engelhardt P(2002) Slipped capital femoral epiphysis and the "healthy" opposite hip. Orthopade 31:888–893

Engelhardt P, Roesler H (1987) Radiometry of epiphyseolysis capitis femoris. A comparison of conventional roentgen study with axial computerized tomography. Z Orthop Ihre Grenzgeb 125:177–182

Exner GU, Schai PA et al (2002) Treatment of acute slips and clinical results in slipped capital femoral epiphysis. Orthopade 31:857–865

Freyschmidt J, Brossmann J et al (2001) Slipped capital femoral epiphysis. Borderlands of normal and early pathological findings in skeletal radiography, vol 1. Freyschmidt, Stuttgart / Thieme, New York, pp 834–836

Gekeler J (2002) Radiology and measurement in adolescent slipped capital femoral epiphysis. Orthopade 31:841–850

Guzzanti V, Falciglia F et al (2003) Slipped capital femoral epiphysis: physeal histologic features before and after fixation. J Pediatr Orthop 23:571–577

Hackenbroch MH, Kumm DA et al (2002) Dyamic screw fixation for slipped capital femoral epiphysis. Treatment results. Orthopade 31:871–879

Harland U, Krappel FA (2002) Value of ultrasound, CT, and MRI in the diagnosis of slipped capital femoral epiphysis (SCFE). Orthopade 31:851–856

Hughes LO, Aronson J et al (1999) Normal radiographic values for cartilage thickness and physeal angle in the pediatric hip. J Pediatr Orthop 19:443–448

Jofe MH, Lehman W et al (2004) Chondrolysis following slipped capital femoral epiphysis. J Pediatr Orthop B 13:29–31

Kallio PE, Lequesne GW et al (1991) Ultrasonography in slipped capital femoral epiphysis. Diagnosis and assessment of severity. J Bone Joint Surg Br 73:884–889

Kallio PE, Paterson DC et al (1993) Classification in slipped capital femoral epiphysis. Sonographic assessment of stability and remodeling. Clin Orthop 294:196–203

Kaplan PA, Helms CA et al (2001). Vascular abnormalities of bone. Musculoskeletal MRI, vol 1. Saunders, Philadelphia, pp 334–339

Kelsey JL (1971) The incidence and distribution of slipped capital femoral epiphysis in Connecticut. J Chronic Dis 23:567–578

Kelsey JL, Keggi KJ et al (1970) The incidence and distribution of slipped capital femoral epiphysis in Connecticut and Southwestern United States. J Bone Joint Surg Am 52:1203–1216

Klein A, Joplin RJ et al (1951) Roentgenographic features of slipped capital femoral epiphysis. Am J Roentgenol 66:361–374

Kocher MS, Bishop JA et al (2004) Delay in diagnosis of slipped capital femoral epiphysis. Pediatrics 113:e322–e325

Lalaji A, Umans H et al (2002) MRI features of confirmed "pre-slip" capital femoral epiphysis: a report of two cases. Skeletal Radiol 31:362–365

Leunig M, Fraitzl C. R et al (2002) Early damage to the acetabular cartilage in slipped capital femoral epiphysis. Therapeutic consequences. Orthopade 31:894–899

Loder RT (1996a) The demographics of slipped capital femoral epiphysis. An international multicenter study. Clin Orthop 322:8–27

Loder RT (1996b) A worldwide study on the seasonal variation of slipped capital femoral epiphysis. Clin Orthop 322:28–36

Loder RT, Aronson DD et al (1993a) The epidemiology of bilateral slipped capital femoral epiphysis. A study of children in Michigan. J Bone Joint Surg Am 75:1141–1147

Loder RT, Richards BS et al (1993b) Acute slipped capital femoral epiphysis: the importance of physeal stability. J Bone Joint Surg Am 75:1134–1140

Loder RT, Mehbod AA et al (2003) Acetabular depth and race in young adults: a potential explanation of the differences in the prevalence of slipped capital femoral epiphysis between different racial groups? J Pediatr Orthop 23:699–702

Lubicky JP (1996) Chondrolysis and avascular necrosis: complications of slipped capital femoral epiphysis. J Pediatr Orthop B 5:162–167

Mandell GA, Keret D et al (1992) Chondrolysis: detection by bone scintigraphy. J Pediatr Orthop 12:80–85

Milz S, Boszczyk A et al (2002) Development and functional structure of the epiphyseal plate. Orthopade 31:835–840

Oppenheim WL, Bowen RE et al (2003) Outcome of slipped capital femoral epiphysis in renal osteodystrophy. J Pediatr Orthop 23:169–174

Poussa M, Schlenzka D et al (2003) Body mass index and slipped capital femoral epiphysis. J Pediatr Orthop B 12:369–371

Schai PA, Exner GU (2002) Indication for and results of intertrochanteric osteotomy in slipped capital femoral epiphysis. Orthopade 31:900–907

Schultz WR, Weinstein JN et al (2002) Prophylactic pinning of the contralateral hip in slipped capital femoral epiphysis: evaluation of long-term outcome for the contralateral hip with use of decision analysis. J Bone Joint Surg Am 84A:1305–1314

Smergel EM, Harcke HT et al (1987) Use of bone scintigraphy in the management of slipped capital femoral epiphysis. Clin Nucl Med 12:349–353

Southwick WO (1967) Osteotomy through the lesser trochanter for slipped capital femoral epiphysis. J Bone Joint Surg Am 49:807–835

Stabler A, Genz K et al (1992) MRT of epiphyseolysis capitis femoris. Bildgebung 59:133–135

Sternlicht AL, Ehrlich MG et al (1992) Role of pin protrusion in the etiology of chondrolysis: a surgical model with radiographic, histologic, and biochemical analysis. J Pediatr Orthop 12:428–433

Stover B, Sigmund G et al (1994) Early changes in the hip joint following epiphysiolysis of the femoral head. Results of an MRT study. Radiologe 34:46–51

Tokmakova KP, Stanton RP et al (2003) Factors influencing the development of osteonecrosis in patients treated for slipped capital femoral epiphysis. J Bone Joint Surg Am 85A:798–801

Tudisco C, Caterini R et al (1999) Chondrolysis of the hip complicating slipped capital femoral epiphysis: long-term follow-up of nine patients. J Pediatr Orthop B 8:107–111

Umans H, Liebling MS et al (1998) Slipped capital femoral epiphysis: a physeal lesion diagnosed by MRI, with radiographic and CT correlation. Skeletal Radiol 27:139–144

Warner WC Jr, Beaty JH et al (1996) Chondrolysis after slipped capital femoral epiphysis. J Pediatr Orthop B 5:168–172

Weiner D (1996) Pathogenesis of slipped capital femoral epiphysis: current concepts. J Pediatr Orthop B 5:67–73

13 Osteonecrosis and Transient Osteoporosis of the Femoral Head

Bruno C. Vande Berg, Frederic E. Lecouvet, Baudouin Maldague, and Jacques Malghem

CONTENTS

13.1 Introduction

Osteonecrosis and transient osteoporosis are two clinically significant conditions that involve the femoral head (Figs. 13.1, 13.2). Osteonecrosis has been extensively investigated because of its poor prognosis, its complex physiopathogenesis and the numerous therapeutic approaches (Mankin 1992; Chang et al. 1993; Jones 1993; Malghem and Maldague 1981). Transient osteoporosis remains an even more mysterious condition (Vande Berg et al. 1993a) and the link between both conditions is still debated.

Magnetic resonance (MR) imaging definitely contributed to increase the detection and staging of those lesions by improving the depiction of specific and non-specific lesion components and by providing new insights into their natural history.

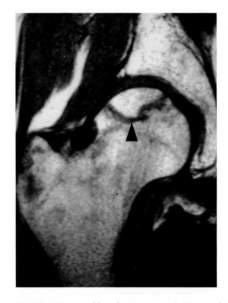

Fig. 13.1. Femoral head osteonecrosis. Coronal T1-weighted SE MR image shows a subchondral fat-like signal intensity lesion surrounded by a low signal intensity rim (*arrowhead*). This geographic or segmental pattern is specific for an infarct of the femoral head

B. C. Vande Berg, MD; F. E. Lecouvet, MD;
B. Maldague, MD; J. Malghem, MD
Department of Radiology and Medical Imaging, Université Catholique de Louvain, University Hospital St Luc, 10 Av. Hippocrate, 1200 Brussels, Belgium

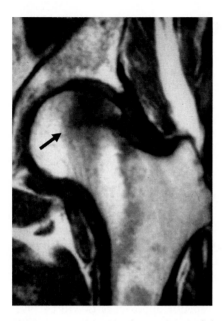

Fig. 13.2. Bone marrow edema pattern of the femoral head. Coronal T1-weighted SE MR image shows a subchondral low signal intensity lesion (*arrow*). Signal change predominates in the subchondral area and there is no clear margin around the lesion. This lesion pattern in non-specific and can be observed in numerous conditions including transient osteoporosis and insufficiency fracture of the femoral head

13.2
Femoral Head Osteonecrosis

13.2.1
Definition

Three different terms will be used in the current chapter; each of them corresponds to a different level of involvement, namely cellular, tissue and organ levels (GLIMCHER and KENZORA 1979)(Table 13.1). Necrosis is the sum of the morphologic cellular changes that follow cell death in a living tissue or organ (ROBBINS et al. 1984a). In bones, coagulation necrosis is the most common pattern of necrosis and results in complete absence of osteocytes within the bone trabeculae, loss of adipocyte nuclei with lipid cysts formation, and death of hematopoietic cells (GLIMCHER and KENZORA 1979; SWEET and MADEWELL

1988). An infarct is a localized area of necrosis in tissue resulting from reduction from either its arterial supply or venous drainage (ROBBINS et al. 1984b). The type of vessels and their spatial arrangement dictate the histopathologic changes that occur in response to ischemia. In yellow marrow, arterial occlusion produces a bloodless or white infarct, whereas in red marrow, hemorrhagic or red infarcts may develop (ROBBINS et al. 1984b)(Fig. 13.3). The term "bone infarct" is generally used to describe a metaphyseal or diaphyseal ischemic lesion, and not an epiphyseal lesion, most likely for historical and not for medical reasons. Epiphyseal osteonecrosis is used to describe a radio-clinical condition characterized by symptoms and functional disability of the joint as an organ, related to an irreversible spontaneous fracture of the femoral head, generally associated with an epiphyseal infarct (Fig. 13.4).

13.2.2
Epidemiology

In the US, the rate of epiphyseal osteonecrosis of the hip is 2–4.5 cases per patient-year with approximately 15,000 new cases reported each year. Epiphyseal osteonecrosis accounts for more than 10% of total hip replacement surgeries performed in the US (KOVAL 2002). A Japanese survey estimated that 2500–3300 cases of epiphyseal osteonecrosis of the hip occur each year (ITO et al. 1999).

Age at onset of femoral head osteonecrosis depends on the underlying cause. Idiopathic epiphyseal osteonecrosis most often develops in male subjects aged between 35 and 55 years and is bilateral in 40%–80% of cases. On average, women present almost 10 years later than men. The male-to-female ratio also depends on the underlying cause, although idiopathic epiphyseal osteonecrosis is more common in men, with an overall male-to-female ratio ranging from 4 to 8:1. There is no racial predilection, except for epiphyseal osteonecrosis associated with sickle cell disease and hemoglobin S and SC disease, which predominantly occur in people of African and Mediterranean descent.

Table 13.1. Terminology

Terms	Target	Imaging modality	definition	Clinic	Outcome
Necrosis	Cells	Microscope	Empty lacunae, death adipocytes	?	?
Infarct	Tissue	MR, X-ray	Well delimited marrow lesion	Variable	Variable
Osteonecrosis	Organ	X-ray, MR	Subchondral bone fracture		
Epiphyseal collapse	Pain	Osteoarthritis			

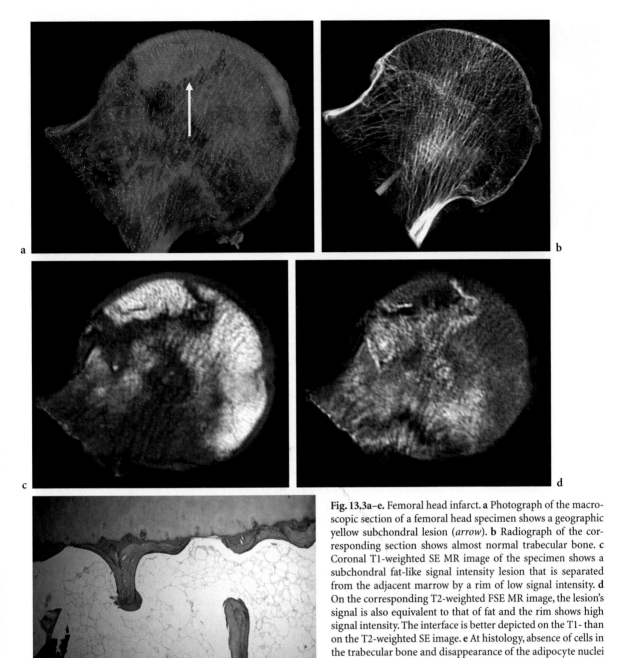

Fig. 13.3a–e. Femoral head infarct. **a** Photograph of the macroscopic section of a femoral head specimen shows a geographic yellow subchondral lesion (*arrow*). **b** Radiograph of the corresponding section shows almost normal trabecular bone. **c** Coronal T1-weighted SE MR image of the specimen shows a subchondral fat-like signal intensity lesion that is separated from the adjacent marrow by a rim of low signal intensity. **d** On the corresponding T2-weighted FSE MR image, the lesion's signal is also equivalent to that of fat and the rim shows high signal intensity. The interface is better depicted on the T1- than on the T2-weighted SE image. **e** At histology, absence of cells in the trabecular bone and disappearance of the adipocyte nuclei indicate bone and marrow necrosis. The architecture of fatty marrow is preserved and the overlying cartilage is normal

13.2.3
Pathophysiology and Natural History

The pathophysiology of epiphyseal osteonecrosis is poorly understood, except when it is due to disruption of blood supply after femoral neck fracture or hip dislocation given the terminal blood supply of the femoral head. In other situations, impaired perfusion with subsequent necrosis of bone and marrow can be caused by several mechanisms including thrombotic or embolic occlusion of blood vessel (e.g., fat embolism, sickle cell crisis, caisson disease), injury to vessel wall (e.g., vasculitis, connective-tissue diseases such as systemic lupus erythematosus, radiation, infection) and increased pressure on vessel wall (e.g., extravasated blood in marrow, inflammation caused by lipid accumulation in osteocytes, intraosseous hypertension from proliferating Gaucher cells in Gaucher disease).

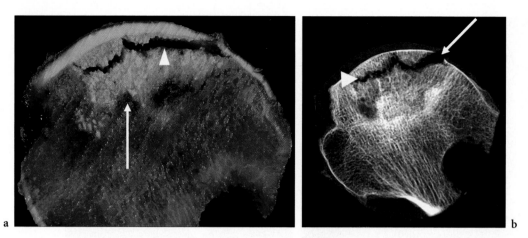

Fig. 13.4a,b. Femoral head osteonecrosis. **a** Photograph of the macroscopic section of a resected femoral head shows a geographic yellow subchondral lesion (*arrow*) with a fracture (*arrowhead*) that runs parallel to the subchondral bone plate. **b** Radiograph of the femoral head specimen with osteonecrosis shows a relatively well delimited subchondral lesion with mild peripheral sclerosis and fracture of the subchondral bone plate (*arrow*) that extends horizontally (*arrowhead*)

Epiphyseal osteonecrosis occurs in several clinical conditions, although it is frequently idiopathic or primary. The etiological factors that have been identified include systemic corticosteroid use, Cushing disease, alcohol abuse, sickle cell disease, other hemoglobinopathies, vasculitis, trauma, renal transplantation and osteodystrophy, radiation therapy, pancreatitis, gout, Gaucher disease, connective-tissue diseases (e.g., SLE), caisson disease and cytotoxic agents (e.g., vinblastine, vincristine, cisplatin, cyclophosphamide, methotrexate, bleomycin, 5-fluorouracil). Several diseases including AIDS and SRAS seem to be associated with an increased prevalence of femoral head osteonecrosis, although epiphyseal lesions (Tehranzadeh et al. 2004) are more likely related to the treatments of the diseases than to the diseases themselves. A Japanese survey estimated that 34.7% were due to corticosteroid use, 21.8% to alcohol abuse, and 37.1% to idiopathic mechanisms (Ito et al. 1999).

An understanding of the natural history of epiphyseal osteonecrosis is important for predicting the fate of a hip, in choosing the appropriate treatment and in evaluating the results of various treatments. Numerous historic reviews of the natural progression of epiphyseal osteonecrosis in symptomatic patients who were conservatively treated (partial non-weight bearing ambulation), documented on 85%–92% risk of progression (Musso et al. 1986; Patterson et al. 1964; Sugano et al. 1992; Zizic and Hungerford 1985). Conversely, recent studies of the natural progression of femoral head lesions in asymptomatic patients screened by using in whom MR imaging showed a 15%–20% risk of appearance of symptoms,

the majority of lesions remaining silent at follow-up (Kopecky et al. 1991; Tervonen et al. 1992; Mulliken et al. 1994; Shimizu et al. 1994; Vande Berg et al. 1994) (Fig. 13.5). Clearly, natural histories of femoral head infarct and osteonecrosis totally differ and largely depend on the selection criteria of the study population.

In addition, the rate at which the femoral head will collapse is related among other things to the cause of the lesion, the stage of the lesion at the initial diagnosis and to the size and location of the lesion in the femoral head. Quantitative determination of the extent and location of femoral head lesions on MR images enabled to estimate the fracture risk (Kopecky et al. 1991; Shimizu et al. 1994; Beltran et al. 1988; Chan et al. 1991; Lafforgue et al. 1993; Takatori et al. 1993). Femoral heads in which the infarct is either limited or involves a limited proportion of the weight-bearing area are less likely to collapse than those with large lesions, whatever the treatment. Signal changes in lesions could also indicate impending fractures because infarcts with fat-like signal intensity show a collapse-free survival much longer than those with heterogeneous signal (Shimizu et al. 1994).

13.2.4
Classification Systems and Treatment

Over the years, numerous different classification systems have been developed to evaluate patients with femoral head osteonecrosis. Although there is no standard unified classification system used by all investigators, there is general agreement that

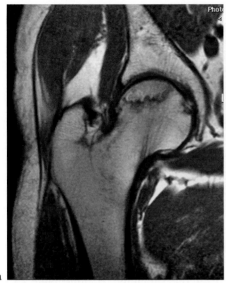
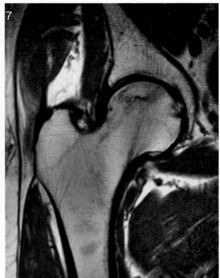

a
b

Fig. 13.5a,b. Natural history of femoral head infarct. **a** Coronal T1-weighted SE MR image shows a well-delimited infarct of the femoral head without collapse. **b** Coronal T1-weighted SE MR image obtained 1 year later shows a similar lesion without fracture. The patient remains asymptomatic 5 years later

the presence of fracture of the subchondral bone represents a pivotal position in all classification systems (generally at stage III, whatever the classification system). Ficat and Arlet originally developed a four-stage classification system based on radiographic changes and the functional exploration of bone (intraosseous phlebography and measurement of bone marrow pressure; Table 13.2) (FICAT 1985). Steinberg's and Arco's classification systems included MRI evaluation, allowing for quantification and topography of the epiphyseal lesion (STEINBERG et al. 1995; Table 13.3). Mitchell's classification system (MITCHELL et al. 1987) included signal pattern of necrotic lesion (A, fat; B, blood; C, edema; D, fibrosis) but it showed limited utility because of the variability of signal intensity of the lesion within the same lesion.

Medical management of symptomatic femoral head osteonecrosis has not proved to be effective in preventing or arresting the disease process (LIEBERMAN et al. 2002). Pain control is usually achieved by non-steroidal analgesics and patients should be advised to use crutches or other supports to avoid weight bearing. Several drugs or other therapeutic methods can be applied.

Several surgical procedures have been tried with variable success. Core decompression of the hip with or without bone graft is the most common procedure currently used to treat the early stages of femoral head osteonecrosis, and it is effective in pain control. Although this procedure has been used for

Table 13.2. Ficat staging system of avascular necrosis of the hip (clinic and radiographs)

Stage	Clinical and radiologic findings
Stage I	• Normal radiographs
	• Decreased or increased uptake on bone scan
	• No pain
	• Increased medullary pressure
Stage II	• Variable change in trabecular bone appearance (sclerosis, delimited area of sclerosis, cyst changes) but preserved femoral head shape
	• Variable pain
Stage III	• Specific changes on radiographs include collapse of subchondral bone and/or crescent sign due to subchondral bone fracture
	• Pain
Stage IV	• Marked collapse of subchondral bone with preserved joint space
Stage V	• Secondary osteoarthritis

approximately three decades and there are numerous publications analyzing its efficacy, there is no general consensus among investigators regarding either the indication for this procedure or its effect on the fate of the femoral head (LIEBERMAN 2004). In late stages, characterized by collapse, femoral head deformity, and secondary osteoarthritis, total hip arthroplasty is the most appropriate treatment, although several osteotomy procedures have been tried with variable success.

Table 13.3. Staging system based on the consensus of the Subcommittee of Nomenclature of the International Association on Bone Circulation and Bone Necrosis (ARCO)

Stage	Clinical and laboratory findings
Stage 0	• No symptoms
	• Normal radiographs and MR images
	• Osteonecrosis at histology
Stage I	• Presence or absence of symptoms
	• Normal radiographs
	• Abnormal MR images
	• Osteonecrosis at histology
Stage II	• Symptoms
	• Trabecular bone changes on radiographs without subchondral bone changes. Preserved joint space
	• Diagnostic MR findings
Stage III	• Symptoms
	• Variable trabecular bone changes with subchondral bone fracture (crescent sign and/or subchondral bone collapse). Preserved shape of femoral head and preserved joint space
	• Subclassification based on extent of crescent, as follows:
	· Stage IIIa: Crescent is less than 15% of the articular surface
	· Stage IIIb: Crescent is 15%–30% of the articular surface
	· Stage IIIc: Crescent is more than 30% of the articular surface
Stage IV	• Symptoms
	• Altered shape of femoral head with variable joint space
	• Subclassification depends on the extent of collapsed surface, as follows:
	· Stage IVa: Less than 15% of surface is collapsed
	· Stage IVb: Approximately 15%–30% of surface is collapsed
	· Stage IVc: More than 30% of surface is collapsed

13.2.5
Radiographs of Femoral Head Osteonecrosis

13.2.5.1
Precollapse Stage – Femoral Head Infarct

Radiographs are insensitive to the detection of early infarcts of the femoral head for two reasons: (a) dead bone remains normal on radiographs and (b) the reactive interface that separates the infarct from the adjacent viable bone cannot be detected before it calcifies (Figs. 13.6, 13.7). Initial radiographic changes include mild sclerosis that tends to delineate a subchondral area with preserved joint space (Fig. 13.6). Bone resorption is generally limited and cystic change is generally lacking in non-collapsed femoral head. Given the spherical shape of the head and the serpiginous organization of the interface, CT may better display the spatial organization of the bone changes than conventional radiographs (Fig. 13.7).

13.2.5.2
Epiphyseal Fracture

The fracture of the subchondral bone plate can show two radiographic patterns: (a) frank and abrupt depression of the subchondral bone plate with subsequent loss of epiphyseal sphericity or (b) a crescentic radiolucent line parallel to the subchondral bone plate (Figs. 13.8, 13.9). These two patterns may coexist in the same femoral head although they usually involve different areas of the femoral head. They may also depend on the hip position, the crescent sign being more frequent in the frog-leg position due to release of the compression forces on the collapsed segment. Epiphyseal collapse generally predominates in the weight-bearing area of the head, underneath the lateral margin of the femoral head.

13.2.5.3
Postcollapse Stages – Femoral Head Osteonecrosis

Radiographs are generally sensitive for the detection of collapsed femoral head osteonecrosis, and they may suffice if conservative therapy is planned. They usually show marked changes in epiphyseal trabecular bone (mixed sclerosis and resorption) with epiphyseal collapse and eventual loss of joint space (Fig. 13.9). Generally the rate of development of osteoarthritis is coherent with the degree of epiphyseal deformity. In the end-stage, it may be impossible (and without clinical significance) to differentiate advanced osteoarthritis from advanced osteonecrosis. In the former, the sequence of event is loss of cartilage followed by epiphyseal deformity. In the latter, epiphyseal deformity occurs first and is followed by loss of joint space.

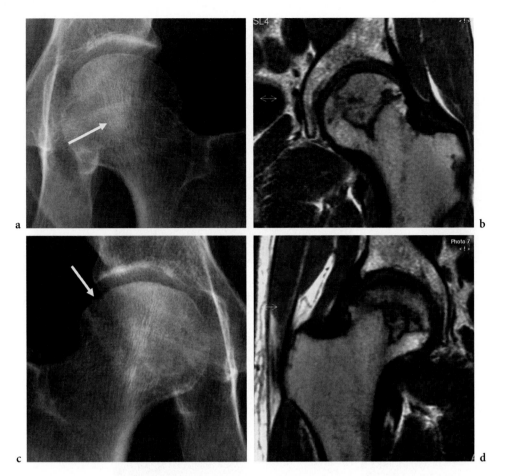

Fig. 13.6a–d. Femoral head infarct and osteonecrosis. **a** Radiograph of the asymptomatic left hip shows normal epiphyseal contour and subtle trabecular bone sclerosis (*arrow*). **b** Coronal T1-weighted SE image shows a subchondral fat-like signal intensity lesion surrounded by a low signal intensity rim that corresponds to a non-collapsed infarct. **c** Radiograph of the symptomatic right hip shows mild trabecular bone sclerosis with fracture of the subchondral bone plate underneath the lateral aspect of the acetabular roof (*arrow*) that indicates epiphyseal osteonecrosis. **d** Coronal T1-weighted SE image shows a well-delimited lesion with abnormal signal intensity in the subchondral area. The lesion is better seen on the MR image than on the radiograph, but the radiograph best depicts the femoral head deformity

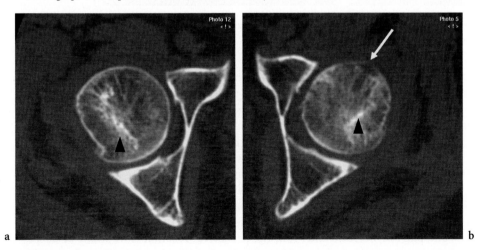

Fig. 13.7a,b. CT images of femoral head osteonecrosis. **a** Axial CT image of the asymptomatic right hip shows a rim of sclerosis (*arrowhead*) that delineates the infarct. The shape of the femoral head is normal. **b** Axial CT image of the symptomatic left femoral head shows altered contour (*arrow*) with prominence of the anterior aspect of the epiphysis. A sclerotic rim surrounds the lesion (*arrowhead*)

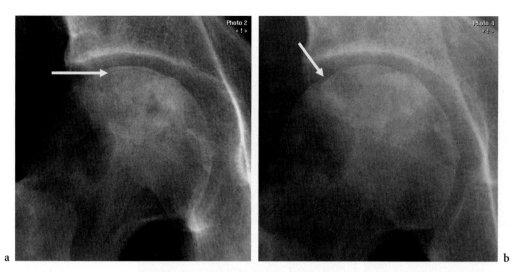

Fig. 13.8a,b. Epiphyseal fracture in femoral head osteonecrosis. **a** Anteroposterior radiograph shows a subchondral cleft fracture (*arrow*) with trabecular bone sclerosis and resorption. **b** Anteroposterior radiograph obtained with an ascending X-ray beam and external rotation of the leg shows focal depression of the subchondral bone plate (*arrow*)

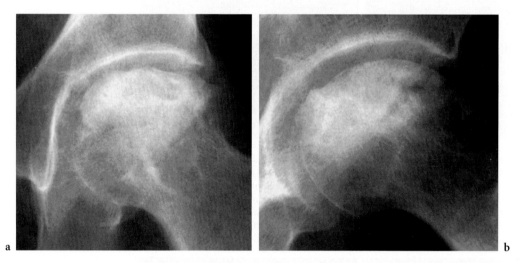

Fig. 13.9a,b. Femoral head osteonecrosis. **a** AP radiograph shows femoral head collapse and sclerosis. **b** Lateral radiograph better depicts the segmental pattern of the lesion

13.2.6
MR Imaging of Femoral Head Osteonecrosis

13.2.6.1
Precollapse Stages – Infarct of the Femoral Head

MR imaging is sensitive for the detection of early marrow infarct (Fig. 13.6). The time delay between the development of bone and marrow necrosis and its appearance on MR images is unknown but probably ranges between 1 to 4 months (KOPECKY et al. 1991). The signal of necrotic yellow marrow remains normal on MR images (LANG et al. 1988; JERGESEN et al. 1990; VANDE BERG et al. 1992; EHMAN et al. 1996; HAUZEUR et al. 1989). The development of marrow changes at the periphery of the necrotic lesion allows its detection. The MR appearance of a yellow marrow infarct is that of an area of normal fatty signal intensity delineated by a rim of low signal intensity on T1-weighted images representing the peripheral reaction (MITCHELL et al. 1987; MARKISZ et al. 1987). In 65%–80% of cases, this peripheral interface shows the double-line sign pattern on T2-weighted images with an outer low and inner high signal intensity line (MITCHELL et al. 1987; COLEMAN et al. 1988; DUDA et al. 1993). This double line pattern probably results from chemical-shift misregistration artifact (VANDE BERG et al. 1993a; DUDA et al. 1993; SUGIMOTO et al. 1989) related to the fact that there is fat on both sides of a water-like equivalent component (the interface).

Differential diagnosis of epiphyseal marrow infarct include subchondral cyst and healed fracture. In subchondral cyst, the overlying cartilage is abnormal and the lesion signal is generally fluid like, although fat can also be present. A healed fracture can show a band-like pattern on T1-weighted images with a double-line sign on T2-weighted images. The line does not completely circumscribe a marrow area and is perpendicular to the trabeculae. In case of doubt, MR imaging of the distal femur can show more typical lesions (infarct or fracture). This pattern is observed in condition in which the healing process in impaired, such as in osteomalacia or patients treated by glucocorticoids.

13.2.6.2
Fracture

The fracture of the subchondral bone plate can show two patterns at MR imaging: (a) frank and abrupt depression of the subchondral bone plate with subsequent loss of epiphyseal sphericity or (b) a high signal intensity line on T2-weighted images extending under the subchondral bone plate (Fig. 13.10). These two patterns may coexist in the same collapsed femoral head but generally in different areas. Contour depression, more prevalent in the weight-bearing area, is more easily detected on coronal images whereas subchondral cleft fracture more prevalent in the non-weight bearing area is more easily detected on sagittal or transverse images. Only T2-weighted and other fluid sensitive images can depict the fracture cleft as a high signal intensity line near to the subchondral bone plate. This line represents fluid accumulating in the subchondral fracture. Recent studies suggested that marrow

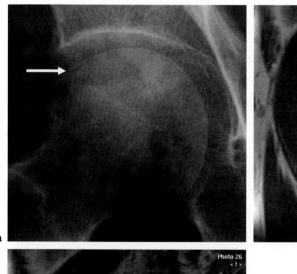

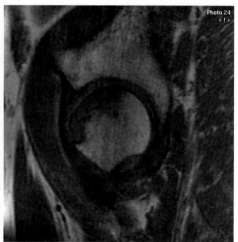

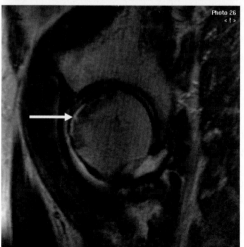

Fig. 13.10a–c. Femoral head osteonecrosis; geographic or segmental pattern. **a** Radiograph of the right femoral head with abduction of the femur shows subtle change of the bone architecture with subchondral cleft fracture (*arrow*). **b** Sagittal T1-weighted SE MR image shows a relatively well-delimited subchondral lesion and flattening of the epiphyseal contour near the acetabular roof with relative prominence of the anterior aspect of the femoral head. **c** The corresponding T2-weighted SE MR image shows a high signal intensity line in the femoral head (*arrow*) corresponding to the fracture of the subchondral bone plate filled by articular fluid. The interface is visible on the T1-weighted SE image only and that there is no double-line sign on the T2-weighted SE image

edema around an apparently uncollapsed ischemic lesion may indicate incipient fracture (Koo et al. 1999; IIDA et al. 2000; HUANG et al. 2003). Histopathologically, edema around the infarct consists of serous exudate, focal interstitial hemorrhage, and mild fibrosis (KUBO et al. 2000). It may result from the development of subchondral fracture, rather than from extension of osteonecrosis (STEVENS et al. 2003).

MR imaging best depicts the ischemic lesion but it shows limitations in the depiction of epiphyseal fracture. Radiographs or best, CT may better display subchondral fracture of the femoral head than MR imaging (STEVENS et al. 2003) (Fig. 13.7).

13.2.6.3
MR Imaging of Epiphyseal Osteonecrosis

Epiphyseal osteonecrosis of the femoral head may show two patterns of involvement based on T1-weighted SE image. The segmental pattern is by far the most frequent pattern. It is observed in patients with known risk factors for marrow infarcts and marrow infarcts can be observed in other regions of the skeleton. The ill-delimited diffuse pattern is less frequent, is observed in patients without risk factors and is usually not associated with marrow infarcts in other bones. This pattern represented about 10% of symptomatic femoral head osteonecrosis (VANDE BERG et al. 1993a; MITCHELL et al. 1987; TURNER et al. 1989; THICKMAN et al. 1986).

13.2.6.3.1
Segmental Pattern

On T1-weighted SE images, the segmental pattern of femoral head osteonecrosis is that of a well-demarcated lesion with necrotic tissue of variable signal intensity, generally including some high signal intensity areas in the subchondral lesion (Figs. 13.3, 13.6, 13.9). Specific imaging features include the reactive interface and subchondral bone fracture. The reactive interface shows the same MR appearance as in noncollapsed lesions, but it is frequently blurred by adjacent reactive changes (COLEMAN et al. 1988). The subchondral bone fracture appears as frank and abrupt depression of the subchondral bone plate with subsequent loss of epiphyseal sphericity or as high signal intensity lines on T2-weighted images extending under the subchondral bone plate. Necrotic and repair tissue, marrow edema, and joint effusion do not

show specific signal intensity patterns. The signal intensity of the necrotic tissue is either equivalent to that of fat or is low on T1-, T2-, and enhanced T1-weighted images reflecting the presence of mummified fat or eosinophilic necrosis, respectively (LANG et al. 1988; JERGESEN et al. 1990; VANDE BERG et al. 1992; HAUZEUR et al. 1989). Reactive changes that surround the lesion show low signal intensity on T1-weighted images and intermediate to high signal intensity on T2-weighted images, depending on the balance among fibrous, sclerotic, and cellular components (LANG et al. 1988; JERGESEN et al. 1990; HAUZEUR et al. 1989; KOO et al. 1999; SAKAI et al. 2000). These changes that are more frequent in symptomatic lesions (KOO et al. 1999) have been generally attributed to the presence of marrow necrosis itself. However, the demonstration of a higher frequency of reactive changes around necrotic lesions in which fracture recently developed than in fracture-free lesions and in collapsed lesions suggests that reactive changes are transient and could partly result from the epiphyseal fracture (SAKAI et al. 2000).

13.2.6.3.2
Ill-Delimited Pattern

On T1-weighted SE images, the ill-delimited pattern of epiphyseal osteonecrosis lacks a detectable interface and demonstrates ill-delimited extensive decreased signal intensity of the epiphyseal marrow that may also involve the femoral neck (Figs. 13.11, 13.12). The lesion shows intermediate to high signal intensity on T2-weighted images. Careful analysis of the subchondral area is of the utmost importance to detect necrotic tissue, the extent of which is strictly limited to the subchondral area. Subchondral necrotic tissue shows low signal intensity on all sequences including T1-, T2- and enhanced T1-weighted SE images (VANDE BERG et al. 1992, 1993a; LANG et al. 1995; BJORKENGREN et al. 1990). The semiology of this ill-delimited pattern is similar to that observed in spontaneous osteonecrosis of the knee (LECOUVET et al. 1998).

The clear demonstration with MR imaging of two different patterns of epiphyseal osteonecrosis suggests that femoral head osteonecrosis with a non-reparable epiphyseal fracture represents a common end-point common to two different pathways (MITCHELL 1989; VANDE BERG 2001). In one sequence, vascular failure of the bone marrow is the triggering event and leads to marrow infarct with subsequent epiphyseal fracture. In the other

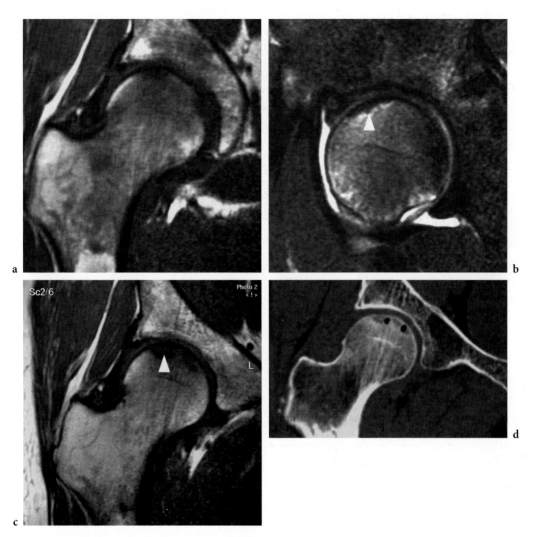

Fig. 13.11a–d. Femoral head osteonecrosis; ill-delimited pattern. **a** Coronal T1-weighted SE image shows diffuse alteration of the signal intensity of the femoral head that extends in the femoral neck. There is no residual fat in the subchondral area and no peripheral rim (diffuse pattern). **b** Sagittal fat-saturated intermediate-weighted FSE image shows high signal intensity in the lesion. In the subchondral area, there is a crescentic and relatively thick low signal intensity area (*arrowhead*) that indicates necrotic tissue. **c** Follow-up coronal T1-weighted SE image obtained 6 months later shows regression of the lesion with residual low signal intensity area near the subchondral bone plate (also visible on the T2-weighted FSE images; not shown). **d** Corresponding coronal CT reformation shows subchondral bone resorption and subchondral vacuum phenomenon that indicates fracture of the subchondral bone plate

sequence, mechanical failure of bone with sub-chondral bone plate fracture is the initial event with subsequent development of necrosis at the interface between the broken osteocartilaginous plate and the epiphysis (MALGHEM and MALDAGUE 1981; GLIMCHER and KENZORA 1979). Mechanical failure of the articular cartilage with rapidly pro-gressive and destructive osteoarthritis can also lead to subchondral bone plate fracture and sub-sequent osteonecrosis (RYU et al. 1997; BOUTRY et al. 2002).

13.2.6.3
Differential Diagnosis of Epiphyseal Osteonecrosis

The segmental pattern of epiphyseal osteonecrosis must be differentiated from other well-delimited lesions including subchondral cysts and sequelae of osteochondritis dissecans. Analysis of the overly-ing cartilage is of the utmost importance: cartilage lesions are generally predominant in subchondral cysts whereas cartilage remains relatively preserved

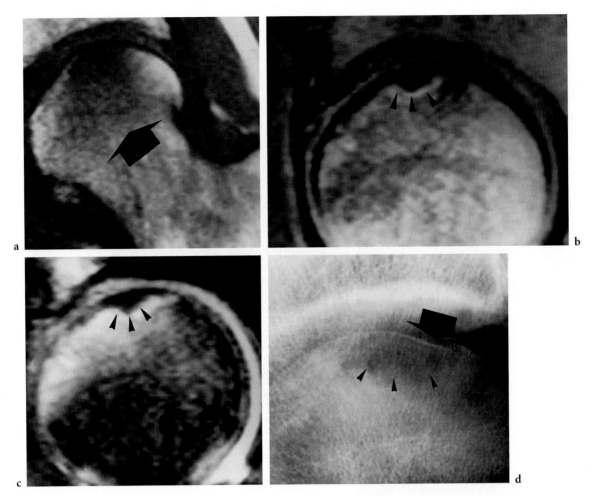

Fig. 13.12a–d. Femoral head osteonecrosis; ill-delimited pattern. **a** Coronal T1-weighted SE MR image of the left hip shows an ill-delimited subchondral area of low signal intensity (*arrow*). **b** On the sagittal T2-weighted FSE MR image and (**c**) fat-saturated intermediate-weighted MR image, the lesion shows high signal intensity. However, a short but thick low signal intensity subchondral area (*arrowheads*) is depicted in the superior pole of the femoral head. This focal subchondral change suggests an irreversible lesion. **d** Radiograph obtained 4 months later shows an abrupt fracture of the subchondral bone plate (*arrow*) and subchondral bone resorption (*arrowheads*). Total hip replacement was performed 9 months later

in non-collapsed osteonecrosis. Cystic changes with high signal intensity on T2-weighted images generally involve the subchondral area in osteoarthritis and involve the interface between the necrotic lesion and the adjacent bone in osteonecrosis.

The ill-delimited pattern of epiphyseal osteonecrosis must be differentiated from lesions that cause edema-like changes in the epiphysis, including transient osteoporosis, the bone marrow edema syndrome, epiphyseal fracture, synovial disease and osteoarthritis. On radiographs and CT images, marked rarefaction of cancellous bone and subchondral bone plate is virtually pathognomonic of transient osteoporosis, whereas evidence of subchondral bone fracture indicates epiphyseal osteonecrosis.

At MR imaging, careful analysis of the subchondral bone plate area on either T2- or enhanced T1-weighted images enables relatively confident differentiation between spontaneously transient and irreversible lesions in the femoral head or condyle (MALDAGUE et al. 1995; LECOUVET et al. 1996).

Previous statements apply to epiphyseal lesions that show normal articular cartilage. If cartilage lesions are present, prognosis is poor and does no more depend on the associated subchondral changes. Degenerative disease of the cartilage shows a wide variety of associated lesions including bone marrow edema. The rapidly progressive form of osteoarthritis can show subchondral necrosis, fracture and edema (RYU et al. 1997; BOUTRY et al. 2002).

13.2.7
Epiphyseal Osteonecrosis in Peculiar Situations

13.2.7.1
Posttraumatic Osteonecrosis

Femoral head osteonecrosis related to displaced sub-capital femoral neck fracture shows the segmental pattern after some time delay. Initially, the fracture causes most marrow and soft tissue changes and the signal of the epiphysis remains normal. Later, the reactive interface appears within the femoral head, at some distance above the fracture level (Fig. 13.13). According to some investigations, fat-suppressed enhanced T1-weighted sequences could enable depiction of the infarcted area (LANG et al. 1993), but, according to our experience, it remains difficult to differentiate normal fatty marrow from avascular fatty marrow.

After hip dislocation, femoral head osteonecrosis is usually not evident and bone marrow edema due to impaction fracture of the femoral head may be a predominant feature. The infarcted area may become more evident at a time delay of 1–3 months after hip dislocation.

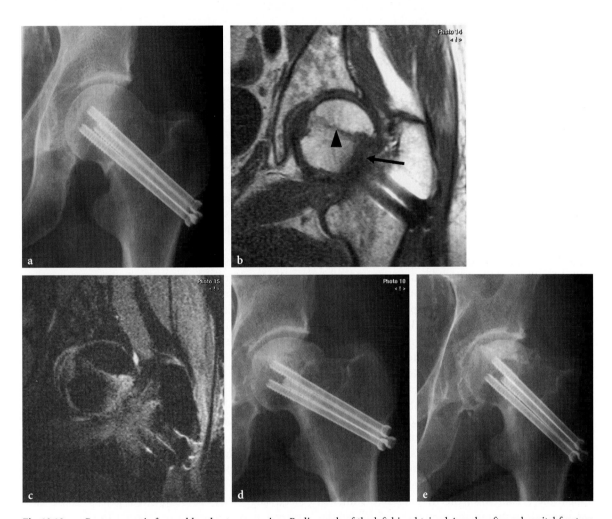

Fig. 13.13a–e. Post-traumatic femoral head osteonecrosis. **a** Radiograph of the left hip obtained 4 weeks after subcapital fracture and osteosynthesis shows a normal femoral head and a vertical fracture of the femoral neck. **b** Coronal T1-weighted SE MR image obtained 2 months after the fracture shows a horizontal line in the femoral head (*arrowhead*) that does not correspond to the fracture (*arrow*). The upper part of the femoral head shows normal high signal intensity and the lower part shows mild decrease in signal intensity. **c** Corresponding STIR image shows fat-like signal intensity in the upper part and mild increase in signal intensity in the lower part of the head. Presence of marrow infiltration in the lower part of the head indicates persistent vascularization whereas absence of edema in the upper part of the epiphysis suggests impaired perfusion. **d** Follow-up radiograph obtained 1 year later shows flattening of the femoral head and subtle sclerosis of its upper pole. **e** Follow-up radiograph obtained 10 years later, before total hip replacement, shows progressive flattening of the femoral head and narrowing of the joint space

13.2.7.2
Osteonecrosis in Patient with Systemic Marrow Diseases

Femoral head osteonecrosis developing in patients with marrow disease including chronic anemia (Sickle-cell disease, thalassemia) or marrow infiltration (Gaucher disease) frequently show the bone marrow edema syndrome, even in the lack of epiphyseal fracture. Most likely, the infarct develops in a red-marrow equivalent area (RAO et al. 1986; BONNEROT et al. 1994; CREMIN et al. 1990; VANDE BERG et al. 1993b) and not in fatty marrow. At a later stage, several other patterns will develop that differ from those observed in yellow marrow infarcts (VANDE BERG et al. 1993b).

13.3
Transient Osteoporosis – the "Bone Marrow Edema Syndrome"

13.3.1
Definitions

Transient osteoporosis is an uncommon epiphyseal disorder that can be recognized on plain radiographs and CT images based on non-specific radiological features in a patient with spontaneous hip pain (Fig. 13.14). The unique feature typical for this disease is the spontaneous time course of the clinical and radiographic changes. Hip pain begins spontaneously, may be rapid or gradual in onset and is aggravated by weight bearing. Then, pain progressively decreases until complete regression by 6–12 months after the onset, without residual sequelae. Initial radiographs are normal, but marked osteoporosis of the femoral head with preserved joint space is seen on follow-up radiographs obtained several weeks after symptoms onset. Radionuclide studies with bone-seeking agents reveal abnormal accumulation of isotope in the femoral head. Follow-up radiographs demonstrate a return to a normal appearance. Therefore, the diagnosis of transient osteoporosis remains presumptive, until demonstration of complete resolution of clinical and radiological changes.

The "bone marrow edema syndrome" is a sign detected at MR imaging characterized by altered marrow signal intensity within the epiphysis suggestive of medullary infiltration by interstitial edema. In this bone marrow edema syndrome, there is no evidence of a reactive interface that is considered specific for osteonecrosis (MITCHELL et al. 1987; HAYES et al. 1993) at MR imaging. Transient osteoporosis is only one of the conditions that show the bone marrow edema syndrome on MR images. By analogy with transient osteoporosis, the term "transient bone marrow edema" may be used to characterize a femoral head lesion in which marrow edema is seen on MR images and spontaneously vanishes at follow-up MR investigation.

13.3.2
Epidemiology

Epidemiological data on transient osteoporosis and transient bone marrow edema are sparse. Transient osteoporosis typically involves middle-aged male patients, although the condition was initially described in women during the third trimester of pregnancy. In a series of 60 patients with transient bone marrow edema at MR imaging, there were 37 male and 23 female patients with a mean age of 49 and 48 years, respectively (VANDE BERG et al. 1999).

In the same series, about half of the lesions was observed in association with various medical conditions including pregnancy, glucocorticoid therapy, alcohol abuse, and metabolic bone diseases (VANDE BERG et al. 1999). The small number of patients with each disorder and the lack of systematic assessment for metabolic bone disease in all patients do not allow to draw any conclusion on the association between these medical conditions and the bone marrow edema syndrome.

13.3.3
Pathophysiology, Histology and Histomorphometry

The pathophysiology of transient osteoporosis remains unknown. Links with ischemia, fractures and reflex sympathetic dystrophy syndrome have been suggested. Several investigators noted that transient osteoporosis on plain films is observed in some but not all cases of bone marrow edema syndrome at MR imaging. Whether this discrepancy between the radiological and MR findings is due to time changes in the same conditions, to relative insensitivity of conventional radiographs to osteopenia or really to different diseases remains unknown.

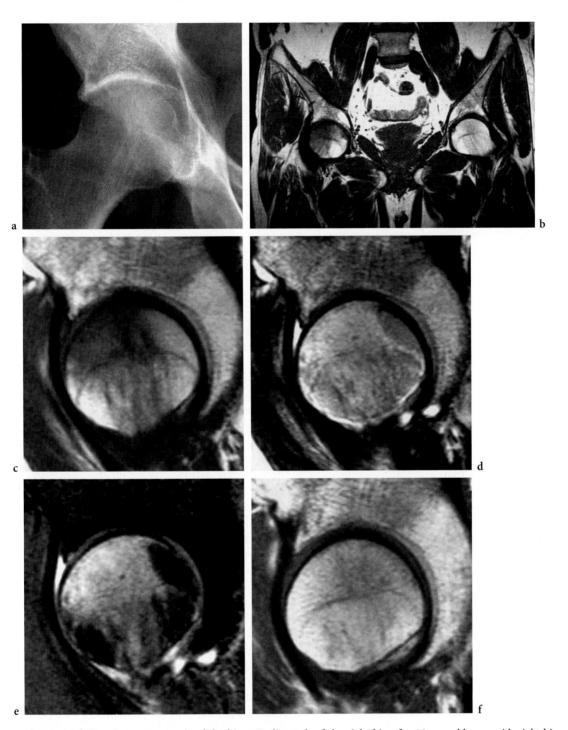

Fig. 13.14a–f. Transient osteoporosis of the hip. **a** Radiograph of the right hip of a 46-year-old man with right hip pain of 3 months duration shows marked rarefaction of the trabecular and subchondral bone. **b** Comparative coronal T1-weighted MR image shows decreased signal intensity in the right femoral head. There is no clear delineation of the lesion and the physis should not be confused with an interface. **c** Sagittal T1-weighted SE MR image of the right femoral head shows ill-delimited marrow infiltration without additional changes. **d** Corresponding sagittal T2-weighted FSE MR image shows high signal intensity in the corresponding area. **e** Fat-saturated intermediate-weighted SE image shows high signal intensity in the femoral head with mild joint effusion. The articular joint space is preserved. **f** Follow-up MR image obtained 5 months later shows almost complete normalization of the signal intensity of the femoral head

At histology, the most characteristic feature of bone marrow edema syndrome of the femoral head is focal area of thin and disconnected bone trabeculae covered by osteoid seams and active osteoblast with formation of irregular woven bone (microcallus) (YAMAMOTO et al. 1999). The surrounding bone marrow tissue shows edematous changes and mild fibrosis, frequently associated with fat cell destruction, vascular congestion and/or interstitial hemorrhage. No osteonecrotic region is observed in either the bone trabeculae or the bone marrow tissue. In addition to increased osteoid volume, a decreased maximal hydroxyl apatite content and a shift to undermineralized bone can be found by mineral densitometry (PLENK et al. 1997).

13.3.4
Natural History

Transient osteoporosis is by definition a transient condition characterized by a return to complete normal clinical and radiological status within 6–12 months.

The "bone marrow edema" syndrome shows a more variable course, depending on the underlying cause that include transient osteoporosis of the hip, transient bone marrow edema of the hip, epiphyseal stress fracture, osteoarthritis and epiphyseal osteonecrosis (VANDE BERG et al. 1993a, 1994; MITCHELL et al. 1987; TURNER et al. 1989; THICKMAN et al. 1986; HAYES et al. 1993; BLOEM 1988; WILSON et al. 1988; HIGER et al. 1989; RAFII et al. 1997; MITCHELL and KRESSEL 1988)). The distinction between these conditions is crucial because of their considerable differences in treatment and prognosis (CONWAY et al. 1996). Actually, the first three conditions are self-limited and generally resolve with conservative treatment. On the contrary, osteoarthritis and epiphyseal osteonecrosis are not reversible and can lead to joint failure (SHIMIZU et al. 1994; LAFFORGUE et al. 1993; TAKATORI et al. 1993).

13.3.5
Classification Systems and Treatment

There is no available classification system for transient osteoporosis or bone marrow edema syndrome. Initially, the bone marrow edema syndrome was included in the ARCO classification system for femoral head osteonecrosis. This concept is more and more disputed mainly because the bone marrow edema syndrome was never shown to convert to a non-collapsed marrow infarct in a femoral head (KIM et al. 2000).

Pain control is usually achieved by non-steroidal analgesics and partial weight-bearing should be recommended. Several surgical procedures have been tried with excellent success. Core decompression consistently provides a rapid relief of pain (CALVO et al. 2000). Whether, core decompression is able to alter the natural history of transient osteoporosis remains debated. In a unique investigation comparing medical treatment versus core decompression in patients with the bone marrow edema syndrome, more rapid resolution of symptoms after core decompression than with conservative treatment was shown, without any effect on the final outcome.

13.3.6
Radiographs of Transient Osteoporosis and Bone Marrow Edema Syndrome

Transient osteoporosis of the femoral head is characterized by the presence of trabecular bone resorption that involves a segment of or the entire femoral head. On radiographs, the subchondral bone plate may focally become indistinct (Fig. 13.14). However, the joint space remains normal, which differentiates TO from septic arthritis although the joint space may remain normal in tuberculous arthritis. Osteophytes and marginal erosions are absent.

The radiographic features observed in transient bone marrow edema of the hip are variable. In a series of 60 patients with transient bone marrow edema at MR imaging, radiographs obtained at the diagnosis were normal ($n=20$), showed osteoporosis ($n=22$), mild sclerosis ($n=7$) or mixed osteoporosis and sclerosis ($n=11$). The mean time delay between onset of symptoms and diagnosis was longer in patients with mild sclerosis than in patients with osteoporosis or normal radiographs, suggesting an evolving process over time (VANDE BERG et al. 1999).

The radiographic features observed in the bone marrow edema syndrome seen on MR images depend on the underlying cause. In the bone marrow edema syndrome associated with osteoarthritis, focal joint space narrowing can be seen on radiographs, mainly if comparative off-lateral views are obtained. In the bone marrow edema syndrome associated with epiphyseal osteonecrosis, epiphyseal collapse or osteochondral fracture can be seen on radiographs, mainly if antero-posterior radiographs are taken with an ascending X-ray beam on the limb in external rotation.

13.3.7
MR Imaging of the Bone Marrow Edema Syndrome

On T1-weighted MR images, the bone marrow edema syndrome of the femoral head is characterized by an ill-delimited area of decreased signal intensity that consistently involves the femoral head and predominates in the subchondral area, frequently in the anterosuperior segment of the femoral head. The extent of the marrow changes is variable both in the head and in the cervical region although epiphyseal involvement is the rule. Rarely, subtle marrow changes can be detected in the posterior aspect of the acetabulum.

On T2-weighted SE images, signal of the lesions becomes equivalent or higher than that of adjacent normal fatty marrow. The lesion lacks well-delimited lesions or margins (MITCHELL et al. 1987; HAYES et al. 1993). On fat-saturated intermediate-weighted FSE images, the signal of the lesion is elevated and homogeneous. On T1-weighted SE images obtained after intravenous contrast material injection, enhancement of the lesion signal is homogeneous. Joint effusion may be present or absent and infiltration of the adjacent muscles has occasionally been reported

13.3.8
Differential Diagnosis

Careful analysis of the articular cartilage, the subchondral bone plate and the subchondral marrow on high-resolution coronal and sagittal T2-weighted FSE images or fat-saturated intermediate-weighted FSE images is mandatory for the differential diagnosis of the bone marrow edema syndrome. Actually, the bone marrow edema syndrome can be observed in numerous conditions, some of which are spontaneously reversible (transient osteoporosis, transient bone marrow edema, and epiphyseal stress fracture) or irreversible (osteoarthritis, femoral head osteonecrosis).

13.3.8.1
Transient Osteoporosis – Transient Marrow Edema–Femoral Head Insufficiency Fracture

The bone marrow edema syndrome can be the unique changes, without any additional subchondral feature. In this case, the bone marrow edema syndrome must be considered to be idiopathic. In our experience, transient osteoporosis as seen on radiographs lacks additional subchondral changes or may show subchondral bands on MR images. Other investigators have noted subchondral changes in all cases of transient osteoporosis (MIYANISHI et al. 2001).

Several features orientate toward the diagnosis of insufficiency fracture, although they can also be observed in transient osteoporosis. Thin low signal-intensity bands or more globular speckled areas of low signal intensity can be seen within the diffuse marrow changes on T2- or enhanced T1-weighted SE images near the subchondral bone area. The linear areas are running parallel to the subchondral bone plate at the variable distance from the epiphyseal surface. These bands can occasionally be more prominent on T2-weighted or fat saturated intermediate weighted spin echo images than on T1-weighted images in opposition to the reactive interface of marrow infarct, which is generally best depicted on T1-weighted images. These bands are generally located near the subchondral plate, they do not show the double line sign on T2-weighted spin echo images and they do not delineate a large marrow area (YAMAMOTO et al. 2001).

Subtle focal deformity of the subchondral bone plane is occasionally visible in the anterosuperior or lateral aspects of the femoral head, just below the acetabular roof margin. The focal and subtle depression of the subchondral bone plate remains limited and is not as abrupt or as marked than fracture in epiphyseal osteonecrosis. They can be better seen on intermediate-weighted SE images or contrast enhanced T1-weighted SE images probably due to a high signal contrast between marrow and cartilage. On T2-weighted SE images, there is no high signal intensity line underneath this depression as observed in subchondral cleft in osteonecrosis.

13.3.8.2
Femoral Head Osteonecrosis

Femoral head osteonecrosis may show a diffuse pattern on T1-weighted SE MR images. Detection and determination of the size of low signal intensity subchondral areas on either T2-weighted images, fat-saturated intermediate-weighted or enhanced T1-weighted SE images help to differentiate osteonecrosis from transient lesions. A low signal intensity subchondral area with a thickness equal or superior to 4 mm or with a length equal or superior to

12.5 mm on T2-weighted images suggested an irreversible lesion with a specificity superior to 92% in a series of 72 femoral head lesions that included 15 irreversible osteonecrosis. Magnitude of epiphyseal contour deformity also helped to recognize irreversible lesions, frank deformity being more frequently associated with irreversible than transient lesions. However, reproducibility of determination of degree of deformity was fair. However, not all irreversible lesions correspond to osteonecrosis or osteoarthritis. Actually, in this series of 15 irreversible femoral head lesions that showed a bone marrow edema syndrome on initial MR investigation without sign of cartilage lesions, only nine showed epiphyseal

osteonecrosis at follow-up investigations. Six lesions showed small subchondral irregularities at follow-up MR that were clinically well tolerated. Therefore there seems to be a continuum between totally reversible lesions, lesions with small residual subchondral sequelae and epiphyseal collapse or osteonecrosis.

13.3.8.3
Osteoarthritis

Osteoarthritis can be associated with bone marrow edema (Figs. 13.15). Marrow changes can be limited

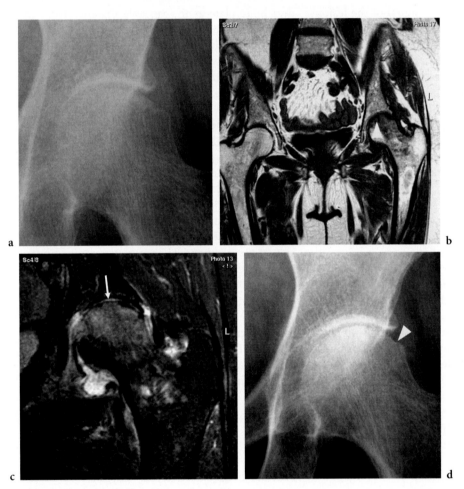

Fig. 13.15a–d. Rapidly destructive osteoarthritis. **a** Radiograph of the left hip of a 65-year-old man with recent onset left hip pain shows moderate joint space narrowing joint space and normal bone structure. **b** Coronal T1-weighted SE MR images show ill-delimited femoral head marrow infiltration without additional subchondral changes (*arrowhead*). (**c**) Coronal fat-saturated intermediate-weighted MR image shows homogeneous increase in signal intensity of the epiphyseal marrow with limited subchondral bone changes. However, the cartilage shows increased signal intensity (*white arrow*). Because of the presence of cartilage alteration, a transient lesion should no more be considered. **d** Follow-up radiograph obtained 2 months later shows progression of joint space narrowing and femoral head collapse (*arrowhead*). This time course of joint space changes indicates a rapidly progressive form of osteoarthritis, a case in which the pattern of marrow involvement at MR imaging lacks prognostic significance

to the subchondral area, near the cartilage lesion. These changes frequently involve the anterosuperior pole of the femoral head and are best seen on sagittal images. Presence of small cyst-like changes in the acetabulum further orientates toward osteoarthritis. Extensive edema in the head and neck appears to be associated with a rapid and destructive form of osteoarthritis (BOUTRY et al. 2002; SUGANO et al. 2001; WATANABE et al. 2002).

13.3.9
Features Observed on Follow-Up MR Investigations

In difficult cases, follow-up MR investigations obtained a few months after the initial study may contribute to assess the outcome of the lesion (Fig. 13.16). In the bone marrow edema syndrome associated with osteoarthritis or osteonecrosis, the

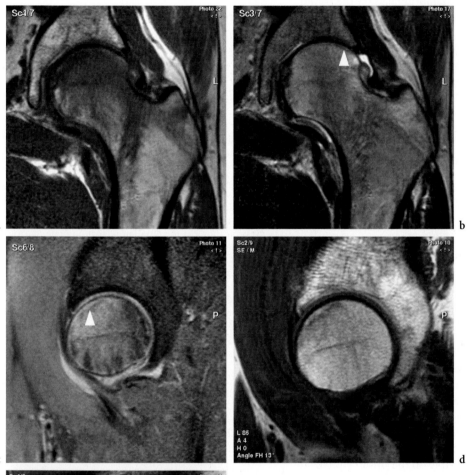

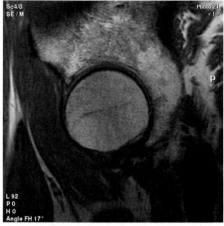

Fig. 13.16a–e. Insufficiency stress fracture of the femoral head. a Coronal T1-weighted MR image of the left hip shows ill-delimited low signal intensity area without peripheral rim. b Corresponding T2-weighted FSE MR image shows high signal intensity within the lesion. A subtle subchondral line (*arrowhead*) indicates a stress fracture. c Corresponding sagittal fat-saturated intermediate-weighted FSE MR image shows marrow infiltration without clear delineation and a low signal intensity line (*arrowhead*). d Follow-up MR image obtained 6 months later shows almost complete normalization of the signal intensity of the lesion with only small residual subchondral changes. In opposition to the interface of osteonecrosis, this line does not completely delineate a marrow area, it is almost adjacent to the subchondral bone plate and does not migrate overtime. e Follow-up MR image obtained 18 months after the initial study shows complete normalization of the signal

bone marrow edema may regress at follow-up but focal subchondral changes persist.

In transient osteoporosis and transient bone marrow edema of the hip, follow up MR investigations demonstrate a complete return to normal marrow appearance within a range of time delay that varies from 3 to 12 months. Generally, by 3 months follow-up, a significant change in marrow alteration distribution has occurred. If marrow alteration completely involved the femoral head on the initial MR study, the amplitude of the marrow infiltration decreases at follow-up MR investigation. If marrow signal intensity change was initially focal (generally in the anterosuperior segment of the femoral head), it usually regresses in that area and migrates in the posterior aspect of the femoral head. Rarely subtle marrow change also develops in the acetabular region. Occasionally, bone marrow edema may regress more rapidly than additional findings and low signal intensity bands in the subchondral area may transiently become prominent.

13.4
Practical Recommendations

The workup of a symptomatic hip with a suspected femoral head lesion begins with a complete radiographic examination with multiple views of the joint to detect subchondral bone fractures or changes in epiphyseal bone architecture. In the setting of a patient with a primary epiphyseal disorder with a preserved joint space, the initial radiographic examination may clearly demonstrate epiphyseal osteonecrosis, may suggest transient osteoporosis or is considered non contributive. Repeat radiographs obtained 4–6 weeks later can show more advanced lesions that were not visible on the initial equivocal plain films including subchondral bone plate fracture (epiphyseal osteonecrosis), marked rarefaction of epiphyseal bone (transient osteoporosis) or focal joint space narrowing (rapidly progressive osteoarthritis). This cost-effective approach is justified as long as no urgent diagnosis is needed or no treatment of proven efficacy can be offered to the patient.

If a definite diagnosis is urged at the initial presentation or if repeated radiographs remain normal or equivocal, MR imaging is the procedure of choice because it provides accurate depiction of femoral head lesions. It should be emphasized that MR images should never be interpreted without the corresponding radiographs that can best depict degenerative disease of the cartilage or subchondral bone fracture. Coronal comparative T1-weighted SE images best depict marrow changes and enable classification between ill-delimited and well-delimited lesions. Sagittal T2-weighted FSE or fat-saturated intermediate-weighted images best depict subchondral fracture in femoral head osteonecrosis.

References

Beltran J et al (1988) Femoral head avascular necrosis: MR imaging with clinical-pathologic and radionuclide correlation. Radiology 166:215–220

Bjorkengren AG et al (1990) Spontaneous osteonecrosis of the knee: value of MR imaging in determining prognosis. AJR 154:331–336

Bloem JL (1988) Transient osteoporosis of the hip: MR imaging. Radiology 167:753–755

Bonnerot V et al (1994) Gadolinium-DOTA enhanced MRI of painful osseous crises in children with sickle cell anemia. Pediatr Radiol 24:92–95

Boutry N et al (2002) Rapidly destructive osteoarthritis of the hip: MR imaging findings. AJR 179:657–663

Calvo E, Fernandez-Yruegas D, Alvarez L (2000) Core decompression shortens the duration of pain in bone marrow oedema syndrome. Int Orthop 24:88–91

Chan TW et al (1991) MRI appearance of femoral head osteonecrosis following core decompression and bone grafting. Skeletal Radiol 20:103–107

Chang CC, Greenspan A, Gerschwin ME (1993) Osteonecrosis: current perspectives on pathogenesis and treatment. Semin Arthritis Rheumat 23:47–69

Coleman BG et al (1988) Radiographically negative avascular necrosis: detection with MR imaging. Radiology 168:525–528

Conway WF, Totty WG, McEnery KW (1996) CT and MR imaging of the hip. Radiology 198:297–307

Cremin BJ, Davey H, Goldblatt J (1990) Skeletal complications of type I Gaucher disease: the magnetic resonance features. Clin Radiol 41:244–247

Duda SH et al (1993) The double-line sign of osteonecrosis: evaluation on chemical shift MR images. Eur J Radiol 16:233–238

Ehman RL et al (1996) Magnetic resonance. Radiology 198:920–926

Ficat RP (1985) Idiopathic bone necrosis of the femoral head. Early diagnosis and treatment. J Bone Joint Surg Br 67:3–9

Glimcher MJ, Kenzora JE (1979) Nicolas Andry award. The biology of osteonecrosis of the human femoral head and its clinical implications. 1. Tissue biology. Clin Orthop 138:284–309

Glimcher MJ, Kenzora JE (1979) The biology of osteonecrosis of the human femoral head and its clinical implications. III. Discussion of the etiology and genesis of the pathological sequelae; comments on treatment. Clin Orthop 140:273–312

Hauzeur JP et al (1989) The diagnostic value of magnetic resonance imaging in non- traumatic osteonecrosis of the femoral head. J Bone Joint Surg Am 71:641–649

Hayes CW, Conway WF, Daniel WW (1993) MR imaging of bone marrow edema pattern: transient osteoporosis, transient bone marrow edema syndrome, or osteonecrosis. Radiographics 13:1001–1011

Higer HP et al (1989) Transitorische osteoporose oder Femurkopfnekrose? Frühdiagnose mit der MRT. Fortschr Röntgenstr 150:407–412

Huang GS et al (2003) MR imaging of bone marrow edema and joint effusion in patients with osteonecrosis of the femoral head: relationship to pain. AJR 181:545–549

Iida S et al (2000) Correlation between bone marrow edema and collapse of the femoral head in steroid-induced osteonecrosis. AJR 174:735–743

Ito H, Kaneda K, Matsuno T (1999) Osteonecrosis of the femoral head. J Bone Joint Surg 81B:969–974

Jergesen HE et al (1990) Histologic correlation in magnetic resonance imaging of femoral head osteonecrosis. Clin Orthop 253:150–163

Jones JP (1993) Osteonecrosis. Arthritis and allied conditions. Lea and Febiger, Philadelphia, pp 1677–1696

Kim YM, Oh HC, Kim HJ (2000) The pattern of bone marrow oedema on MRI in osteonecrosis of the femoral head. J Bone Joint Surg Br 82:837–841

Koo KH et al (1999) Bone marrow edema and associated pain in early stage osteonecrosis of the femoral head: prospective study with serial MR images. Radiology 213:715–722

Kopecky KK et al (1991) Apparent avascular necrosis of the hip: appearance and spontaneous resolution of MR findings in renal allograft recipients. Radiology 179:523–527

Koval KJ (2002) Orthopaedic knowledge update. Am Acad Orthop Surg 17:421–425

Kubo T et al (2000) Histological findings of bone marrow edema pattern on MRI in osteonecrosis of the femoral head. J Orthop Sci 5:520–523

Lafforgue P et al (1993) Early-stage avascular necrosis of the femoral head: MR imaging for prognosis in 31 cases with at least 2 years of follow-up. Radiology 187:199–204

Lang P et al (1988) Avascular necrosis of the femoral head: high-field-strength MR imaging with histologic correlation. Radiology 169:517–524

Lang P et al (1993) Acute fracture of the femoral neck: assessment of femoral head perfusion with gadopentetate dimeglumine-enhanced MR imaging. AJR 160:335–341

Lang P et al (1995) Spontaneous osteonecrosis of the knee joint: MRT compared to CT, scintigraphy and histology. Rofo Fortschr Rontgenstr 162:469–477

Lecouvet FE et al (1996) Nontraumatic bone marrow edema of the femoral condyles: natural history and prognostic value of initial MR findings. Radiology 201:431

Lecouvet FE et al (1998) Early irreversible osteonecrosis versus transient lesions of the femoral condyles: prognostic value of subchondral bone and marrow changes on MR imaging. AJR 170:71–77

Lieberman JR (2004) Core decompression for osteonecrosis of the hip. Clin Orthop 418:29–33

Lieberman JR et al (2002) Osteonecrosis of the hip: management in the twenty-first century. J Bone Joint Surg 84A:834–853

Maldague BE et al (1995) Avascular necrosis, transient osteoporosis, and presumed stress fractures of the femoral head: imaging approach and differential diagnosis. In: Baert AL, Grenier P, Willi UV, Bloem JL, editors. Musculo-

skeletal imaging: an update. Springer, Berlin Heidelberg New York, pp 45–56

Malghem J, Maldague B (1981) Radiologic aspects of epiphyseal necrosis and pathogenetic implications. Acta Orthop Belg 47:200–224

Mankin HJ (1992) Nontraumatic necrosis of bone (osteonecrosis). N Engl J Med 326:1473–1479

Markisz JA et al (1987) Segmental patterns of avascular necrosis of the femoral heads: early detection with MR imaging. Radiology 162:717–720

Mitchell DG (1989) Using MR imaging to probe the pathophysiology of osteonecrosis. Radiology 171:25–26

Mitchell DG, Kressel HY (1988) MR imaging of early avascular necrosis. Radiology 169:281–282

Mitchell DG et al (1987) Femoral head avascular necrosis: correlation of MR imaging, radiographic staging, radionuclide imaging, and clinical findings. Radiology 162:709–715

Miyanishi K et al (2001) Subchondral changes in transient osteoporosis of the hip. Skeletal Radiol 30:255–261

Mulliken BD et al (1994) Prevalence of previously undetected osteonecrosis of the femoral head in renal transplant recipients. Radiology 192:831–834

Musso ES et al (1986) Results of conservative management of osteonecrosis of the femoral head. A retrospective review. Clin Orthop 207:209–215

Neuhold A et al (1993) Bone marrow edema - an early form of femur head necrosis. Rofo Fortschr Rontgenstr 159:120–125

Patterson RJ, Bickel WH, Dahlin DC (1964) Idiopathic avascular necrosis of the head of the femur. A study of fifty-two cases. J Bone Joint Surg Am 46:267–282

Plenk H et al (1997) Histomorphology and bone morphometry of the bone marrow edema syndrome of the hip. Clin Orthop Rel Res 334:73–84

Rafii M et al (1997) Insufficiency fracture of the femoral head: MR imaging in three patients. AJR 168:159–163

Rao VM et al (1986) Painful sickle cell crisis: bone marrow patterns observed with MR imaging (published erratum appears in Radiology 1987, 162:289). Radiology 161:211–215

Robbins SL, Cotran RS, Kumar V (1984a) Cellular injury and adaptation. In: Robbins SL, Cotran RS, Kumar V (eds) Pathologic basis of disease. Saunders, Philadelphia, pp 1–39

Robbins SL, Cotran RS, Kumar V (1984b) Fluid and hemodynamic derangements. In: Robbins SL, Cotran RS, Kumar V (eds) Pathologic basis of disease. Saunders, Philadephia, pp 85–117

Ryu KN et al (1997) Ischemic necrosis of the entire femoral head and rapidly destructive hip disease: potential causative relationship. Skeletal Radiol 26:143–149

Sakai T et al (2000) MR findings of necrotic lesions and the extralesional area of osteonecrosis of the femoral head. Skeletal Radiol 29:133–141

Shimizu K et al (1994) Prediction of collapse with magnetic resonance imaging of avascular necrosis of the femoral head. J Bone Joint Surg Am 76:215–223

Steinberg ME, Hayken GD, Steinberg DR (1995) A quantitative system for staging avascular necrosis. J Bone Joint Surg Br 77:34–41

Stevens K et al (2003) Subchondral fractures in osteonecrosis of the femoral head: comparison of radiography, CT, and MR imaging. AJR 180:363–368

Sugano N et al (1992) Rotational osteotomy for non-traumatic avascular necrosis of the femoral head. J Bone Joint Surg Br 74:734–739

Sugano N et al (2001) Early MRI findings of rapidly destructive coxopathy. Magn Reson Imaging 19:47–50

Sugimoto H, Tanaka O, Ohsawa T (1989) MR imaging of femoral head avascular necrosis with STIR sequence. Nippon Igaku Hoshasen Gakkai Zasshi 49:1067–1069

Sweet DE, Madewell JE (1988) Pathogenesis of osteonecrosis. In: Resnick D (ed) Diagnosis of bone and joint disorders. Saunders, Philadelphia, pp 3188–3237

Takatori Y et al (1993) Avascular necrosis of the femoral head. Natural history and magnetic resonance imaging. J Bone Joint Surg Br 75:217–221

Tehranzadeh J, Ter Oganesyan RR, Steinbach LS (2004) Musculoskeletal disorders associated with HIV infection and AIDS, part I. Infectious musculoskeletal conditions. Skeletal Radiol 33:249–259

Tervonen O et al (1992) Clinically occult avascular necrosis of the hip: prevalence in an asymptomatic population at risk. Radiology 182:845–847

Thickman D et al (1986) Magnetic resonance imaging of avascular necrosis of the femoral head. Skeletal Radiol 15:133–140

Turner DA et al (1989) Femoral capital osteonecrosis: MR finding of diffuse marrow abnormalities without focal lesions. Radiology 171:135–140

Vande Berg BC et al (1992) Avascular necrosis of the hip: comparison of contrast-enhanced and nonenhanced MR imaging with histologic correlation. Radiology 182:445–450

Vande Berg BC et al (1993a) MR imaging of avascular necrosis and transient marrow edema of the femoral head. Radiographics 13:501–520

Vande Berg BC et al (1993b) Apparent focal bone marrow ischemia in patients with marrow disorders: MR studies. J Comput Assist Tomogr 17:792–797

Vande Berg BC et al (1994) Transient epiphyseal lesions in renal transplant recipients: presumed insufficiency stress fractures. Radiology 191:403–407

Vande Berg BC et al (1999) Idiopathic bone marrow edema lesions of the femoral head: predictive value of MR imaging findings. Radiology 212:527–535

Vande Berg BC et al (2001) Magnetic resonance imaging and differential diagnosis of epiphyseal osteonecrosis. Semin Musculoskelet Radiol 5:57–67

Watanabe W, Itoi E, Yamada S (2002) Early MRI findings of rapidly destructive coxarthrosis. Skeletal Radiol 31:35–38

Wilson AJ et al (1988) Transient osteoporosis: transient bone marrow edema? Radiology 167:757–760

Yamamoto T et al (1999) A clinicopathologic study of transient osteoporosis of the hip. Skeletal Radiol 28:621–627

Yamamoto T, Schneider R, Bullough PG (2001) Subchondral insufficiency fracture of the femoral head: histopathologic correlation with MRI. Skeletal Radiol 30:247–254

Zizic TM, Hungerford DS (1985) Avascular necrosis of bone. In: Kelly WN, Harris ED, Ruddy S, Sledge CB (eds) Textbook of rheumatology. Saunders, Philadelphia, pp 1689–1710

14 Bony Trauma 1: Pelvic Ring

Philip Hughes

CONTENTS

14.1
Introduction

Major pelvic ring and acetabular fractures are predominantly high energy injuries and consequently are not infrequently associated with injury to the pelvic viscera and vascular structures. Mortality and morbidity related to these injuries primarily results from haemorrhage, the outcomes have however improved through the use of external fixation devices and other compression devices. Recognition of the type and severity of injuries, particularly those involving the pelvic ring, is essential to the application of corrective forces during external or internal fixation techniques. The pattern and severity of injury also predict the probability of pelvic

P. HUGHES, MD
Consultant Radiologist, X-Ray Department West, Derriford Hospital, Derriford Road, Plymouth, PL6 8DH, UK

haemorrhage and visceral injury which can prove influential when assessing the likely site of haemorrhage and the appropriateness of further cross-sectional imaging or operative intervention.

Acetabular fractures can be classified into simple and complex patterns which require a thorough understanding of the regional anatomy and the associated radiological correlates. The patterns of fracture determine the operative approach and although predominantly determined by plain film views (AP and Judet obliques) are often supplemented by CT (2D, MPR and 3D surface reconstructions). CT is also required to identify intra-articular fragments that are not usually identifiable on plain films and secondly to assess postoperative alignment of articular surfaces. MR may also be performed following femoral head dislocations or acetabular fracture-dislocations where viability of the femoral head is questioned and would alter management.

The final group exhibiting a distinctive pattern of pelvic fractures to be considered include avulsion injuries which are encountered predominantly in individuals following sporting activity and are more frequent in the immature skeleton. Stress fractures and pathological fractures of the pelvis are covered in Chaps. 16 and 22, respectively.

14.2
Pelvic Ring Fractures

14.2.1
Anatomy

The pelvic ring comprises the sacrum posteriorly and paired innominate bones, each formed by the bony fusion of the ilium, ischium and pubic bones, each having evolved from independent ossification centres. The sacrum and innominate bones meet at the sacroiliac articulations, and the pubic bones at the fibrous symphysis pubis. The integrity of the bony ring is preserved by ligaments, an appreciation of which is essential to the understanding of patterns of injury and the assessment of stability of injured pelvic ring.

Anteriorly the symphysis is supported predominantly by the superior symphyseal ligaments (Fig. 14.1a). Posteriorly the sacroiliac joints are stabilised by the anterior and posterior sacroiliac ligaments (Fig. 14.1b). The posterior ligaments are amongst the strongest ligaments in the body, running from the posterior inferior and superior iliac spines to the sacral ridge. The superficial component of the posterior sacroiliac ligament runs inferiorly to blend with the sacrotuberous ligaments. The sacrospinous and sacroiliac ligaments support the pelvic floor and oppose the external rotation of the lilac blade. The iliolumbar ligaments extend from the transverse processes of the lower lumbar vertebrae to the superficial aspect of the anterior sacroiliac ligaments and can avulse transverse processes in association with pelvic fractures.

Important arterial structures vulnerable to injury include the superior gluteal artery in the sciatic notch which may be disrupted by shearing forces exerted during sacroiliac joint diastasis. The obturator and pudendal arteries are not uncommonly injured during lateral compression injuries resulting in comminution of the anterior pubic arch. Other commonly injured vessels include the median and lateral sacral, and iliolumbar arteries.

Urogenital injuries are also commonly associated with pelvic ring injury consequent upon the close association of the urethra and symphysis and pubic rami and bladder. Anterior compression forces are more commonly responsible for urethral injury, usually affecting the fixed membranous portion of the urethra.

14.2.2
Techniques

The AP pelvic radiograph is one of the three basic radiographs performed as part of the ATLS protocol in the setting of major trauma, the other radiographs including views of the cervical spine and chest. The AP views demonstrate the majority of pelvic fractures, excepting intra-articular fragments (RESNIK et al. 1992). The pelvic inlet and outlet views supplement the AP view in pelvic ring fractures, the former demonstrating rotation of the pelvis, additional fractures of the pubic rami and compression fractures of the sacral margins while the latter assesses craniocaudal displacement particularly in vertical shear injuries. The widespread use of CT in trauma cases in general and its invariable use in pelvic fractures to assess both severity and requirement for operative fixation have essentially eliminated the requirement for inlet and outlet views. CT technique will vary with the type of scanner used but should include section thicknesses between 2.5–5.0 mm. The mAs can be reduced when the scan is purely performed for the purposes of bony anatomy from the standard around 120 mAs to 70 mAs.

14.2.3
Classification of Pelvic Fractures

The classification of pelvic fractures has changed during the last two decades to more accurately reflect the mechanism of injury and quantify the degree of instability. Malgaine, straddle and open-book fractures, used as descriptive terms prior to the 1980s in most standard texts, failed to provide

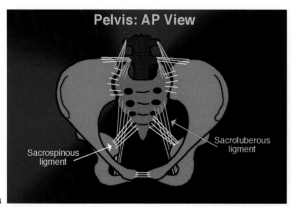

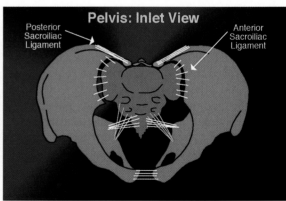

a   b

Fig. 14.1. a AP view of pelvic ligaments and (**b**) pelvic inlet perspective demonstrating anterior and posterior sacroiliac ligaments

precise detail relating to pelvic injury and did not emphasise the importance of the unseen ligamentous structures.

Penall et al. (1980) first described the correlation between the pattern of fracture and the direction of the applied traumatic force. They proposed the forced vector classification of pelvic fractures, identifying anteroposterior compression (AP), lateral compression (LC) and vertical shear as pure bred forces responsible for specific patterns of injury. Tile (1984) subsequently documented the high risk of pelvic haemorrhage particularly in injuries to the posterior pelvis and the advantage of this systematic classification when applying external fixation devices.

Young et al. (1986) further refined the classification identifying a constant progression or pattern to pelvic injury within each vector group which was both easily remembered and more importantly accurately reflected the degree of instability based predominantly on the imaging appearances. Later studies also linked probability of pelvic haemorrhage and bladder injury to the pattern of fracture allowing an element of risk stratification to be undertaken in relation to haemodynamically unstable patients with pelvic injury (Ben-Menachem et al. 1991).

14.2.4
Force Vector Classification of Pelvic Ring Injury

There are three primary vectors responsible for pelvic injuries, Young et al. (1986) identified an LC pattern in 57% of patients, AP compression in 15% and a vertical shear pattern in 7%. The remainder, 22%, demonstrated hybrid features as a result of oblique or combined multidirectional forces which are referred to as 'complex' fractures.

14.2.4.1
Anteroposterior Compression Injuries

These injuries are commonly the result of head on road traffic accidents or compressive forces applied in the AP plain. The effect of this force is to externally rotate the pelvis, the posterior margin of the sacroiliac joint acting as the pivot.

This force will initially result in fractures of the pubic rami or disruption of the symphysis and symphyseal ligaments. Progressive force will further externally rotate the pelvis disrupting the sacrotuberous, sacrospinous and anterior sacroiliac liga-

ments. The final phase if further force is applied is disruption of the posterior sacroiliac ligaments effectively detaching the innominate bone from the axial skeleton. The extent of posterior pelvic injury allows AP injuries to be stratified into one of three groups reflecting increasing severity and instability.

14.2.4.1.1
AP Type 1

This is the commonest type of AP compression injury, the impact of the trauma is confined to the anterior pubic arch and the posterior ligaments are intact. Radiographs demonstrate either fractures of the pubic rami which characteristically have a vertical orientation (Fig. 14.2) or alternatively disruption and widening of the symphysis. Integrity of the posterior ligaments restricts the symphyseal diastasis to less than 2.5 cm. Compression devices can however re-oppose the margins of a diastased symphysis, caution should therefore be exercised in ruling out injury on the basis of a normal AP radiograph without correlation to the clinical examination. In practice this eventuality occurs rarely. CT scans can occasionally over-estimate the extent of injury of a true type 1 injury by demonstrating minor widening of the anterior component of the sacroiliac joint, which it is postulated, results from stretching rather than disruption of the anterior sacroiliac ligaments (Young et al. 1986). These injuries are essentially stable and require non-operative management.

14.2.4.1.2
AP Type 2

These comprise anterior arch disruption as described above with additional diastasis of the anterior aspect

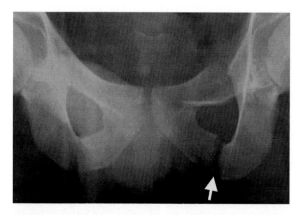

Fig. 14.2. AP type 1 injury characterised by vertical fracture line in inferior pubic ramus typical of AP compression injury

of the sacroiliac joint space commonly referred to as an "open book" injury or "sprung pelvis"(Fig. 14.3). Sacroiliac diastasis is more accurately assessed by CT than plain film (Fig. 14.4). These injuries exhibit partial instability being stable to lateral compressive forces (internal rotation) but unstable to AP compressive forces (external rotation).

14.2.4.1.3
AP Type 3

This pattern of injury result in total sacroiliac joint disruption (Fig. 14.5). Features described in the less severe types 1 and 2 injuries are present but in addition the sacroiliac joint is widely diastased posteriorly as well as anteriorly due to the posterior sacroiliac ligament rupture (Fig. 14.6). The hemipelvis is unstable to all directions of force, and usually requires operative stabilisation. Variants on the type three pattern include preservation of the sacroiliac joint integrity at the expense of sacral or iliac fracture (Fig. 14.7).

Complications of AP compression injuries include bladder rupture, usually intra-peritoneal type, which requires cystography for confirmation (Fig. 14.8) and vascular injury, particularly affecting the superior gluteal artery due to shear forces in the sciatic notch.

14.2.4.2
Lateral Compression Injuries

The commonest pattern of pelvic injury is discussed in the review of Young et al. (1986). Most patients with this mechanism of injury demonstrate pubic rami fractures. Exceptions are encountered when the symphysis is disrupted and overlaps. Three types of LC fracture are recognised.

14.2.4.2.1
LC Type 1

This represents the least severe injury pattern and is sustained by lateral force applied over the posterior pelvis causing internal rotation of the innominate bone which pivots on the anterior margin of the sacroiliac joint (Fig. 14.9). Radiographic features include pubic rami fractures, which are oblique, segmental (Fig. 14.10), frequently comminuted and rarely overlapping (Fig. 14.11) in contrast to the vertical fractures of AP compression injuries. Compression fractures of the anterior margin of the sacrum

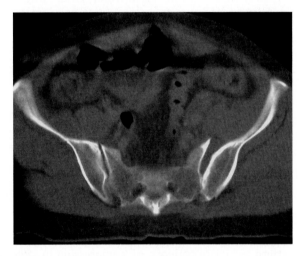

Fig. 14.4. CT scan demonstrating AP type 2 injury (open-book). Diastasis of the anterior part of the left sacroiliac hinged on its posterior margin as the posterior sacroiliac ligament remains intact

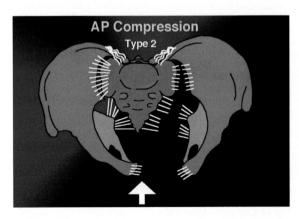

Fig. 14.3. AP type 2 injury

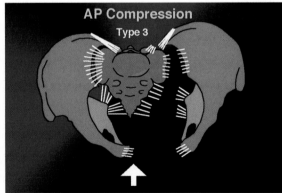

Fig. 14.5. AP type 3 injury

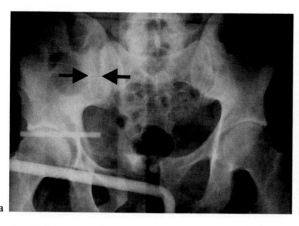
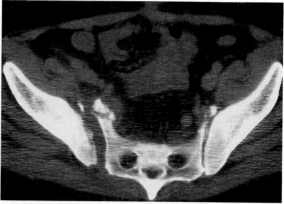

a   b

Fig. 14.6a,b. a AP type 3 injury comprising wide diastasis of the symphysis (> 2.5 cm) and diastased sacroiliac joint (*black arrows*). **b** CT demonstrating AP type 3 injury, wide diastasis throughout right sacroiliac joint, anterior and posterior sacroiliac ligaments are disrupted

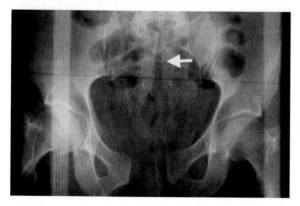

Fig. 14.7. AP type 3 variant. Symphyseal diastasis, intact sacroiliac joints but midline sacral fracture (*arrow*)

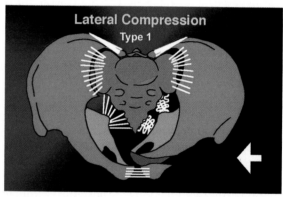

Fig. 14.9. LC type 1

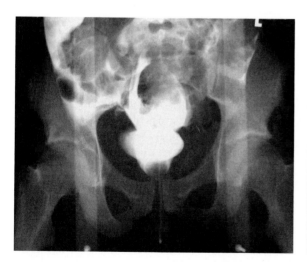

Fig. 14.8. Cystogram demonstrating intraperitoneal bladder rupture. The compression device has reduced the pelvic diastasis, pelvic instability cannot be excluded by a normal radiograph

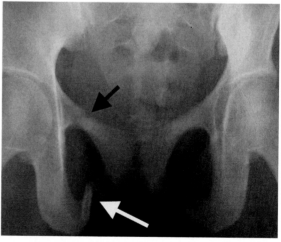

Fig. 14.10. LC type 1 injury demonstrating oblique (*black arrow*) and buckle fracture (*white arrow*) indicative of lateral compression

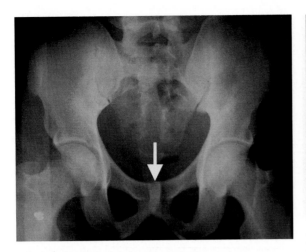

Fig. 14.11. LC type 1 injury overlapping pubic rami

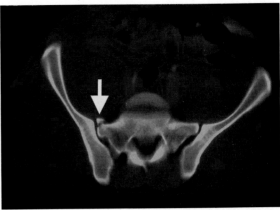

Fig. 14.12. CT demonstrating LC type 1 injury, compression fracture of the anterior sacral margin (*white arrow*)

are better demonstrated by CT than plain films (Fig. 14.12) (RESNIK et al. 1992). These injuries have little resultant instability and do not require operative management.

14.2.4.2.2
LC Type 2

The lateral compressive force in type 2 injuries is usually applied more anteriorly (Fig. 14.13). The pubic rami injuries are as described for type 1 but as the pelvis internally rotates pivoting on the anterior margin of the sacroiliac joint the posterior sacroiliac ligaments are disrupted. An alternative outcome if the strong posterior ligaments remain intact is for the ilium to fracture. This latter pattern is referred to as a type 2a injury (Fig. 14.14) as it was the first recognised but in reality the posterior sacroiliac joint diastasis, type 2b injury (Fig. 14.15), is the more commonly encountered pattern.

14.2.4.2.3
LC Type 3

This pattern of injury often referred to as the "wind-swept" pelvis (Fig. 14.16), results from internal rotation on the side of impact and external rotation on the other, and is often the result of a roll-over injury. The associated ligamentous injury and radiographic features combine lateral compression injuries on one side and AP compression on the other, as described in the preceding text.

Recognition of lateral compression injuries is important as external fixation devices and other methods of stabilisation tend to exert internal compressive forces that could exacerbate deformity and

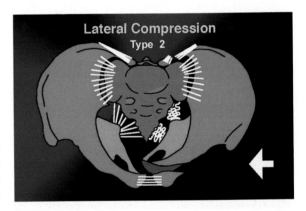

Fig. 14.13. LC type 2

increase the risk of progressive haemorrhage in this group.

14.2.4.3
Vertical Shear

Vertical shear injuries are usually the result of a fall or jump from a great height but loads transmitted through the axial skeleton from impacts to the head and shoulders can have identical consequences. The injury is typically unilateral comprising symphyseal diastasis or anterior arch fracture and posterior disruption of the sacroiliac joint with cephalad displacement of the pelvis on the side of impact (Fig. 14.17). Variants include disruption of the sacroiliac joint opposite to the side of impact or fracture of the sacrum.

Vertical shear injuries are invariably severe in that all ligaments are disrupted, the pelvis being totally unstable. There are no subcategories in this

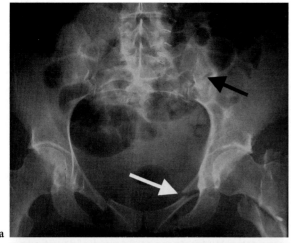

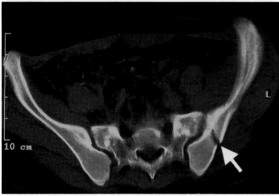

Fig. 14.14a,b. Pelvic radiograph (**a**) and CT scan (**b**) demonstrating LC type 2a injury. Oblique superior ramus fracture and iliac blade fracture on plain film (*white* and *black arrows*, respectively). CT demonstrates intact sacroiliac joint and fractured ilium

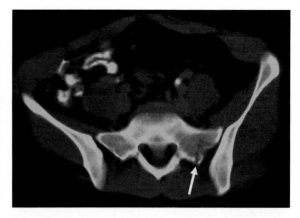

Fig. 14.15. CT demonstrating avulsion fracture of the posterior ilium by the posterior sacroiliac ligament (LC type 2b injury)

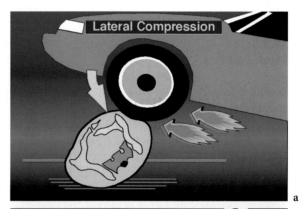

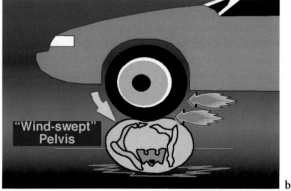

Fig. 14.16a,b. LC type 3 injury: Windswept pelvis. LC injury on side of impact (**a**) and AP injury on the "roll-over" side (**b**)

injury type. Radiographs demonstrate ipsilateral or contralateral pubic rami fractures, which have a vertical orientation similar to that described in AP compression injuries. The sacroiliac joint is also disrupted but the main differentiating feature from AP injuries is cephalad displacement of the pelvis on the side of impact. Careful attention to the relative positions of the sacral arcuate lines and lower border of the sacroiliac joint is a good guide to malalignment.

14.2.4.4
Complex Injuries

Complex patterns are not uncommon and when reviewed the majority will demonstrate a predominate pattern usually an LC type. Recognition of the complexity is important as external fixation devices and operative intervention will have to apply the appropriate corrective forces.

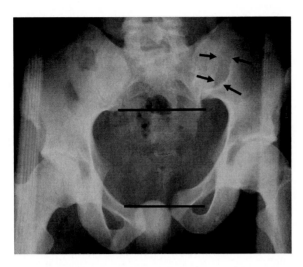

Fig. 14.17. Vertical shear pattern of injury. Disrupted symphysis and sacroiliac joint (*black arrows*), lines drawn through sacral foramen and symphysis highlight the extent of cephalad displacement on the side of impact

14.2.5
Pelvic Stability

Stability depends on integrity of the bony ring and supporting ligaments. TILE (1984) demonstrated that in AP compression disruption of the symphysis and its ligaments will allow up to 2.5 cm of diastasis. Widening of the symphysis by more than 2.5 cm is only achieved by disruption of the sacrotuberous, sacrospinous and anterior sacroiliac ligaments. Total pelvic instability only results if the posterior sacroiliac ligaments are also disrupted. It can be appreciated therefore that stability or more precisely instability of the pelvis represents a spectrum dependent on the extent of disruption of the bony ring and ligaments. A sequential graded pattern of instability also applies to lateral compression injuries

14.2.6
Diagnostic Accuracy of Plain Film and Computed Tomography in Identification of Pelvic Fractures

Considerable variation exists in the accuracy of plain radiographic evaluation of pelvic fractures. A 6-year retrospective review identified that plain films failed to diagnose 29% of sacroiliac joint disruptions, 34% of vertical shear injuries, 57% of sacral lip fractures and 35% of sacral fractures (MONTANA et al. 1986). Computed tomography (CT) was used as the gold standard and considerably improved diag-

nostic accuracy. When the films were re-reviewed by this group applying the force vector classification, with particular attention to sacral alignment and detail, their accuracy increased, the vertical shear injuries benefited most, accuracy of identification increasing to 93%.

RESNIK et al. (1992) prospectively evaluated a similar number of patients with pelvic fractures presenting over an 8-month period. In all, 160 fractures were identified in total with CT, of these only 9% were not identified prospectively. This group included sacroiliac joint diastasis, sacral lip fractures, iliac and pubic rami fractures, but all were subtle and none altered the management decision. Acetabular fractures were also evaluated, 80% of intra-articular fractures could not be identified on plain film indicating the essential requirement of CT in this subset of patients.

These studies identify firstly the importance of an understandable system of classification as an adjunct to improving performance and secondly the benefits of regular exposure to pelvic trauma in the latter study, which improves familiarity with injury pattern and subtle signs associated with pelvic trauma. Plain films will always remain the initial assessment in the emergency room, and should allow most fractures to be appreciated. CT is essential preoperatively and should also be considered earlier in the diagnostic work-up if there are clinical doubts or if trauma exposure and expertise is limited.

14.2.7
Risk Analysis and the Force Vector Classification

BEN-MENACHEM (1991) analysed the outcomes of patients with pelvic trauma. In type 1 injuries due to either lateral or AP compression the risk of severe haemorrhage was less than 5%. Conversely the risk of severe haemorrhage in the AP type 3 injury was 53%, 60% in LC type 3, 75% in vertical shear and 56% in complex injuries. This probability data, whilst not an absolute, enables an informed judgement on the likelihood of pelvic haemorrhage as an alternative to other visceral injury.

14.3
Acetabular Fractures

Acetabular injuries have complex fracture lines and in order to accurately describe these injuries according to the classification described by JUDET et al. (1964) and LETOURNEL (1980), a comprehensive understanding of the three-dimensional acetabular anatomy is required. It is inadequate to report an acetabular injury as "complex fracture as shown" as an accurate description using the aforementioned classification determines the requirement for surgery and the operative approach.

14.3.1
Acetabular Anatomy

The acetabulum comprises two columns (posterior and anterior) and two walls (posterior and anterior) which are connected to the axial skeleton by the sciatic buttress (Fig. 14.18). The anterior column is long and comprises the superior pubic ramus continuing cephalad into the iliac blade. The posterior column is shorter and more vertical extending cephalad from the ischial tuberosity into the ilium.

14.3.2
Radiographic Anatomy

Several important lines are identifiable on the anteroposterior radiograph, these include the iliopectineal (iliopubic) line, the ilioischial line and the margins of the anterior and posterior walls of the acetabulum (Fig. 14.19). The integrity of the obturator ring is also an important factor in fracture classification. The iliopectineal line runs along the superior margin of the superior pubic ramus towards the greater sciatic notch. It defines the anterior part of the pelvis which includes the anterior column, disruption of this line as will be discussed can result from fractures other than anterior column injury. The ilioischial line runs vertically from the greater sciatic notch past the cotyloid recess through the ischial tuberosity and comprises the posterior supportive structures of the acetabulum including the posterior column.

The anterior wall crosses the acetabulum obliquely and is less substantial and more medially positioned than the posterior wall which is lateral and more vertically orientated. The obturator ring if intact or not breached at two points excludes the

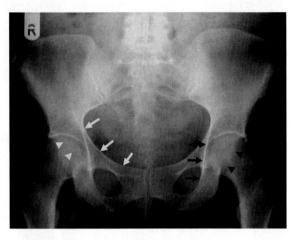

Fig. 14.19. Radiographic lines essential to identification and classification of acetabular fractures. Iliopectineal (iliopubic) line (*white arrows*), ilioischial line (*black arrows*), posterior acetabular wall (*black arrowhead*), anterior acetabular wall (*white arrowhead*) and obturator ring circled

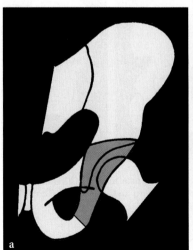
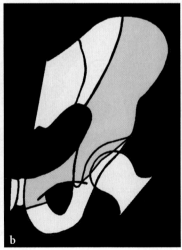
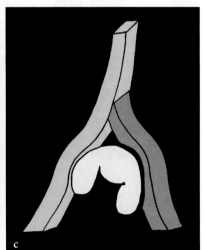

Fig. 14.18a–c. Acetabular (column) anatomy. *Pink shaded area* represents short posterior column (a), anterior column *shaded blue* (b) and enclosing roof, anterior and posterior walls supported between the columns (c)

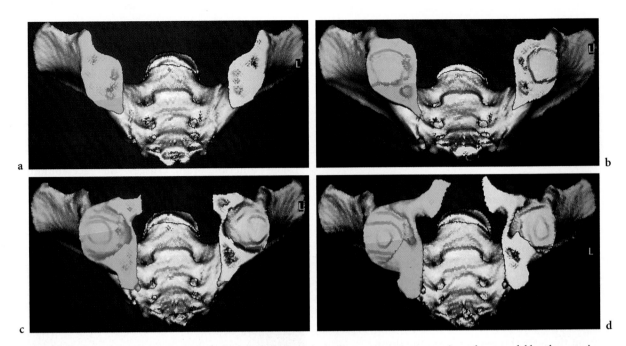

Fig. 14.20a–d. Serial CT sections through the acetabulum, *pink shading* representing posterior column and *blue* the anterior column

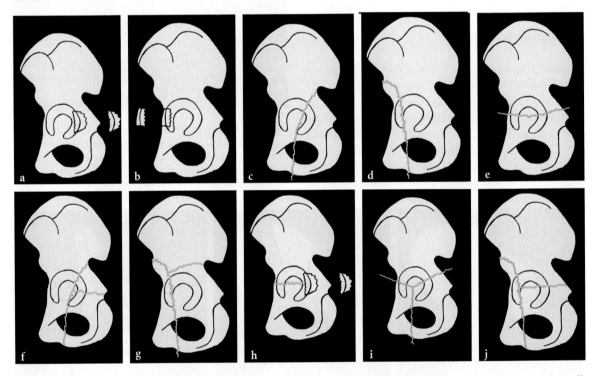

Fig. 14.21a–k. Elementary and complex patterns of acetabular fracture. Elementary group: (**a**) posterior wall; (**b**) anterior wall; (**c**) posterior column; (**d**) anterior column; (**e**) transverse. Complex group: (**f**) posterior column and posterior wall; (**g**) both columns; (**h**) transverse and posterior wall; (**i**) T-shaped; (**j**) anterior column and posterior hemi-transverse

possibility of a column fracture irrespective of disruption to the iliopectineal or ilioischial lines.

Oblique radiographic views (Judet pair) are often requested to gain additional detail. These views are referred to as the iliac oblique (IO) view which demonstrates the ilium en face and the obturator oblique (OO) view. The IO view improves evaluation of the anterior wall, posterior column and blade of the ilium. The OO view demonstrates the posterior wall, anterior column (lower part), obturator ring and the "spur" sign in double column injuries.

CT can provide additional detail regarding intra-articular fragments and supportive data regarding column involvement and interruption of the obturator ring. Figure 14.20 demonstrates the corresponding CT locations of the column anatomy.

14.3.3
Classification

The Judet and Letournel classification is widely accepted and is based on interpretation of the mor-

Table 14.1. Diagnostic check list in acetabular fractures

1. Obturator ring (OR) fracture
   (a) Anterior column (OR and iliopectineal line disruption)
   (b) Posterior column (OR and ilioischial line disruption)
   (c) T-shaped (OR and transverse acetabular fracture)
2. Iliopectineal line disrupted
   (a) Anterior column (coronal fracture plane)
   (b) Transverse and posterior wall
3. Ilioischial line disrupted
   (a) Posterior column (coronal fracture plane)
   (b) Anterior column and posterior hemi-transverse
4. Both iliopectineal and ilioischial lines disrupted
   (a) Transverse (splits acetabulum into upper and lower halves)
   (b) T-shaped (as above with vertical fracture disrupting OR)
   (c) Bi-column (Sciatic strut disconnected from acetabulum, Spur sign)
5. Posterior wall fracture
   (a) Posterior wall (Isolated, if ilioischial and iliopectineal lines intact)
   (b) Posterior wall and column (as above and disrupted ilioischial line)
6. Anterior wall fracture
   (a) Anterior wall (Isolated, if ilioischial and iliopectineal lines intact)
7. Fracture orientation
   (a) Coronal, splitting acetabulum into anterior and posterior segments
       Column fracture (anterior or posterior)
   (b) Transverse, splitting acetabulum into upper and lower segments
       Transverse or T-shape fracture
8. Spur sign
   Bi-column fracture
9. Fragments
   Not specific to type of fracture most common in posterior wall fractures

phological patterns of fracture using AP and Judet views. CT provides additional information regarding fracture orientation and intra-articular fragments. CT multiplanar reformats and surface reconstructions improve diagnostic accuracy particularly for inexperienced observers but systematic analysis of plain films and transverse CT images alone should allow most fractures to be classified (BRANDSER and MARSH 1998)

The acetabular classification divides fractures into a basic or elementary group, which include a single main fracture line and a complex or associated group representing combinations of the elementary patterns (Fig. 14.21). There are five elementary fracture patterns, posterior column, anterior column, posterior wall, anterior wall and transverse. Complex patterns most commonly encountered include posterior column and posterior wall, both column, and transverse with posterior wall fracture. The less common complex patterns include anterior column with posterior hemi-transverse and T-shaped. Variations including degree of comminution and extension into the ilium require separate description. Table 14.1 provides a diagnostic check list facilitating accurate assessment and classification of acetabular fractures.

14.3.4
Basic Patterns

14.3.4.1
Posterior Wall Fracture

Posterior wall fractures are one of the commonest acetabular injuries, either as an isolated injury (Fig. 14.22) or in combination with other fractures. They are sustained most frequently through direct compression of the posterior wall by the femoral head a situation encountered in a "dash-board" injury resulting from a frontal impact and are not uncommonly associated with posterior dislocation of the femoral head. The posterior wall fracture can be appreciated on AP radiographs but the OO view often improves visualisation. The size and comminution of the posterior fracture determines the prognosis and risk of re-dislocation or instability. CT is invaluable therefore in assessing the size of the posterior wall defect relative to the overall posterior wall depth. Fractures which constitute greater than 40% of the posterior wall represent an indication for operative reduction and internal fixation (KEITH et al. 1988) (Fig. 14.23).

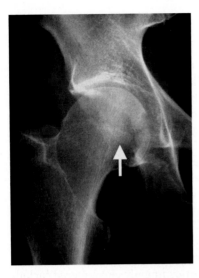

Fig. 14.22. Posterior wall fracture: AP radiograph demonstrating posterior wall fracture (*white arrow*)

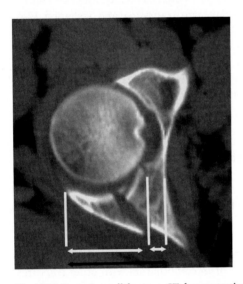

Fig. 14.23. Posterior wall fracture: CT demonstrating posterior wall fracture, with approximately 80% (*white arrow*) involvement of the posterior wall; operative repair is indicated

14.3.4.2
Anterior Wall Fractures

This is an uncommon fracture that infrequently requires surgical fixation. The displacement in this elementary pattern is often minor and this region of the acetabulum is not as heavily loaded as the roof and posterior wall. The fracture is identified on the AP view by disruption of the iliopectineal line but unlike anterior column or transverse fractures, the inferior pubic ramus and ilioischial lines respec-

tively remain intact. CT excludes significant steps in the cortex or intra-articular fragments which would indicate a requirement for open reduction.

14.3.4.3
Anterior Column Fractures

Column fractures cross the acetabulum in a coronal oblique orientation dividing the acetabulum into anterior and posterior elements (Fig. 14.24). The cephalad end of the fracture exits anteriorly disrupting the iliopectineal line and extends into the iliac blade a variable distance. The obturator ring is invariably fractured in column injuries, this therefore forms an important observation in classification, as a 'T-shaped' fracture is the only other acetabular fracture to disrupt the ring. Iliopectineal line and obturator ring disruption are pivotal features in this pattern and may be better demonstrated on the OO view than the AP radiograph. CT elegantly demonstrates the coronal fracture line distinguishing the injury from a transverse injury which splits the acetabulum into upper and lower halves.

14.3.4.4
Posterior Column Fractures

The orientation of the primary fracture line splits the acetabulum into anterior and posterior components and disrupts the ring, this is similar to that of an anterior column injury but the cephalad exit point of the fracture line in posterior column injuries is posteriorly sited disrupting the ilioischial line (Fig. 14.25). Posterior column injuries although commonly encountered in their elementary form are also common in association with anterior column (bi-column) and posterior wall injuries.

14.3.4.5
Transverse Fractures

The transverse fracture is a common pattern of injury, the fracture line traverses the acetabulum in an axial or oblique axial orientation dividing the acetabulum into upper and lower halves. The upper half includes the roof of the acetabulum which maintains its continuity with the acetabular strut (Fig. 14.26). This distinguishes transverse and 'T-shaped' fractures from bi-column injuries as the latter disrupt the roof and sciatic strut decoupling the acetabulum in its entirety from the axial

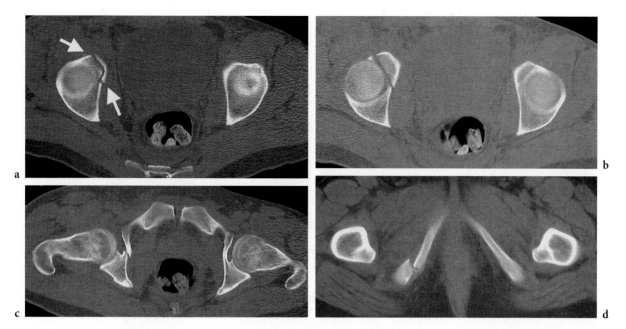

Fig. 14.24a–d. Anterior column fracture: CT demonstrating anterior column fracture with coronal fracture plane extending through the anterior aspect of the roof of the acetabulum (**a**), splitting the acetabulum into anterior and posterior halves (**b,c**) and disruption of the obturator ring (**d**)

skeleton. The 'T-shaped' variant of the transverse injury comprises an additional vertical fracture line extending through the obturator foramen.

14.3.5
Complex or Associated Fracture Patterns

14.3.5.1
Posterior Column and Posterior Wall Fractures

One of the commoner complex patterns, posterior wall disruption, is most easily recognised, but interrogation of plain film and CT will also demonstrate disruption of the obturator ring (Fig. 14.27), a feature not present in elementary posterior wall fractures.

14.3.5.2
Bi-column Fractures

In the case of this fracture, the spur sign distinguishes it from a 'T-shaped' fracture. The spur represents the sciatic strut's detachment from the acetabulum and is demonstrated on the obturator oblique view as a fragment projecting into the gluteal musculature. Evaluation using CT in these cases reveals a lack of continuity between the acetabulum and the sciatic strut (Fig. 14.28).

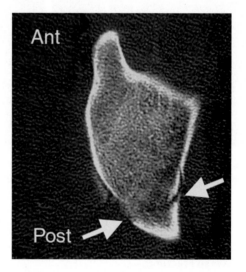

Fig. 14.25. Posterior column fracture: CT demonstrating coronal fracture plane exiting posteriorly typical of posterior column injury

14.3.5.3
T-Shaped Fractures

This fracture includes disruption of the obturator ring and both the ilioischial and iliopectineal lines (Fig. 14.29). These features are also common to bi-column injuries, but, in the 'T'-shape injury pattern the roof remains in continuity the sciatic strut and axial skeleton.

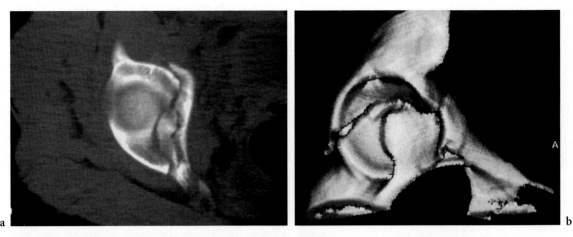

Fig. 14.26a,b. Transverse fracture: axial CT (**a**) and 3D reconstruction (**b**) demonstrating transverse fracture plane dividing acetabulum into upper and lower halves. No fracture through acetabular roof or into obturator ring

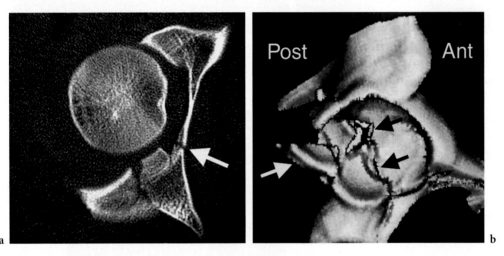

Fig. 14.27a,b. Posterior column and posterior wall fracture: CT demonstrating column type fracture plane (*white arrow*) and posterior wall fracture (**a**) and 3D CT confirms posterior column (*black arrows*) and posterior wall fracture (*white arrow*) (**b**)

14.3.5.4
Anterior Column and Posterior Hemi-transverse Fractures

A rare pattern of injury. A classic anterior column fracture pattern, with a further transverse fracture plane extending through the ilioischial line below the roof.

14.3.5.5
Transverse and Posterior Wall Fractures

A common pattern of fracture, characterised by disruption of the iliopectineal line, intact obturator ring (distinguishing from anterior column) and posterior wall involvement (Fig. 14.30).

14.3.6
Relative Accuracy of the AP Radiograph, Oblique Radiographs and Computed Tomography

While useful in predicting outcomes the Letournel classification is prone to considerable variation in interpretation. HUFNER et al. (2000) found that only 11% of fractures were correctly diagnosed by trainees when compared with a consensus diagnosis rising to 61% in acetabular surgical specialists, these diagnoses relating to plain film interpretation. They also noted a 20% divergence in classification amongst experts.

The finding of increasing reliability with experience is further supported by the work of PETRISOR et al. (2003). This latter group improved accuracy

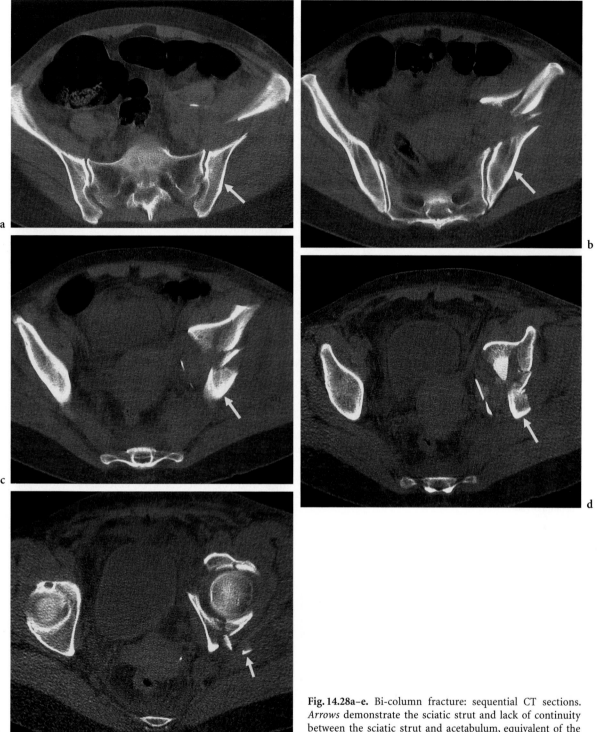

Fig. 14.28a–e. Bi-column fracture: sequential CT sections. *Arrows* demonstrate the sciatic strut and lack of continuity between the sciatic strut and acetabulum, equivalent of the spur sign on oblique film when strut protrudes posteriorly

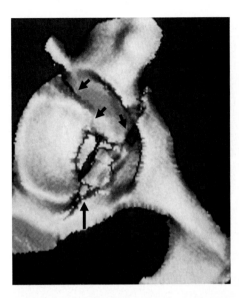

Fig. 14.29. T-shaped fracture: 3D CT demonstrating horizontal fracture plane (*short black arrows*) dividing acetabulum into upper and lower halves, the vertical fracture line (*long arrow*) disrupting the obturator ring distinguishes the T-shaped fracture from a simple transverse fracture

Table. 14.2. Radiographic lines fundamental in acetabular classification

Ilioischial
Iliopectineal
Anterior wall
Posterior wall
Acetabular roof
Tear drop disruption

and inter-observer agreement by emphasising the importance of six lines (Table 14.2), they also failed to demonstrate improved accuracy with additional oblique (Judet) views.

The effect of CT on diagnostic accuracy of classifying acetabular fractures is widely debated and disputed. Many early publications refer to single slice CT which has been superseded by spiral and multislice CT with increased speed, reduced section thickness and improved reconstructions. Publications also vary greatly in observer expertise ranging from orthopaedists to radiologists and trainees through generalists to specialist orthopaedists and musculoskeletal radiologists. There is, however, little doubt that CT is essential to the identification of intra-articular fragments (RESNIK et al. 1992) and although 2D images demonstrate basic fracture data enabling classification, inexperienced orthopaedists and radiologists can improve the accuracy of their classification by employing 3D surface reconstructions (GUY et al. 1991).

Recent articles by HARRIS et al. (2004a) have sought to redefine the anterior column relying heavily on CT based anatomy and the embryological derivation of the acetabulum. The redefined anterior column is proposed to lie below a line joining the iliopectineal line and arcuate line (true pelvic) and not as classically described by Letournel extending into the iliac blade (HARRIS et al. 2004a). This observation maintains that fractures extending high into the iliac blade be considered more precisely as anterior column with superior extension rather than a simple anterior column (Letournel). A further article by the same authors sets out a new classification which relies on cross-sectional identification of column involvement and defines four

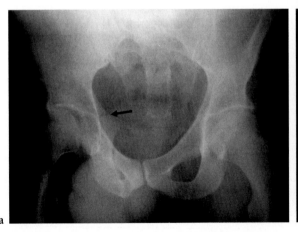

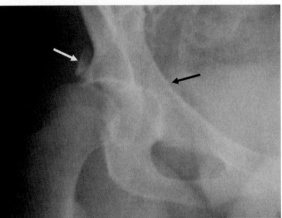

a   b

Fig. 14.30. Transverse and posterior wall fracture: AP (**a**) and obturator oblique (**b**) demonstrating transverse fracture line (*black arrows*) and posterior wall fragment (*white arrow*)

groups, Group 0 represent wall fractures; Group 1 single column fractures, Group 2 bi-column involvement and Group 3 floating acetabulum (Harris et al. 2004b). Groups 1 and 2 may have associated wall involvement and Group 2 is further subdivided according to extension beyond the acetabulum: 'A' no extension beyond acetabulum, 'B' extension into the iliac blade and 'C' extension into the inferior pubic rami or ischium. The redefinition of the anterior column seems justifiable but it remains to be seen whether the Letournel classification will be supplanted, as Harris' classification requires to prove in practice its advantages over the Judet and Letournel classification, its reproducibility and applicability across orthopaedic practices involved in acetabular reconstruction.

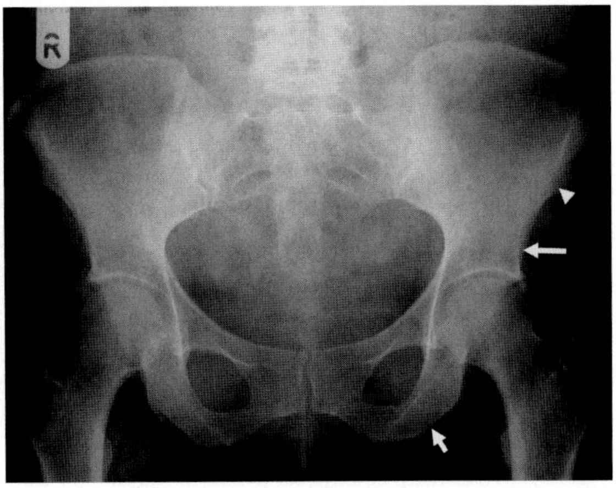

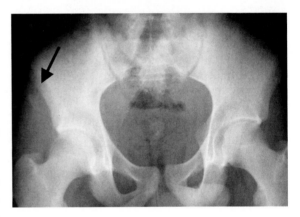

Fig. 14.31. Sites of common pelvic avulsion injuries. Origins of Sartorius (*arrowhead*) from anterior superior iliac spine, rectus femoris from anterior inferior iliac spine (*long arrow*) and the hamstrings from the ischial tuberosity (*short arrow*)

14.4
Avulsion Fractures

Avulsion injuries of the pelvic ring usually occur in young or skeletally immature individuals, commonly athletes. The injuries follow isometric muscle contraction and affect three main sites (Fig. 14.31): the anterior superior iliac spine (origin of Sartorius) (Fig. 14.32); the anterior inferior iliac spine (origin of Rectus Femoris); the ischial tuberosity (origin of the Hamstrings) (Fig. 14.33).

Plain radiographic evaluation is usually adequate to establish the diagnosis, but diagnostic difficulty can be encountered in the skeletally immature individual where ossification at the origins of these muscles is limited. Both MRI and US can establish a positive diagnosis in these cases, but the option is dependent on there being local US expertise. US is usually immediately available and well tolerated by young children (Fig. 14.34) but MRI is often preferred as it provides a more comprehensive evaluation in relation to more subtle muscle injuries or occult fractures in and around the pelvis which are part of the working differential diagnosis in such cases.

Chronic avulsions may present as either hypertrophic ossification simulating a mass lesion (Fig. 14.35) or localised erosion suggesting an adjacent mass lesion. In both cases the site of the lesion should suggest the diagnosis, in the latter scenario MRI can exclude a mass lesion (Fig. 14.36). MRI can also identify co-existent pathology which can contribute to symptoms in avulsion injuries, a common example is the association of sciatic neuritis with ischial tuberosity injury (Fig. 14.37)

Fig. 14.32. Sartorius avulsion: anterior superior iliac spine avulsion (*arrow*)

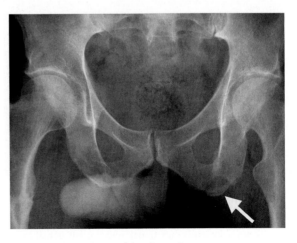

Fig. 14.33. Hamstring avulsion (*arrow*)

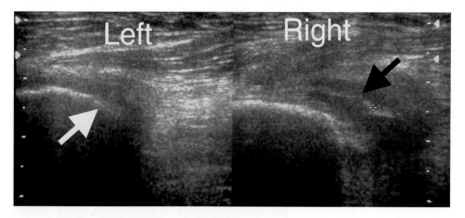

Fig. 14.34. Hamstring apophyseal avulsion: sagittal US of hamstring origin in a 12-year-old boy. Normal left side, cortical line (*white arrow*) capped with cartilaginous growth zone. Cortical avulsion (*black arrow*) on right side with surrounding hypoechoic haematoma

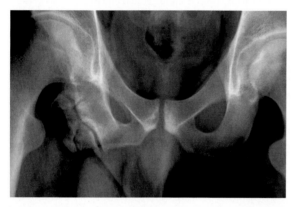

Fig. 14.35. Hypertrophic ossification adjacent to right ischial tuberosity indicative of previous avulsion, not a recent injury

14.5
Conclusion

There are a wide variety of bony pelvic injuries that occur as a result of differing forces, in a wide spectrum of ages. In the old and young the skeleton is relatively weak and predisposed to injury. In adults injuries usually result from high energy collisions or falls. It is important for reporting radiologists appreciate the mechanism of injury and systematically analyse the pattern of fracture, reporting fully complex pelvic ring and acetabular injury.

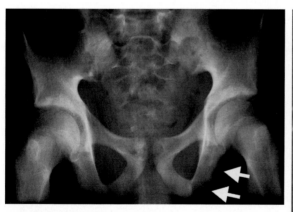

a

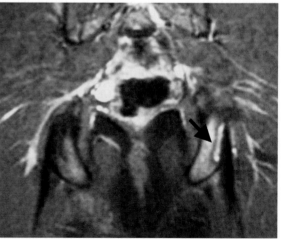

b

Fig. 14.36a,b. Repetitive tractional injury of left ischial tuberosity. Bony resorption demonstrated on AP radiograph (a) and granulating hyperaemic interface on coronal STIR image (b)

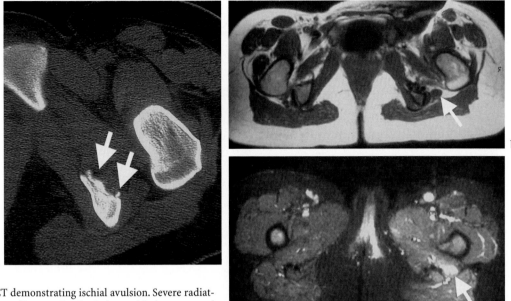

Fig. 14.37. a CT demonstrating ischial avulsion. Severe radiating leg pain caused by associated sciatic neuritis demonstrated on axial T1-SE (*arrow*) (**b**) and STIR (*arrow*) (**c**)

References

Ben-Menachem Y, Coldwell DM, Young JW, Burgess AR (1991) Haemorrhage associated with pelvic fractures: causes, diagnosis, and emergent management. AJR 157:1005–1014

Brandser E, Marsh JL (1998) Acetabular fractures: easier classification with a systematic approach. AJR 171:1217–1228

Guy RL, Butler-Manuel PA, Holder P, Brueton RN (1991) The role of 3D CT in assessment of acetabular fractures. Br J Radiol 65:384–389

Harris JH Jr, Coupe KJ, Lee JS, Trotscher T (2004a) Acetabular fractures revisited, part 2. A new CT-based classification. AJR 182:1367–1375

Harris JH Jr, Lee JS, Coupe KJ, Trotscher T (2004b) Acetabular fractures revisited, part I. Redefinition of the Letournel Anterior Column. AJR 182:1367–1375

Hufner T, Pohlemann T, Gasslen A, Assassi P, Prokop M, Tscherne H (2000) Classification of acetabular fractures. A systematic analysis of the relevance of computed tomography. Unfallchirurg 102:124–131

Judet R, Judet J, Letournel E (1964) Fractures of the acetabulum: classification and surgical approaches for open reduction. J Bone Joint Surg Am 46:1615–1638

Keith JE, Brasher HR, Guilford WB (1988) Stability of posterior wall fracture dislocations of the hip: quantitative assessment using computed tomography. J Bone Joint Surg Am 70A:711–714

Letournel E (1980) Acetabular fractures: classification and management. Clin Orthop 151:12–21

Montana MA, Richardson ML, Kilcoyne RF, Harley JD, Shuman WP, Mack LA (1986) CT of sacral injury. Radiology 161:499–503

Pennal GF, Tile M, Waddell JP, Garside H (1980) Pelvic disruption: assessment and classification. Clin Orthop 151:12–21

Petrisor BA, Bandari M, Orr R, Mandel S, Kwok DC, Schemitsch EH (2003) Improving reliability in the classification of fractures of the acetabulum. Arch Orthop Trauma Surg 123:228–233

Resnik CS, Stackhouse DJ, Shanmuganathan K, Young JW (1992). Diagnosis of pelvic fractures in patients with acute pelvic trauma: efficacy of plain radiographs. AJR 158:109–112

Tile M (1984) Fractures of the pelvis and acetabulum. Williams and Wilkins, Baltimore, pp 70–96

Young JW, Burgess AR, Brumback RJ, Poka A (1986) Pelvic fractures: value of plain radiography in early assessment and management. Radiology 160:445–451

15 Bony Trauma 2: Proximal Femur

Jeffrey J. Peterson and Thomas H. Berquist

CONTENTS

15.1
Introduction

Fractures of the hip are significant injuries occurring in both young and old patients. Proximal femoral fractures have a significant effect on lifestyle and morbidity as well as a tremendous effect on the health care system. The worldwide incidence of proximal femoral fractures continues to rise parallel to the average increase in the age of the population (Maniscalo et al. 2002). Frandsen and Kruse (1983) predict the number of proximal femoral fractures will triple by the year 2050.

Fractures most commonly occur after falls and are more common in elderly women (Frandsen and Kruse 1983). The propensity for femoral fractures to occur in the elderly is multifactorial including osteoporosis, decreased physical activity, malnutrition, decreased visual acuity, neurologic defects, altered reflexes, and equilibrium problems (Maniscalo et al. 2002). It is estimated that by age 80, 10% of Caucasian women and 5% of Caucasian men will

J. J. Peterson, MD; T. H. Berquist, MD
Department of Radiology, Mayo Clinic, 4500 San Pablo Road, Jacksonville, FL 32224-3899, USA

sustain a hip fracture. These figures double to 20% and 10% respectively by age 90 (Manister et al. 2002).

Proximal femoral fractures are best categorized by their location, either intracapsular or extracapsular. Intracapsular fractures can be further subdivided into capital, subcapital, transcervical, or basocervical fractures. Extracapsular fractures can be subdivided into intertrochanteric or subtrochanteric.

15.2
Intracapsular

15.2.1
Classification

Intracapsular fractures can be subdivided into capital, subcapital, transcervical, or basocervical fractures. Subcapital fractures are most common, while capital and basocervical fractures are less frequent. Transcervical fractures are rare. As a generalization the more proximal the fracture line the greater severity of the fracture and the greater risk of nonunion and avascular necrosis (Manister et al. 2002).

Several classification schemes have been proposed for intracapsular proximal femoral fractures; however, two classifications have proven clinically relevant. Both account for factors which determine stability of the fracture and are therefore applicable to both management and prognosis.

The first classification was described by Pauwels in 1935 (Table 15.1). Pauwels classified subcapital femoral fractures based on the obliquity of the fracture line in relation to the horizontal (Fig. 15.1). Type I fractures formed an angle of 30° or less; type II fractures formed an angle between 30° and 70°, and type III fractures formed an angle of greater than 70°. According to Pauwels' classification, the angle of the fracture determined the ultimate prognosis of the fracture with more vertical

Table 15.1. Classification of intracapsular proximal femoral fractures

Pauwels' classification

Type I	Femoral neck fracture with an angle of 30° or less
Type II	Femoral neck fracture with an angle of between 30° and 70°
Type III	Femoral neck fracture with an angle greater than 70°

Garden's classification

Stage I	Incomplete or impacted fracture of the femoral neck with no displacement of the medial trabeculae
Stage II	Complete fracture of the femoral neck with no displacement of the medial trabeculae
Stage III	Complete fracture of the femoral neck with varus angulation and displacement of the medial trabeculae
Stage IV	Complete fracture with the femoral neck with total displacement of the fragments

fractures being inherently less stable and therefore more prone to nonunion. More horizontal fractures (type I) tend to impact and impart some degree of stability increasing the ability of the fracture to heal. With more vertical fractures (type III) axial loading with weight bearing creates varus shearing and instability hindering the fractures ability to heal. Pauwels' classification was based on obliquity and alignment on post-reduction radiographs.

The more commonly utilized classification scheme was elaborated by GARDEN (1964) (Table 15.1). Garden's classification is based on alignment on prer-

eduction radiographs and relates to displacement of the fracture and the ability to obtain stability on post-reduction radiographs. A four-stage classification scheme was described by GARDEN with instability and nonunion seen more frequently in stages III and IV. Stage I fractures consisted of incomplete fractures with valgus positioning of the femoral neck. Stage II fractures in contrast are non-displaced complete fractures with varus angulation (Fig. 15.2). Stage III fractures represent complete fractures with varus angulation of the femoral head and displacement of the fracture (Fig. 15.3). Stage IV fractures are complete displaced fractures in which the femoral head fragment returns to normal position (BERQUIST 1992). Assessment of the position of the femoral head with subcapital fractures is helpful as valgus position indicates a stage I fracture, while varus position indicates stage II or III. Anatomic position of the femoral head is typically seen with stage IV fractures (MANISTER et al. 2002).

Incomplete fractures (stage I) or subtle nondisplaced fractures (stage II) require careful examination of the radiographic studies and may require additional cross sectional imaging for full characterization. Occasionally degenerative changes about the proximal femur with linear osteophyte formation may be seen mimicking fracture. Cross sectional imaging is of great value in such cases. MR imaging is preferable to CT for evaluation of equivocal proximal femoral fractures as MR will detect associated marrow edema and subtle trabecular fractures which may not be appreciable with radiographs or CT. CT is very helpful, however, in complete fractures and can be useful in assessing alignment and preoperative planning.

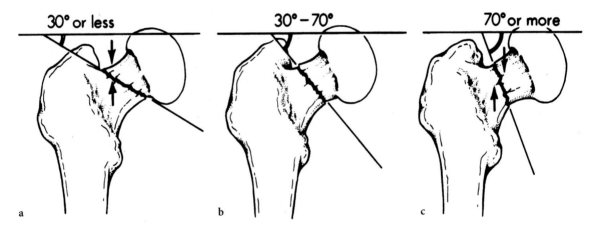

Fig. 15.1a–c. Pauwels' classification of femoral neck fractures. **a** Class I, fracture line 30° or less from vertical. **b** Class II, fracture line 30°–70°. **c** Class III, fracture line greater than 70°

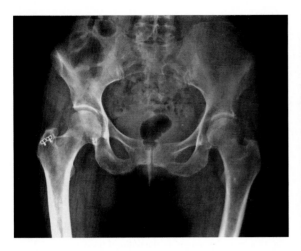

Fig. 15.2. An 85-year-old female status post fall with impacted Garden type II fracture of the left femoral neck

15.2.2
Treatment

Choice of treatment options for femoral neck fractures varies depending on several factors, the most important of which being stability of the fractures. Unstable fractures include Garden III and IV fractures while stable fractures consist of Garden type I and II fractures. Adequate reduction is the first and most important step in the treatment of displaced intracapsular proximal femoral fractures. No internal fixation device can compensate for malreduction (Bosch et al. 2002).

The primary aim of treatment of intracapsular fractures of the femur is to restore function of the hip to preinjury levels with a little comorbidity as possible (Bosch et al. 2002). Conservative nonoperative treatment of femoral fractures as commonly utilized in the early 19th century are quite debilitating and disabling. In 1931, Smith-Petersen reported open reduction and internal fixation of femoral neck fractures, while Leadbetter in 1933 described a closed reduction technique with a guide wire and cannulated implants. In 1943 Moore and Bohlman first reported the use of endoprosthesis replacement of the femoral head and an alternative to internal fixation. In the latter half of the last century hemiarthroplasty and total hip replacement has proven to be an additional alternative. Today the options for treatment of intracapsular fractures are many and continue to evolve. Currently the most common method for internal fixation are with cannulated screws placed in parallel. Cannulated screws allow axial compression across the fracture line aiding stability.

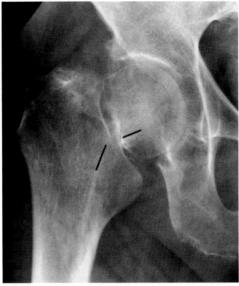

Fig. 15.3. Garden stage III fracture of the femoral neck with displacement of the fracture and varus angulation with malalignment of the medial trabeculae (*black lines*)

A major factor in dictating treatment of proximal femoral fractures is the age of the patient. In older patients proximal femoral fractures are common most frequently related to osteoporosis and falls. In contrast in the younger age population proximal femoral fractures are more commonly the result of high-energy trauma. In younger patients (< 50 years) preservation of the femoral head is ideal. The outcome of their treatment may have long-term effect on the function of their hip and may have a large impact on work and disability (Verattas et al. 2002). Femoral head-preserving procedures are the method of choice in compliant young active individuals who are able to perform the demands of postoperative rehabilitation (Krischak et al. 2003). Use of cannulated cancellous screws are most commonly utilized. Patients who do not achieve adequate function following internal fixation may have a satisfactory result with subsequent conversion of a total hip arthroplasty. In older patients (> 50 years) hemiarthroplasty and total hip replacement is becoming an increasingly popular treatment option.

Timing of surgery is another factor in treatment options. Urgent reduction of proximal femoral fractures has been suggested to minimize the risk of complications (Iorio et al. 2001; Jeanneret and Jacob 1985). After 48 h following a fracture, there is a progressive risk of healing complications with intracapsular femoral fractures (Bosch et al. 2002). Evidence from experimental studies indicate that early reduction relieves compression of the surrounding vascular structures and restores blood flow to the femoral head (BOSCH et al. 2002). MANNINGER et al. (1985) also reported a significantly lower incidence of articular collapse of the femoral head with prompt (< 6 h) reduction and internal fixation of intracapsular femoral fractures.

15.2.3
Complications

Although reduction in anatomic orientation is achieved in less than 30% of cases of intracapsular femoral fractures fixed with cancellous screws (WEINROBE et al. 1998), clinical studies show that uneventful fracture healing occurs in 62%–72% of cases (CHIU et al. 1994; COBB and GIBSON 1986; GERBER et al. 1993).

It has been reported that in patients with displaced hip fractures, an average rate of nonunion of 33% is expected (KYLE et al. 1994) and a 28% re-operation rate should be expected for failures of internal fixation of proximal femoral fractures (LU-YAO et al. 1994).

It is generally agreed that the optimal reduction of proximal femoral fractures should be as anatomic as possible (KRISCHAK et al. 2003). Although some authors prefer slight valgus orientation secondary to both impaction of the fragments during weight bearing, and the increased bony stability at the fracture site (KRISCHAK et al. 2003). Slight valgus angulation may also decrease the risk of developing a less favorable varus angulation. Stability of internal fixation depends upon both the accuracy of reduction, the technique utilized, and the density of the cancellous bone in the femoral head (JACKSON and LEARMONTH 2002). Nonunion may develop where stability of the fixation has been compromised by poor surgical technique or by the inability to achieve compression because of severe osteoporosis. The exact rate of nonunion is difficult to estimate and is related to numerous factors including patient demographics, severity of injury, degree of mineralization of the bone, and surgical technique (JACKSON and LEARMONTH 2002).

Because of the morphologic features of proximal femoral fractures there is significant risk of vascular injury to the femoral head with the potential risk of avascular necrosis (JACKSON and LEARMONTH 2002). The primary circulation to the femoral head is through the retinacular artery, which ends as the lateral epiphyseal artery (BERQUIST 1992) (Fig. 15.4).

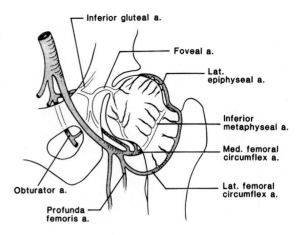

Fig. 15.4. Vascular supply to the femoral head

Additional blood supply to the femoral head included the medial retinacular artery which is a branch of the inferior retinacular artery, and the foveal artery. Poor contact, unstable reduction, and disruption of the retinacular arteries are the most prominent factors leading to avascular necrosis (BERQUIST 1992), which typically presents 9–12 months following the fracture, but can present as early as 3 months or as late as 3 years following the fracture (Fig. 15.5). In younger populations, there is a higher incidence of avascular necrosis and nonunion with TOOK and FAVERO (1985) reporting an incidence of 33% and 5.5% nonunion of nondisplaced intracapsular fractures (VERATTAS et al. 2002). SWIONTKOWSKI et al. (1984), in a series of 27 displaced intracapsular femoral fractures, also reported a 20% incidence of avascular necrosis with no nonunions. Prompt reduction appears to have an effect as all cases in SWIONTKOWSKI et al.'s 1984 study were reduced within 12 h. GAUTAM et al. (1998) also reported that emergent open reduction and screw fixation in 25 patients revealed only one nonunion at 32 months.

Treatment variables play a key role in achieving good outcome with proximal femoral fractures. Accurate reduction and stable fixation are prerequisites for satisfactory union. Tissue variables also play a role in the success of treatment of intracapsular hip fractures. Many fractures are associated with osteoporosis. Adequate reduction is often difficult with significant deficiencies in bone mineralization contributing to nonunion. It has also been found that patients with abnormal bone such as Paget's disease have up to a 75% risk of nonunion (DOVE 1980) prompting treatment with prosthetic replacement in these patients. This has also been reported to be a concern in patients with fibrous dysplasia and

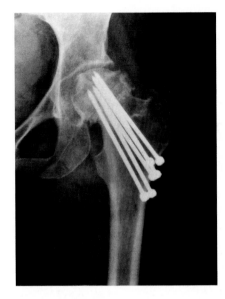

Fig. 15.5. A 49-year-old patient status post fall with closed reduction and internal fixation of a left femoral neck fracture 2 years previously with subsequent development of vascular necrosis and collapse of the articular surface of the femoral head

osteopetrosis (Steinwalter et al. 1995; Tsuchiya et al. 1995).

Imaging can be helpful in evaluating for nonunion. With conventional radiographs, a change in fracture or screw position, backing out of screws, or penetration of the femoral head by a screw suggest unstable internal reduction and nonunion. Recent advances in CT allow precise visualization of the hardware and surrounding bone with very little metallic artifact and can be quite helpful in equivocal cases or in preoperative planning when revision is needed.

In cases of nonunion several options are available for achieving union and the decision must be tailored to the individual patient. Prosthetic replacement is the most obvious option but in cases in which prosthesis replacement is deemed unsuitable there are many femoral head sparing options for achieving union of the fracture (Jackson and Learmonth 2002). Several procedures including vascularized fibular grafting, additional compression fixation, and femoral neck osteotomy augmented by muscle pedicle grafting are options (Jackson and Learmonth 2002). Simple removal of the cancellous screws with larger screws may be successful in uncomplicated cases with no significant malalignment of foreshortening. Dynamic hip screws may also be considered especially in cases of foreshortening (Wu et al. 1999). Bone grafting with

free vascularized or nonvascularized fibular grafts may also utilized (Hou et al. 1993; Nagi et al. 1998). Treatment of nonunion with total hip arthroplasty typically represents the best option in older patients with low functional demands and in complicated cases, although studies have shown a slightly higher failure rate with arthroplasty following nonunion for hip fracture as opposed to those for osteoarthritis (Franzen et al. 1990; Skeide et al. 1996). It is generally accepted that hip arthroplasty should be reserved for older patients, noncompliant patients, and for patients with significant preexisting acetabular disease (Rodriguez-Marchan 2003).

15.3
Extracapsular

15.3.1
Classification

Extracapsular fractures are those fractures occurring below the hip joint involving the trochanters and the subtrochanteric femur and fittingly can be divided into intertrochanteric fractures and subtrochanteric fractures. Avulsion fractures of the greater and lesser trochanters can also occur and represent a third category of extracapsular proximal femoral fractures.

15.3.2
Intertrochanteric Fractures

Fracture lines occur with variable obliquities but typically extend between the greater and lesser trochanters. Comminution with detachment of the greater and lesser trochanters are common (Maniscalco et al. 2002). Intertrochanteric fractures are most commonly the result of a fall. The musculature about the hip plays a role in the fracture morphology. The external rotators of the hip tend to remain with the proximal fragment while the internal rotators tend to remain attached to the distal fracture fragment (Berquist 1992).

Various classification schemes have been suggested based on location, angulation, fracture plane, and degree of displacement. Delee (1984) classified fractures as stable or unstable with fractures considered stable if, when reduced, there was adequate cortical contact medially and posteriorly at the fracture site, the medial cortex of the femur was not comminuted, and the lesser trochanter was intact. Vertically oriented fractures, or fractures with comminution of the medial cortex were considered unstable.

ENDER (1978) proposed a classification scheme (Table 15.2) for intertrochanteric fractures based on mechanism of injury, either eversion fracture (type 1), impaction fracture (type 2), or ditrochanteric fracture (type 3). Probably the most widely used classification scheme today is the Evans system, modified by JENSEN and MICHAELSON in 1975 (Table 15.2). This classification scheme is based on the prognosis for anatomic reduction and the likelihood of post-reduction instability. The scheme classified fractures by the degree of comminution of the calcar region and the greater trochanter (Fig. 15.6). Involvement of these structures increases the risk of instability following reduction. Fracture obliquity is also important. Stable fractures follow the intertrochanteric line which fracture orientation perpendicular to this leads to greater instability. Type 1 fractures are nondisplaced two part fractures which follow the intertrochanteric line while type 2 fracture are similarly oriented fractures with displacement. Type 1 and type 2 fractures can be successfully reduced in 94% of cases (JENSEN 1980) and are considered stable. Type 3 fractures are three part fractures with displacement of the greater trochanter. These fractures are unstable and can be successfully reduced in 33% of cases. Type 4 is a three part fracture with displacement of the lesser trochanter or involvement of the trochanter and can be reduced in only 21% of cases. Type 5 fractures are four part fractures and represent a combination of type 3 and 4 fractures with both medial and lateral comminution and involvement of both of the trochanters (Fig. 15.7).

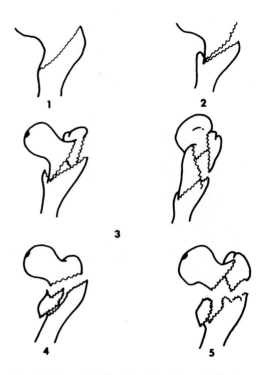

Fig. 15.6. Evans classification of trochanteric fractures modified by Jansen and Michaelson. Type *1*, nondisplaced two-part fracture. Type *2*, displaced two-part fracture. Type *3*, three-part fracture with greater trochanteric fragment. Type *4*, three-part fracture with lesser trochanteric or calcar fragment. Type *5*, four-part fracture with lesser and greater trochanteric fragments

Table 15.2. Classification of extracapsular intertrochanteric proximal femoral fractures

Ender classification	
Type I	Eversion fracture
Type II	Impaction fracture
Type III	Ditrochanteric fracture
Evans classification	
Type I	Undisplaced two-part fracture
Type II	Displaced two-part fracture
Type III	Three-part fracture with greater trochanteric fragment
Type IV	Three-part fracture with lesser trochanteric or calcar fragment
Type V	Four-part fracture with greater and lesser trochanteric fragments

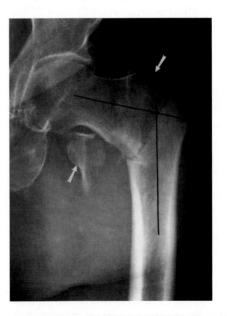

Fig. 15.7. Evans classification type 5 fracture with varus angulation (*black lines*) and both lesser and greater trochanteric fracture fragments (*white arrows*)

15.3.3
Subtrochanteric Fractures

Subtrochanteric fractures occur below the level of the trochanters; however, extension distally into the femoral shaft and proximally into the intertrochanteric region is not uncommon. Subtrochanteric fractures tend to occur in younger patients with significant trauma or in patients with underlying pathologic bone.

There are three major classification schemes for subtrochanteric fractures. Fielding proposed a simple classification of subtrochanteric fractures based on location (Table 15.3). Zone 1 includes the lesser trochanter, zone 2, 1–2 in. distal to the lesser trochanter, and zone 3, 2–3 in. below the lesser trochanter (Fig. 15.8). With zone 2 and zone 3 there is progressive involvement of cortical bone which heals slower and occurs in higher stress regions which makes treatment more difficult (BERQUIST 1992).

Seinsheimer further classified subtrochanteric fractures utilizing anatomical considerations such as the number of fracture lines, the location and shape of the fracture lines and the degree of comminution (Table 15.3). There are eight different categories. Three part spiral fractures which compose group III have the highest rate of failure following internal fixation (WEISSMAN and SLEDGE 1986).

Boyd and Griffin's classification is based on clinical information rather than anatomic considerations (Table 15.3). Their classification scheme is based on prognosis of obtaining and maintaining reduction of the extracapsular fracture (Fig 15.9). Zone 1 fractures are linear intertrochanteric in which reduction

Table 15.3. Classifications of extracapsular subtrochanteric proximal femoral fractures

Fielding classification	
Zone 1	Fracture includes the lesser trochanteric region
Zone 2	Fracture 1–2 in. distal to the lesser trochanter
Zone 3	Fracture 2–3 in. distal to the lesser trochanter

Boyd and Griffen classification	
Type I	Linear intertrochanteric fracture
Type II	Comminuted fracture with main fracture line along the intertrochanteric line
Type III	Subtrochanteric fracture with at least one fracture line passing through or just below the lesser trochanter
Type IV	Comminuted trochanteric fracture extending into the shaft with fracture lines in at least two planes

Seinsheimer classification	
Group I	Undisplaced fracture (less than 2 mm)
Group II	Two-part fracture:
	A. Transverse fracture
	B. Spiral fracture
	C. Spiral fracture with lesser trochanteric involvement
Group III	Three-part fracture:
	A. Spiral fracture with lesser trochanteric involvement
	B. Spiral fracture with butterfly fragment
Group IV	Four-part fracture
Group V	Subtrochanteric fractures with extension into the intertrochanteric region and involvement of the greater trochanter

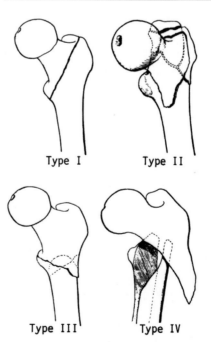

Fig. 15.9. The Boyd and Griffen classification

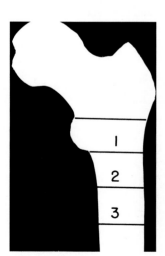

Fig. 15.8. The Fielding classification of subtrochanteric fractures

is less difficult. Type 2 is a subtrochanteric fracture with multiple fracture lines with the main fracture occurring along the intertrochanteric line. Type 2 fractures are more difficult to achieve lasting reduction than type 1 fractures. Type 3 consist of subtrochanteric fracture lines that coexist with fractures of type 1 and 2. Type 4 fractures are comminuted with trochanteric extension of the fracture lines and extension into the shaft (Fig. 15.10). Type 4 fractures have fracture lines extending in at least two planes. Type 3 and 4 fractures are more difficult to treat and loss of reduction is not uncommon.

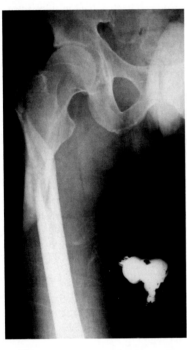

Fig. 15.10. Boyd and Griffen classification type IV fracture with comminuted proximal femoral fracture with fracture lines in at least two planes and extension into the proximal femoral shaft

15.3.4
Avulsion Fractures

Abrupt muscular contraction can lead to greater or lesser trochanteric fractures which compose the third category of extracapsular proximal femoral fractures. Greater trochanteric avulsion fractures are not uncommon and are typically seen in elderly populations, while lesser trochanteric fractures are uncommon and mostly seen in younger athletic individuals (DELEE 1984; EPSTEIN 1973). Pathologic fractures of the lesser trochanter are actually more common than traumatic avulsions (ROGERS 1982). Several muscle groups attach to the greater trochanter and can result in avulsions, while the iliopsoas tendon attaches to the lesser trochanter. Treatment of trochanteric fractures as with intracapsular femoral fractures depends on stability (BERQUIST 1992).

15.3.5
Treatment

A successful reduction will align the fracture fragments, obtain bone-to-bone contact of the calcar and medial cortex, and avoid varus angulation Reduction and fixation are fluoroscopically monitored. The variety of implants available for the treatment of extracapsular proximal femoral fractures continues to evolve. Sliding hip screws are most commonly utilized and allow impaction at the fracture site favoring healing (BOLDIN et al. 2003) (Fig. 15.11). The sliding nail also decreases the probability of cut-out or acetabular protrusion (MANISCALO et al. 2002). Fixed nail plates should not be used as stresses at the angle of the nail plate have been found to be significant which can lead to failure (BERQUIST 1992). From the biomechanical perspective, there are two main options, the

a
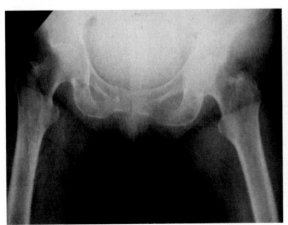

b
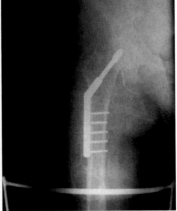

Fig. 15.11a,b. A 63-year-old female status post motor vehicle accident with type 1 trochanteric fracture (**a**). Internal fixation was performed with a sliding-screw and plate (**b**)

sliding neck screw or bolt connected to a plate on the lateral femoral cortex or a sliding neck screw or bolt stabilized by an intramedullary nail (BOLDIN et al. 2003). The choice remains controversial. The use of intramedullary fixation minimizes soft tissue dissection and surgical trauma, blood loss, infection, and wound complications; however, the Gamma nail, the most commonly utilized intramedullary device, has a high learning curve and has been reported to have technical and mechanical failure rates of about 10% (BOLDIN et al. 2003). The most widely used method is currently the dynamic hip screw (DHS) (BOLDIN et al. 2003), which utilizes a sliding screw and a lateral side plate. There are reportedly lower complications rates with extramedullary implants compared to intramedullary devices (BOLDIN et al. 2003). Often in the final analysis it is the experience of the surgeon that becomes the determining factor in the choice of treatment of trochanteric fractures (DAVIS et al. 1990). For markedly comminuted intertrochanteric fractures in older populations, treatment with an endoprosthesis may be the proper choice (LORD et al. 1977).

15.3.5
Complications

Common complications are typically easily seen with routine conventional radiographs and include fracture of the fixation devices, loss of reduction, and migration of the devices (Fig. 15.12). Loss of reduction with cutting out of the fixation is the most common complication especially in those patients with osteopenia. Unlike intracapsular fractures, extracapsular proximal femoral fractures rarely injure the vascular supply to the femoral head and therefore avascular necrosis is less common (BERQUIST 1992). Trochanteric fractures have a low incidence of nonunion with approximately 1%–2% for intertrochanteric fractures and 5% for subtrochanteric fractures (VERATTAS et al. 2002).

References

Berquist TH (1992) Imaging of orthopedic trauma, 2nd edn. Raven, New York

Boldin C, Seibert FJ, Fankhauser F et al (2003) The proximal femoral nail (PFN) – a minimal invasive treatment of unstable proximal femoral fractures. Acta Orthop Scand 74:53–58

Bosch U, Schreiber T, Krettek C (2002) Reduction and fixation of displaced intracapsular fractures of the proximal femur. Clin Orthop 399:59–71

Chiu KY, PunWK, Luk KDK et al (1994) Cancellous screw fixation for subcapital femoral neck fractures. J R Coll Surg Edinb 39:130–132

Cobb AG, Gibson PH (1986) Screw fixation of subcapital fractures of the femur – a better method of treatment? Injury 17:259–264

Davis TRC, Sher JL, Horsman A et al (1990) Intertrochanteric femoral fractures. Mechanical failure after internal fixation. J Bone Joint Surg [Br] 61:342–346

Delee JC (1984) Fractures and dislocations of the hip. In: Rockwood CA, Green DP (eds) Fractures in adults, vol 2. Lippincott, Philidelphia, pp 1211–1356

a 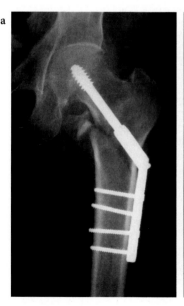 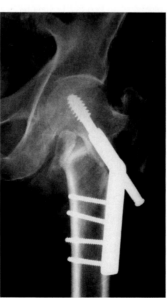 b

Fig 15.12a,b. Dynamic hip screw failure. **a** Unstable subtrochanteric fracture with sliding-screw and plate internal fixation. **b** At 1 month following surgery the fragments have collapsed and the screw has backed out

Dove J (1980) Complete fractures of the femur in Paget's disease of bone. J Bone Joint Surg 63B:12–17

Ender HG (1978) Treatment of trochanteric and subtrochanteric fractures of the femur with Ender pins. The hip. Proceedings of the sixth open scientific meeting of the hip society. Mosby, St Louis

Epstein HC (1973) Traumatic dislocation of the hip. Clin Orthop 92:116–142

Frandsen PA, Kruse T (1983) Hip fractures in the county of Funen, Denmark. Implications of demographic aging and changes in incidence rates. Acta Orthop Scand 54:681–686

Franzen H, Nilsson LT, Stromqvist B et al (1990) Secondary total hip replacement after fractures of the femoral neck. J Bone Joint Surg 72B:784–787

Garden RS (1964) Low angle fixation in fractures of the femoral neck. J Bone Joint Surg (Br) 43:630–647

Gautam VK, Anand S, Dhaon BK (1998) Treatment of displaced femoral neck fractures in young adults. Injury 29:215–218

Gerber C, Strehle J, Ganz R (1993) The treatment of fractures of the femoral neck. Clin Orthop 292:77–86

Hou SM, Hang YS, Liu TK (1993) Ununited femoral neck fractures by open reduction and vascularized iliac bone graft. Clin Orthop 294:176–180

Iorio R, Healy W, Lemos DW et al (2001) Displaced femoral neck fractures in the elderly. Clin Orthop 383:229–242

Jackson M, Learmonth D (2002) Treatment of nonunion after intracapsular fracture of the proximal femur. CORR 399:119–128

Jeanneret B, Jacob RP (1985) Konservative versus operative, Therapie der Abduktions-schenkelhalsfrakturen. Unfallchirurg 88:270–273

Jensen JS (1980) Classification of trochanteric fractures. Acta Orthop Scand 51:803–810

Jensen JS, Michaelson M (1975) Trochanteric fractures treated with McLaughlin osteosynthesis. Acta Orthop Scand 46:795–803

Krischak G, Beck A, Wachter N et al (2003) Relevance of primary reduction for the clinical outcome of femoral neck fractures. Arch Orthop Trauma Surg 123:404–409

Kyle RF, Schmidt AH, Campbell SJ (1994) Complications of treatment of fractures and dislocations of the hip. In: Epps CH Jr (ed) Complications in orthopaedic surgery. Lippincott, Philidelphia, pp443–486

Leadbetter GW (1933) A treatment for fracture of the neck of the femur. J Bone Joint Surg 15:931–941

Lord G, Marotte JH, Blantard JP et al (1977) Head and neck arthroplasty in treatment of intertrochanteric fractures after age 70. Rev Chir Orthop 63:135–148

Lu-Yao G, Keller R, Littenberg B et al (1994) Outcomes after displaced fractures of the femoral head: a meta-analysis of one hundred and six published reports. J Bone Joint Surg 76A:15–18

Maniscalo P, Rivera F, Bertone C et al (2002) Compression hip screw nail-plate system for intertrochanteric fractures. Panminerva Med 44:135–139

Manninger J, Kazac C, Fekete C (1985) Avoidance of avascular necrosis of the femoral head, following fracture of the femoral neck, by early reduction and internal fixation. Injury 16:437–448

Manister BJ, Disler DG, May DA (2002) Musculoskeletal Imaging: the requisites, 2nd edn. Mosby, St Louis

Moore AT, Bohlman HR (1943) Metal hip joint: a case report. J Bone Joint Surg 25:688–692

Nagi ON, Dhillon MS, Goni VG (1998) Open reduction, internal fixation and fibular autografting for neglected fracture of the femoral neck. J Bone Joint Surg 80B:798–804

Pauwels F (1935) Der Schenkelausbruch: ein mechanishes problem. Grundlagen des Heilungsvorganges: Prognose und kausale Therapie. Enke, Stuttgart

Rodriguez-Marchan EC (2003) Displaced intracapsular hip fractures: hemiarthroplasty or total hemiarthroplasty? CORR 399:72–77

Rogers LF (1982) Radiology of skeletal trauma. Churchill Livingstone, New York

Skeide BI, Lie SA, Havelin LI et al (1996) Total hip arthroplasty after femoral neck fractures: results from the national registry on joint prosthesis. Tidsskr Nor Laegeforen 116:1449–1451

Smith-Petersen MN (1931) Intracapsular fractures of the neck of the femur: Treatment by internal fixation. Arch Surg 23:715–759

Steinwalter G, Hosny GA, Koch S et al (1995) Bilateral nonunited femoral neck fracture in a child with osteopetrosis. J Pediatr Orthop 44:213–215

Swiontkowski MF, Winquist RA, Hansen ST (1984) Fractures of the femoral neck in patients between the ages of twelve and forty-nine years. J Bone Joint Surg 66:837–846

Took MT, Favero KJ (1985) Femoral neck fractures in skeletally mature patients, 50 years old or less. J Bone Joint Surg 67:1255–60

Tsuchiya H, Tomita K, Masumoto T et al (1995) Shepard's crook deformity with an intracapsular femoral neck fracture in fibrous dysplasia. Clin Orthop 310:160–164

Verattas D, Galanis B, Kazakos K et al (2002) Fractures of the proximal part of the femur in patients under 50 years of age. Injury 33:41–45

Weinrobe M, Stankevich CJ, Mueller B et al (1998) Predicting the mechanical outcome of femoral neck fractures fixed with cancellous screws: and in vivo study. J Orthop Trauma 12:27–37

Weissman BN, Sledge CB (1986) Orthopedic radiology. Saunders, Philadelphia

Wu CC, Shih CH, Chen WJ et al (1999) Treatment of femoral neck nonunions with a sliding compression screw: comparison with and without subtrochanteric valgus osteotomy. J Trauma 46:312–317

16 Bone Trauma 3: Stress Fractures

WILFRED C. G. PEH and A. MARK DAVIES

CONTENTS

16.1
Introduction

Stress fractures affecting the bony structures in and around the pelvic ring are being increasingly diagnosed in clinical practice. They contribute to patient disability and morbidity, particularly if they fail to be recognized and managed early. These fractures are usually classified into fatigue and insufficiency fractures, and are associated with a wide variety of etiological factors. Signs of fractures may be nonspecific on physical examination, particularly as a wide range of patients may be afflicted – ranging from young military recruits to elderly post-meno-

W. C. G. PEH, MD, MBBS, FRCP, FRCR
Clinical Professor and Senior Consultant Radiologist, Programme Office, Singapore Health Services, 7 Hospital Drive, #02-09, Singapore 169611, Republic of Singapore
A. M. DAVIES, MBChB, FRCR
Consultant Radiologist, The MRI Centre, Royal Orthopaedic Hospital, Birmingham B31 2AP, UK

pausal women. Imaging, therefore, has an important role in the detection, diagnosis, and management of patients suspected of having stress fractures of the pelvic ring and proximal femora.

16.2
Classification of Stress Fractures

Conventional traumatic fractures are caused by sudden external trauma to normal or locally-diseased bone (pathological fractures). In contrast, stress fractures result from repeated and prolonged muscular action upon bone that has not accommodated itself to such forces. Stress fractures may develop as a result of three mechanisms, namely: (1) direct repeated impact of the weight of the body; (2) repeated contractions of antagonistic muscles; and (3) direct and repeated trauma to bone (CHEVROT 1992). They can also be regarded as "over-use" injuries of bone. Stress fractures can be classified into fatigue and insufficiency fractures (PENTECOST et al. 1964; DAVIES 1990; DAFFNER and PAVLOV 1992; PERIS 2003), although a minority favored using the term "pathological fractures" in place of, or together with, insufficiency fractures (CALANDRUCCIO 1983; SEO et al. 1996).

Fatigue fractures occur when normal bone is subjected to excessive repetitive stress. This category of stress fracture has long been widely recognized, with the first clinical description of the "march fracture" being made by Breithaupt, a Prussian army surgeon, in 1855. The location of fatigue fractures depends on the type of activity which produces them. Although these fractures may affect virtually every bone in the body, the lower limbs are most commonly involved (Fig. 16.1). Examples of predisposing activities include: excessive walking, marching, running, jumping, dancing, and gymnastics (DAFFNER and PAVLOV 1992).

In contrast to fatigue fractures, insufficiency fractures are caused by the effects of normal or

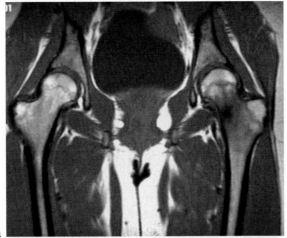

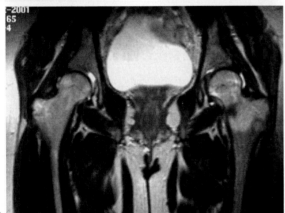

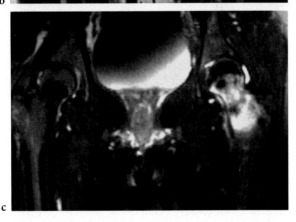

Fig. 16.1a–c. Fatigue fracture left femoral neck. Radiographs were normal. **a** Coronal T1-weighted MR image shows a dark linear fracture line with surrounding hypointense oedema. **b** Coronal T2-weighted fast spin echo shows the fracture line but with poor conspicuity between the marrow oedema and normal marrow fat. **c** Coronal STIR image shows both the fracture line and the oedema. (Images courtesy of Dr. R Whitehouse)

physiological stresses upon weakened bone, in which elastic resistance is decreased (PENTECOST et al. 1964; DAVIES 1990). These fractures occur most

frequently in elderly women with post-menopausal osteoporosis. The commonest site involved is the thoracic vertebra, with other typical sites being the femur, fibula, and talus (DAFFNER and PAVLOV 1992). The pelvic ring is another typical site of insufficiency fractures. Some patients develop fractures that are due to a combination of "fatigue" and "insufficiency" components.

16.3
Causative Factors and Clinical Features

16.3.1
Fatigue Fractures

The following clinical triad is associated with fatigue fractures; activity that is: (1) new or different for the person, (2) strenuous, and (3) repeated with a frequency that produces signs and symptoms (WILSON and KATZ 1969; MATHESON et al. 1987; DAFFNER and PAVLOV 1992). The location of fatigue fractures, and hence the clinical presentation, is dependent on the type of activity that produces them. For example, in the region of the bony pelvis, dancers are particularly susceptible to fractures of the femoral neck (Fig. 16.1) (SCHNEIDER et al. 1974). The distribution of bone injuries also depends on the patient population, e.g. distribution in athletes differs from that in military recruits (MCBRYDE 1975).

Although fatigue fractures of the pelvic ring normally involve just one site, a minority of patients have multiple sites of fractures. KIURU and coworkers (2003), in a study of military conscripts, found that almost one-quarter of their patients with fatigue stress fractures of the pelvic bones and proximal femur had multiple injuries. Bone injuries were found in 40% of cases, of which 60% were located in the proximal femur and 40% in the pelvic bones. In athletes, stress changes to the symphysis pubis are associated with sacral fatigue fractures or degenerative changes to the sacroiliac joint (MAJOR and HELMS 1997).

Fatigue fractures of the pelvis most often affect the pubic ramus (Fig. 16.2) (MATHESON et al. 1987). In the bony pelvis, obturator ring fractures may be caused by bowling and gymnastics, while pubis ramus fractures and symphysis pubis stress injury (osteitis pubis) have been reported in runners and soccer players (Fig. 16.3) (KOCH and JACKSON 1981; TEHRANZADEH et al. 1982; NOAKES et al. 1985; MAJOR and HELMS 1997). Female army recruits are prone

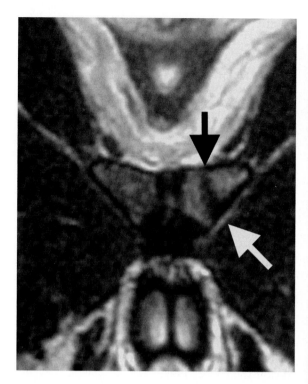

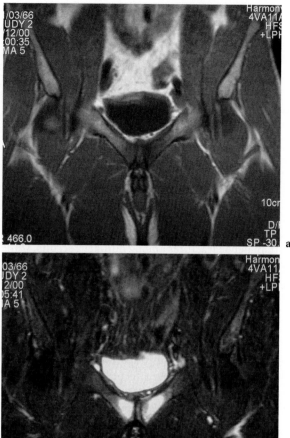

Fig. 16.2. Coronal T2-weighted image of a fatigue fracture of the left superior pubic ramus in an athlete. The fracture is visible as a dark vertical line (*black arrow*). There is some juxtacortical oedema (*white arrow*). (Image courtesy of Dr. Philip Hughes)

Fig. 16.3a,b. A 34-year-old male enthusiastic soccer player with a stress injury of the pubic symphysis. **a** Coronal T1-weighted and (**b**) Coronal STIR images showing marrow oedema in the pubic bones adjacent to the symphysis

to inferior pubic ramus fractures (HILL et al. 1996; KIURU et al. 2003). Acetabular fractures occurring in military endurance athletes and recruits have been recently identified as a rare and poorly-recognized cause of activity-related hip pain (WILLIAMS et al. 2002).

Fatigue fractures may occur in the sacrum. In contrast to sacral insufficiency fractures, they present in much younger patients and result from a variety of activities. These fractures are very rare and appear in physically-active people. Sacral fatigue fractures may be caused by running (CZARNECKI et al. 1988; BOTTOMLEY 1990; HAASBEEK and GREEN 1994; ELLER et al. 1997), aerobics (RAJAH et al. 1993) and volleyball playing (SHAH and STEWART 2002). Military recruits may also develop fatigue fractures of the sacrum during basic training (VOLPIN et al. 1989; AHOVUO et al. 2004).

Fatigue fractures of the sacrum have also very rarely been reported in children. These children are not elite sports persons but are fit and active. This diagnosis needs to be considered in healthy children presenting with unexplained low back and buttock pain (RAJAH et al. 1993; GRIER et al. 1993; MARTIN

et al. 1995; LAM and MOULTON 2001). Women may develop fatigue fractures during pregnancy or in the post-partum period. It is uncertain whether these fractures are true fatigue fractures that arise as a result of unaccustomed stress related to rapid excessive weight gain during advanced pregnancy, or whether they actually represent insufficiency fractures related to osteoporosis associated with pregnancy (BREUIL et al. 1997; THIENPONT et al. 1999). Signal changes of the pubic cartilage and small bruises of the pubic bones have also been demonstrated on MR imaging of asymptomatic postpartum women (WURDINGER et al. 2002).

In female athletes, disruption of the normal hormonal balance may predispose to fractures that are probably a combination of fatigue and insufficiency mechanisms. Women may rarely develop an inter-related problem of disordered eating, amenorrhea and osteoporosis, the so-called female athlete triad. The female athlete triad is a serious problem that may result in permanent loss of bone mass (MILLER et al. 2003).

Fatigue fractures of the femoral neck are uncommon injuries that are seen in young, healthy, active individuals such as recreational runners, endurance athletes and military recruits (Fig. 16.1) (EGOL et al. 1998). Fatigue fractures of the femoral neck are not uncommon in the military population (MILGROM et al. 1985). MILGROM et al. (1985) reported that proximal femur fractures were seven times commoner than pelvic fractures among military recruits, while KIURU et al. (2003) found fractures of the femoral neck and proximal shaft to be 50% more common than pelvic injuries. Subchondral fatigue fractures of the femoral head have been recently reported among military recruits (SONG et al. 2004).

The femoral neck is affected in approximately 1% of fatigue fractures due to sports activities (HA et al. 1991). They particularly affect long distance runners (HA et al. 1991; KUPKE et al. 1993; KERR and JOHNSON 1995; CLOUGH 2002). The biomechanical cause of this injury in long distance runners may be related to reduction in shock absorption of the running shoe due to sole erosion (KUPKE et al. 1993). Femoral neck fractures present with insidious onset of exertional groin pain or anterior thigh pain, and pain at the extremes of hip motion. Patients may also present with pain and stiffness around the hip. These clinical features are non-specific. Diagnosis requires a high index of clinical suspicion. Initial radiographs are often normal (Fig. 16.1). Clinical and imaging differential diagnosis include groin strain, inguinal hernia, osteoid osteoma, osteosarcoma, and osteomyelitis (KALTSAS 1981; MILGROM et al. 1985; CLOUGH 2002).

Diagnostic delay for femoral neck fractures is common, averaging 14 weeks. Although most fractures are initially undisplaced, a delay in diagnosis can lead to fracture displacement, with resultant collapse and varus angulation (FULLERTON 1990; JOHANSSON et al. 1990; CLEMENT et al. 1993; KUPKE et al. 1993; KERR and JOHNSON 1995). Femoral neck displacement is the main determinant of prognostic outcome, with a 30% incidence of osteonecrosis (JOHANSSON et al. 1990).

Patients with fatigue fractures usually present with an insidious onset of pain. In the pelvis, patients complain of pain in the hip, buttock or groin region during or after physical exercise. Physical examination findings are typically non-specific. It is often difficult to differentiate between fatigue fractures of the femoral neck from other fractures of the pelvis, based on the patient's history and physical examination findings alone (SALLIS and JONES 1991; SHIN et al. 1996). In athletes, groin pain may be produced by fatigue fractures of the femoral neck and osteitis pubis (Fig. 16.3). Differential diagnoses of apophyseal avulsion fractures, sports-related hernias, and adductor muscle strains need to be considered in athletes (LYNCH and RENSTROM 1999).

The typical history of pubic symphysis stress injury is gradually increasing discomfort or pain in the pubic region, one or both adductor regions of the groin, and in the area of the lower rectus abdominis muscle. Certain movements such as running or pivoting on one leg typically aggravate the pain. Pubic symphysis stress injury may also be associated with an acute episode of forced hip abduction or rotation, kicking, or fall (Fig. 16.3) (SCHNEIDER et al. 1976; LA BAN et al. 1978; WILEY 1983; ALBERTSEN et al. 1994; MAJOR and HELMS 1997).

In sacral fractures, patients may develop buttock pain or low back pain that mimics sciatica. Among young military recruits, sacral fatigue fractures occur more frequently among women. These fractures are associated with stress-related hip pain, and other injuries of the pelvis may be seen simultaneously with the sacral fractures. Compared to men, women have to carry the same type of military equipment on their backs, with greater resultant vertical loads relative to their physical size (AHOVUO et al. 2004). During mixed training of male and female recruits, women have to increase their stride length when marching, predisposing them to fatigue fractures of the inferior pubic ramus (HILL et al. 1996). Altered mechanical forces from hip extensors in the female pelvis have been proposed as contributing to pelvic fatigue fractures in women (KELLY et al. 2000; MAJOR and HELMS 2000).

Female navy recruits undergoing basic military training who developed pelvic fatigue fractures were found to be significantly shorter and lighter, and were more frequently Asian or Hispanic (KELLY et al. 2000). In a study of female army recruits, fatigue fractures were more likely to occur in those who smoke, drink heavily, use corticosteroids, and have a lower adult weight. A history of regular exercise was protective against fractures, as was a longer history of exercise (LAPPE et al. 2001).

A history of recent increased physical activity is essential for diagnosis of fatigue fractures. Typically, these fractures are seen in beginners who have recently embarked on an over-rigorous training program or an athlete who has suddenly increased his or her training program (LYNCH and RENSTROM 1999). Pain also typically occurs after unusual or prolonged activity, and usually resolves with rest. If physical activity is continued, the pain will increase.

16.3.2
Insufficiency Fractures

The most common cause of insufficiency fracture is post-menopausal osteoporosis. Other important causes are senile osteoporosis, pelvic irradiation (LUNDIN et al. 1990; ABE et al. 1992; BLOMLIE et al. 1993; FU et al. 1994; PEH et al. 1995a,b; MAMMONE and SCHWEITZER 1995; BLISS et al. 1996; MUMBER et al. 1997; MORENO et al. 1999; HUH et al. 2002; OGINO et al. 2003), and rheumatoid arthritis (GODFREY et al. 1985; CRAYTON et al. 1991; PEH et al. 1993; WEST et al. 1994). Prolonged corticosteroid therapy, osteomalacia (Fig. 16.4), Paget's disease, fibrous dysplasia, scurvy, osteopetrosis (Fig. 16.5), osteogenesis imperfecta (Fig. 16.6), primary biliary cirrhosis, lung transplantation, tabes dorsalis, vitamin D deficiency, and fluoride therapy are other rarer reported causes (DORNE and LANDER 1985; VAN LINTHOUDT and OTT 1987; TARR et al. 1988; DAVIES 1990; SCHNITZLER et al. 1990; EASTELL et al. 1991; TOUNTAS 1993; COOPER 1994; CHARY-VALCKENAERE et al. 1997; MARC et al. 1997; SCHULMAN et al. 1997; ADKINS and SUNDARAM 2001; SOUBRIER et al. 2003).

Mechanical failure from large bony defects such as TARLOV cysts or bony tumors has been postulated to be an additional predisposing factor to the development of sacral insufficiency fractures (PEH and EVANS 1992; PEH et al. 1997; OLIVER and BEGGS 1999). Sacral fractures occurring secondary to instability due to septic arthritis of the symphysis pubis have also been reported (ALBERTSEN et al. 1995). Total hip replacement may also contribute to fracture development due to combined fatigue and insufficiency mechanisms. Surgical treatment from various procedures in and around the pelvic ring may also cause alteration of the distribution of weight-bearing forces, with resultant fractures (LAUNDER and HUNGERFORD 1981; CARTER 1987; TAUBER et al. 1987; DAVIES 1990; MATHEWS et al. 2001; CHRISTIANSEN et al. 2003; NOCINI et al. 2003). Femoral neck fractures have also been reported in association with surgical procedures such as hip

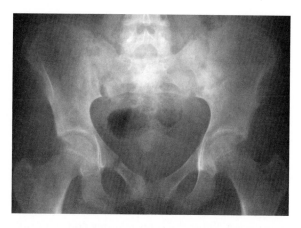

Fig. 16.4. AP radiograph of teenage Asian immigrant with severe osteomalacia. There is generalized osteopenia with insufficiency fractures (Looser's zones) affecting the pubic and left iliac bones

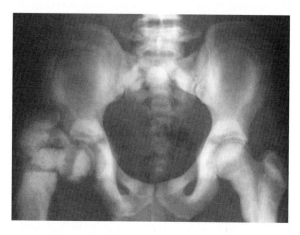

Fig. 16.5. AP radiograph of osteopetrosis. Typical bone-within-a-bone appearance with healing insufficiency fractures of the right proximal femur

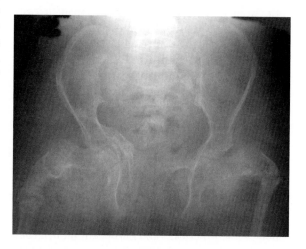

Fig. 16.6. AP radiograph of osteogenesis imperfecta. Marked deformity due to bone softening and insufficiency fractures of the proximal femora

arthroplasty, internal fixation for trochanteric fracture, intramedullary nailing, and knee arthroplasty (ESCHENROEDER and KRACKOW 1988; HARDY et al. 1992; BUCIUTO et al. 1997; ARRINGTON and DAVINO 1999; KITAJIMA et al. 1999; KANAI et al. 1999).

LOURIE (1982) was credited for first recognizing insufficiency fractures of the sacrum. In the bony pelvis, insufficiency fractures of the os pubis were identified by GOERGEN et al. in 1978. These pubic fractures were later found to be frequently associated with sacral insufficiency fractures (Fig. 16.7) (COOPER et al. 1985b; DE SMET and NEFF 1985). This strong association is now well accepted as a diagnostic criterion. Pubic fractures may develop as a result of increased anterior arch strain secondary to initial failure of the posterior arch (sacrum).

Other typical sites of insufficiency fractures are the femoral head (BANGIL et al. 1996; RAFII et al. 1997; VISURI 1997) and the femoral neck (Fig. 16.8) (AITKEN 1984; DORNE and LANDER 1985; TARR et al. 1988; SCHNITZLER et al. 1990; TOUNTAS 1993). Recently, the entity of subchondral femoral head insufficiency fractures has been recognized as a distinct clinical entity. These fractures present with an acute onset of pain around the hip, usually in elderly osteoporotic women. These fractures may also be associated with insufficiency fractures at other sites (YAMAMOTO and BULLOUGH 1999, 20001; HAGINO et al. 1999; YAMAMOTO et al. 2000; BUTTARO et al. 2003; LEGROUX GEROT et al. 2004; DAVIES et al. 2004).

Insufficiency fractures of the femoral neck typically present with persistent hip pain but without a history of significant trauma. AITKEN (1984) hypothesized that postural instability was the major determinant for femoral neck fractures in osteoporotic women. Besides osteoporosis, insufficiency fractures of the femoral neck may also occur in association with chronic renal failure (TARR et al. 1988), rheumatoid arthritis (PULLAR et al. 1985), and fluoride therapy (SCHNITZLER et al. 1990). Femoral neck fractures are very rare in children but have been described in Gaucher's disease (GOLDMAN and JACOBS 1984).

The true incidence of pelvic insufficiency fractures is unknown, but is estimated to occur in 1%–5%, depending on the referral population (ABE et al. 1992; WEBER et al. 1993; WEST et al. 1994; PEH et al. 1995a; BLISS et al. 1996). No racial predilection exists. Although this entity has been predominantly reported among white Americans and Europeans (SCHNEIDER et al. 1985; WEBER et al. 1993; GRANGIER et al. 1997), it also afflicts Australians (GOTIS-GRAHAM et al. 1994), Japanese (ABE et al. 1992), and Chinese (PEH

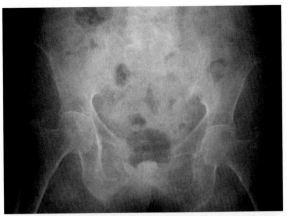

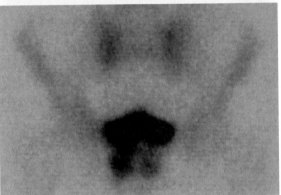

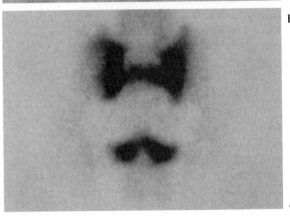

Fig. 16.7a–c. Concomitant sacral and parasymphyseal insufficiency fractures. **a** AP radiograph showing generalized osteopenia and a displaced right parasymphyseal fracture. **b** Anterior bone scintigraphy revealing increased activity in the right pubis. **c** Posterior bone scintigraphy showing the typical "H-shaped" pattern of increased activity in the sacrum

et al. 1995a). The vast majority of patients are elderly women, typically over the age of 60 years, with mean ages ranging from 62 to 74 years among various studies (ABE et al. 1992; NEWHOUSE et al. 1992; WEBER et al. 1993; GOTIS-GRAHAM et al. 1994; PEH et al. 1995a; BLOMLIE et al. 1996; FINIELS et al. 1997; SOUBRIER et al. 2003). The occurrence of insufficiency fractures

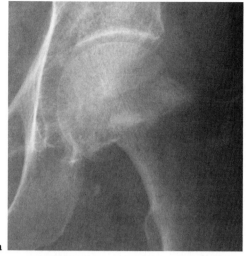

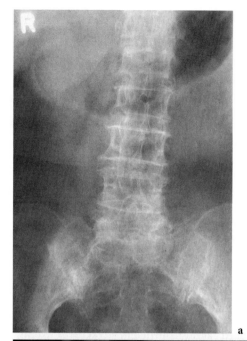

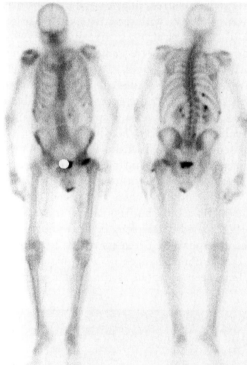

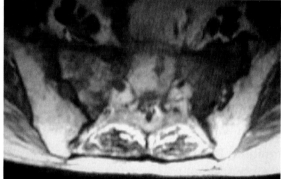

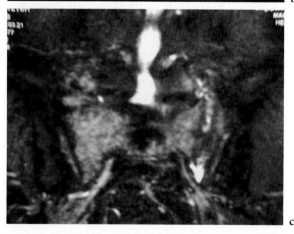

Fig. 16.8a,b. Insufficiency fracture femoral neck. **a** AP radiograph showing linear sclerosis. **b** Whole-body bone scintigraphy showing linear increased activity in the left femoral neck corresponding to the fracture. There are further insufficiency fractures of the ribs

among younger patients is extremely uncommon and is usually due to bone loss secondary to underlying disease (GRANGIER et al. 1997).

Patients with pelvic insufficiency fractures typically present with a history of groin, low-back, or buttock pain (Fig. 16.9). One-quarter of patients have multiple sites of pain. In most patients, pain

Fig. 16.9a–c. Sacral insufficiency fractures in a 62-year-old female presenting with low back pain. **a** AP radiograph shows lumbar spondylosis and ill-defined sclerosis in the right sacral ala. **b** Axial T1-weighted MR image shows broad band-like areas of hypointense signal in both sacral ala. **c** Coronal fat-suppressed T2-weighted image shows areas of hyperintense signal in the ala with fluid in the left-sided fracture

is severe enough to render the patient non-ambulatory. Usually, patients present with either no history of trauma or a history of low-impact trauma. On physical examination, the signs of insufficiency fracture are usually nonspecific or nonexistent. The most common physical signs are sacral or groin tenderness, and restricted lumbar and hip movement (DAVIES et al. 1988; RAWLINGS et al. 1988; NEWHOUSE et al. 1992; WEBER et al. 1993; GOTIS-GRAHAM et al. 1994; PEH et al. 1995a). Neurologic deficit is rare but has been reported in a few patients (LOURIE 1982; RIES 1983; JONES 1991; LOCK and MITCHELL 1993; BEARD et al. 1996). In patients who have undergone pelvic irradiation, local soft-tissue complications, especially affecting the rectum and producing bleeding, are frequently encountered. The same factors that determine the therapeutic effects upon the tumor also contribute to complications in the bone and soft tissues, resulting in prostatitis and cystitis (PEH et al. 1995b). Radiation-induced sacral insufficiency fractures usually occur approximately 12 months post-irradiation (PEH et al. 1995b; BLOMLIE et al. 1996). In patients with insufficiency fractures, there is typically discordance between the severe symptoms and the mild or absent physical signs.

16.4
Imaging Techniques

As clinical assessment by itself may not provide a definitive diagnosis of stress fracture, imaging has an important role in the detection and diagnosis of these fractures, particularly of insufficiency fractures. The imaging findings are very variable and depend on many factors such as the type of activity, site of fracture, and timing of imaging in relation to injury (PENTECOST et al. 1964; SAVOCA 1971). Radiography should be the first form of imaging obtained and can be used to confirm the diagnosis at a low cost (ANDERSON and GREENSPAN 1996). In the sacrum, radiographs may be difficult to interpret due to overlying bowel gas, bladder shadow and the normal curved sacral angulation. In an adequately-taken anteroposterior radiograph, the sacral arcuate lines that outline the sacral foramina should be visible. Even so, sacral stress fractures are not easily detected on radiographs (Fig. 16.10). If taken during the early stages of stress injuries, radiographs may not be very sensitive, with sensitivities being as low as 15% (GREANEY et al. 1983; NIELSEN et al. 1991). A delay in appearance of radiographic findings may result in false-negatives, and delay appropriate therapy. False-positive results are less common but if there is aggressive periostitis or reactive new bone formation, stress fractures may mimic malignancy, with resultant unnecessary biopsy.

Bone scintigraphy is a sensitive technique for the detection of both fatigue and insufficiency fractures (Figs. 16.1, 16.7, 16.8) (SCHNEIDER et al. 1985; RIES 1983). Technetium (Tc)-99m methylene diphosphonate (MDP) scintiscans show stress fractures as areas of increased uptake long before radiographic changes are apparent. Given its ability to demonstrate these subtle changes in bone metabolism, it has long been accepted as the imaging modal-

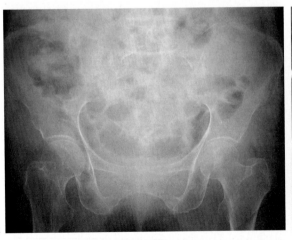
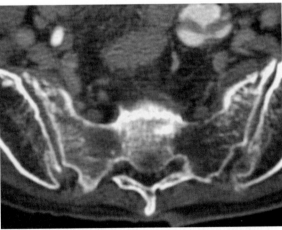

a   b

Fig. 16.10a,b. Bilateral sacral insufficiency fractures in an 82-year-old female who had previously undergone radiotherapy for carcinoma of the rectum. **a** AP radiograph shows generalized osteopenia with no obvious fracture. **b** CT shows bilateral fractures through the sacral ala anteriorly

ity of choice for the assessment of stress fractures (AMMANN and MATHESON 1991). Abnormal uptake on Tc-99m MDP scintigraphy may be seen from 6 to 72 hours of injury, with degree of uptake being dependent upon factors such as bone turnover rate and local blood flow (GREANEY et al. 1983). The sensitivity of bone scintigraphy approaches 100%, with false-negative scans being very rare (MILGROM et al. 1984; KEENE and LASH 1992). Normal bone scintigraphy virtually excludes the diagnosis of a stress fracture (ROSEN et al. 1982; ZWASS et al. 1987). Bone scintigraphy relies on accurate interpretation of the uptake pattern. Although it is highly sensitive, atypical uptake patterns may sometimes be difficult to interpret.

As stress fractures tend to be positive on all three phases, the sensitivity of bone scintigraphy can be improved by using the three-phase technique (STERLING et al. 1992). The first phase correlates to increased blood flow in the arterial phase, the second phase to tissue hyperemia, and the third phase to increased osteoblastic activity in response to the stress fracture. With healing of stress fractures, there is a progressive decrease in radionuclide uptake. Abnormal uptake may however persist for several months (RUPANI et al. 1985; AMMANN and MATHESON 1991).

Magnetic resonance imaging (MR) imaging is a very sensitive method for the detection of occult bone injuries, being positive before fractures are radiographically apparent (LEE and YAO 1988; BERGER et al. 1989; BRAHME et al. 1990; NEWHOUSE et al. 1992; BLOMLIE et al. 1993, 1996; MAMMONE and SCHWEITZER 1995). Early stress reactions are seen as areas of low signal intensity within marrow on T1-weighted images, and high signal intensity on T2-weighted and short tau inversion recovery (STIR) images (Figs. 16.1, 16.2, 16.9) (MINK and DEUTSCH 1989; MEYERS and WIENER 1991). The application of fat-suppression is recommended to enhance the conspicuity of associated medullary edema or hemorrhage, particularly on fast spin-echo T2-weighted images (ANDERSON and GREENSPAN 1996). The possibility of stress fractures needs to be considered when there is marrow edema on MR images. Detection of a fracture line is a helpful feature that aids the diagnosis. The fracture line is seen as a linear area of low signal intensity on both T1- and T2-weighted images, and represents callus and new bone formation at the fracture site (Figs. 16.1, 16.9) (LEE and YAO 1988; DAFFNER and PAVLOV 1992). MR imaging is currently the modality of choice for the detection and anatomical delineation of soft tissue and marrow

abnormalities. MR imaging also has the advantage of distinguishing stress fractures from other causes of increased scintigraphic uptake, such as inflammatory arthritis and osteomyelitis. However, it suffers from having a limited ability to detect subtle cortical changes, small calcifications and cortical fragments. MR imaging findings may be positive within 24 h of onset of symptoms, in comparison with bone scintigraphy which takes longer to become positive. In a comparative study, MR imaging has been found to be more sensitive than two-phase bone scintigraphy for the assessment of stress injuries to the pelvis and lower limb (KIURU et al. 2002). As it is highly sensitive, MR images need to be correlated with findings obtained with other modalities in order to optimize image interpretation and diagnosis.

Patients with stress fractures of the pelvis may present with contralateral pain and develop multiple bone stress injuries. In such circumstances, using just a single surface coil for MR imaging may result in an increased number of false-negatives. It is recommended that the entire pelvis and both proximal femurs be simultaneously imaged in patients with stress-related hip or groin pain in order to optimize detection of fractures, and avoid delay in diagnosis and appropriate treatment (KIURU et al. 2003). Application of dynamic contrast-enhanced MR imaging may be useful to show increased tissue perfusion in patients with pelvic stress injuries in which the fracture line, callus and muscle edema are seen on pre-contrast MR images (KIURU et al. 2001). Sacral insufficiency fractures are often not clinically suspected and patients are instead referred for routine lumbar spine MR imaging instead of a dedicated sacral study. Signal changes of these fractures may only be seen on the lateral images of the sagittal sequences and on the scout images (BLAKE and CONNORS 2004).

Computed tomography (CT) provides further definition of the fracture, especially if MR imaging is unavailable or if bone scintigraphy is inconclusive. CT allows an accurate anatomical display of stress fractures in and around the pelvis, and aids in differentiating fractures from metastases (Fig. 16.10) (COOPER et al. 1985b; DE SMET and NEFF 1985; DAVIES et al. 1988; PEH et al. 1995a, 1997). Appropriate windowing needs to be employed for optimal visualization of the fracture line and callus (YOUSEM et al. 1986; DAVIES et al. 1988). Perifracture edema may sometimes be seen with adjustment of soft tissue settings (SOMER and MEURMAN 1982). CT may not accurately detect fractures that are oriented transversely (DAVIES 1990). This problem may be overcome by utilization of the direct coronal CT technique (Peh et al. 1995a), or by image reconstruction in the coronal and sagittal planes from fine-cut axial images on spiral or multidetector CT scanners.

16.4.1
Imaging Features of Fatigue Fractures

On radiographs, a fatigue fracture typically appears as a sclerotic focus that is linearly-oriented. A cortical break or focal periosteal reaction may be seen (Savoca 1971). Determination of the fracture age may sometimes be possible. An acute fracture is often seen as a fine lytic line while subacute or chronic fractures are wholly sclerotic.

Radiographic appearances of fatigue fractures can be divided into two types, depending on location. Cortical fractures typically involve the diaphyses of long bones. They are seen initially as subtle ill-definition of the cortex, the so-called "gray cortex sign", or faint intra-cortical striations due to osteoclastic tunneling (Daffner 1984; Ammann and Matheson 1991; Mulligan 1995). These radiographic changes become more apparent with formation of new bone periosteally or endosteally, and when a true fracture line develops (Savoca 1971; Martin and Burr 1982; Greaney et al. 1983). In athletes, stress injuries of the pubic symphysis may manifest radiographically as sclerosis, erosions, or offset at the pubic symphysis (Major and Helms 1997). Cancellous fractures are seen at sites consisting primarily of medullary bone, for example, at the ends of long bones. Cancellous fractures are often detected, being seen radiographically as subtle blurring of trabecular margins and faint areas of sclerosis secondary to peri-trabecular callus. A more apparent linear sclerotic band may subsequently be more radiographically visible, with fracture progression (Greaney et al. 1983; Anderson and Greenspan 1996). In complex-shaped bones such as the pelvis, both cortical and cancellous fractures may be present.

The typical scintigraphic pattern of a stress fracture is the presence of a sharply-marginated focus of increased uptake confined to the cortex of bone (Collier et al. 1984; Davies et al. 1989). Foci of less intense uptake, presumably representing pre-fracture areas of remodeling, have been called "indeterminate bone stress lesions" and "stress reactions" (Rupani et al. 1985; Floyd et al. 1987). Generally, high-grade lesions seen on scintiscans correlate

with increased stress and higher likelihood of positive radiographs (Zwas et al. 1987; Nielsen et al. 1991). The hyperemia present in the early part of the three-phase bone scintiscan is most intense during the first 2 weeks. With fracture healing, there is a progressive decrease in radionuclide uptake. The increased uptake observed in the third phase of the scintiscan remains positive much longer. Although gradual uptake diminution occurs, abnormal uptake may persist for several months, with variability in scintigraphic detectability of lesions (Rupani et al. 1985; Ammann and Matheson 1991). In children, the physiological increase in radionuclide uptake in the epiphyseal region may mask the abnormal uptake caused by osteoblastic activity due to fatigue fractures.

On MR imaging, a fatigue fracture appears as a band of low signal intensity that arises from the cortex of bone and extends perpendicular to the bone surface (Figs. 16.1, 16.2). Areas of high signal intensity are often present on T2-weighted images, particularly within 4 weeks after symptom onset. These areas represent edema or hemorrhage. MR imaging is particularly useful in patients with severe osteoporosis. In such circumstances, bone scintigraphy may produce false-negatives due to generalized poor uptake of radionuclides.

In a study of military conscripts with stress-related hip pain, Ahovuo et al. (2004) found that 8% of patients had signal changes in MR images of the cranial part of the sacrum that extended to the first and second sacral foramina. This pattern of involvement differs from that of insufficiency fractures. These changes were isointense on T2-weighted images and hyperintense on T2-weighted and STIR images. A linear signal void fracture line is seen in advanced fractures on all MR imaging sequences (Featherstone 1999; Major and Helms 2000). In contrast to insufficiency fractures, sacral fatigue fractures most commonly appear unilaterally (Ahovuo et al. 2004).

Bone marrow edema has been detected in MR imaging of asymptomatic, physically-active persons (Lazzarini et al. 1997; Lohman et al. 2001). Kiuru et al. (2003) found bone marrow edema, as well as fracture line and callus, on the asymptomatic side of military conscripts with fatigue fractures of the pelvis and proximal femur. These authors stress the importance of diagnosing asymptomatic injuries of the femoral neck as complications can occur. Subchondral fatigue fractures of the femoral head have been reported in military recruits. MR imaging shows a localized or diffuse pattern of marrow edema in the femoral head, with a subchondral fracture line. MR imaging is useful in monitoring the clinical course. Bone scintigraphy is non-specific, showing increased uptake in the femoral head (SONG et al. 2004).

In a MR imaging study of symptomatic and asymptomatic postpartum patients, as well as nulliparous non-pregnant volunteers, both the postpartum groups were found to have increased inter-pubic gap and increased signal intensity of the symphysis pubis cartilage on T2-weighted images. The majority of postpartum women also had bruises of the parasymphyseal pubic bones. Other findings were pubic symphysis rupture and sacral fracture (WURDINGER et al. 2002).

16.4.2
Imaging Features of Insufficiency Fractures

16.4.2.1
Parasymphyseal and Pubic Ramus Fractures

Parasymphyseal and pubic ramus fractures may have an aggressive appearance that depends on the stage of fracture maturity (Fig. 16.7). Findings include sclerosis, lytic fracture line, bone expansion, exuberant callus, and osteolysis. The most common radiographic finding is a sclerotic band or line (Fig. 16.11). A lytic fracture line or cortical break is rarely observed (GOERGEN et al. 1978; DE SMET and NEFF 1985; DAVIES et al. 1988). Before

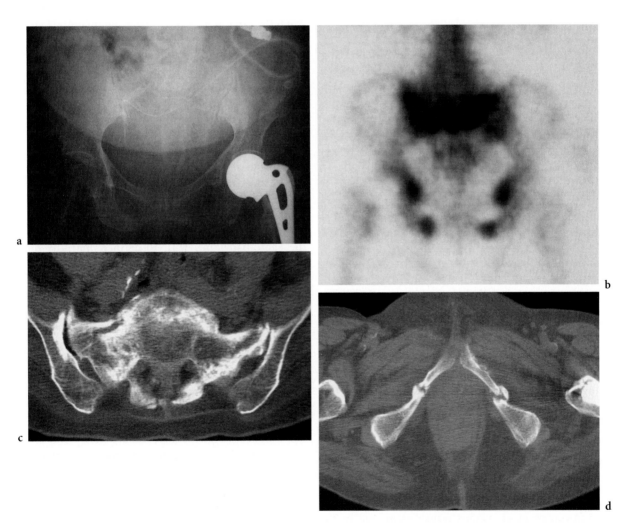

Fig. 16.11a–d. Multiple sacral and pubic insufficiency fractures in a 71-year-old female with chronic renal failure and a left hemiarthroplasty. **a** AP radiograph showing fractures of both superior pubic rami and a peritoneal dialysis catheter. **b** Posterior bone scintigraphy shows sacral fractures as an asymmetric "H-shaped" pattern and bilateral pubic rami fractures. **c** CT confirms the bilateral sacral fractures. **d** Follow-up CT obtained 5 months later shows callus formation around ununited pubic rami fractures

these pubic fractures were fully recognized, many patients presenting with these lesions were subjected to unnecessary biopsies. The marked cellular proliferation involved in the bony repair sequence may also present a diagnostic dilemma to the histopathologist, sometimes making a healing fracture difficult to distinguish from malignancy, particularly osteosarcoma (GOERGEN et al. 1978; CASEY et al. 1984; HALL et al. 1984).

Pubic fractures are seen as a focal area of intense uptake on bone scintigraphy (Fig. 16.11). CT shows the fracture line, usually having poorly-defined margins with adjacent sclerosis. Typically, a soft-tissue mass is absent, bone destruction is lacking, and adjacent fascial planes are preserved (DAVIES et al. 1988). Parasymphyseal fractures are seen on MR imaging as a hyperintense mass with a hypointense rim on T2-weighted images. The lesions are iso- to hypointense on T1-weighted images, and display peripheral enhancement. These MR imaging features were considered to be distinctive enough for the diagnosis of parasymphyseal fractures in patients with osteoporosis and previous irradiation (HOSONO et al. 1997). MR imaging may show a hematoma between the fracture ends and marrow edema in the contralateral pubic ramus (GIBBON and HESSION 1997).

16.4.2.2
Sacral Fractures

Sacral insufficiency fractures often are difficult to detect on radiographs (Figs. 16.9–16.11). These fractures may occasionally be seen as sclerotic bands, cortical disruption, or even fracture lines (COOPER et al. 1985b; DE SMET and NEFF 1985; DAVIES et al. 1988). In most instances, however, these sacral fractures are either not detectable radiographically or are obscured by overlying bowel gas. Other imaging techniques such as bone scintigraphy and CT are therefore necessary for the detection of these radiographically-occult insufficiency fractures (Figs. 16.7, 16.10)

The "H"- or butterfly-shaped scintigraphic uptake pattern of sacral insufficiency fractures was first described by RIES (1983), and subsequently and rapidly confirmed by others (Figs. 16.7, 16.11) (SCHNEIDER et al. 1985; COOPER et al. 1985b; DE SMET and NEFF 1985). The vertical limbs of the "H" lie within the sacral ala, parallel to the sacroiliac joints, while the transverse bar of the "H" extends across the sacral body. The horizontal linear dot

pattern of scintigraphic uptake was reported by BALSEIRO et al. (1987). Other variant incomplete patterns of uptake have since been described, with the typical "H"-shaped pattern being seen in only approximately one-half of cases. These variant patterns include bilateral sacral uptake without the horizontal bar, unilateral sacral uptake, and bilateral sacral uptake with a partial horizontal bar (DAVIES et al. 1988; WEBER et al. 1993; BAKER and SIEGEL 1994; GOTIS-GRAHAM et al. 1994; PEH et al. 1995a; GRANGIER et al. 1997; FINIELS et al. 1997).

CT is considered the definitive imaging method for confirming insufficiency fractures of sacrum. Sacral fractures are typically oriented vertically and are located parallel to the sacroiliac joint (Figs. 16.10, 16.11). A linear fracture line with surrounding sclerosis is observed. CT is indicated particularly when the bone scintiscans display an incomplete or variant pattern. CT is also useful for detecting large bony defects in the sacrum, such as Tarlov cysts (PEH and EVANS 1992), and for the diagnosis of coexisting malignant lesions (PEH et al. 1997; OLIVER and BEGGS 1999). The detection of an additional metastatic lesion may have management and prognostic implications. CT is also the optimal imaging modality for detecting intra-fracture gas which may have originated from the adjacent sacroiliac joint (STABLER et al. 1995; PEH and OOI 1997).

BRAHME et al. (1990) first reported the MR imaging appearances of sacral insufficiency fractures. These fractures were located on the iliac side of the sacroiliac joint, with ill-defined margins on all imaging sequences (Fig. 16.9). They were T1-hypointense, T2-hyperintense, and demonstrated enhancement (MAMMONE and SCHWEITZER 1995). The fracture line may be detected within the zone of surrounding hyperintense marrow edema on T2-weighted images. The fracture line is typically located parallel to the sacroiliac joint (GRANGIER et al. 1997). A transient bone marrow edema pattern has been reported as a variant pattern of sacral insufficiency fractures (PEH et al. 1998). The presence of intra-fracture fluid has been proposed as a new diagnostic sign for sacral insufficiency fracture (PEH 2000). There is consensus among some authors that the MR imaging characteristics of these fractures are sufficiently characteristic for differentiation from metastatic disease, particularly in postradiotherapy patients (MAMMONE and SCHWEITZER 1995; BLOMLIE et al. 1996). However, if the fracture line is not demonstrated, MR imaging appearances can be non-specific and may be misinterpreted as malignant disease (BLAKE and CONNORS 2004).

16.4.2.3
Iliac Fractures

Iliac fractures may occur at three locations, namely: supra-acetabular, oblique iliac (Fig. 16.12), and superomedial iliac (Davies and Bradley 1991). Supra-acetabular fractures may be seen on radiographs as hazy bands of sclerosis located immediately above and parallel to the acetabular roof (Cooper et al. 1985a). They appear as areas of linear or focal uptake on bone scintiscans. Oblique iliac fractures extend diagonally across the iliac ala from the greater sciatic notch while superomedial iliac fractures are located adjacent to the sacroiliac joint (Davies and Bradley 1991). On radiographs, the fracture line may be seen extending from the upper ilium into the bone (Gaucher et al. 1986). Iliac fractures have a linear configuration and may also be seen as slanting lines of uptake across the iliac wing on bone scintigraphy (Cooper et al. 1985b; Gaucher et al. 1986).

CT is useful in confirming the presence of suspected fractures, revealing further fractures, and excluding the likelihood of malignancy (Davies and Bradley 1991). MR imaging shows iliac fractures as areas of low signal intensity on T1-weighted images and high signal intensity on T2-weighted images (Mumber et al. 1997). Imaging in the sagittal plane may be useful on depiction of iliac fractures (Grangier et al. 1997). On MR imaging, supra-acetabular insufficiency fractures are seen as a characteristic linear area of low signal intensity on both T1- and T2-weighted images, with adjacent edema being depicted as diffuse bands of high T2 signal (Otte et al. 1997).

16.4.2.4
Femoral Head and Neck Fractures

Initial radiographs of subchondral femoral head insufficiency fractures may be normal. This may progress to a subchondrally-located focal area of sclerosis or a radiolucent linear area that represents a fracture line. A focal depression, discrete step or femoral head collapse may then occur. The weight-bearing and supero-lateral areas of the femoral head are most commonly involved. Although these radiographic changes may resemble those of osteonecrosis, histological examinations have shown these entities to be distinctly different (Yamamoto and Bullough 1999, 2000a; Hagino et al. 1999; Yamamoto et al. 2000, 2001; Davies et al. 2004).

On bone scintigraphy of subchondral insufficiency fractures, there is focal increased radionuclide uptake in the femoral head. These findings are considered non-specific although the presence of increased uptake at other typical sites of occurrence of insufficiency fractures may be a helpful clue. On MR imaging, a curvilinear band that is hypointense on both T1- and T2-weighted images is seen in the subchondral region, parallel or convex to the articular surface. There may be associated contour femoral head abnormality and adjacent bone marrow edema. These changes may resolve on follow-up MR imaging (VandeBerg et al. 1994; Bangil et al. 1996; Rafii et al. 1997; Yamamoto and Bullough 1999, 2000a; Hagino et al. 1999; Yamamoto et al. 2000, 2001; Davies et al. 2004).

MR imaging findings may resemble those of osteonecrosis of the femoral head. Bone marrow edema is found in both conditions, and is also a non-specific finding for transient osteoporosis of the hip (Watson et al. 2004). The typical band of low signal intensity in the subchondral location is considered specific for an insufficiency fracture, in contrast to the well-defined zonal pattern of signal abnormality found in osteonecrosis (Lang et al.

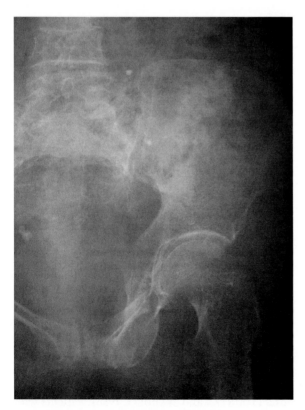

Fig. 16.12. AP radiograph in an 89-year-old osteoporotic female showing pubic and oblique iliac insufficiency fractures

1988; VandeBerg et al. 1993; Watson et al. 2004). In early osteonecrosis, the subchondral bone segment proximal to the low-intensity band does not show a high signal on T2-weighted images as the proximal segment is totally necrotic. This differs from subchondral insufficiency fracture where the proximal segment consists of marrow edema and repair tissue, hence producing high signal intensity on T2-weighted images (Yamamoto et al. 2001).

Diffuse bone marrow edema with contrast enhancement effect has been described in both proximal and distal segments of the low-signal intensity band of the subchondral insufficiency fracture, features that are distinct from those of osteonecrosis (Uetani et al. 2003). In the late stage where there is advanced femoral head collapse, differentiation of subchondral insufficiency fracture from osteonecrosis may be difficult (Davies et al. 2004). Subchondral fractures have been identified in patients with transient osteoporosis of the hip and are hypothesized to result from osteoporosis associated with this entity (Miyanishi et al. 2001).

Yamamoto and Bullough (2000b) have suggested that insufficiency fracture of the femoral head is associated with and gives rise to rapidly-destructive hip disease. Others have supported this hypothesis (Watanabe et al. 2002; Davies et al. 2004). Joint space narrowing, and a diffuse pattern of low signal intensity on T1-weighted and high signal intensity on T2-weighted images, may be early signs of rapid-destructive hip disease (Sugano et al. 2001).

Insufficiency fractures of the femoral neck can be missed easily. In spite of persistent hip pain with no history of significant antecedent trauma, patients with these fractures often have normal radiographs or display subtle changes. Early radiographic changes include osteoporosis, minor trabecular malalignment, mild cortical or endosteal sclerosis, and lucent fracture lines (Fig. 16.8). Undiagnosed and untreated fractures may progress to displaced subcapital fracture, angular deformity and osteonecrosis of the femoral head (Dorne and Lander 1985; Tountas 1993).

16.4.2.5
Concomitant Fractures in and Around the Pelvis

The association between sacral and os pubis fractures was first identified in 1995 (Cooper et al. 1985b; de Smet and Neff 1985). This and other combinations of insufficiency fractures in and around the bony pelvis is now recognized as being diagnos-

tic (Fig. 16.7) (Davies et al. 1988; Rawlings et al. 1988; Davies and Bradley 1991; Peh et al. 1995a, 1996; Soubrier et al. 2003). Lakhanpal et al. (1986) reported a total of 32 insufficiency fractures occurring in a 51-year-old woman with long-standing rheumatoid arthritis.

There are two radiographic patterns of insufficiency fractures in the pelvic region, namely: aggressive and occult types. The parasymphyseal and pubic ramus fractures fall into the aggressive category while the occult group includes fractures of the sacrum and ilium (Peh et al. 1996). Bone scintigraphy is helpful for detecting all sites of insufficiency fractures. Concomitant findings of two or more areas of uptake in the sacrum and at another pelvic site are considered diagnostic of insufficiency fractures of the pelvis. The degree of confidence is considered high as bone scintiscans are highly sensitive and highly specific, when concomitant sacral and pubic uptake is observed. If a typical pattern of abnormality is not present, bone scintigraphy is much less specific and may need to be supplemented by CT.

16.5
Management of Stress Fractures

16.5.1
Fatigue Fractures

Sacral fatigue fractures are treated with prolonged rest, during which physical activity is not permitted (Volpin et al. 1989; Ahovuo et al. 2004). Symphysis pubis fatigue injury is a self-limiting condition that may take several months to resolve. Administration of corticosteroid injections may help in the rehabilitation process (Lynch and Renstrom 1999). Fatigue fractures of the femoral neck are often initially missed. Early recognition and regular clinical and imaging review are required to prevent progress of the fracture to a displaced fracture. Outcome and prognosis are dependent on femoral neck displacement which may lead to development of osteonecrosis (Johansson et al. 1990; Clough 2002). Patients may either be treated conservatively or with internal fixation. Transverse fractures are potentially unstable and may require prompt internal fixation, while compression fractures have a benign prognosis (Tountas and Waddell 1986). Patients who develop complications require major surgery, such as hip replacement (Johansson et al. 1990).

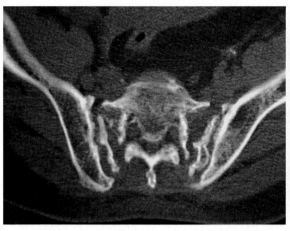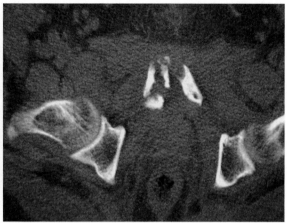

a   b

Fig. 16.13a,b. CT sacrum (**a**) and CT pubis (**b**) showing non-union bilateral sacral and right parasymphyseal insufficiency fractures in a 64-year-old female who had undergone radiotherapy for carcinoma of the uterus

16.5.2
Insufficiency Fractures

Management of insufficiency fractures of the pelvic ring is conservative and consists initially of enforced bed rest, reduced weight- bearing, and then followed by gradual mobilization. Delayed healing is common and nonunion recognized (Figs. 16.11d, 16.13). The administration of subcutaneous calcitonin has been suggested (Peh et al. 1993; Weber et al. 1993; West et al. 1994). Non-narcotic analgesics for pain relief are considered helpful (Newhouse et al. 1992; Weber et al. 1993). Graded exercises are started once symptomatic improvement is observed. Prognosis is good, with healing being expected within 4–6 months (Rawlings et al. 1988; Crayton et al. 1991; Weber et al. 1993; Gotis-Graham et al. 1994; Peh et al. 1996). For patients who are undergoing radiation therapy for pelvic malignancies, reduction of dose contribution to the sacrum and sacroiliac joint has been suggested, as it may help prevent insufficiency fractures in postmenopausal women with multiple deliveries or low body weight (Ogino et al. 2003). It is also useful to identify and specifically treat the underlying causes of reduced bone mineralization.

Surgery is sometimes required to stabilize pelvic ring fractures. In a study of insufficiency fractures that developed secondary to altered biomechanics following iliac bone graft harvesting, Nocini et al. (2003) divided the iliac crest fractures into two groups, depending on region of bone graft harvesting. Fractures resulting from anterior graft harvesting remain stable and heal spontaneously without further complications, while fractures due to posterior iliac crest harvesting often develop pelvic ring

instability, require complex surgical treatments, and are prone to permanent disability. Sacroplasty, a procedure in which polymethylmethacrylate is injected into the fracture, has recently been described for treatment of sacral insufficiency fractures. This technique appears to be useful in providing symptomatic relief and may be an alternative mode of therapy (Garant 2002; Pommersheim et al. 2003).

For subchondral insufficiency fractures of the femoral head, the prognosis depends on the fracture extent, degree of osteoporosis, body weight and initial treatment (Yamamoto et al. 2000). Fractures that are identified early are treated conservatively with a period of non-weight bearing. Underlying osteoporosis should also be treated. Patients who have already developed rapidly-destructive hip disease at presentation are expected to have a poor clinical outcome and may require early hip surgery (Legroux Gerot et al. 2004; Davies et al. 2004).

16.6
Summary

Stress fractures of the bony pelvis and hips can affect a wide spectrum of patients, with variable causative factors and clinical presentations. Classification into fatigue and insufficiency categories of fractures is useful. Diagnosis of these fractures requires a high index of clinical suspicion. Imaging has an important role in the early diagnosis of stress fracture which in turn, has a major impact on management of affected patients, and prevention of further morbidity and potential complications.

References

Abe H, Nakamura M, Takahashi S et al (1992) Radiation-induced insufficiency fractures of the pelvis: evaluation with 99m Tc-methylene diphosphonate scintigraphy. Am J Roentgenol 158:599-602

Adkins MC, Sundaram M (2001) Radiologic case study. Insufficiency fracture of the acetabular roof in Paget's disease. Orthopedics 24:1019-1020

Ahovuo JA, Kiuru MJ, Visuri T (2004) Fatigue stress fractures of the sacrum: diagnosis with MR imaging. Eur Radiol 14:500-505

Aitken JM (1984) Relevance of osteoporosis in women with fracture of the femoral neck. Br Med J 288:597-601

Albertsen AM, Egund N, Jurik AG (1994) Post-traumatic osteolysis of the pubic bone simulating malignancy. Acta Radiol 35:40-44

Albertsen AMB, Egund N, Jurik AG (1995) Fatigue fractures of the sacral bone associated with septic arthritis of the symphysis pubis. Skeletal Radiol 24:605-607

Ammann W, Matheson GO (1991) Radionuclide bone imaging in the detection of stress fractures. Clin J Sports Med 1:115-122

Anderson MW, Greenspan A (1996) Stress fractures. Radiology 199:1-12

Arrington ED, Davino NA (1999) Subcapital femoral neck fracture after closed reduction and internal fixation of an intertrochanteric hip fracture: a case report and review of the literature. Am J Orthop 28:517-521

Baker RJ, Siegel A (1994) Sacral insufficiency fracture: half of an "H". Clin Nucl Med 19:1106-1007

Balseiro J, Brower AC, Ziessman HA (1987) Scintigraphic diagnosis of sacral insufficiency fractures. Am J Roentgenol 148:111-113

Bangil M, Soubrier M, Dubost JJ et al (1996) Subchondral insufficiency fracture of the femoral head. Rev Rhum Engl Ed 63:859-861

Beard JP, Wade WH, Barber DB (1996) Sacral insufficiency stress fracture as etiology of positional autonomic dysreflexia: case report. Paraplegia 34:173-175

Berger PE, Ofstein RA, Jackson DW et al (1989) MRI demonstration of radiographically occult fractures: what have we been missing? Radiographics 9:407-436

Blake SP, Connors AM (2004) Sacral insufficiency fracture. Br J Radiol 77:891-896

Bliss P, Parsons CA, Blake PR (1996) Incidence and possible aetiological factors in the development of pelvic insufficiency fractures following radical radiotherapy. Br J Radiol 69:548-554

Blomlie V, Lien HH, Iversen T et al (1993) Radiation-induced insufficiency fractures of the sacrum: evaluation with MR imaging. Radiology 188:241-244

Blomlie V, Rofstad EK, Talle K et al (1996) Incidence of radiation-induced insufficiency fractures of the female pelvis: evaluation with MR imaging. Am J Roentgenol 167:1205-1210

Bottomley AM (1990) Sacral stress fracture in a runner. Br J Sports Med 24:243-244

Brahme SK, Cervilla V, Vint V et al (1990) Magnetic resonance appearance of sacral insufficiency fractures. Skeletal Radiol 19:489-493

Breuil V, Brocq O, Euller-Ziegler L et al (1997) Insufficiency fracture of the sacrum revealing a pregnancy associated osteoporosis. Ann Rheum Dis 56:278-279

Buciuto R, Hammer R, Herder A (1997) Spontaneous subcapital femoral neck fracture after healed trochanteric fracture. Clin Orthop 342:156-163

Buttaro M, Della Valle AG, Morandi A et al (2003) Insufficiency subchondral fracture of the femoral head: report of four cases and review of the literature. J Arthroplasty 18:377-382

Calandruccio RA (1983) Classification of femoral neck fractures in the elderly as pathologic fractures. Hip 8-33

Carter SR (1987) Stress fractures of the sacrum: brief report. J Bone Joint Surg (Br) 69:843-844

Casey D, Mirra J, Staple TW (1984) Parasymphyseal insufficiency fractures of the os pubis. Am J Roentgenol 142:581-586

Chary-Valckenaere I, Blum A, Pere P et al (1997) Insufficiency fractures of the ilium. Rev Rhum Engl Ed 64:542-548

Chevrot A (1992) Stress fractures. In: Resnick D, Petterson H (eds) Skeletal Radiology. Merit Communications, London, pp 173-190

Christiansen CG, Kassim RA, Callaghan JJ et al (2003) Pubic ramus insufficiency fractures following total hip arthroplasty. A report of six cases. J Bone Joint Surg (Am) 85:1819-1822

Clement DB, Amman W, Taunton JE et al (1993) Exercise induced stress injuries to the femur. Int J Sports Med 14:347-352

Clough TM (2002) Femoral neck stress fracture: the importance of clinical suspicion and early review. Br J Sports Med 36:308-309

Collier D, Johnson RP, Carrera GF et al (1984) Scintigraphic diagnosis of stress induced incomplete fracture of the proximal tibia. J Trauma 24:156-160

Cooper KL (1994) Insufficiency stress fractures. Curr Prob Diagn Radiol 23:29-68

Cooper KL, Beabout JW, McLeod RA (1985a) Supraacetabular insufficiency fractures. Radiology 157:15-17

Cooper KL, Beabout JW, Swee RG (1985b) Insufficiency fractures of the sacrum. Radiology 156:15-20

Crayton HE, Bell CL, de Smet AA (1991) Sacral insufficiency fractures. Semin Arthritis Rheum 20:378-384

Czarnecki DJ, Till EW, Minikel JL (1988) Unique sacral stress fracture in a runner. Am J Roentgenol 151:1255

Daffner RH (1984) Anterior tibial striations. Am J Roentgenol 143:651-653

Daffner RH, Pavlov H (1992) Stress fractures: current concepts. Am J Roentgenol 159:245-252

Davies AM (1990) Stress lesions of bone. Curr Imaging 2:209-216

Davies AM, Bradley SA (1991) Iliac insufficiency fractures. Br J Radiol 64:305-309

Davies AM, Evans NS, Struthers GR (1988) Parasymphyseal and associated insufficiency fractures of the pelvis and sacrum. Br J Radiol 61:103-108

Davies AM, Carter SR, Grimer RJ et al (1989) Fatigue fractures of the femoral diaphysis in the skeletally immature simulating malignancy. Br J Radiol 62:893-896

Davies M, Cassar-Pullicino VM, Darby AJ (2004) Subchondral insufficiency fractures of the femoral head. Eur Radiol 14:201-207

De Smet AA, Neff JR (1985) Pubic and sacral insufficiency fractures: clinical course and radiologic findings. Am J Roentgenol 145:601-606

Dorne HL, Lander PH (1985) Spontaneous stress fractures of the femoral neck. Am J Roentgenol 144:343-347

Eastell R, Dickson ER, Hodgson SF et al (1991) Rates of vertebral bone loss before and after liver transplantation in women with primary biliary cirrhosis. Hepatology 14:296-300

Egol KA, Koval KJ, Kummer F et al (1998) Stress fractures of the femoral neck. Clin Orthop 348:72-78

Eller DJ, Katz DS, Bergman AG et al (1997) Sacral stress fractures in long-distance runners. Clin J Sports Med 7:222-225

Eschenroeder HC Jr, Krackow KA (1988) Late onset femoral stress fracture associated with extruded cement following hip arthroplasty. A case report. Clin Orthop 236:210-213

Featherstone T (1990) Magnetic resonance imaging in the diagnosis of sacral stress fracture. Br J Sports Med 33:276-277

Finiels H, Finiels PJ, Jacquot JM et al (1997) Fractures of the sacrum caused by bone insufficiency. Meta-analysis of 508 cases. Presse Med 26:1568-1573

Floyd WN Jr, Butler JE, Clanton T et al (1987) Roentgenologic diagnosis of stress fractures and stress reactions. South Med J 80:433-439

Fu AL, Greven KM, Maruyama Y (1994) Radiation osteitis and insufficiency fractures after pelvic irradiation for gynecologic malignancies. Am J Clin Oncol 17:248-254

Fullerton LR (1990) Femoral neck stress fractures. J Sports Med 9:192-197

Garant M (2002) Sacroplasty: a new treatment for sacral insufficiency fracture. J Vasc Interv Radiol 13:1265-1267

Gaucher A, Pere P, Bannwarth B et al (1986) Unusual features of stress fractures of the pelvic girdle. J Rheumatol 13:826-827

Gibbon WW, Hession PR (1997) Diseases of the pubis and pubic symphysis: MR imaging appearances. Am J Roentgenol 169:849-853

Godfrey N, Staple TW, Halter D et al (1985) Insufficiency os pubis fractures in rheumatoid arthritis. J Rheumatol 12:176-179

Goergen TG, Resnick D, Riley RR (1978) Post-traumatic abnormalities of the pubic bone simulating malignancy. Radiology 126:85-87

Goldman AB, Jacobs B (1984) Femoral neck fractures complicating Gaucher disease in children. Skeletal Radiol 12:162-168

Gotis-Graham I, McGuigan L, Diamond T et al (1994) Sacral insufficiency fractures in the elderly. J Bone Joint Surg (Br) 76:882-886

Grangier C, Garcia J, Howarth NR et al (1997) Role of MRI in the diagnosis of insufficiency fractures of the sacrum and acetabular roof. Skeletal Radiol 26:517-524

Greaney RB, Gerber FH, Laughlin RL et al (1983) Distribution and natural history of stress fractures in US Marine recruits. Radiology 146:339-346

Grier D, Wardell S, Sarwark J et al (1993) Fatigue fractures of the sacrum in children: two case reports and a review of the literature. Skeletal Radiol 22:515-518

Ha KI, Hahn SH, Chung MY et al (1991) A clinical study of stress fractures in sports activities. Orthopaedics 14:1089-1095

Haasbeek JF, Green NE (1994) Adolescent stress fractures of the sacrum: two case reports. J Pediatr Orthop 14:336-338

Hagino H, Okano T, Teshima R et al (1999) Insufficiency fracture of the femoral head in patients with severe osteoporosis: report of two cases. Acta Orthop Scand 70:87-89

Hall FM, Goldberg RP, Kasdon EJ et al (1984) Post-traumatic osteolysis of the pubic bone simulating a malignant lesions. J Bone Joint Surg (Br) 66:121-126

Hardy DC, Delince PE, Yasik E et al (1992) Stress fracture of the hip. An unusual complication of total knee arthroplasty. Clin Orthop 281:140-141

Hill PF, Chatterji S, Chambers D et al (1996) Stress fracture of the pubic ramus in female recruits. J Bone Joint Surg (Br) 78:383-386

Hosono M, Kobayashi H, Fujimoto R et al (1997) MR appearance of parasymphyseal insufficiency fractures of the os pubis. Skeletal Radiol 26:525-528

Huh SJ, Kim B, Kang MK et al (2002) Pelvic insufficiency fracture after pelvic irradiation in uterine cervical cancer. Gynecol Oncol 86:264-268

Johansson C, Ekenman I, Tornkvist H et al (1990) Stress fractures of the femoral neck in athletes. The consequence of a delay in diagnosis. Am J Sports Med 18:524-528

Jones JW (1991) Insufficiency fracture of the sacrum with displacement and neurologic damage: a case report and review of the literature. J Am Geriatr Soc 39:280-283

Kaltsas DS (1981) Stress fractures of the femoral neck in young adults: a report of seven cases. J Bone Joint Surg (Br) 63:33-37

Kanai H, Igarashi M, Yamamoto S et al (1999) Spontaneous subcapital femoral neck fracture complicating a healed intertrochanteric fracture. Arch Orthop Trauma Surg 119:271-275

Keene JS, Lash EG (1992) Negative bone scan in a femoral neck stress fracture: a case report. Am J Sports Med 20:234-236

Kelly EW, Jonson SR, Cohen ME et al (2000) Stress fractures of the pelvis in female navy recruits: an analysis of possible mechanisms of injury. Mil Med 165:142-146

Kerr PS, Johnson DP (1995) Displaced femoral neck stress fracture in a marathon runner. Injury 26:491-493

Kitajima I, Tachibana S, Mikami Y et al (1999) Insufficiency fracture of the femoral neck after intermedullary nailing. J Orthop Sci 4:304-306

Kiuru MJ, Pihlajamaki HK, Perkio JP et al (2001) Dynamic contrast-enhanced MR imaging in symptomatic bone stress of the pelvis and the lower extremity. Acta Radiol 42:277-285

Kiuru MJ, Pihlajamaki HK, Hietanen HJ et al (2002) MR imaging, bone scintigraphy, and radiography in bone stress injuries of the pelvis and the lower extremity. Acta Radiol 43:207-212

Kiuru MJ, Pihlajamaki HK, Ahuvuo JA (2003) Fatigue stress injuries of the pelvic bones and proximal femur: evaluation with MR imaging. Eur Radiol 13:605-611

Koch R, Jackson D (1981) Pubic symphysitis in runners: a report of two cases. Am J Sports Med 9:62-63

Kupke MJ, Kahler DM, Lorenzoni MH et al (1993) Stress fracture of the femoral neck in a long distance runner: biomechanical aspects. J Emerg Med 11:587-591

La Ban M, Merschaert J, Taylor R et al (1978) Symphyseal and sacroiliac joint pain associated with pubic symphysis instability, Arch Phys Med Rehab 59:470-472

Lakhanpal S, McLeod RA, Luthra HS (1986) Insufficiency type stress fractures in rheumatoid arthritis: report of an interesting case and review of the literature. Clin Exp Rheumatol 4:151-154

Lam KS, Moulton A (2001) Stress fracture of the sacrum in a child. Ann Rheum Dis 60:87

Lang P, Jegesen HE, Moseley ME et al (1988) Avascular necrosis of the femoral head: high-field strength MR imaging with histological correlation. Radiology 169:517-524

Lappe JM, Stegman MR, Recker RR (2001) The impact of lifestyle factors on stress fractures in female Army recruits. Osteoporosis Int 12:35-42

Launder WJ, Hungerford DS (1981) Stress fractures of the pubis after total hip arthroplasty. Clin Orthop 159:183-185

Lazzarini KM, Troiano RN, Smith RC (1997) Can running cause the appearance of marrow edema on MR images of the foot and ankle? Radiology 202:540-542

Lee JK, Yao L (1988) Stress fractures: MR imaging. Radiology 169:217-220

Legroux Gerot I, Demondion X, Louville AB et al (2004) Subchondral fractures of the femoral head: a review of seven cases. Joint Bone Spine 71:131-135

Lock SH, Mitchell SCM (1993) Osteoporotic sacral fracture causing neurological deficit. Br J Hosp Med 49:210

Lohman M, Kivisaari A, Vehmas T et al (2001) MRI abnormalities of foot and ankle in asymptomatic, physically active individuals. Skeletal Radiol 30:61-66

Lourie H (1982) Spontaneous osteoporotic fracture of the sacrum. An unrecognized syndrome of the elderly. JAMA 248:715-717

Lundin B, Bjorkholm E, Lundell M et al (1990) Insufficiency fractures of the sacrum after radiotherapy for gynaecological malignancy. Acta Oncol 29:211-215

Lynch SA, Renstrom PA (1999) Groin injuries in sport: treatment strategies. Sports Med 28:137-144

Major NM, Helms CA (1997) Pelvic stress injuries: the relationship between osteitis pubis (symphysis pubis stress injury) and sacroiliac abnormalities in athletes. Skeletal Radiol 26:711-717

Major NM, Helms CA (2000) Sacral stress fractures in long-distance runners. Am J Roentgenol 174:727-729

Mammone JF, Schweitzer ME (1995) MRI of occult sacral insufficiency fractures following radiotherapy. Skeletal Radiol 24:101-104

Marc V, Dromer C, Sixou L et al (1997) A new case of insufficiency fracture in a patient with tabes dorsalis. Rev Rhum Engl Ed 64:271-273

Martin J, Brandser EA, Shin MJ et al (1995) Fatigue fracture of the sacrum in a child. Can Assoc Radiol J 46:468-470

Martin RB, Burr DB (1982) A hypothetical mechanism for the stimulation of osteonal remodeling by fatigue damage. J Biomech 15:137-139

Matheson GO, Clement DB, McKenzie DC et al (1987) Stress fractures in athletes. A study of 320 cases. Am J Sports Med 15:46-58

Mathews V, McCance SE, O'Leary PF (2001) Early fracture of the sacrum or pelvis: an unusual complication after multilevel instrumented lumbosacral fusion. Spine 26: E571-E575

McBryde AM Jr (1975) Stress fractures in athletes. J Sports Med 3:212-217

Meyers SP, Wiener SN (1991) Magnetic resonance imaging features of fractures using the short tau inversion recovery (STIR) sequence: correlation with radiographic findings. Skeletal Radiol 20:499-507

Milgrom C, Chisin R, Giladi M et al (1984) Negative bone scans in impending tibial stress fractures. Am J Sports Med 12:488-491

Milgrom C, Giladi M, Stein M et al (1985) Stress fractures in military recruits: a prospective study showing an unusually high incidence. J Bone Joint Surg (Br) 67:732-735

Miller C, Major N, Toth A (2003) Pelvic stress injuries in the athlete: management and prevention. Sports Med 13:1003-1012

Mink JH, Deutsch AL (1989) Occult osseous and cartilaginous injuries about the knee: MR assessment, detection, and classification. Radiology 170:823-829

Miyanishi L, Yamamoto T, Nakashima Y et al (2001) Subchondral changes in transient osteoporosis of the hip. Skeletal Radiol 30:255-261

Moreno A, Clemente J, Crespo C et al (1999) Pelvic insufficiency fractures in patients with pelvic irradiation. Int J Radiat Oncol Biol Phys 44:61-66

Mulligan ME (1995) The "gray cortex": an early sign of stress fracture. Skeletal Radiol 24:201-203

Mumber MP, Greven KM, Haygood TM (1997) Pelvic insufficiency fractures associated with radiation atrophy: clinical recognition and diagnostic evaluation. Skeletal Radiol 26:94-99

Newhouse KE, El-Khoury GY, Buckwalter JA (1992) Occult sacral fractures in osteoporotic patients. J Bone Joint Surg (Am) 74:1472-1477

Nielsen MB, Hansen K, Holmes P et al (1991) Tibial periosteal reactions in soldiers: a scintigraphic study of 29 cases of lower leg pain. Acta Orthop Scand 62:531-534

Noakes TD, Smith JA, Lindenberg G et al (1985) Pelvic stress fractures in long distance runners. Am J Sports Med 13:120-123

Nocini PF, Bedogni A, Valsecchi S et al (2003) Fractures of the iliac crest following anterior and posterior bone graft harvesting. Review of the literature and case presentation. Minerva Stomatol 52:441-452

Ogino I, Okamoto N, Ono Y et al (2003) Pelvic insufficiency fractures in postmenopausal woman with advanced cervical cancer treated by radiotherapy. Radiother Oncol 68:61-67

Oliver TB, Beggs I (1999) Defects in the pelvic ring as a cause of sacral insufficiency fractures. Clin Radiol 54:852-854

Otte MT, Helms CA, Fritz RC (1997) MR imaging of supra-acetabular insufficiency fractures. Skeletal Radiol 26:279-283

Peh WCG (2000) Intrafracture fluid: a new diagnostic sign of insufficiency fractures of the sacrum and ilium. Br J Radiol 73:895-898

Peh WCG, Evans NS (1992) Tarlov cysts: another cause of sacral insufficiency fractures? Clin Radiol 46:329-330

Peh WCG, Ooi GC (1997) Vacuum phenomena in the sacroiliac joints and in association with sacral insufficiency fractures. Incidence and significance. Spine 22:2005-2008

Peh WCG, Gough AK, Sheeran T et al (1993) Pelvic insufficiency fractures in rheumatoid arthritis. Br J Rheumatol 32:319-324.

Peh WCG, Khong PL, Ho WY et al (1995a) Sacral insufficiency fractures. Spectrum of radiological features. Clin Imaging 19:92-101

Peh WCG, Khong PL, Sham JST et al (1995b) Sacral and pubic insufficiency fractures after irradiation of gynaecological malignancies. Clin Oncol (R Coll Radiol) 7:117-122

Peh WCG, Khong PL, Yin Y et al (1996) Imaging of pelvic insufficiency fractures. Radiographics 16:335-348

Peh WCG, Khong PL, Ho WY (1997) Sacral insufficiency fractures masking malignancy. Clin Radiol 52:71-72

Peh WCG, Cheng KC, Ho WY et al (1998) Transient bone marrow oedema: a variant pattern of sacral insufficiency fractures. Australas Radiol 42:102-105

Pentecost RL, Murray RA, Brindley HH (1964) Fatigue, insufficiency, and pathological fractures. JAMA 187:1001-1004

Peris P (2003) Stress fractures. Best Pract Res Clin Rheumatol 17:1043-1061

Pommersheim W, Huang-Hellinger F, Baker M et al (2003) Sacroplasty: a treatment for sacral insufficiency fractures. Am J Neuroradiol 24:1003-1007

Pullar T, Parker J, Capell HA (1985) Spontaneous fractured neck of femur in rheumatoid arthritis: absence of radiographic changes on initial X-ray. Scot Med J 30:178-180

Rafii M, Mitnick H, Klug J et al (1997) Insufficiency fracture of the femoral head: MR imaging in three patients. Am J Roentgenol 168:159-163

Rajah R, Davies AM, Carter SR (1993) Fatigue fracture of the sacrum in a child. Pediatr Radiol 23:145-146

Rawlings CE III, Wilkins RH, Martinez S et al (1988) Osteoporotic sacral fractures: a clinical study. Neurosurgery 22:72-76

Ries T (1983) Detection of osteoporotic sacral fractures with radionuclides. Radiology 146:783-785

Rosen PR, Michell LJ, Treves S (1982) Early scintigraphic diagnosis of bone stress and fractures in athletic adolescents. Pediatrics 70:11-15

Rupani HD, Holder LE, Espinola DA et al (1985) Three-phase radionuclide bone imaging in sports medicine. Radiology 156:187-196

Sallis RE, Jones K (1991) Stress fractures in athletes. How to spot this underdiagnosed injury. Postgrad Med 89:185-188, 191-192

Savoca CJ (1971) Stress fractures. A classification of the earliest radiographic signs. Radiology 100:519-524

Schneider HJ, King AY, Bronson JL et al (1974) Stress injury and developmental change of lower extremities in ballet dancers. Radiology 113:627-632

Schneider R, Kaye J, Ghelman B (1976) Adductor avulsion injuries near the symphysis pubis. Radiology 120:567-569

Schneider R, Yacovone J, Ghelman B (1985) Unsuspected sacral fractures: detection by radionuclide bone scanning. Am J Roentgenol 144:337-341

Schnitzler CM, Wing JR, Mesquita JM et al (1990) Risk factors for the development of stress fractures during fluoride therapy for osteoporosis. J Bone Mineral Res 5 [Suppl]: S195-S200

Schulman LL, Addesso V, Staron RB et al (1997) Insufficiency fractures of the sacrum: a cause of low back pain after lung transplantation. J Heart Lung Transplant 16:1081-1085

Seo GS, Aoki J, Karakida O et al (1996) Stress fractures. Radiology 201:879

Shah MK, Stewart GW (2002) Sacral stress fractures: an unusual cause of low back pain in an athlete. Spine 27: E104-E108

Shin AY, Morin WD, Gorman JD et al (1996) The superiority of magnetic resonance imaging in differentiating the cause of hip pain in endurance athletes. Am J Sports Med 24:168-176

Somec K, Meurman KOA (1982) Computed tomography of stress fractures. J Comput Assist Tomogr 6:109–115

Song WS, Yoo JJ, Koo KH et al (2004) Subchondral fatigue fracture of the femoral head in military recruits. J Bone Joint Surg (Am) 86:1917-1924

Soubrier M, Dubost JJ, Boisgard S et al (2003) Insufficiency fracture. A survey of 60 cases and review of the literature. Joint Bone Spine 70:209-218

Stabler A, Beck R, Bartl R et al (1995) Vacuum phenomena in insufficiency fractures of the sacrum. Skeletal Radiol 24:31-35

Sterling JC, Edelstein DW, Calvo RD et al (1992) Stress fracture in the athlete: diagnosis and management. Sports Med 14:336-346

Sugano N, Ohzono K, Nishii T et al (2001) Early MRI findings of rapidly destructive coxopathy. Magn Reson Imaging 19:47-50

Tarr RW, Kaye JJ, Nance EP Jr (1988) Insufficiency fractures of the femoral neck in association with chronic renal failure. South Med J 81:863-866

Tauber C, Geltner D, Noff M et al (1987) Disruption of the symphysis pubis and fatigue fractures of the pelvis in a patient with rheumatoid arthritis. A case report. Clin Orthop 215:105-108

Tehranzadeh J, Kurth L, Elyaserani M et al (1982) Combined pelvic stress fracture and avulsion of the adductor longus in a middle-distance runner: a case report. Am J Sports Med 10:108-111

Thienpont E, Simon JP, Fabry G (1999) Sacral stress fracture during pregnancy: a case report. Acta Orthop Scand 70:525-526

Tountas AA (1993) Insufficiency stress fractures of the femoral neck in elderly women. Clin Orthop 292:202-209

Tountas AA, Waddell JP (1986) Stress fracture of the femoral neck. A report of seven cases. Clin Orthop 210:160-165

Uetani M, Hashmi R, Ito M et al (2003) Subchondral insufficiency fracture of the femoral head: magnetic resonance imaging findings correlated with micro-computed tomography and histopathology. J Comput Assist Tomogr 27:189-193

Van Linthoudt D, Ott H (1987) Supraacetabular and femoral head stress fracture during fluoride treatment. Gerontology 33:302-306

VandeBerg BE, Malghem JJ, Labaisse MA et al (1993) MR imaging of avascular necrosis and transient bone marrow edema of the femoral head. Radiographics 13:501-520

VandeBerg B, Malghem J, Goffin EJ et al (1994) Transient epiphyseal lesions in renal transplant recipients: presumed insufficiency stress fractures. Radiology 191:403-407

Visuri T (1997) Stress osteopathy of the femoral head: 10 military recruits followed for 5-11 years. Acta Orthop Scand 68:138-141

Volpin G, Milgrom C, Goldsher D et al (1989) Stress fractures of the sacrum following strenuous activity. Clin Orthop 243:184-188

Watanabe W, Itoi E, Yamada S (2002) Early MRI findings of rapidly destructive coxarthrosis. Skeletal Radiol 31:35-38

Watson RM, Roach NA, Dalinka MK (2004) Avascular necrosis and bone marrow edema syndrome. Radiol Clin North Am 42:207-219

Weber M, Hasler P, Gerber H (1993) Insufficiency fractures of the sacrum. Twenty cases and review of the literature. Spine 18:2507-2512

West SG, Troutner JL, Baker MR et al (1994) Sacral insufficiency fractures in rheumatoid arthritis. Spine 19:2117-2121

Wiley J (1983) Traumatic osteitis pubis: the gracilis syndrome. Am J Sports Med 11:360-363

Williams TR, Puckett ML, Denison G et al Acetabular stress fractures in military endurance athletes and recruits: incidence and MRI and scintigraphic findings. Skeletal Radiol 31:277-281

Wilson ES, Katz FN (1969) Stress fractures: an analysis of 250 consecutive cases. Radiology 92:481-486

Wurdinger S, Humbsch K, Reichenbach JR et al (2002) MRI of the pelvic ring joints postpartum: normal and pathological findings. J Magn Reson Imaging 15:324-329

Yamamoto T, Bullough PG (1999) Subchondral insufficiency fracture of the femoral head: a differential diagnosis in acute onset of coxarthrosis in the elderly. Arthritis Rheum 42:2719-2723

Yamamoto T, Bullough PG (2000a) Subchondral insufficiency fracture of the femoral head and medial femoral condyle. Skeletal Radiol 29:40-44

Yamamoto T, Bullough PG (2000b) The role of subchondral insufficiency fracture in rapid destruction of the hip joint: as preliminary report. Arthritis Rheum 43:2423-2427

Yamamoto T, Schneider R, Bullough PG (2000) Insufficiency subchondral fracture of the femoral head. Am J Surg Pathol 24:464-468

Yamamoto T, Schneider R, Bullough PG (2001) Subchondral insufficiency fracture of the femoral head: histopathologic correlation with MRI. Skeletal Radiol 30:247-254

Yousem DM, Magid D, Fishman EK et al (1986) Computed tomography of stress fractures. JCAT 10:92-95

Zwas ST, Elkanovitch R, Frank G (1987) Interpretation and classification of bone scintigraphic findings in stress fractures. J Nucl Med 28:452-457

17 Soft Tissue Injuries

George Koulouris and David Connell

CONTENTS

17.1
Introduction

Soft tissue injury in the hip region is a not an uncommon complaint in both the elite and recreational athlete. Furthermore, degenerative soft tissue conditions in this region occur with increasing frequency in the elderly, particularly with a history of athletic activity in their youth (Sadro 2000). In order to interpret the acute and degenerative soft tissue disorders that occur around the hip and pelvis, the musculoskeletal radiologist must be familiar with both the regional anatomy and the type of injuries that commonly occur (see Table 17.1).

MR imaging has emerged as a sensitive imaging modality with superb soft tissue contrast and multiplanar capability. It is able to image the hip articulation, surrounding musculature as well as adjacent pelvic and abdominal viscera, which may refer pain to this region. The use of a surface coil placed over the region of clinical concern will afford superior image quality and detect subtle muscle and tendon pathologies that may be missed with the use of a body coil alone. A STIR or proton density/T2-weighted fat suppressed image are sensitive sequences for the detection of soft tissue injury, while either a high resolution T1 or proton density weighted sequence will help to accurately assess the regional anatomy and also be useful for the detection of fibrosis and scar tissue.

Ultrasound offers superior spatial resolution for soft tissue injury and affords the advantage of both

G. Koulouris, MD
MRI Fellow, The Alfred Hospital, Commercial Road, Melbourne, Victoria 3004, Australia
D. Connell, MD
Consultant Musculoskeletal Radiologist, Royal National Orthopaedic Hospital, Stanmore, HA7 4LP, UK

Table 17.1. Categorisation of soft tissue injuries around the hip/pelvis

Anterior soft tissues
Iliopsoas tendinopathy (iliopsoas syndrome)
Iliopsoas bursitis
"Snapping hip" syndrome
Rectus femoris injury
Groin pain
Osteitis pubis
Sportsman's hernias
Adductor enthesopathy
Lateral soft tissues
Greater trochanteric pain syndrome
Gluteus tendinopathy
Trochanteric bursitis
Tensor fascia lata tendinopathy
Posterior soft tissues
Hamstring muscle complex
Sciatic nerve pathology
Piriformis syndrome

dynamic assessment and guidance for intervention. Other imaging modalities play a complimentary role. As the causes of hip pain are so diverse, it comes as no surprise that the use of more than one modality may be necessary to make a formative diagnosis. Furthermore, it is prudent to be vigilant following discovering an abnormality, as there is a high incidence of synchronous causes for a patient's symptoms.

17.1.1
Muscle Injury

As skeletal muscle is the largest single tissue in the body, familiarity with the imaging features of injury is crucial. Muscle injury can manifest in many ways, principally in the form of strain, contusion and avulsion (Bencardino et al. 2000; Farber and Buckwalter 2002).

Muscle strain is the end of a continuum of muscle stretching, of which eccentric contraction and delayed onset muscle soreness (DOMS) are the mildest forms (El-Khoury et al. 1996). Mild (grade 1) strain injury manifests clinically as pain with activity, however relative preservation of function. MR imaging usually manifests as oedema at the musculotendinous junction (where most strain injuries occur). This region is therefore hyperintense on T2 weighted imaging and normal on T1. With increasing injury, loss of function ensues, resulting in a moderate or grade 2 strain. The principal feature is that of macroscopic myofibrillar disruption and discrete haematoma formation, thus again T2 hyperintense and a variable T1 weighted appearance. Finally, severe (grade 3) strain manifests as avulsion of the muscle-tendon-bone unit. In the adolescent, this is in the form of an apophyseal disruption (bone–bone interface) compared to the adult, where this has united. In the skeletally mature, avulsion occurs at the muscle-tendon or tendon-bone junction. Significant haematoma formation is present, often of quite variable T1 and T2 appearance, depending on its age, size and the presence of re-bleeding (Tuite and de Smet 1994; Bush 2000).

17.1.2
Tendinopathy

Recent advances in the ultra-structural examination of the morphological changes which tendons undergo has altered the way in which tendon disease, or tendinopathy, is classified. Tendinopathy most commonly manifests as tendinosis, a term previously mistakenly referred to as tendonitis. The hallmark of tendinosis is essentially degeneration and not what was thought to be inflammation. Findings associated with tendinosis include the loss of normal collagen orientation, increased fibre separation and the accumulation of mucoid ground substance. Further to this is the presence of type III collagen (Mafulli et al. 2003) and the distinct absence of an inflammatory response. Thus the previously used term tendonitis (the suffix –itis implying inflammation) for this pathology is now no longer used. The latter is specifically reserved in the setting of actual tendon tearing with associated vascular disruption, which in turn evokes a true inflammatory response and is thus appropriately termed as tendonitis (Khan and Cook 2003).

17.2
Anterior Soft Tissues

17.2.1
Iliopsoas Tendinopathy ("Iliopsoas Syndrome")

The iliopsoas compartment is comprised of three muscles: psoas major, iliacus and psoas minor (present in 60% of the population). Unlike the former two, psoas minor inserts separately onto the iliopectineal eminence. The psoas major muscle arises from the transverse processes of the twelfth thoracic and all lumbar vertebrae (its minor counterpart originating from only the two most superior of these vertebral bodies). It fuses with the iliacus (which gains origin from the iliac wing) to insert on the lesser trochanter.

Like any tendinopathy, disease of the iliopsoas tendon manifests as T2 weighted signal hyperintensity usually at its insertion, often with peri-tendinous fluid collections and thickening. On ultrasound, this manifests as discrete foci of hypoechogenicity, in keeping with collagen disruption and loss of uniform tendon fibrillar echotexture. Associated iliopsoas bursitis may be present, the two processes making up the "iliopsoas syndrome" (Johnston et al. 1998), which may result in crepitus, the "snapping hip syndrome". Rarely, the patient may present with tearing of the iliopsoas muscle, usually at the musculotendinous junction (Fig. 17.1). This usually occurs in the acute athletic setting with resistance against extremes of eccentric flexion.

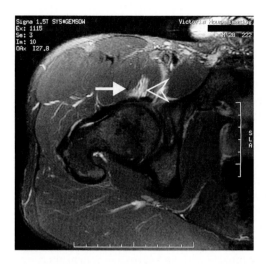

Fig. 17.1. Axial fat saturated proton density (PD) images through the hip of a 28-year-old male professional tennis player demonstrating hyperintensity at the musculotendinous junction of the iliopsoas muscle consistent with strain injury

et al. 2002a), and given that the differential diagnostic possibilities for a mass in this area is broad, imaging is a useful adjunct to clinical examination. Inguinal hernia, lymphadenopathy, vascular lesions and undescended testis are but a few of the diverse pathological processes represented in this anatomical region. Iliopsoas bursitis importantly must not be confused with a paralabral cyst. Thus careful exclusion of an associated labral tear is warranted (SCHNARKOWSKI et al. 1996; STEINER et al. 1996). Again, for this reason, MR imaging is the diagnostic procedure of choice (KOZLOV and SONIN 1998). Uncommon presentations of iliopsoas bursitis include femoral nerve (YOON et al. 2000) or vein compression (LEGAYE and REDIER 1995) and retroperitoneal extension of the bursa along the iliopsoas muscle (probably via neural pathways), where gas may be present to cause confusion with an abscess (COULIER and COOTS 2003).

17.2.2
Iliopsoas Bursitis

The iliopsoas bursa is the largest in the human body, present in 98% of individuals (VARMA et al. 1991). It lies deep to the tendon of iliopsoas, bordered medially by the iliopectineus muscle and laterally by the anterior inferior iliac spine. The bursa lies anterior to the hip joint, with which it communicates in 15% of normal asymptomatic individuals by way of a defect between the pubofemoral and iliofemoral ligaments. The incidence of this communication, and thus bursitis, is higher in the setting of hip derangement, and is usually secondary to synovitis and/or increased intracapsular pressures, which ultimately result in capsular thinning (ROBINSON et al. 2004). MR imaging is clearly superior to ultrasound and CT in demonstrating this communication (100% compared with approximately 40% for the latter two), which is specific for confident discrimination of the iliopsoas bursa from other foci of fluid within this area (WUNDERBALDINGER et al. 2002). Additional specificity is obtained by noting contrast enhancement of the synovial wall.

Iliopsoas bursitis is most commonly secondary to overuse syndromes, trauma, impingement and arthropathies (typically rheumatoid) (KATAKOA et al. 1995). Due to its frequent communication with the hip, iliopsoas bursitis may herald the presence of any intra-articular pathology which results in synovitis and subsequent decompression into it. Clinically, bursitis may present as a mass (BIANCHI

17.2.3
"Snapping Hip" Syndrome

This condition (also referred to as coxa saltans) is characterised by the complaint of a painful snapping or clicking sensation of the hip during motion, which is often palpable or audible snap. Causes for this are classified into extra- and intra-articular processes and discussed below.

17.2.3.1
Intra-articular

Internal derangement of the hip joint, such as labral tear, intra-articular loose bodies, post fracture/dislocation or synovial osteochondromatosis, are just a few of the causes which require careful exclusion and are best diagnosed with MR imaging (JANZEN et al. 1996). Such pathology may warrant surgical intervention, and warrants early and accurate detection.

17.2.3.2
Extra-articular

In the setting of a negative study for intra-articular pathology, attention should then be turned to outside the hip joint, focusing on the surrounding tendons to exclude a friction syndrome with adjacent soft tissue or osseous structures. The snapping hip syndrome is further divided into the tendon groups involved – external (lateral) (gluteus maximus or iliotibial band, and the greater trochanter), internal (medial) (iliopsoas and the iliopectineal eminence) or less commonly posterior (biceps femoris and the ischial tuberosity) (BOUTIN and NEWMAN 2003). Less commonly reported is an impingement syndrome affecting the iliofemoral ligament and the femoral neck.

As the condition is intermittent, highest diagnostic yield is achieved with dynamic testing; as such ultrasound is the investigation of choice (JACOBSON 2002). Unlike modalities previously utilised (bursography and tenography), the non-invasive and specific clinical correlation achieved with ultrasound is more acceptable in the athletic setting. Owing to its high spatial resolution, ultrasound has a high sensitivity for detecting bursitis, tendinopathy or synovitis which may result in the snapping hip syndrome. Examining the contralateral tendon is useful, as a baseline, carefully evaluating and comparing each for thickness and echogenicity. This is not entirely reliable, as for example, iliopsoas tendinopathy is bilateral in over 50% as well as painless in a similar number (PELSSER et al. 2001). Other associated abnormalities include focal tears, which manifest as hypoechoic clefts on ultrasound and increased intra-tendinous signal on MR imaging (JANZEN et al. 1996).

Ultrasound has one advantage in that imaging can be performed dynamically during hip motion in order to elicit a patient's symptoms (JOHNSTON et al. 1998). By instructing the patient to reproduce their symptom with the necessary provocative manoeuvre, the examiner can palpably or audibly detect a snap whilst examining for transient subluxation, pathognomonic features of this condition. Combined passive hip flexion, abduction and external rotation is a common clinical provocative test for eliciting snapping of the iliopsoas tendon. Movement in a medial to lateral direction or of a rotational nature should not occur and the suspected muscle/tendon should be mobile and glide normally over its adjacent osseous relations. Infrequently, impingement is a recognised complication post total hip joint replacement, the tendon being irritated by an area of focal prominence created by the acetabular component (REZIG et al. 2004).

17.2.4
Rectus Femoris

The rectus femoris has two origins, a bipennate straight (direct or superficial) head, which gains origin from the anterior inferior iliac spine and the deep (indirect or reflected) head, arising above the hip joint from the superior acetabular ridge groove. The two converge to contribute to the superficial layer of the quadriceps tendon (ZEISS et al. 1992).

The rectus femoris is more commonly injured than the other quadriceps muscles because of its bi-articular heads. Distal tears of the musculotendinous junction are more common, with proximal tears usually involving the central aponeurotic portion, which is contributed to by the deep head (BIANCHI et al. 2002b) (Fig. 17.2). The latter may present as a thigh mass, simulating a mesenchymal neoplasm, especially when the T1 and T2 inhomogeneity of haemorrhage and an inflammatory response provide the muscle with an aggressive appearance.

Avulsion fractures are exclusive to adolescents, as the fracture occurs through the provisional zone of calcification of the apophyseal plate. The powerful forces generated by the weight bearing muscles of the lower limbs account for the high incidence of this type of injury, combined with the later age of physeal plate closure. The rectus femoris is second to only the ischial tuberosity, as the commonest avulsion fracture of the developing pelvis (ROSSI and DRAGONI 2001). Similarly, as with complex tears of the muscles, chronic avulsion fractures, or healing acute avulsion fractures of the anterior inferior iliac spine may be confused with more aggressive processes, such as an osteosarcoma (RESNICK et al. 1996). This is especially the case if the reaction is florid; however, attention paid to the characteristic site and clinical history should avoid unnecessary biopsy and also false interpretation by the pathologist as osteosarcoma.

17.3
Groin Pain

Groin injuries make up 2%–5% of sporting injuries (MORELLI and SMITH 2001) and are seen most frequently in kicking sports (SCHLEGEL et al. 1999). Though having a relatively low incidence, the potentially prolonged recovery period makes the groin pain significant, as it is often a chronic and debilitating complaint, posing a major diagnostic and therapeutic challenge. As pain syndromes in this region have been an area of dynamic research, the terminology is confusing and rapidly changing. It is apparent now that not all groin complaints are the result of osteitis pubis, a condition now less

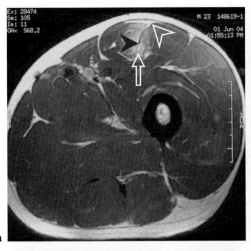

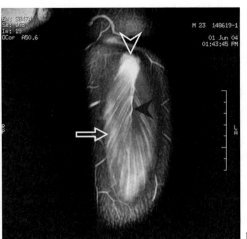

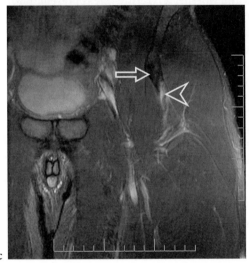

Fig. 17.2a–c. Axial PD (**a**) and coronal fat saturated PD sequences (**b**) through the right thigh of an elite 23-year-old male footballer who complained of a sudden tearing sensation during kicking, resulting in the inability to continue to take part in competition. Hyperintensity (*open arrow*) adjacent to the tendon (*black arrow*) is in keeping with a musculotendinous junction strain; however, free fluid, in keeping with haematoma (*open arrowhead*) pools around the muscle, limited by the fascia, in keeping with extension to the muscle epimysium. **c** Coronal fat saturated PD sequences through the left hip of another footballer reveals hyperintensity (*open arrowhead*) without muscle strain at the anterior inferior iliac spine (*open arrow*) in keeping with apophysitis of the proximal insertion of the rectus femoris muscle

common than previously thought. Importantly, multiple causes for groin pain have been found in approximately a quarter of patients (LOVELL 1995). As such, care must be made to consider non-musculoskeletal causes, as abdominal, pelvic, genitourinary disease, as well as referred pain, from the lumbar spine may all present with discomfort to this area.

17.3.1
Osteitis Pubis ("Pubic Symphysitis")

The pubic symphysis is composed of a fibrocartilaginous disk complex interposed between hyaline lined pubic bones and reinforced by capsular ligaments anteriorly, posteriorly and inferiorly. Additional support is provided by the arcuate ligaments, cruciate extension of the inguinal ligaments and aponeurosis of the adjacent adductor muscles and rectus abdominis.

Osteitis pubis is a poorly defined and understood disabling chronic condition of the pubic symphysis, with a strong male and kicking sport predominance (HOLMICH et al. 1999). Secondary involvement of adjacent myofascial and aponeurotic structures commonly co-exists. It is the result of repetitive microtrauma, most likely due to forces created by contraction of the agonist-antagonist of this joint, the adductor muscle and rectus abdominis (BRIGGS et al. 1992). Biomechanical theories point to an imbalance between these forces and an increased or unaccustomed training load. Ultimately, alteration in biomechanical distribution of forces through the pelvic ring leads to an inadequate bone remodelling in response to this increased stress (RODRIGUEZ et al. 2001). Whether the condition is degenerative or inflammatory (or a combination) is currently a point of debate. Management is controversial, ranging simply from complete rest to arthrodesis.

The most severe forms of osteitis pubis result in symphyseal instability, which can be demonstrated on flamingo views of the pelvis. Movement greater than 2 mm on single leg standing, or widening of the symphyseal space of more than 7 mm, is diagnostic. Other plain film and CT features include bone resorption, symphyseal widening, sclerosis, stamp erosions, insertional spurs and periarticular calcifications. Though useful initial tests, plain radiographs and CT may be negative or non-specific (BARILE et al. 2000). MR imaging similarly demonstrates the above findings, with the additional advantage of depicting changes such as extrusion of the fibrocartilaginous disc (usually superiorly and posteriorly), para-articular marrow and soft tissue/muscle oedema (GIBBON and HESSION 1997) (Fig. 17.3). Pubic bone marrow oedema, the hallmark feature of osteitis pubis, is accurately depicted with MR imaging, with its severity and extent correlating well clinically with the presence of symptoms (VERRALL et al. 2001a). Later, with healing, low signal on both T1 and T2 is reflective of sclerosis and disease quiescence (TUITE and DESMET 1994). MR imaging may also detect other soft tissue sources of the athlete's pain, such as inguinal wall defects or hernias.

Additional tests include CT or fluoroscopically guided symphyseal cleft injection, which may be utilised to confirm that the pubic symphysis is the source of an athlete's pain, as it may reproduce symptoms, with relief obtained following local anaesthetic infiltration. Contrast may extravasate into venous and lymphatic channels, potentially due to an increase in vascularity thought to be representative of an inflammatory component to this disease. Importantly, symphyseal injection allows for the injection of corticosteroid, proven to be a useful adjunct to conservative therapy, as it has been shown to hasten recovery and return to athletic competition (HOLT et al. 1995; O'CONNELL et al. 2002).

Potential clinical and radiological pitfalls exist, with significant prognostic and therapeutic ramifications. Pubic rami stress or insufficiency fractures (HOSONO et al. 1997) and adductor tendon avulsion injury needs to be carefully differentiated from osteitis pubis. Careful attention must be paid to the clinical history, the region and pattern of bone oedema and whether a fracture line is present. Both of these conditions have a markedly better prognosis than osteitis pubis and are treated with rest and a graduated rehabilitation program. Further to this, the sacroiliac joints require specific attention. As the pelvis acts as a functional ring through which forces are distributed, an increased load borne by the sacroiliac joint may occur secondary to pubic symphyseal dysfunction, resulting in premature degenerative change and thus symptoms (MAJOR and HELMS 1997).

17.3.2
Sportsman's Hernia

The hallmark of this condition (also referred to as pubalgia, Gilmore's groin, posterior inguinal wall

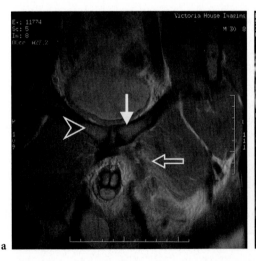
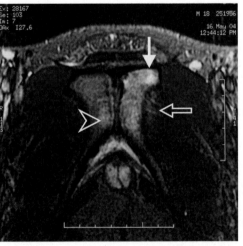

Fig. 17.3a,b. Axial (**a**) and coronal (**b**) PD fat saturated sequences through the pubic symphysis in two footballers, 30 and 18 years of age, respectively, who present with long standing groin pain. Oedema is noted of both the left (*arrow*) and right (*open arrow*) pubic rami with associated hyperintensity of the proximal insertion of the left adductor muscles (*open arrow*) most likely reactive. The findings are compatible with osteitis pubis

deficiency, pre-hernia complex, incipient hernia and groin disruption) is weakness of the posterior inguinal ring (MacLeod and Gibbon 1999). Most patients are male (98%), with 70% of symptoms being chronic and usually unilateral. Adductor soreness is present in slightly less than half (Gilmore 1998). This attenuation of the abdominal wall musculature is felt to represent the earliest manifestation of a continuum of inguinal wall dehiscence, of which hernia formation is the most severe end of the spectrum. It is usually diagnosed clinically, examination revealing focal tenderness, bulging and a dilated external (superficial) inguinal ring, in the absence of a hernia.

The condition is secondary to increased forces through the region and can be understood once appreciating the complex anatomy of the groin. The conjoint tendon is formed by the aponeurosis of the internal oblique and transversus abdominis muscles and contrary to popular thinking, the two leaves are not fused (in 97% of the population). Furthermore, they insert more frequently onto the rectus sheath (in three quarters) and not the pubic tubercle (Gibbon 1999a). As the rectus abdominis and adductor muscles are antagonists, they form a single functional unit, exerting forces through their inseparable attachment at the pubis. Thus, forces transmitted via the adductor muscles (as with increased training loads in the athlete) in turn are passed onto the rectus abdominis and therefore its sheath (Fig. 17.4). Given the anatomic relationship described above (between the conjoint tendon and the rectus sheath), if forces generated through the adductors are severe enough, disruption of the conjoint tendon eventually occurs and hence integrity of the superficial inguinal ring, developing finally as the "sportsman's hernia".

Ultrasound findings are those of a dynamic increase in the cross sectional area of the superficial inguinal ring, often associated with a convex anterior bulge of the posterior wall during stress. Pain correlates well with bilateral findings and increasing age (Orchard et al. 1998). MR imaging demonstrates attenuation (seen in 90%) or bulging of the abdominal wall musculofascial layers, as well as increased signal in one or both pubic bones or groin muscles (Albers et al. 2001). The diagnosis is important to make, as these patients were probably previously diagnosed with osteitis pubis and clearly respond to inguinal surgical repair as opposed to an osteitis pubis rehabilitation regimen (Gilmore 1991). A differential diagnoses for this condition which may confuse the clinician and a common, yet

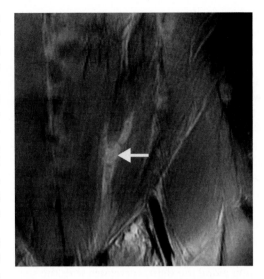

Fig. 17.4. Coronal PD images through the left rectus abdominis in a professional female tennis player following an injury sustained during serving whilst competing demonstrates hyperintensity of the distal rectus abdominis (*arrowheads*) with some retraction of fibres consistent with a high degree of strain

unrecognised, cause of chronic groin pain is enthesopathy of the pubic attachment of the inguinal ligament. Unlike the sportsman's hernia, this responds well to conservative treatment and direct corticosteroid injection (Ashby 1994).

17.3.3
Adductor Muscles

The pectineus, adductor brevis and longus muscles attach onto the posteromedial aspect of the femur (including the linea aspera) in descending order. The attachment of the adductor magnus is most extensive, spanning nearly the entire length of the femur to the level of the adductor tubercle. Gracilis is the only muscle of this group to cross two joints, a factor thought to contribute to an increased rate of strain injury.

Apart from the sportsman's hernia/overt hernia spectrum of injury, strain to the adductor musculature is the most common cause of groin pain in the athlete (Lovell 1995), present in nearly a quarter of soccer players in one playing season, with up to nearly a third recurring in that same year (Gibbon 1999b). Like any muscle injury, strain may be detected with MR imaging and ultrasound, typically occurring at the musculotendinous junction. Such injury in the adductor group is usually proximal (and anteriorly placed), mostly involving the adductor longus muscle, with secondary involvement of surrounding musculature, such as the rectus femoris and abdominis (TUITE et al. 1998). Plain radiographs have a limited role in adductor strain, but are important if an acute avulsion is suspected (to determine whether an ossified fragment is present), or to detect the presence of myositis ossificans (CETIN et al. 2004). Avulsion injury most commonly occurs distally at the femoral insertion, with milder forms of this spectrum of injury manifesting as a chronic avulsive enthesopathy, otherwise known as "thigh splints" or the adductor insertion avulsion syndrome. Technetium 99m labelled bone scintigraphy demonstrates linear scintigraphic uptake consistent with a periosteal reaction along the medial proximal femoral shaft (SINGH et al. 2001) and depending on its position along the shaft, correlates with the specific adductor involved; proximally (brevis), middle (longus) and posterior (magnus). Corresponding changes on MR imaging include cortical thickening and marrow oedema. MR also has the advantage of depicting soft tissue T2 hyperintensity, again secondary to oedema (ANDERSON et al. 2001). Ultrasound had also been employed in this region with success, with the advantage of eliciting point tenderness (WEAVER et al. 2003). Proximal enthesopathy is less common and is felt to be at least in part secondary to a poor blood supply and the small area from which the adductors gain their origin (LYNCH and RENSTROM 1999). Pathology such as exercise induced and chronic compartment syndromes of the adductor compartment have been rarely reported (LEPPILAHTI et al. 2002).

17.4
Lateral Soft Tissues

17.4.1
Greater Trochanteric Pain Syndrome

The greater trochanteric pain syndrome is a recently coined term which encompasses the broad range of pathology that may result in lateral hip pain (BIRD et al. 2001). In essence, it involves tendinosis of the gluteal musculature, and bursa-related pathology, with the two often co-existing. The condition is not restricted to the soft tissues, as more potentially incapacitating conditions of the femur, such as avascular necrosis, can cause pain to be referred laterally. Thus careful exclusion of osseous pathology is paramount, with the superiority of MR imag-

ing in this respect having been well established (DE PAULIS et al. 1998).

17.4.2
Gluteus Tendinopathy

Particular emphasis recently has focused on the function and disorders of the gluteus minimus and medius muscle. The two act as abductors and medial rotators of the hip (GOTTSCHALK et al. 1989; KUMAGAI et al. 1997), gluteus medius being the main abductor, with minimus assuming an additional role in stabilising the femoral head within the acetabulum (BECK et al. 2000). Given the similarities with the stabilising role that supraspinatus provides the shoulder, the two gluteals are best conceptualised as the "rotator cuff of the hip" (BUNKER et al. 1997). Like supraspinatus, pathology of the gluteus medius and minimus most commonly manifests as tendinosis, the result of chronic and repetitive micro-trauma. Unlike the rotator cuff of the shoulder, no acromial equivalent exists to provide osseous impingement (KAGAN 1999). Tension within the iliotibial band (ITB) may result in a form of soft tissue impingement, akin to acromial impingement.

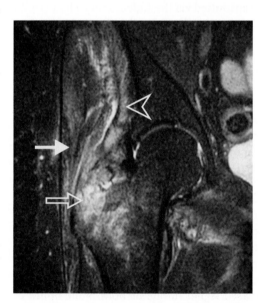

Fig. 17.5. An aerial skier presented for assessment following a training mishap resulting from falling on his right side. Coronal fat saturated PD sequences reveal the presence of underlying bone oedema of the greater trochanter (*open arrow*) consistent with bone bruising. Further, lateral to this, haemorrhage manifesting as hyperintensity within the gluteus medius (*arrow*) and minimus (*open arrowhead*) muscle fibres is also noted

MR imaging of gluteal tendinopathy is typically seen as thickening and abnormal T2 weighted hyperintensity of the conjoint tendon (Fig. 17.5). Ultrasound examination demonstrates enlargement of the gluteal tendon and loss of the normal organised fibrillar echotexture, secondary to hypoechoic change. Tendon tears manifest as focal areas of tendon discontinuity, as evidenced by linear hypoechoic defects, either involving only a portion of the tendon (partial tearing) or extending from one side to the other (full thickness). The deepest and most anterior aspects of the gluteus medius tendon is most commonly affected by partial tears (CONNELL et al. 2003). The frequency of co-existent gluteus minimus tears is variable, ranging from 20% (KINGZETT-TAYLOR et al. 1999) to 100% (CVITANIC et al. 2004). Most tears on MR imaging are roughly two thirds partial strain and one third full thickness tears, with the latter mainly being focal (1 cm or less) (CVITANIC et al. 2004). When full thickness tears extend across the entire length of the tendon, retraction results to form the so called "bald trochanter" (KINGZETT-TAYLOR et al. 1999). Ultimately, by virtue of the loss of the critical stabilising role these muscles afford the hip, irrespective of the pathology, a Trendelenburg gait ensues.

The condition is important to identify, as radiologists play an important role in conservative management of gluteal tendinopathy, by performing ultrasound guided corticosteroid injection. Failing that, and other conservative measures, primary open surgical repair and tendon re-attachment to the tro-chanter is indicated (KAGAN 1999). A specific subgroup exists, where chronic disruption of the gluteal musculature must also be brought to the attention of the orthopaedic surgeon. Alteration of the surgical approach in total hip arthroplasty is necessary to gain access to the gluteal medius and minimus tendons if a tear exists and the aim is for repair and/or re-attachment (SCHUH and ZEILER 2003). The presence of fat infiltration and atrophy of the normally large gluteal musculature, consistent with disuse, should alert the interpreting radiologist to possible gluteal tendon pathology or muscle disruption (WALSH and ARCHIBALD 2003). In the setting of contact sports, discrete haematoma may form within the gluteal muscles, one of the most commonly contused muscles (Fig. 17.6). This usually resolves after 6–8 weeks, however, rarely, a seroma may form (BENCARDINO and PALMER 2002). Knowledge of the clinical history and the variable appearances of haemorrhage prevents misinterpreting a simple contusion with a more aggressive process, such as a sarcoma.

17.4.3
Trochanteric Bursitis

Over 20 bursae have been identified in the trochanteric region (HELLER 2003); however, three are noteworthy: the trochanteric, subgluteus medius and subgluteus minimus bursae (PFIRMANN et al. 2001). The trochanteric bursa is located deep to the gluteus

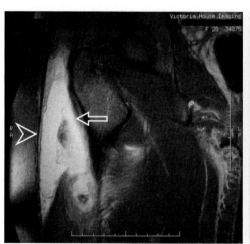
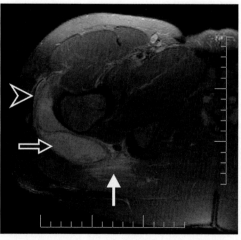

a   b

Fig. 17.6a,b. A 28-year-old aerial ski Olympic gold medallist presented with buttock pain following a fall during competition. **a** Coronal fat saturated PD images demonstrate a hyperintense collection in keeping with a haematoma (*arrow*) limited laterally by the investing fascia of the lower limb (*arrowhead*). Contusion to the overlying gluteus maximus muscle (*arrow*) on the axial images (**b**) is appreciated

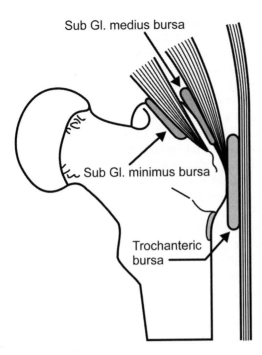

Sub Gl. medius bursa

Sub Gl. minimus bursa

Trochanteric bursa

Fig. 17.7. Diagrammatic representation of the anatomy depicting the major bursae related to the hip

maximus and ITB, covering the posterior facet of the greater trochanter and the lateral aspect of the insertion of the gluteus medius. The subgluteus medius bursa lies between the tendon and its attachment at the lateral facet of the trochanter. Similarly, the subgluteus minimus bursa lies deep to the attachment of the gluteus minimus, at the anterior facet of the greater trochanter (Fig. 17.7).

Associated trochanteric bursitis has been demonstrated to co-exist with gluteal tendinosis in up to 40% of patients (KINGZETT-TAYLOR et al. 1999). Interestingly, the condition is usually unilateral and has a middle aged to elderly female predominance (CHUNG et al. 1999), probably secondary to biomechanical differences due to a wider pelvis resulting in a mechanical disadvantage. Bursitis manifests as homogenous T2 hyperintensity of the involved bursa, which may be distended, with contrast enhancement of the wall, which poses a synovial lining (Figs. 17.8 and 17.9).

Pathology resulting in the greater trochanteric pain syndrome is not necessarily chronic and degenerative. Again, like the supraspinatus, calcific tendonitis can result in acute symptoms, and has been described in the gluteus maximus (KARAKIDA et al. 1995) and medius (YANG et al. 2002). In such instances, plain radiographs or computed tomography (CT) are best at demonstrating the amorphous cloud-like calcifications characteristic of this condition. Prominent oedema may also extend into the surrounding musculature as well as trochanteric marrow (YANG et al. 2002). However, calcification lateral to the trochanter is most commonly related to bursitis and is seen in 40% of such cases. This is to be distinguished from calcific tendonitis, where the calcified foci follow the course of the involved gluteal tendon and extend to its osseous insertion. Similarly, trochanteric bursitis can be acute, often following direct contusion, as seen in contact sports (BENCARDINO and PALMER 2002), with the irritation being post-haemorrhagic

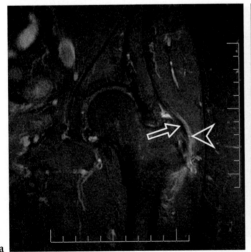

a

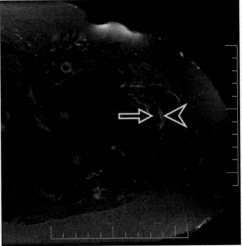

b

Fig. 17.8a,b. Coronal (**a**) and axial (**b**) fat saturated proton density images of the left hip of a middle-aged female patient reveals thickening and hyperintensity of the gluteus medius distal tendon (*arrow*) with secondary trochanteric bursal thickening and irregularity (*arrowhead*)

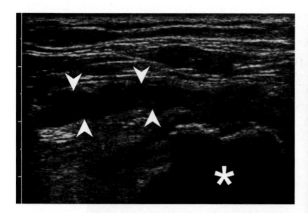

Fig. 17.9. Ultrasound of the greater trochanter (*asterisk*) in a 65-year-old female demonstrates no normal gluteus medius tendon, consistent with a complete full thickness tear and retraction associated with bursal distension (*arrowheads*)

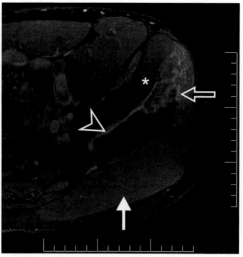

Fig. 17.10. Axial fat saturated PD images of a 22-year-old professional male tennis player following acute onset of buttock pain during competition. Hyperintensity within the muscle fibres of the gluteus medius muscle (*open arrow*) is consistent with strain injury with extension through the epimysium in keeping with free haematoma (*open arrowhead*). Anterior lies the gluteus minimus (*asterisk*) and posteriorly, the gluteus maximus muscle (*arrow*)

in nature. Less common is septic bursitis, which importantly, may be iatrogenic in aetiology (such as secondary to radiologically guided corticosteroid injection).

Other acute causes of the greater trochanteric pain syndrome include the less commonly encountered acute muscle injury, such as strain (Fig. 17.10) and even rupture of the gluteals. Though the gluteals are not as frequently strained as other nearby muscles, such as the hamstrings, early recognition is imperative, so that early primary surgical repair is carried out in complete disruption in order to ensure an optimal and functional outcome. The mechanism of injury is probably secondary to hyperadductive hip motion (KINGZETT-TAYLOR et al. 1999); however, it can also occur spontaneously, in previously abnormal tendons or even healthy individuals (LONNER and VAN KLUENEN 2002).

17.4.4
Tensor Fascia Lata

The tensor fascia lata (TFL) is a fan shaped muscle which gains origin from the outer aspect of the iliac crest and adjacent portions of the anterior inferior iliac spine. It inserts into the iliotibial tract (or band – ITB), usually in the upper half of the thigh. The TFL is at a distinct mechanical advantage in the role of hip abduction, when compared with the two gluteals (medius and minimus), which are more vertically orientated. Just as the supraspinatus pulls the humeral head into the glenoid fossa to increase stability, and initiate abduction, so too do the gluteals. With abduction initiated, the

action is then completed by the TFL (GOTTSCHALK et al. 1989).

TFL tendinopathy usually manifests as pain over the anterior iliac crest. The condition is more common in females and this may be due to the wider pelvis, placing the muscle in excessive stress with some activities. Its predominance in a younger age group suggests that tendinosis is the result of repetitive micro-trauma as opposed to degeneration. Due to its superficial location, the TFL is an ideal muscle to examine with ultrasound, with increase in the size of its origin (up to 2.5 times) and tendon (greater than 20%) when compared with the contralateral size in keeping with tendinosis (BASS and CONNELL 2003). Tears of the deep fibres are a typical finding, with more severe disease corresponding with coexistent involvement of the more superficially placed fibres (Fig. 17.11). Asymmetrical hypertrophy rarely may occur and present clinically as a mass. Enlargement is either the result of increase muscle fibre content (true hypertrophy) or accumulation of connective tissue, including fat (pseudo-hypertrophy). This uncommon condition is seen in patients following pelvic/hip surgery or suffering from an underlying myopathy or neurological disorder (ILASLAN et al. 2003).

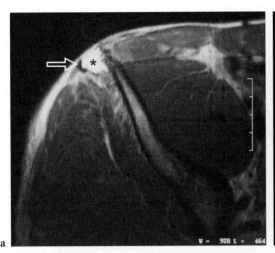
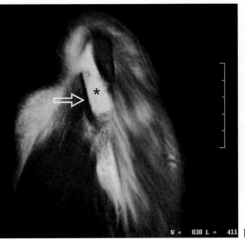

a   b

Fig. 17.11a,b. Axial (**a**) and coronal (**b**) PD sequences demonstrate avulsion of the origin of the tensor fascia lata from the cortex (*open arrowhead*) associated with haemorrhage (hyperintense collection) medially (*asterisk*)

17.5
Posterior Soft Tissues

17.5.1
The Hamstring Muscle Complex

The hamstring muscles (long head of biceps femoris, semimembranosus and semitendinosus) arise from the ischial tuberosity and the short head of biceps from the linea aspera of the femur. The latter joins the long head approximately midway down the calf to insert on the fibular head along with the lateral collateral ligament of the knee. Semitendinosus inserts, along with gracilis and sartorius, as the pes anserinus and the semimembranosus has extensive, multiple and complex attachments into the medial structures of the knee (BELTRAN et al. 2003).

Injuries to the hamstring muscle complex are the most common of all muscle strains. The hamstring muscles are predisposed to strain as they cross two joints, their antagonists (iliopsoas and quadriceps) are significantly larger and are composed of fast twitch fibres. Also they play an important role in preventing anterior tibial translation during the gait cycle and thus constantly concentrically and eccentrically contract during the gait cycle, a further predisposing factor. Increasing age and a past history of osteitis pubis are further documented risk factors (VERRALL et al. 2001b). The most common muscle injured is the long head of biceps femoris and is typically a strain injury, though haemorrhage and avulsion may occur and are usually proximal (Fig. 17.12).

Strain injury is usually at the musculotendinous junction in approximately two-thirds to three quarters of cases (KOULOURIS and CONNELL 2003; SLAVOTINEK et al. 2002).

Recent active research has focused on the role of imaging and prognostication that it may provide, in order to confidently guide the clinician, since recurrence rates are high and result in significantly prolonged periods out of competition. Though hamstring strain is usually diagnosed clinically without the need for imaging, the presence of MR signal abnormality (or positive ultrasound demonstration of a tear) and the increasing length of disruption has been shown to be associated with an increased recovery period (VERRALL et al. 2003; CONNELL et al. 2004; in print).

17.5.2
Sciatic Nerve

The sciatic nerve descends into the lower limb after passing through (in most cases) the piriformis muscle and exiting the pelvis via the greater sciatic foramen (formed by the greater sciatic notch anteriorly, sacrotuberous ligament posteriorly and sacrospinous ligament inferiorly). It then courses vertically deep to gluteus maximus, between the greater trochanter and ischial tuberosity to terminate at the superior apex of the popliteal fossa as the tibial (more direct continuation) and common peroneal nerves.

By far the most common cause of sciatic nerve pathology is secondary to lumbar spine disease,

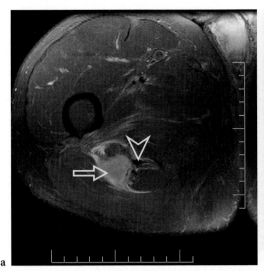 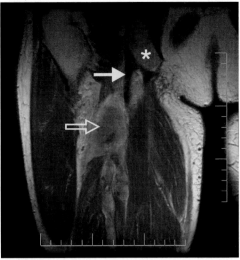

a   b

Fig. 17.12a,b. Axial fat saturated PD (**a**) and coronal PD (**b**) images of the right hip in an amateur footballer demonstrates hyperintensity and retraction (*open arrow*) in keeping with avulsion of the conjoint tendon of the biceps femoris and semitendinosus from the ischial tuberosity (*asterisk*). The uniform hypointense signal of the normal semimembranosus tendon is noted (*arrow*) as is the retracted tendon (*open arrowhead*)

particularly intervertebral disc impingement, canal stenosis and facet joint degenerative arthropathy. Other causes are less frequently encountered, usually the result of direct compression. Juglard et al. (1991) and Sherman et al. (2003) described paralabral cysts arising from the hip compressing the nerve. In such cases, excluding a causative labral tear is paramount. Tumours arising from the nerve are rarer causes of pathology; benign nerve sheath tumours being most common (Yamamoto et al. 2001) though the less common malignant counterpart have been reported (Sharma et al. 2001). Even muscle injury, usually involving the hamstring muscle complex, resulting in haematoma can exert mass effect to result in sciatica in the athletic setting. Post-haemorrhage fibrosis and scar tissue formation may cause ongoing symptoms, presumably the result of impaired mobility and glide of the sciatic nerve (Koulouris and Connell 2003) to result in the "intersection syndrome". The nerve may also become entrapped at the level of the ischial tuberosity by fibromuscular aponeurotic bands (McCrory and Bell 1999). Identifying fatty replacement and/ or atrophy of the muscles supplied by the sciatic nerve are important clues to detecting the location of disease. In cases where the spine is deemed as having no significant mass to account sciatica, or the symptoms are unremitting, a high index of suspicion should exist for excluding pathology of the sciatic nerve.

17.5.3
Piriformis Syndrome

The piriformis muscle has a pyramidal morphology, arising from the three digitations between the sacral foramina as well as possessing a fascial attachment to the sacroiliac joint capsule. It exits along with the sciatic nerve via the greater sciatic foramen, where the nerve roots converge at the inferior aspect of the muscle. Piriformis inserts on to the superior aspect of the greater trochanter, by way of a rounded tendon superficial to and occasionally blending with the tendon of gluteus medius.

Piriformis syndrome is an entrapment neuropathy secondary to mechanical compression or irritation of the sciatic nerve by the adjacent piriformis muscle. The site of pathology occurs inferior to the greater sciatic notch. The condition is controversial, as objective data is often lacking. MR imaging is the imaging modality of choice (Jroundi et al. 2003), being more sensitive than CT in detecting muscle pathology (Fig. 17.13), with other modalities being rarely of use, such as technetium labelled bone scintigraphy (Karl et al. 1985). Assessment is made as to the presence of hypertrophy, at least a reliable and objective sign, often in conjunction with effaced fat within the foramen, and anterior displacement of the sciatic nerve (Rossi et al. 2001; Jankiewicz et al. 1991). In the setting of T2 weighted hyperintensity, an inflammatory, neoplastic or infective cause should be sus-

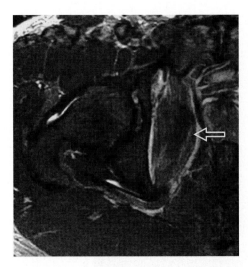

Fig. 17.13. Axial PD images demonstrate asymmetrical thickening of the right piriformis muscle (*arrow*) accounting for a 28-year-old female's symptoms of sciatica

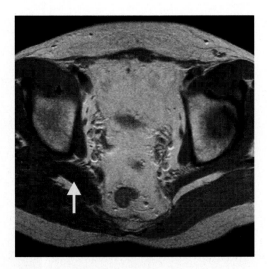

Fig. 17.14. Axial PD images through the right hip in a 27-year-old male rugby player reveals thickening and hyperintensity of the obturator internus muscle (*arrow*), in keeping with strain injury, sustained after an unusual twisting injury

pected. The condition is thought to arise from overuse, trauma, repetitive strain or any combination of the above. It is associated with asymmetric leg length and pelvic instability. Rarely, myositis ossificans may cause the syndrome (Beauchesne and Schutzer 1997). Prolonged sitting is a risk factor for bilateral disease and overall the condition has a strong female predominance. In the setting of negative radiological examination but a strong clinical history, intermittent spasm is thought to be the underlying aetiology, though this is controversial (McCrory 2001; Read 2002). Other, rare causes of the piriformis syndrome include pseudoaneurysm of the inferior gluteal artery, sacro-ileitis and compensatory hypertrophy secondary to altered biomechanics. Recently, treatment has focused on using fluoroscopic guidance to inject the muscle with botulinum toxin (Beck et al. 2002) with fair to excellent results in 90% of cases (Lang 2004). Similarly, the obturator internus muscle may demonstrate pathology, such as oedema due to strain injury (Fig. 17.4), which in turn may compress and/or irritate the adjacent obturator nerve to result in referred pain to the hip.

References

Albers SL, Spritzer CE, Garrett WE Jr et al (2001) MR findings in athletes with pubalgia. Skeletal Radiol 30:270-277

Anderson MW, Kaplan PA, Dussault RG (2001) Adductor insertion avulsion syndrome (thigh splints); spectrum of MR imaging features. AJR Am J Roentgenol 177:673-675

Ashby EC (1994) Chronic obscure groin pain is commonly caused by enthesopathy: 'tennis elbow' of the groin. Br J Surg 81:1162-1164

Barile A, Erriquez D, Cacchio A et al (2000) Groin pain in athletes: role of magnetic resonance. Radiol Med (Torino) 100:216-222

Bass CJ, Connell DA (2003) Sonographic findings of the tensor fascia lata tendinopathy: another cause of anterior groin pain. Skeletal Radiol 31:143-148

Beauchesne RP, Schutzer SF (1997) Myositis ossificans of the Piriformis muscle: an unusual cause of Piriformis syndrome: a case report. J Bone Joint Surg 79:906-910

Beck M, Sledge JB, Gautier E et al (2000) The anatomy and function of the gluteus minimus muscle. J Bone Joint Surg [Br] 82-B:358-363

Beck PV, Mahajan G, Wilsey BL et al (2002) Fluoroscopic and electromyographic guided injection of the piriformis muscle with Botulinum toxin type B. Pain Med 3:179

Beltran J, Matityahu A, Hwang K et al (2003) The distal semimembranosus complex: normal MR anatomy; variants, biomechanics and pathology. Skeletal Radiol 32:435-445

Bencardino JT, Palmer WE (2002) Imaging of hip disorders in athletes. Radiol Clin North Am 40:267-287

Bencardino JT, Rosenberg ZS, Brown RB et al (2000) Traumatic Musculotendinous Injuries of the Knee: diagnosis with MR Imaging. Radiographics 20:S103-S120

Bianchi S, Martinoli C, Keller A et al (2002a) Giant iliopsoas bursitis: sonographic findings with magnetic resonance correlation. J Clin Ultrasound 30:437-441

Bianchi S, Martinoli C, Peiris Waser N et al (2002b) Central aponeurosis tears of the rectus femoris: sonographic findings. Skeletal Radiol 31:581-586

Bird PA, Oakley SP, Shnier R et al (2001) Prospective evaluation of magnetic resonance imaging and physical examination findings in patients with greater trochanteric pain syndrome. Arthritis Rheum 44:2138-2145

Boutin RD, Newman JS (2003) MR imaging of sports-related

hip disorders. Magn Reson Imaging Clin North Am 11:255-281

Briggs RC, Kolbjornsen PH, Southall RC (1993) Osteitis pubis, Tc-99m MDP, and professional hockey players. Clin Nucl Med 17:861-863

Bunker TD, Esler CAN, Leach WJ (1997) Rotator-cuff tear of the hip. J Bone Joint Surg [Br] 79B:618-620

Bush CH (2000) The magnetic resonance imaging features of musculoskeletal hemorrhage. Skeletal Radiol 29:1-9

Cetin C, Sekir U, Yildiz Y et al (2004) Chronic Groin pain in an amateur soccer player. Br J Sports Med 38:223-224

Chung CB, Robertson E, Cho GJ et al (1999) Gluteus medius tendon tears and avulsive injuries in elderly women: imaging findings in six patients. AJR Am J Roentgenol 173:351-353

Connell DA, Bass C, Sykes CA et al (2003) Sonographic evaluation of gluteus medius and minimus tendinopathy. Eur Radiol 13:1339-47

Connell DA, Schneider-Kolsky, Hoving JL et al (2004) Longitudinal study comparing sonographic and MRI assessments of acute and healing hamstring injuries. AJR Am J Roentgenol 183:975-984

Coulier B, Cloots V (2003) Atypical retroperitoneal extension of iliopsoas bursitis. Skeletal Radiol 32:298-301

Cvitanic O, Henzie G, Skezas N et al (2004) MRI diagnosis and tears of the hip abductor tendons (gluteus medius and gluteus minimus). AJR Am J Roentgenol 182:137-143

De Paulis F, Cacchio A, Michelini O et al (1998) Sports injuries in the pelvis and hip: diagnostic imaging. Eur J Radiol 27:S29-S59

El-Khoury GY, Brandser EA, Kathol MH et al (1996) Imaging of muscle injuries. Skeletal Radiol 25:3-11

Farber JM, Buckwalter KA (2002) MR imaging in nonneoplastic muscle disorders of the lower extremity. Radiol Clin North Am 40:1013-1031

Gibbon WW (1999a) Groin pain in athletes. Lancet 24:1444-1445

Gibbon WW (1999b) Groin pain in professional soccer players: a comparison of England and the rest of Western Europe. Br J Sports Med 33:435

Gibbon WW, Hession PR (1997) Diseases of the pubis and pubic symphysis: MR imaging appearances. AJR Am J Roentgenol 169:849-853

Gilmore OJA (1991) Gilmore's groin: ten years experience of groin disruption – a previously unsolved problem in sportsmen. Sports Med Soft Tissue Trauma 3:12-14

Gilmore OJA (1998) Groin pain in the soccer athlete: fact, fiction and treatment. Clin Sports Med 17:787-793

Gottschalk F, Kourosh S, Leveau (1989) The functional anatomy of tensor fasciae latae and gluteus medius and minimus. J Anat 166:179-189

Heller A (2003) Anatomy of the trochanteric bursae (letter). Radiology 226:921-922

Holmich P, Uhkstrou P, Ulnits L et al (1999) Effectiveness of active physical training as treatment for long-standing adductor-related groin pain in athletes: randomised trial. Lancet 353:439-443

Holt MA, Keen JS, Graf BK et al (1995) Treatment of osteitis pubis in athletes: results of corticosteroids injections. Am J Sports Med 23:601-606

Hosono M, Kobayashi H, Fujimoto R et al (1997) MR appearances of parasymphyseal insufficiency fractures of the os pubis. Skeletal Radiol 26:525-528

Ilaslan H, Wenger DE, Shives TC et al (2003) Unilateral hypertrophy of the tensor fascia lata: a soft tissue simulator. Skeletal Radiol 32:628-632

Jacobson JA (2002) Ultrasound in sports medicine. Radiol Clin North Am 40:363-386

Jankiewicz JJ, Hennrikus WL, Houkom JA (1991) The appearance of the piriformis muscle syndrome in computed tomography and magnetic resonance imaging. A case report and review of the literature. Clin Orthop 262:205-209

Janzen DL, Partridge E, Logan PM et al (1996) The snapping hip: clinical and imaging findings in transient subluxation of the iliopsoas tendon. Can Assoc Radiol J 47:202-208

Johnston CA, Wiley JP, Lindsay DM et al (1998) Iliopsoas bursitis and tendonitis. A review. Sports Med 25:271-283

Jroundi L, El Quessar A, Chakir N et al (2003) The piriformis syndrome: a rare cause of non discogenic sciatica: a case report. J Radiol 84:715-717

Juglard G, Le Nen D, Lefevre C et al (1991) Synovial cyst of the hip with revealing neurological symptoms. J Chir (Paris) 128:424-427

Kagan A 2nd (1999) Rotator cuff tears of the hip. Clin Orthop 368:135-140

Karakida O, Aoki J, Fujioka F et al (1995) Radiological and anatomical investigation of calcific tendinitis of the gluteus maximus tendon. Nippon Igaku Hoshasen Gakkai Zasshi 55:483-487

Karl RD, Yedinak MA, Hartshorne MF et al (1985) Scintigraphic appearance of the piriformis muscle syndrome. Clin Nucl Med 10:361-363

Kataoka M, Torisu T, Nakamura et al (1995) Iliopsoas bursa of the rheumatoid hip joint. A case report and review of the literature. Clin Rheumatol 14:358-364

Khan K, Cook J (2003) The painful nonruptured tendon: clinical aspects. Clin Sports Med 22:711-725

Kingzett-Taylor A, Tirman PF, Feller J et al (1999) Tendinosis and tears of gluteus medius and minimus muscles as a cause of hip pain: MR imaging findings. AJR Am J Roentgenol 173:1123-1126

Koulouris G, Connell D (2003) Evaluation of the hamstring muscle complex following acute injury. Skeletal Radiol 32:582-589

Kozlov DB, SoninAH (1998) Iliopsoas bursitis: diagnosis by MRI. J Comput Assist Tomogr 22:625-628

Kumagai M, Shiba N, Higuchi F et al (1997) Functional evaluation of hip abductor muscles with use of magnetic resonance imaging. J Orthop Res 15:888-893

Lang AM (2004) Botulinum toxin type B in piriformis syndrome. Am J Phys Med Rehabil 83:198-202

Legaye J, Redier S (1995) Synovial cyst of the hip. Report of a case with venous compression. Acta Orthop Belg 61:140-1433

Leppilahti J, Trevonen O, Herva R et al (2002) Acute bilateral exercise-induced medial compartment syndrome of the thigh. Correlation of repeated MRI with clinicopathological findings. Int J Sports Med 23:610-615

Lonner JH, van Kleunen JP (2002) Spontaneous rupture of the gluteus medius and minimus tendons. Am J Orthop 31:579-581

Lovell G (1995) The diagnosis of chronic pain in athletes; a review of 189 cases. Aust J Sci Med Spotr 27:76-79

Lynch SA, Renstrom PA (1999) Groin injuries in sport: treatment strategies. Sports Med 28:137-144

MacLeod DA, Gibbon WW (1999) The sportsman's groin. Br J Surg 86:849-850

Mafulli N, Wong J, Alkeminders LC (2003) Types and epidemiology of Tendinopathy. Clin Sports Med 22:675-692

Major NM, Helms CA (1997) Pelvic stress injuries: the relationship between osteitis pubis (symphysis pubis stress injury) and sacroiliac abnormalities in athletes. Skeletal Radiol 26:711-717

McCrory P (2001) The "piriformis syndrome" – myth or reality? Br J Sports Med 35:209-210

McCrory P, Bell S (1999) Nerve entrapment syndromes as a cause of pain in the hip, groin and buttock. Sports Med 27:261-274

Morelli V, Smith V (2001) Groin injuries in athletes. Am Fam Physician 64:1405-1414

O'Connell MJ, Powell T, McCaffrey NM et al (2002) Symphyseal cleft injection in the diagnosis and treatment of osteitis pubis in athletes. AJR Am J Roentgenol 179:955-959

Orchard JW, Read JW, Neophyton J et al (1998) Groin pain associated with ultrasound finding of posterior wall deficiency in Australian Rules footballers. Br J Sports Med 342:134-139

Pelsser V, Cardinal E. Hobden R et al (2001) Extrarticular snapping hip: sonographic findings. AJR Am J Roentgenol 176:67-73

Pfirmann CWA, Chung CB, Theumann NH et al (2001) Greater trochanter of the hip: attachment of the abductor mechanism and a complex of three bursae – MR imaging and MR bursography in cadavers and MR imaging in asymptomatic volunteers. Radiology 221:469-477

Read MT (2002) The "piriformis syndrome" – myth or reality? Br J Sports Med 36:76

Resnick JM, Humberto Carrasco C, Edeiken J et al (1996) Avulsion fracture of the anterior iliac spine with abundant reactive ossification in the soft tissue. Skeletal Radiol 25:580-584

Rezig R, Copercini M, Montet X et al (2004) Ultrasound diagnosis of anterior iliopsoas impingement in total hip replacement. Skeletal Radiol 33:112-116

Robinson P, White LM, Kandel R et al (2004) Primary synovial osteochondromatosis of the hip: extracapsular patterns of spread. Skeletal Radiol 33:210-215

Rodriguez C, Miguel A, Lima H et al (2001) Osteitis pubis syndrome in the professional soccer athlete: a case report. J Athl Train 36:437-440

Rossi F, Dragoni S (2001) Acute avulsion fractures of the pelvis in adolescent competitive athletes: prevalence, location and sports distribution of 203 cases collected. Skeletal Radiol 30:127-131

Rossi P, Cardinali P, Serrao M et al (2001) Magnetic resonance imaging findings in piriformis syndrome; a case report. Arch Phys Med Rehabil 82:519-521

Sadro C (2000) Current concepts in magnetic resonance imaging of the adult hip and pelvis. Semin Roentgenol 35:231-248

Schlegel TF, Boublik M, Ho CP et al (1999) Role of MR Imaging in the management of injuries in professional football players. MR Clin North Am 7:175-190

Schnarkowski P, Steinbach LS, Tirman PFJ et al (1996) Magnetic resonance imaging of labral cysts of the hip. Skeletal Radiol 25:733-737

Schuh A, Zeiler G (2003) Rupture of the gluteus medius tendon. Zentralbl Chir 128:139-142

Sharma RR, Pawar SJ, Mahapatra AK et al (2001) Sciatica due to malignant nerve sheath tumour of sciatic nerve in the thigh. Neurol India 49:188-190

Sherman PM, Matchette MW, Sanders TG et al (2003) Acetabular paralabral cyst: an uncommon cause of sciatica. Skeletal Radiol 32:90-94

Singh AK, Dickinson C, Dworkin HJ et al (2001) Adductor insertion avulsion syndrome. Clin Nucl Med 26:709-711

Slavotinek JP, Verrall GM, Fon GT (2002) Hamstring injury in athletes: using MR imaging measurements to compare extent of muscle injury with amount of time lost from competition. AJR Am J Roentgenol 179:1621-1628

Steiner E, Steinbach LS, Schnarkowski et al (1996) Ganglia and cysts around joints. Radiol Clin North Am 34:395-425

Tuite MJ, DeSmet AA (1994) MR of selected sports injuries: muscle tears, groin pain and osteochondritis dissecans. Semin Ultrasound CT MR 15:318-340

Tuite DJ, Finegan PJ, Saliaris AP et al (1998) Anatomy of the proximal musculotendinous junction of the adductor longus muscle. Knee Surg Sports Traumatol Arthrosc 6:134-137

Varma DG, Richli WR, Charnsangavej C et al (1991) MR appearances of the distended iliopsoas bursa. AJR Am J Roentgenol 156:1025-1028

Verrall GM, Slavotinek JP, Fon GT (2001a) Incidence of pubic bone marrow oedema in Australian rules football players: relation to groin pain. Br J Sports Med 35:28-33

Verrall GM, Slavotinek JP, Barnes PG et al (2001b) Clinical risk factors for hamstring strain injury: a prospective study with correlation of injury by magnetic resonance imaging. Br J Sports Med 35:435–440

Verrall GM, Slavotinek JP, Barnes PG et al (2003) Diagnostic and prognostic value of clinical findings in 83 athletes with posterior thigh injury. Comparison of clinical findings with magnetic resonance imaging documentation of hamstring muscle strain. Am J Sports Med 31:969–973

Walsh G, Archibald CG (2003) MRI in greater trochanter pain syndrome. Australas Radiol 47:85–88

Weaver JS, Jacobson JA, Jamadar DA et al (2003) Sonographic findings of adductor insertion avulsion syndrome with magnetic resonance imaging correlation. J Ultrasound Med 22:403–407

Wunderbaldinger P, Bremer C, Schellenberger M et al (2002) Imaging features of iliopsoas bursitis. Eur Radiol 12:409–415

Yamamoto T, Maruyama S, Mizuno K (2001) Schwannomatosis of the sciatic nerve. Skeletal Radiol 30:109–113

Yang I, Hayes CW, Biermann SJ (2002) Calcific tendinitis of the gluteus medius tendon with bone marrow edema mimicking metastatic disease. Skeletal Radiol 31:359–361

Yoon TR, Song EK, Chung JY et al (2000) Femoral neuropathy caused by enlarged iliopsoas bursa associated with osteonecrosis of femoral head – a case report. Acta Orthop Scand 71:322–324

Zeiss J, Saddemi SR, Ebraheim NA (1992) MR imaging of the quadriceps tendon: normal layered configuration and its importance in tendon rupture. AJR Am J Roentgenol 159:1031–1034

18 Arthritis 1: Hip

Herwig Imhof

CONTENTS

18.1
Degenerative Joint Disease (Osteoarthritis)

18.1.1
Introduction

The noninflammatory arthritides are certainly the most commonly encountered form of arthritis in the Western world, and degenerative osteoarthritis in its many and varied presentations is the most commonly encountered condition in orthopedic practice. Primary degenerative osteoarthritis is a degenerative disease which is clinically associated with age and obesity (body mass index > 30). But there is also a direct relationship with chronic underuse ("no gymnastics") and chronic (repetitive) overuse (Hunder 1998; Brandt et al. 1998; Felson 2004).

Usually two conditions are differentiated:
- Primary nodal osteoarthritis, which results in Heberden and Bouchard nodes in the small joints of the hands, but it does not cause significant loss in hand function and is most commonly found in menopausal women, and primary generalized osteoarthritis, which involves three or more joints, as for instance most commonly the spine, knee or hip (Bullough 2004).
- Secondary degenerative osteoarthritis is based on well-known etiologies and is found in younger patients. They represent about 20% of all cases with degenerative osteoarthritis. Most commonly these etiologies involve minimal chronic or severe acute trauma, acquired and inborn problems as Perthes disease, dysplasia, slipped epiphysis, Gaucher disease, crystal arthropathies, hemoglobinopathies, rheumatoid diseases and inflammatory arthritis, Paget's disease, ischaemic necrosis with or without subchondral insufficiency fractures, osteochondritis dissecans, and other diseases such as diabetes mellitus.

18.1.2
Definition

There is as yet no generally accepted definition of degenerative osteoarthritis, but it seems clear that primary degenerative osteoarthritis is the result of different overlapping diseases with different etiology which involves cartilage, subchondral bone and vessels, synovium, ligaments, the capsule and neighboring muscles (Imhof et al. 2002).

Degenerative osteoarthritis is basically different from aging, but is very often combined with aging. Osteoarthritis shows an increased metabolism in bone and cartilage with production of more tissue (new formation of cartilage, osteophytes, etc.) and a higher amount of tissue water, at least in the early phases. Moreover, characteristically the amount of subchondral vessels is rarefied. In contrast to these osteoarthritis features, aging has a decreased metabolism with less water content, aging pigment (=lipofuscin) and less tissue (e.g. cartilage, vessels and subchondral bone), but no eburnation. Car-

H. Imhof, MD
Professor, Department of Radiology, AKH Vienna, Waehringer Guertel 18–20, 1090 Vienna, Austria

tilage abnormalities are typically found in non-weight-bearing positions.

The "wear and tear" theory of causation for degenerative osteoarthritis has had a stultifying effect on medical opinion with regard to its views on prevention and treatment of the disease. Osteoarthritis seems not to be an inevitable disease. As far as we understand today it has metabolic, mechanical, vascular, inflammatory and genetic components. Searches for a single, all encompassing cause of osteoarthritis seems to not be very successful.

In recent years, the term pre-osteoarthritis has been emphasized. Patients with pre-osteoarthritis have a high probability of developing degenerative osteoarthritis in the involved joint(s) in a very short time. Early diagnosis and treatment of pre-osteoarthritis may prevent, or at least delay, the development of degenerative osteoarthritis.

18.1.3
Pathology and Pathophysiology

Typical findings of degenerative osteoarthritis in the cartilage are edema, local defect (tear, cleft), fibrillation and baldness in a weight-bearing position which is accompanied by cortical thickening ("subchondral" sclerosis) (Fig. 18.1). These are the typical arthroscopic staging findings of chondromalacia, which are paralleled by typical MRI stages (edema; incomplete cartilage tear; complete cartilage tear; localized loss of cartilage). Intrinsic and extrinsic repair mechanisms may lead to (insufficient) cartilage repair with formation of areas of irregular cartilage ("primitive" fibrous cartilage) with less elasticity (Fig. 18.2).

In the subchondral region the bony matrix may be insufficient (Localized osteoporosis? Loss of bone quality?) (Arokoski et al. 2004; Beary 2001) leading to microfractures with new bone formation (sclerosis) or localized micronecrosis (formation of cystoid structures) and vessel rarefaction (Fig. 18.3). There is currently a discussion about whether vessel rarefaction (due to aging, localized overloading, etc.) may be one of the primary etiologies of degenerative osteoarthritis resulting in the formation of abnormal (insufficient) bone (Imhof et al. 2002; Crock 1996). This bony insufficiency raises the likelihood for localized micro-fractures during loading (insufficiency fractures) (Fig. 18.4) (Yamamoto and Bullough 1999, 2000). Those microfractures trigger a localized healing process with new bone formation. But (over)loading could also lead

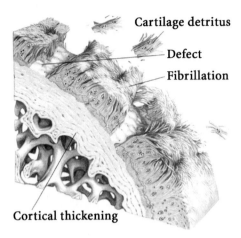

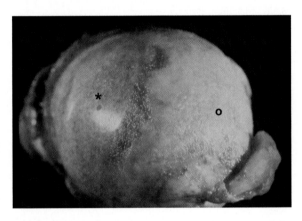

Fig. 18.1. Typical degenerative osteoarthritis with cortical thickening and cartilage abnormalities

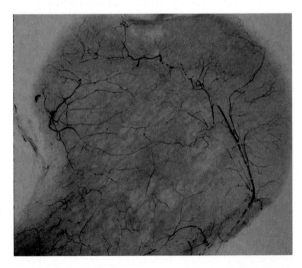

Fig. 18.2. Head of femur with severe degenerative osteoarthritis: baldness (*asterisk*) and cartilage repair (*circle*)

Fig. 18.3. Post-mortem angiography of the femoral head with severe vessel rarefaction in degenerative osteoarthritis

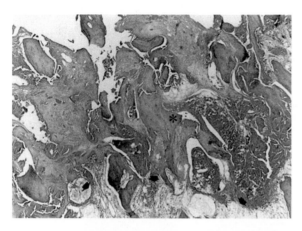

Fig. 18.4. Histologic cut (HE): multiple subchondral insufficiency fractures in a patient with degenerative osteoarthritis

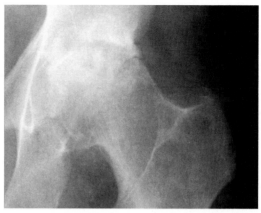

Fig. 18.5. Conventional radiograph (ap): degenerative osteoarthritis of the hip joint (coxarthrosis) with deformity, subchondral sclerosis and cysts, osteophytes and joint space narrowing

to localized micro-bleedings with the development of subchondral "cystoid" structures. Finally, during (over)loading subchondral micro-infarctions may develop, ending up in micronecrosis and in minor bone-deformities. Those deformities, but also the abnormal cartilaginous and subchondral structures in degenerative osteoarthritis will change the physiologic biomechanical loading process (ALTMAN et al. 2004).

Subchondral new bone formation is well known as subchondral sclerosis; the subchondral cystoid structures represent the well-known subchondral "cysts" (Fig. 18.5). The frequently mentioned "intraarticular high pressure theory" as common etiology for the development of subchondral cysts seems to be very unlikely or at least very uncommon. In the majority of cases the subchondral cysts are separated from the joint space by a thin subchondral bone plate. Microscopically, cysts vary from myxomatous to walled-off, fibrous, membranous cavities with or without extension to the surface containing a clear, viscoid fluid. The acetabular cysts are so-called Egger's cyst. Myxomatous "cysts" cannot be differentiated from ganglions.

At the borders of the chondromalacic cartilage new bone formation may take place as a repair mechanism. It is the pathophysiologic response to altered loading and probably initiated by localized adaptive processes (activation of local growth factors, osteoprotegerin, new vessel formation, etc.). This process is also well know as osteophyte formation, buttressing, etc. (Fig. 18.6). All those processes lead to deformity of the articulating joint shape (remodeling), joint support, as well as altered tissue matrices, which may aggravate the above men-

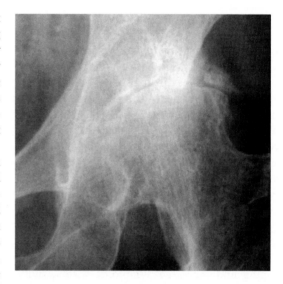

Fig. 18.6. Conventional radiograph (oblique): severe degenerative osteoarthritis with new bone formation around the femoral neck ("buttressing"). Osteophyte formation at the acetabular roof. Additionally joint space narrowing, subchondral sclerosis and "cyst", as well as joint deformity

tioned processes in vicious circles, but may also lead to a functional restoration. It must be stressed that osteophyte formation by no means heralds a symptomatic osteoarthritis.

The hemispherical head of the femur articulates with the cup-shaped acetabulum in a ball and socket configuration. However, the articular cartilage of the acetabulum is horseshoe shaped, rather than hemispherical, because of the presence of the acetabular notch (Fig. 18.7). This deficiency, and the presence of acetabular anteversion, means that car-

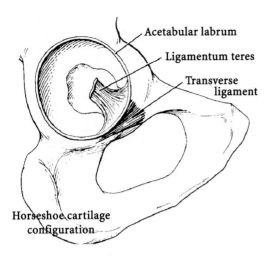

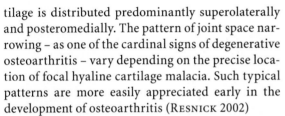

Fig. 18.7. The surface of the acetabulum. Typical horseshoe configuration of the cartilage

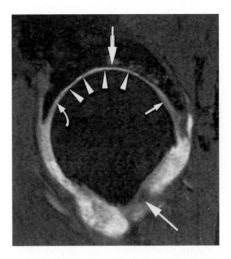

Fig. 18.8. MRI of the hip joint (3D-GRE with fat-suppression, paraxial): irregular thickness of cartilage, subchondral "cyst" (*arrowheads*), synovial effusion and thickening, free intraarticular body (*arrows*) in degenerative osteoarthritis

tilage is distributed predominantly superolaterally and posteromedially. The pattern of joint space narrowing – as one of the cardinal signs of degenerative osteoarthritis – vary depending on the precise location of focal hyaline cartilage malacia. Such typical patterns are more easily appreciated early in the development of osteoarthritis (RESNICK 2002)

Loose intraarticular bodies are also a typical feature of degenerative osteoarthritis. Most commonly, they develop on the basis of small peeled off cartilage pieces or fractured fragments, which may be the trigger mechanism for new chondral, or bone, formation, or they are the result of synovial metaplasia. They may lead to joint locking, pain, clicking, snapping and increased symptoms with activity. Pathologically they are accompanied with effusion and synovitis (Fig. 18.8).

The synovium – as one of the most (immune) reactive structures within the human body, which has no submucosal border – is activated by cytokines of the destroyed (dying) cartilage cells, but also mechanically by cartilage debris (chondral loose bodies). In both cases synovium hyperemia is followed by joint-effusion and mild cellular infiltration of the synovium, increasing the cell-lining of the intimal layer and cellular infiltration of the subintimal layer with new vessel formation, i.e. villous synovial hyperplasia. The activated synovium itself produces cartilage damaging cytokines (e.g. interleukin 1), which enhances the degenerative process. Because patients have clinical signs of an inflamed synovium, this process is called an "activated degenerative osteoarthritis". Not uncommonly, synovial

proliferation also leads to the production of synovial osteochondral bodies (Fig. 18.9) (ISENBERG and RENTON 2003).

Degenerative joint disease affects fibrocartilaginous tissue, as well as ligaments and tendons. This includes myxoid degeneration, microcyst formation, chondroid metaplasia and deposition of calcium pyrophosphate dihydrate crystals. Naturally these structures will lose their biomechanical resistance (Fig. 18.10).

In the last years the labrum acetabuli has received increased clinical and scientific interest. The labrum serves as load distributor, stabilizer and joint "sealer"

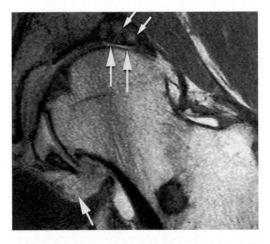

Fig. 18.9. MRI of the hip joint (T1-weighted, coronal): severe degenerative osteoarthritis with loss of cartilage (*long arrows*), subchondral cysts (*short arrows*), deformity, synovial thickening (*inferior arrow*), effusion, osteophyte formation and buttressing

during motion. The labrum is ten times stiffer than the hyaline cartilage and broadens the acetabulum by about 20%. Degeneration of the labrum leads to mucoid/cystic transformations of the labrum matrix (an abnormal intralabral signal), followed by mild free edge blunting (Figs. 18.11, 18.12). Because of the abnormal internal structure labral tears may develop. In 40%–80% of patients with degenerative osteoarthritis labral tears are found (most commonly anteriorly and anterosuperiorly). They have a very low capacity for self healing – very similar to the degenerative tears in the menisci of the knee joint. On the other hand, it is well known that asymptomatic labral tears are found in 42%–58% of all persons over 50 years of age. Labral tears are also found in 72% of patients with dysplasia, in patients with Perthes disease, slipped epiphysis and reduced anteversion (Fig. 18.13) (Farjo et al. 1999).

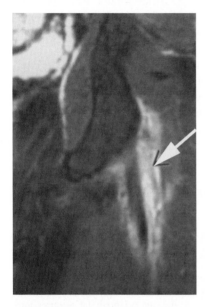

Fig. 18.10. MRI detail of hip joint (proton density-weighted, fat-suppression, coronal): thickened hamstring tendon with surrounding edema (collagenous degeneration)

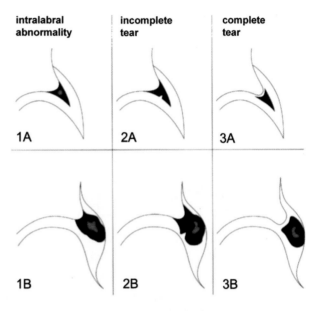

Fig. 18.12. Staging of degenerative labral abnormalities

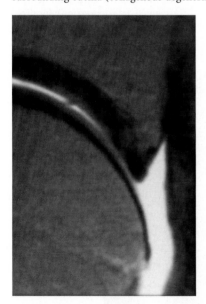

Fig. 18.11. MRI arthrography of the hip joint (T1-weighted, coronal, fat suppression): inhomogeneity of the labrum representing stage 1A

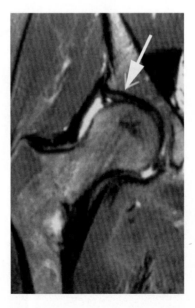

Fig. 18.13. MRI hip joint (coronal, proton density-weighted): labral tear with acetabular dysplasia (*arrow*)

Femoroacetabular impingement (= Pincer impingement) and cam impingement (acetabular rim syndrome) – due to abnormal contact (loading) of the femoral neck (head) on the acetabular labrum during axial loading, flexion and internal rotation in non-dysplastic hips or due to a dysplastic hip joint with a deformed head, respectively – lead to labral damage (edema, blunting, tear, paralabral cyst) and are followed by damage of the neighboring cartilage, ending up in early degenerative osteoarthritis (Figs. 18.14, 18.15). Femoroacetabular impingement might be due to anatomical variations with a reduction in the mean femoral anteversion and mean head-neck offset relative to the anterior aspect of the neck (Fig. 18.16). Moreover, it can be found in persons with a "pistol grip" deformity of the head (asymmetry of the head due to excessive sport) (Fig. 18.17). Controversy surrounds whether these

mechanisms might represent very common etiologies of "primary" degenerative osteoarthritis of the hip joint in patients younger than 50 years (STOLLER 2004; ANDERSON et al. 1998).

Labral tears and internal structural abnormalities may end up in the development of large paralabral cysts (filled with synovial fluid) and/or labral calcifications (Fig. 18.18). It is thought that paralabral tears are connected with and based on labral tears. They cannot be differentiated from ganglion cysts which are filled with mucoid material and may be adjacent to any portion of the fibrocartilaginous labrum.

Another reason for early development of degenerative osteoarthritis is the "snapping hip syndrome", which is characterized by a snapping or clicking sensation upon movement of the hip and is typically found in ballet-dancers (coxa saltans). Its patho-

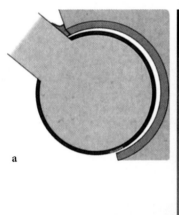

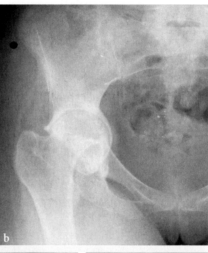

Fig. 18.14a. Schematic drawing of femoroacetabular impingement: during maximal flexion the labrum is compressed and damaged. The femoral counterpart shows bone marrow edema. **b** Conventional radiographs (ap): protrusio acetabuli (axial migration in degenerative osteoarthritis) with labral impingement. **c** MRI of the hip joint (detail, proton density-weighted, fat suppression): femoroacetabular impingement with acetabular edema (*arrow*). **d** MRI of the hip joint (detail, proton density-weighted, fat suppression): localized bone marrow edema in acetabular dysplasia (local overloading during flexion)

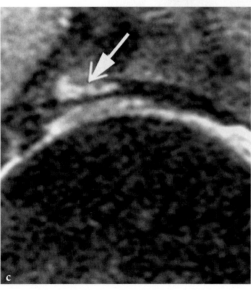

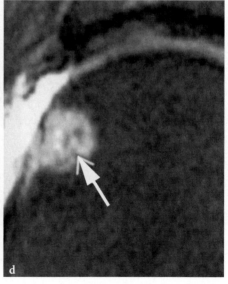

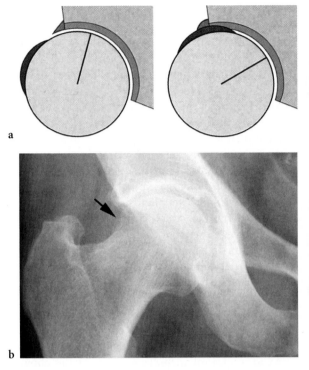

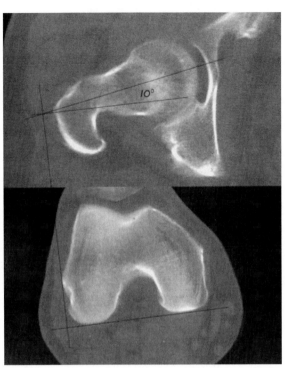

Fig. 18.15a. Schematic drawing of cam impingement syndrome (acetabular rim syndrome): due to the out-of-round configuration of the femoral head the labrum will be damaged during flexion. **b** Conventional radiograph of the hip joint (ap): mild abnormal configuration of the femoral head (*arrow*) with clinically acetabular rim syndrome

Fig. 18.16. CT (axial): measurement of the anteversion of the femoral neck (> 15° = abnormal)

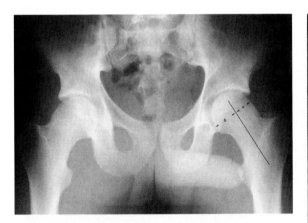

Fig. 18.17. Conventional radiograph of both hip joints: "pistol grip" deformity of the left hip joint, leading to femoroacetabular impingement

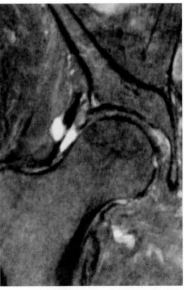

Fig. 18.18. MRI of the right hip joint (coronal, proton density-weighted, fat suppression): paralabral cysts with extension in the surrounding soft tissue

physiology is based on an overuse mechanism leading to a tight and shortened proximal iliotibial band which slides over the greater trochanter during hip extension from a flexed position and/or a tight (and shortened) iliopsoas tendon which moves over the iliopectineal eminence. Both bands are thickened with edematous swelling (tendinitis). The accompanying bursa is inflamed. In the long term this process leads to labral tears/fragments and damage to the neighboring hyaline cartilage (early osteoarthritis).

Finally, degenerative osteoarthritis is combined with migration of the hip (Fig. 18.19) (RESNICK 2002). The superior and superior lateral migration is found in 80% of all hip osteoarthritis patients.

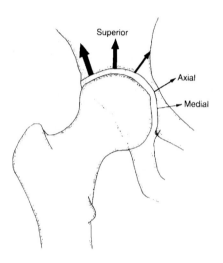

Fig. 18.19. Main migration directions of the hip femoral head in degenerative osteoarthritis

Antero-supero-lateral migration is the most common pattern in both sexes and is usually unilateral (Fig. 18.20). The posteromedial joint space is accordingly widened. Subchondral cyst formation – which can be very large and prominent – may occur on both sides of the joint and is sometimes the earliest feature in the acetabular roof. Calcification may be seen in the acetabular labrum.

Antero-supero-medial migration is much rarer and more commonly seen in women and is often bilateral (Fig. 18.21). Joint space narrowing occurs with resorption along the superolateral aspect of the femoral head and osteophytosis along the femoral neck (Wiberg sign = calcar buttressing) and the medial/inferior aspect of the femoral head.

Posteromedial migration of the femoral head is usually bilateral and more common in women (15% of all osteoarthritis patients) (Fig. 18.22). The etiology in this low stress zone may be based on variations in acetabular design, bone matrix changes, and increased varus angulation of the femoral neck; however, there is no definitive explanation.

Axial migration includes features of the above mentioned patterns and results in concentric loss of the hyaline cartilage. It might be combined with a mild protrusio acetabuli. It is the least common pattern of hip migration in degenerative osteoarthritis (Fig. 18.23). It leads to femoroacetabular impingement (Fig. 18.24).

All these migrations lead to changes in the biomechanical loading process during motion, but it is not clear whether they are a result of an already existing degenerative osteoarthritic process or whether they are forerunners of a degenerative osteoarthritic pro-

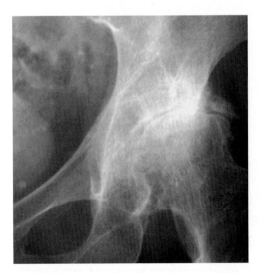

Fig. 18.20. Conventional radiograph of the hip joint: antero-supero-lateral/migration

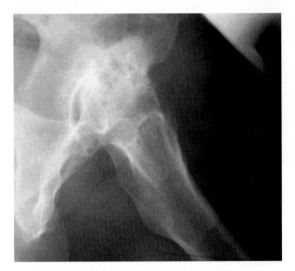

Fig. 18.21. Conventional radiograph of the hip joint: antero-supero-lateral/migration

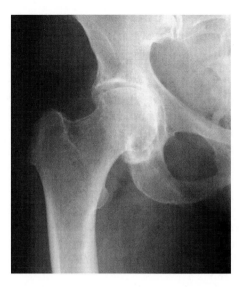

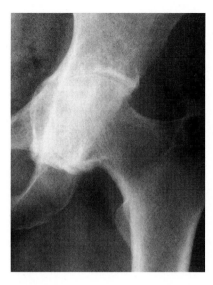

Fig. 18.22. Conventional radiograph of the right hip joint: postero-medial/migration

Fig. 18.23. Conventional radiograph of the left hip joint: axial migration with mild protrusio acetabuli left

cess. It is evident, however, that the localized overloading parallels the migration direction.

During walking the hip joint shows different patterns of motion (Mow and HAYA 1991):

1. During stance there is maximal flexion followed by a middle-sized extension and low sized second flexion during the swing.
2. At the same time but to a much lesser degree an adduction takes place during the stance, while during the swing there are only minimal waveformed adductions. There is normally no abduction.
3. During the stance an internal rotation is followed by an external rotation and again an internal rotation, while during the swing there is almost no rotation.

These motion processes, according to the above mentioned patterns, are "fragile"; in the event of an abnormal rotation axis as in a varus/valgus position, or a shortening of one leg, abnormal femoral anteversion or pelvic rotation, etc., localized chronic overloading may result. But problems may also arise in an imbalance of muscles, tendons or abnormal tissue structures. These also lead to chronic overloading of muscles, tendons and bones and may result in early degenerative osteoarthritis.

The natural history of degenerative osteoarthritis is variable. The disease may stabilize ("heal") or even regress focally or progress.

A special form of osteoarthritis is rapidly destructive joint disease (KHANNA et al. 2004). Typically it is found in the shoulder ("Milwaukee" shoulder)

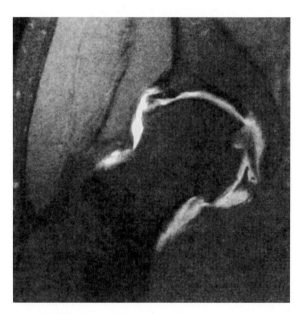

Fig. 18.24. MRI of right hip joint (T2-weighted with fat suppression): severe degenerative osteoarthritis with femoroacetabular impingement and axial migration

and the hip joint (Postel arthritis), but it may also involve other joints. It leads to joint destruction within months with a notable paucity of osteophytes (Fig. 18.25). The condition is much less inflammatory than rheumatoid arthritis. It may represent a subset of degenerative osteoarthritis, but contributing causes may be neuropathic arthropathies, drug-induced arthropathies, crystal disease and newly defined cytokine-mediated disease (LAROCHE et al. 2002).

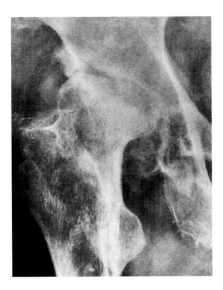

Fig. 18.25. Right hip joint radiograph (ap): within 4 months completely deformed head of the femur with a large lucency and reactive sclerosis. Almost no other reactive changes. This represents rapidly destructive joint disease

Erosive osteoarthritis refers to an unusual presentation of degenerative joint disease that involves mainly middle aged women and has a more acute clinical presentation. They can be confused with inflammatory-type arthritides, such as rheumatoid arthritis. Radiographically, erosive osteoarthritis is usually seen in small joints of the hand, rarely in the hip joint. The involved joints are narrowed, small osteophytes are seen, the subchondral surfaces are irregular, but the cortices are usually well-outlined, at the cartilage borders are well-demarcated.

18.1.4
Imaging

Degenerative osteoarthritis is usually demonstrated on conventional radiographs. These should be performed in an upright position to demonstrate the joint space narrowing in loading conditions.

The well known imaging signs are joint space narrowing with migration, subchondral sclerosis with thickening and cyst formation, osteophytes preferable in non-weightbearing positions, loose bodies, calcifications in the soft tissues (pyrophosphate and hydroxyapatite deposition), soft tissue (muscle) thinning (Fig. 18.26) (EL-KHOURY 2003).

CT will be used in unclear cases, particularly if there is the question of abnormal positioning (anteversion, pelvis torsion, etc.), tiny calcifications (intraarticular loose bodies), or preoperatively to

visualize the joint in 3D format (Fig. 18.27). The best results are achieved with a multi-detector spiral CT, which enables isotropic reconstruction in all planes.

MRI is gaining more and more clinical importance because of its excellent results in cartilage and soft-tissue imaging. It is important to have at least one sequence which visualizes both hips at the same time with similar quality. This allows the comparison of both hips, which could help in the differential diagnosis. Usually one starts with a T1-weighted sequence, followed by a fat-suppressed T2-weighted sequence. Finally, cartilage sequences (fat-suppressed gradient echoes) are applied. The examination should show the hip joint in at least two planes in different sequences (usually coronal and axial) (Figs. 18.8, 18.9).

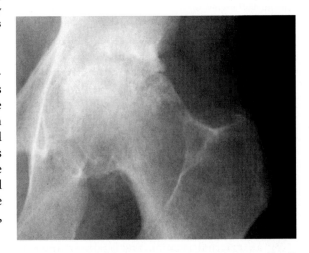

Fig. 18.26. Conventional radiograph of the left hip joint (detail, ap): joint space narrowing superolateral, subchondral sclerosis and "cysts" deformity

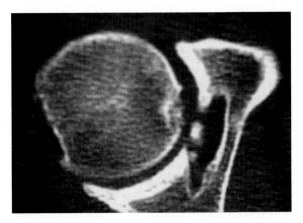

Fig. 18.27. Axial CT with mild degenerative changes (osteophytes) and free fragments

Intravenous contrast application is recommended in cases of unclear hip pain, to rule out (reactive) inflammatory and tumorous processes.

Localized surface coils (or phased array coils), 512 matrix and modern 1.5 Tesla machines with strong gradient fields and a short slew rate represent today's gold standard (VIGNON 2004; DOUGADOS 2004). In the near future 3T machines with special coils and sequences will probably give the best results.

To improve visualization of cartilage and labrum MR arthrography of the hip joint was introduced in clinical practice in 1997 (ELENTUCK and PALMER 2004). It enables visualization of incomplete and complete tears of the labrum and outline cartilage thinning or defects with much higher precision (90% accuracy) (Fig. 18.28). The visualization of different zones of cartilage – similar to those established by histology – is not possible nowadays, because of the thinness of cartilage (maximum 3 mm). Standard imaging is done with T1-weighted gradient echoes in two or three planes (sagittal, coronal, oblique axial). The use of a surface (phased array) coil is mandatory. The oblique axial view best depicts the anterosuperior acetabular labrum. Degenerative labral tears are most commonly found in the lateral (superior) location.

Loose bodies are best visualized with T2-weighted images. Because of the lower intensity of repaired cartilage, it cannot be differentiated from the sclerotic subchondral region and thickened calcified cartilage. All those three parts are hypointense on T1- and T2-weighted images. With MR arthrography the destroyed and reparative cartilage have an irregular surface (Fig. 18.29). Both – repaired and destroyed – cartilages show an abnormal uptake of i.v. applied Gd compounds on late MR images (30–45 min after i.v. administration).

For years bone scintigraphy represented an imaging standard in unclear degenerative osteoarthritis cases. This was particularly helpful in cases with pain. Typically, all cases with degenerative osteoarthritis will show a mild to high uptake in the bone phase of the three-phase bone scintigraphy

Fig. 18.28. a Localization of the trochanter major and the inguinal vessel bundle. Halfway in between direct puncture of the hip joint. **b** Oblique axial orientation of MR planes. **c** MR arthrography of the left hip joint (oblique axial T1-weighted) showing a complete labral tear

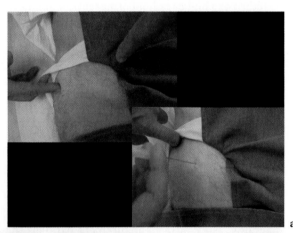

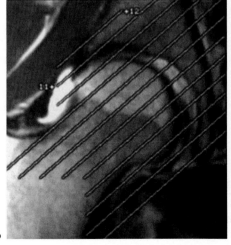

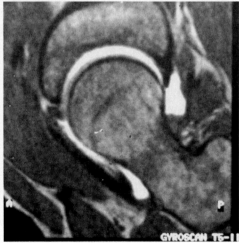

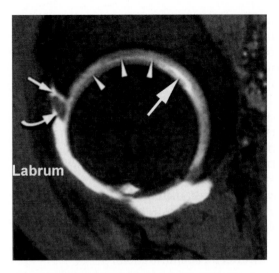

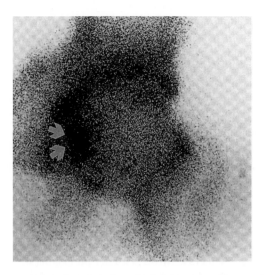

Fig. 18.29. MR arthrography of the right hip joint: abnormal thickness of cartilage with defects (*arrowheads*). Complete labral tear (*arrows*)

Fig. 18.30. Bone scintigraphy left hip joint (Tc-99m diphosphonate, 740 MBq): eccentric tracer uptake in the medial part of the hip joint

(Fig. 18.30). This is based on the higher bony metabolic turnover in these patients and/or the reactive synovialis (BAHK 2000).

If there is a higher radiopharmaceutical uptake in the first two phases, this represents reactive synovial hyperplasia with (pseudo-)inflammation and effusions. These cases are called "activated degenerative osteoarthritis" and will be treated additionally with anti-inflammatory drugs.

As standard for bone scintigraphy double coincidence positron cameras are used. The radiopharmaceuticals in use are commonly Tc-99m-polyphosphate compounds.

Nowadays, bone scintigraphy has been replaced more or less by MRI with i.v. contrast application. MRI has much better detail resolution than bone scintigraphy, enabling a more accurate (differential) diagnosis. The contrast enhancement parallels the higher radio-indicator uptake in the three phases of bone scintigraphy. Currently, PET or PET/CT do not play an important role in the diagnosis of degenerative osteoarthritis.

18.2
Rheumatoid Arthritis

18.2.1
Introduction, Definition and Pathophysiology

Rheumatoid arthritis is a self-perpetuating, inflammatory arthrocentric disease. It is initially charac-

terized clinically by swelling in several joints and stiffness lasting several weeks, ending up in chronic inflammatory destruction of the joint. A diagnosis of rheumatoid serum-negative should be made only if spondyloarthropathies have been excluded. The diagnosis is based on the so-called ARA criteria (four out of seven criteria). It has been estimated that it affects at least 0.5% of the population. It is more prevalent in female patients and there appears to be a steady association with increasing age (HUNDER 1998).

The pathology of rheumatoid arthritis can be described in four basic stages. In the first stage, an unknown antigen reaches the synovial membrane and initiates a local immune response. In the second stage, a chronic synovial inflammation ensues, with numerous cellular infiltrates and cytokines. In the third stage, pannus develop, eventuating in a final fourth stage of bone and cartilage destruction caused by inflammation and proliferation of synovial mesenchymal cells.

Irreversible joint damage and deformity occur. The distribution of lesions is typically symmetric, with involvement of small joint and, to a lesser extent, also the large joints as the hip joint.

18.2.1
Imaging

Standard imaging techniques are conventional radiographs (preferable in upright position), ap and axial.

In unclear cases and for semiquantitative follow-up studies three-phase-bone-scintigraphy or, as more frequently used today, MRI with i.v. application of contrast medium or duplex ultrasound are used. In most cases inflammatory activity is paralleled by the radioindicator uptake, the abnormal Duplex-signal or the contrast-enhancement by MRI, respectively.

The roentgenographic findings depend on the duration of illness, pathologic stage and destructive changes. Of these factors duration of illness is the single most important factor correlating with radiographic lesions.

In the early stages of rheumatoid arthritis there may be no radiologic changes; however, with joint pain and morning sickness, soft-tissue swelling may be roentgenographically evident (Fig. 18.31). With progressive synovitis and due to the periarticular hyperemia, the roentgenographic evidence of periarticular osteopenia is evident. Because the synovium attaches directly at the bone near the borders of the hyaline cartilage, localized bone destruction (erosion) may be seen on conventional radiographs, CT and high-resolution MRI. The latter will also show localized bone marrow edema.

The aggressive newly formed mesenchymal synovial tissue (pannus) and the cartilage destroying cytokines will, in addition, finally destroy the subarticular bone and cartilage.

In MRI this aggressive pannus behaves like a "malignant" tumor, showing T1-weighted hypointensity and T2-weighted hyperintensity. With the long duration of this disease the aging pannus becomes more fibrotic (T2-weighted hypointense) and shows no or less contrast-enhancement.

The final stages of destruction of bone and cartilage are reflected in erosion and narrowing of joint space, and secondary degenerative osteoarthritic changes, such as osteophytes, may develop over the long term. Abnormal shaping of the joint with deformation, subluxation and cyst formations due to multiple tiny aseptic necrosis and/or subchondral erosions are also characteristic changes (Figs. 18.32, 18.33).

Subchondral sclerosis, that is so characteristic of degenerative osteoarthritis is absent. In severe cases the joint destruction may end up (heal) with joint fusion, which is also extremely uncommon in degenerative osteoarthritis.

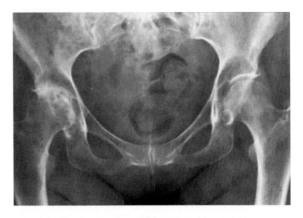

Fig. 18.32. Conventional radiograph of both hip joints (ap): rheumatoid arthritis (right > left) with joint space narrowing, erosions, deformity and reactive sclerosis. No osteophytes!

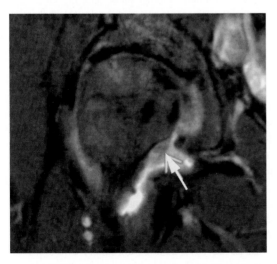

Fig. 18.31. MRI of the right hip joint (coronal, fat suppression, proton density-weighted): hypertrophic synovium (*arrow*) in rheumatoid arthritis

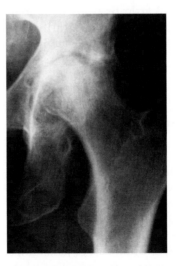

Fig. 18.33. Conventional radiograph of the left hip joint (ap): regional osteopenia and sclerosis, deformity, joint space narrowing in rheumatoid arthritis

Tendons, ligaments, muscles and bursae may be involved in rheumatoid arthritis, usually in the form of a non-specific chronic inflammation. Around the hip joint particularly painful bursitis and insertion tendinitis may develop. Areas of necrosis similar to the fibrinoid necrosis in the central zone of the rheumatoid nodule within the joint may be seen.

Rheumatoid arthritis is the prototype of inflammatory arthritis. However, it can be distinguished from so-called rheumatoid variants only on clinical pathological grounds.

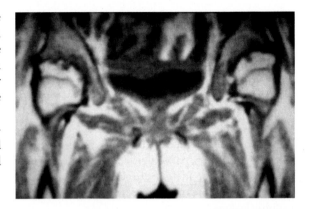

Fig. 18.34. MRI (T1-weighted, coronal): bilateral epiphyseal erosions in juvenile rheumatoid arthritis

18.3
Juvenile Rheumatoid Arthritis

The radiographic presentation of the juvenile form of the disease can mimic the adult form. However, juvenile arthritis often starts in one or even several large joints. Involvement of the hip joint, therefore, is not uncommon (ARGYROPOULOU et al. 2002; FROSCH et al. 2003).

The initial stage of synovitis is followed by erosions in the articular cartilage, resulting in narrowing of the joint space (Fig. 18.34).

Radiographically, on MRI with i.v. contrast medium application and duplex ultrasound joint effusions with synovial thickening and hyperemia are typical. These findings are followed by subchondral erosions and osteopenia. Enlargement of joints – very similar to hemophilia but without hemosiderin deposition – can be seen (LAMER and SEBAG 2000).

Juvenile rheumatoid arthritis tends to be more proliferative than adult rheumatoid arthritis, and fusions across joints are therefore found at times.

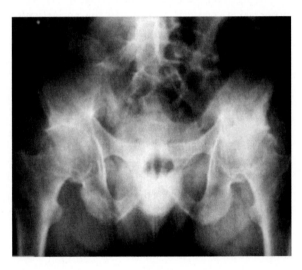

Fig. 18.35. Conventional radiograph of both hip joints (ap): uniform joint space narrowing and moderate subchondral sclerosis in ankylosing spondylitis

18.4
Seronegative Spondyloarthropathies and -Arthritis

Seronegative (rheumatoid factor-negative) spondyloarthropathies represent a spectrum of diverse but radiologically and genetically overlapping medical diseases (HUNDER 1998).

The peripheral joint involvement by ankylosing spondylitis occurs mainly in the large joints (hips, knees, shoulders) with uniform narrowing of the joint spaces, moderate subchondral sclerosis and proliferative synovial changes (Fig. 18.35). In psoriasis hip joint involvement is very rare. Involvement of small distal joints is typical.

Reiter's or "reactive" arthritis is typical oligoarticular, usually involving the distal lower extremity. Hip joint involvement is very common. The "productive" appearance of this arthritis type with new bone formation (ossification) usually enables a differential diagnosis.

Arthritis in inflammatory bowel disease can be seen in about 10%–20% of all cases. The synovial inflammation with thickening is usually transient and not destructive, involving mostly the knees and ankles and rarely the hip joints.

18.5
Granulomatous Arthritis

The differential diagnosis of granulomatous disease in joints includes tuberculosis and very rarely fungi infections (coccidiomycosis, candidiasis).

Non-AIDS-related osseoarticular tuberculosis occurs primarily in the fifth through seventh decade. In underdeveloped countries it is more common in younger patients. The hip and knee joints are fairly common sites, but altogether the osseoarticular system is only involved in 3%–5% of all Tb cases, and in 20% of AIDS patients. The spread of Tb into the joint can be hematogenous, but is very often contiguous from an adjacent osteomyelitis. The latter is particularly true in cases where the joint synovium reaches fairly down alongside the bone, as for instance in the hip joint. In contrast to other arthritides, it is typically monoarticular (BARANTZ et al. 1999; RAMANATH et al. 2002).

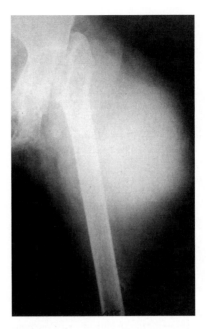

Fig. 18.36. Conventional radiograph left hip joint: severe destructive tuberculous arthritis with extensive destruction of the head, neck and acetabulum, as well as dislocation

18.5.1
Imaging

Clinically, tuberculous arthritis is a subacute/chronic disease with minimal evidence of inflammation over months. Accordingly, narrowed joint spaces are typical in the early phase, and can also last for several months. The articular cartilage tends to be preserved. There is some accompanying effusion and synovial thickening ("soft tissue mass"). These findings are followed by epiphyseal erosions. Osteoporosis is less common in tuberculosis, but it may be seen in early cases (Fig. 18.36).

These imaging findings can also be seen with MRI and CT. Bone-scintigraphy may show a very unspectacular localized uptake.

intraarticular injections of any kind, and prosthetic joint surgery.

Causative agents are *S. aureus* or gonococci. Both joint damage and chronic inflammation have been considered to be contributing predisposing factors. The most commonly involved joints are the knee, hip and shoulder.

Gonococcal arthritis is usually a monoarticular process involving the knee.

However, unlike the other septic arthritides gonococcal arthritis commonly involves other joints such as the wrist and interphalangeal joints in the hand and wrist. It may even be a migratory disease and disseminated, as evidenced by tenosynovitis (HUNDER 1998).

18.6
Septic Arthritis

Septic arthritis is usually a monoarticular infection, most commonly involving the hip in infants and young children, and the knee in older children and adults. Factors predisposing to bacterial arthritis are contiguous osteomyelitis (particularly after closure of the growth plate), contiguous soft tissue infection, penetrating injury into the joint, hematogenous spread from a remote infection, drug addiction with infection at the injection site,

18.6.1
Imaging

Early imaging – particularly in children – should include ultrasound and MRI. Both allow visualization of the effusion and involvement of the synovium (synovial thickening with hyperemia) (Fig. 18.37). In all unclear cases a biopsy with removal of synovium and fluid may prove the diagnosis.

The disease is usually very foudroyant, leading, if left untreated, to early destruction of bone and cartilage, ending up with bony fusion in worst cases.

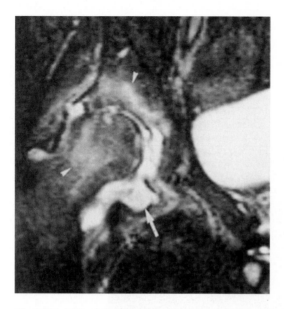

Fig. 18.37. MRI of the right hip joint (coronal, T2-weighted, fat suppression, contrast application): effusion, erosion, bone marrow edema, synovial contrast enhancement in acute granulomatous arthritis

References

Altman RD, Bloch DA, Dougados M, Hochberg M, Lohmander S, Pavelka K, Spector T, Vignon E (2004) Measurement of structural progression in osteoarthritis of the hip: the Barcelona consensus group. Osteoarthritis Cartilage 12:515–524

Anderson J, Read JW, Steinweg J (1998) Atlas of imaging in sports medicine. McGraw-Hill, New York

Argyropoulou MI, Fanis SL, Xenakis T, Efremidis SC, Siamopoulou A (2002). The role of MRI in the evaluation of hip joint disease in clinical subtypes of juvenile idiopathic arthritis. Br J Radiol 75:229–233

Arokoski JP, Arokoski MH, Vainio P, Kroger H, Jurvelin JS (2004) Estimation of femoral head bone density using magnetic resonance imaging: comparison between men with and without hip osteoarthritis. J Clin Densitom 7:183–191

Bahk YW (2000) Combined scintigraphic and radiographic diagnosis of bone and joint disease. Springer, Berlin Heidelberg New York

Baratz ME, Watson AD, Imbreglia JE (1999). Orthopaedic surgery – the essentials. Thieme, New York

Beary JF 3rd (2001) Joint structure modification in osteoarthritis: development of SMOAD drugs. Curr Rheumatol Rep 3:506–512

Brandt KD, Doherty M, Lohmander LS (1998) Osteoarthritis. Oxford University Press, Oxford

Bullough P (2004) Orthopaedic pathology. Mosby/Elsevier, New York

Crock HV (1996) An atlas of vascular anatomy of the skeleton and spinal cord. Dunitz, London

Dougados M (2004) Monitoring osteoarthritis progression and therapy. Osteoarthritis Cartilage 12 [Suppl A]:S55–S60

Elentuck D, Palmer WE (2004) Direct magnetic resonance arthrography. Eur Radiol 14:1956–1967

El-Khoury GE (2003) Essentials of musculo-skeletal imaging. Elsevier Science, New York

Farjo LA, Glick JM, Sampson TG (1999) Hip arthroscopy for acetabular labral tears. Arthroscopy 15:132–137

Felson DT (2004) An update on the pathogenesis and epidemiology of osteoarthritis. Radiol Clin North Am 42:1–9

Frosch M, Foell D, Ganser G, Roth J (2003) Arthrosonography of hip and knee joints in the follow up of juvenile rheumatoid arthritis. Ann Rheum Dis 62:242–244

Hunder GG (1998) Atlas of rheumatology. Blackwell Science, Philadelphia

Imhof H, Czerny C, Gahleitner A, Grampp S, Kainberger F, Krestan C, Sulzbacher I (2002) Koxarthrose. Radiologe 42:416–431

Isenberg DA, Renton P (2003) Imaging in rheumatology. Oxford University Press, Oxford, UK

Khanna AJ, Domb BG, Moshirfar A, Wenz JF Sr (2004) Rapidly destructive osteoarthrography of the hip. Am J Orthop 33:243–247

Laroche M, Moineuse C, Durroux R, Mazieres B, Puget J (2002) Can ischemic hip disease cause rapidly destructive hip osteoarthritis? A case report. Joint Bone Spine 69:76–80

Lamer S, Sebag GH (2000) MRI and ultrasound in children with juvenile chronic arthritis. Eur J Radiol 33:85–93

Mow CV, Haja WC (1991) Basic orthopaedic biomechanics. Raven, New York

Ramanath VS, Damron TA, Ambrose JL, Rose FB (2002) Tuberculosis of the hip as the presenting sign of HIV and simulating pigmented villonodular synovitis. Skeletal Radiol 31:426–429

Resnick D (2002) Diagnosis of bone and joint disorders. Saunders-Elsevier, Philadelphia

Stoller WD (2004) Diagnostic imaging orthopaedics. Amirsys-Elsevier, Salt Lake City, Utah

Vignon E (2004) Radiographic issues in imaging the progression of hip and knee osteoarthritis. J Rheumatol [Suppl] 70:36–44

Yamamoto T, Bullough PG (1999) Subchondral insufficiency fracture of the femoral head: a differential diagnosis in acute onset of coxarthritis the elderly. Arthritis Rheum 42:2719–2723

Yamamoto T, Bullough PG (2000) The role subchondral insufficiency fracture in rapid destruction of the hip joint: a preliminary report. Arthritis Rheum 43:2423–2427

19 Arthritis 2: Sacroiliac Joint

Anne Grethe Jurik

CONTENTS

19.1
Introduction

The sacroiliac joints (SIJ) are centrally placed in the human body and have a rather complex anatomy which allows transmission of all forces from the body to the lower extremities through the joints. The SIJ may be involved in most inflammatory disorders, but predominantly in the group of disorders defined as seronegative spondylarthropathies (SpA). Infectious arthritis is rare, but degenerative or stress induced changes are common and may be the cause of low back pain.

Conventional radiography is widely used to screen for SIJ changes and will detect manifest osseous and/or joint lesions, but not minor abnormali-

ties, partly due to the complex anatomy of the joints. Cross-sectional imaging by CT or MR imaging are necessary for detecting minor SIJ changes and have gained wide acceptance for the diagnosis of inflammatory and infectious lesions, but not for detecting degenerative changes. Other imaging methods such as scintigraphy and ultrasound usually have limited diagnostic value.

19.2
Joint Anatomy

The performance and interpretation of SIJ imaging demand knowledge of the normal anatomy. The SIJs are built to be stable during the transmission of forces from the body to the lower extremities. This stability is obtained by obliquely orientated undulating joint facets (Fig. 19.1), surrounding joint ligaments, and also strong external ligaments and muscles. The joint is composed of two compartments: a C-shaped cartilaginous part that lies inferiorly/anteriorly and a ligamentous part superiorly/ posterior containing strong interosseous ligaments. The cartilaginous joint facets are convex anteriorly and are usually narrower in females than in males, although the joint varies greatly in size, shape and contour (BOWEN and CASSIDY 1981; PUHAKKA et al. 2004a; FRANCOIS et al. 2000).

The sacral cartilage in adults is thick and of low cell density. It rests upon a thin bone end-plate supported by porous, cancellous bone. The iliac cartilage and bone display the converse proportions with thinner cartilage and thicker subchondral bone (FRANCOIS et al. 2000) (Fig. 19.2a). The cartilaginous portion of the joint is without synovia (a symphysis) proximally, whereas there is a small synovial recess at the distal part of the joint (Fig. 19.2b,c). The anatomy of the middle part is rather variable with a variety of normal variations giving rise to pitfalls at MR imaging (FRANCOIS et al. 2000; PUHAKKA et al. 2004a).

A. G. JURIK, MD, DMSc
Associate Professor, Department of Radiology, Aarhus University Hospital, Noerrebrogade 44, 8000 Aarhus C, Denmark

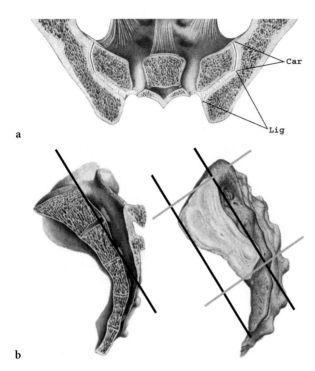

a

b

Fig. 19.1a,b. Macroscopic anatomy of the sacroiliac joints (SIJs). **a** A transverse section of the middle part of the SIJs showing the oblique orientation of the joint facets and the two joint portions, the anterior cartilaginous part (*Car*) and the ligamentous part posterior (*Lig*). **b** A sagittal section at the middle of the sacrum (*left*) and of the cartilaginous sacral joint facet, which is C-shaped with the convex side facing anteriorly. To visualise as much as possible of the cartilaginous part of the joint on relatively few sections, it is necessary to use a semi-coronal scan plane (*black streaks*), obtainable at both CT and MR imaging. The posterosuperior ligamentous portion of the joint is not well visualised in this scan plane, but will be visualised by a semi-axial slice plane (*grey streaks*), which can be obtained at MR imaging (see Fig. 19.7)

19.3
Imaging Modalities

The diagnosis of sacroiliac joint disorders can be obtained by conventional radiography when the disease has resulted in definite abnormalities of the bone or joint facets. However, erosions and joint space alteration in early sacroiliitis may be difficult to assess on radiographs, and symptoms of sacroiliitis often occur 1–9 years before there are manifest changes at radiography (Braun et al. 2000). CT and especially MR imaging have proved superior to radiography for the detection of SIJ changes making it possible to diagnose SpA earlier than at radiography (Fam et al. 1985; Geijer et al. 1998; Blum et al. 1996). The finding of sacroiliitis by imaging

is important for the early diagnosis of ankylosing spondylitis (AS) and to differentiate AS from other forms of arthritis and infectious lesions. Therefore, today, cross-sectional imaging plays a great role in the identification of early SIJ abnormalities.

19.3.1
Conventional Radiography

Conventional radiography is a well-established and widely used method for detecting definite SIJ and/ or osseous alterations. Various methods have been used, but none is ideal as the normal oblique and undulating joint surfaces often cause overprojection of osseous structures in addition to shadows of pelvic soft tissue structures. A frontal projection is usually preferred. It can be performed in the supine position with the tube angulated 20–30° in the cephalic direction (Fig. 19.3) or as a PA projection with 25–30° caudal angulation, so the X-rays diverge in consistence with the joint orientation. In either case both SIJs are exposed on a single film, facilitating comparison of the two joints (Fig. 19.4). To cope with overprojecting bone structures on frontal radiographs, a supplementary oblique projection has been used (Fig. 19.5). These images can be obtained either in the supine or the prone position, and are performed as a separate radiograph of each joint with the side of the body elevated 20–25°. The performance of both frontal and oblique projections does not seem justifiable. It increases the radiation dose to the patient (Jurik et al. 2002) and the diagnostic value is questionable. In an analysis based on nearly 900 joints, the agreement between the findings on an AP view and oblique views was high, and there were no cases in which a normal SIJ on an AP film was found to show unequivocal abnormalities on an oblique view (Battistone et al. 1998).

It has been widely accepted that inflammatory radiographic abnormalities of the SIJs are graded according to the New York criteria in five stages: 0, normal; 1, suspicious changes; 2, minimal abnormality in the form of small areas of erosions or sclerosis without alteration in the joint width; 3, unequivocal abnormality – moderate or advanced sacroiliitis consisting of erosions, sclerosis, widening, narrowing, and/or partial ankylosis; and 4, severe abnormality in the form of total ankylosis (van der Linden 1984) (Fig. 19.4). The inter- and intra-observer variation is, however, considerable for slight changes (Hollingsworth et al. 1983) and

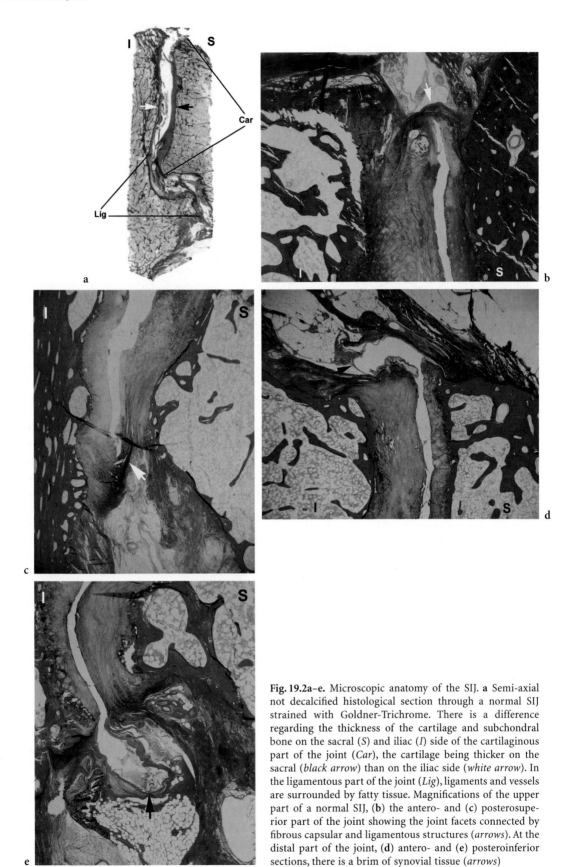

Fig. 19.2a–e. Microscopic anatomy of the SIJ. **a** Semi-axial not decalcified histological section through a normal SIJ strained with Goldner-Trichrome. There is a difference regarding the thickness of the cartilage and subchondral bone on the sacral (*S*) and iliac (*I*) side of the cartilaginous part of the joint (*Car*), the cartilage being thicker on the sacral (*black arrow*) than on the iliac side (*white arrow*). In the ligamentous part of the joint (*Lig*), ligaments and vessels are surrounded by fatty tissue. Magnifications of the upper part of a normal SIJ, (**b**) the antero- and (**c**) posterosuperior part of the joint showing the joint facets connected by fibrous capsular and ligamentous structures (*arrows*). At the distal part of the joint, (**d**) antero- and (**e**) posteroinferior sections, there is a brim of synovial tissue (*arrows*)

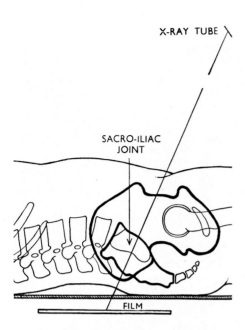

X-RAY TUBE

SACRO-ILIAC
JOINT

FILM

Fig. 19.3. Positioning and tube angulation at AP radiography of the SIJ

train does not seem to improve the ability to analyse radiographs with regard to sacroiliitis (van Tubergen et al. 2003).

19.3.2
Computed Tomography

CT has proved superior to radiography for the detection of SIJ changes in spondylarthropathies (Carrera et al. 1981; Geijer et al. 1998; Mester et al. 2000; Puhakka et al. 2003, van Tubergen et al. 2003), encompassing joint erosion, subchondral bone changes and enthesitis. The better sensitivity of CT can reduce the length of the observation period before a SpA diagnosis is established. Additionally, observer variation may be significantly reduced (Geijer et al. 1998). CT has therefore been widely used for imaging the SIJs. Although MR imaging is diagnostically preferable and without radiation risk, CT still has a place in the diagnosis of SIJ disorders, especially when MR imaging cannot be performed.

In addition to its diagnostic potentials CT can be used to guide joint aspiration or biopsies and corticosteroid injection into the joint.

Diagnostic CT is mostly performed in the supine position either with a semi-coronal or an axial slice orientation. The semi-coronal CT technique described by Carrera et al. (1981) with the gantry angled so the scan plane is as parallel as possible to the long axis of the upper sacrum has gained wide acceptance for evaluation of the SIJs. It is diagnostically preferable to axial CT as it allows an overall view of the cartilaginous joint facets and also visualises the ligamentous part of the SIJ (Fig. 19.6). Moreover, the radiation dose is less than 6–8 contiguous 5 mm slices visualise the joints in adults, whereas visualisation of the whole joint region in the axial plane may demand 14–16 5 mm slices (Jurik et al. 2002). The difference in number of scans is due to the joint anatomy, the cartilaginous joint facets being narrower in the semi-coronal than in the cranio-caudal direction (Fig. 19.1b). The dose reduction gained by a semi-coronal compared to axial slice orientation is important in children and young adults and especially in females where direct radiation to the ovaries is avoided. Therefore, a semi-coronal orientation should be applied also at multislice CT although it may be easier to perform axial slices and view the joints by varying multiplanar reconstructions.

For serial CT, the scan parameters are based on the available literature which recommends 5 mm contiguous slices obtained at high kV (130–140) and as low an mAs as possible. Thinner slices have not been proved to give further diagnostic information (Jurik et al. 2002), and the value of multislice CT of the SIJs has not yet been systematically analysed.

When evaluating CT one should always take into consideration the normal SIJ anatomy corresponding to the slice orientation or reconstruction plane used, including the fact that CT only identifies the two different joint portions by their orientation and position (Carrera et al. 1981). New bone formation corresponding to tendon insertions (entheses) are well visualised on CT (Puhakka et al. 2003), and may be a sign of SpA (Fig. 19.6). It is, however, important not to over-diagnose CT changes due to a better joint visualisation than by radiography and be aware that sclerosis and joint space narrowing have been found to occur in patients without SIJ symptoms (Elgafy et al. 2001). This can explain that the specificity of CT may not be improved compared to radiography (Elgafy et al. 2001; van Tubergen et al. 2003).

Grading of sacroiliitis at CT has mostly been performed as an overall grading in accordance with the New York criteria for radiography. A semi-quantitative grading for CT abnormalities has been proposed by Puhakka et al. (2003) to make MR and CT grading comparable. This grading includes assessment of: (1) erosions, (2) subchondral sclerosis, (3) joint space alteration, and (4) new bone formation at entheses corresponding to both the

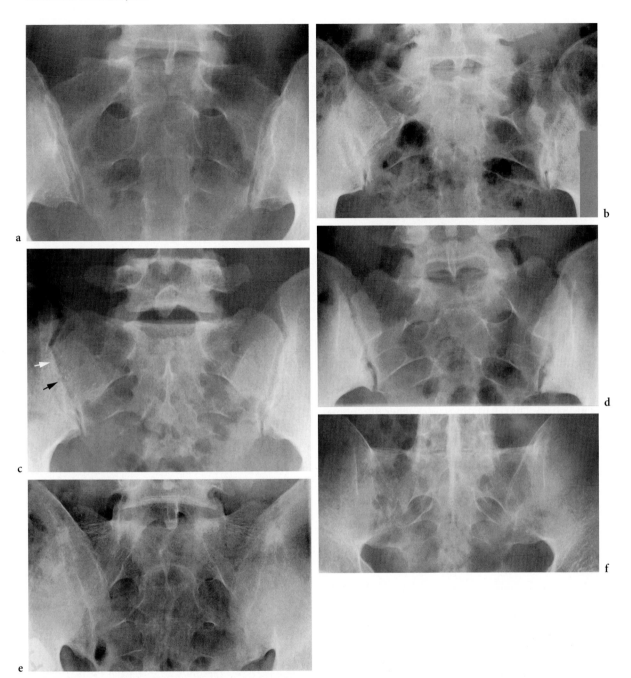

Fig. 19.4a–f. The five grades of sacroiliitis according to New York Criteria. **a** Grade 0, normal joints. **b** Grade 1, suspicious changes of the left SIJ in the form of slight irregularity of the joint facets (26-year-old woman). **c** Grade 2, minimal abnormality in the form of small areas of erosions (*black arrow*) and sclerosis (*white arrow*) without alteration in the joint width (28-year-old man). **d** Grade 3 changes in the form of moderate erosion with subchondral sclerosis and focal joint space widening (25-year-old woman). **e** Grade 3–4, severe abnormality in the form of joint ankylosis, but still visible joint contours (34-year-old man). **f** Grade 4 with homogeneous joint ankylosis including ankylosis corresponding to the ligamentous structures (53-year-old man)

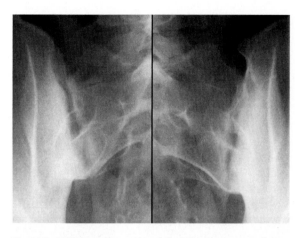

Fig. 19.5. Oblique radiographs of the SIJs demonstrated on a frontal radiograph in Fig. 19.3d. There are less overprojecting osseous structures, but the views give no further diagnostic information

cartilaginous and the ligamentous part of the joint. The findings were graded: 0–3, where 0=normal, 1=minimal, 2=moderate and 3=severe. Using this grading system, CT abnormalities were found to be sensitive to changes at 1-year follow-up (PUHAKKA et al. 2004c). The CT findings were generally comparable to the chronic changes observed at MR imaging, except that CT seems better for evaluating joint space alteration, including a higher inter-observer

agreement, and was able to demonstrate entheseal ossification not always identifiable at MR imaging (PUHAKKA et al. 2003). The reports of CT being superior to MR imaging for detecting sclerosis probably relate to the use of other MR sequences (MURPHEY et al. 1991; YU et al. 1998).

19.3.3
MR Imaging

The advantages of MR imaging compared to CT and radiography are that, in addition to chronic changes, it also visualises soft tissue and can detect active inflammatory changes, making it possible to diagnose sacroiliitis before definite joint destruction is detectable on CT or radiography (BATTAFARANO et al. 1993; BLUM et al. 1996; YU et al. 1998; OOSTVEEN et al. 1999; BRAUN et al. 2000).

There is no doubt that the capability of MR imaging to distinguish between acute and chronic changes and to estimate the degree of disease activity are of great value in the diagnosis of sacroiliitis and for monitoring the disease course, including the effect of pharmacological treatment (BRAUN et al. 2002), and also with regard to classification of the different forms of SpA (MUCHE et al. 2003). When possible MR imaging should therefore be used for

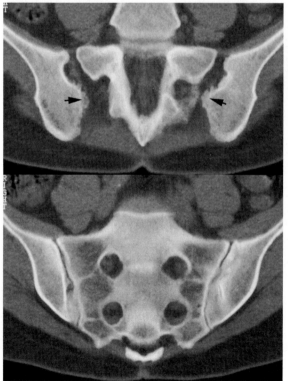

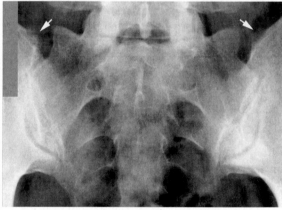

Fig. 19.6a,b. CT scanning. **a** Two semi-coronal CT slices of a patient with Crohn's disease showing narrowing of the cartilaginous joint space and fluffy periosteal new bone formation (*arrows*) at the ligamentous part of the joint. **b** At a preceding radiograph some of the new bone formation was detectable (*arrows*)

evaluating sacroiliitis. MR imaging, however, has disadvantages, including long examination times, relative high cost, requirement for skilled staff and specific contraindications such as pacemakers. The interpretation of MR imaging may also be difficult. It requires thorough knowledge of the normal anatomy and pitfalls at MR imaging to establish the diagnosis of early sacroiliitis (PUHAKKA et al. 2004a). The use of a standardised examination technique may facilitate the evaluation. Most published analyses of the SIJ have been based on semi-coronal MR slices, but a recent MR study with histological comparison has shown that semi-axial slices are important for optimal visualisation of both the cartilaginous and the ligamentous portion of the joint, and especially the transition between the two portions. Semi-axial MR slices clearly delineated the two anatomically different joint portions by revealing fatty tissue in the ligamentous, but not in the cartilaginous portion (PUHAKKA et al. 2004a). Such anatomical differentiation can be difficult on semi-coronal slices (MUCHE et al. 2003), and thereby to obtain a certain anatomical location of joint abnormalities, especially of lesions occurring in the ligamentous part of the joint. However, semi-coronal slices give a better overview of joint erosion and subchondral osseous lesions corresponding to the cartilaginous joint portion, so both slice orientations should be performed. Standard slice orientations including semi-coronal slices obtained parallel to a line joining the upper dorsal aspect of S1 and S3, and semi-axial slices perpendicular to this semi-coronal plane have been proposed (PUHAKKA et al. 2003) (Fig. 19.1b and 19.7). The necessary MR sequences depend on the diagnostic purpose. Screening for sacroiliitis may only require a semi-axial STIR (or T2-weighted sequence with fat suppression, T2 FS), which displays inflammation as areas of high signal intensity, and a semi-coronal T1-weighted sequence, displaying chronic changes such as erosion and fatty bone marrow changes, appearing as areas of increased signal intensity. If they are normal, inflammatory disorders and also infection and malignancies are excluded. If they are equivocal a semi-coronal STIR (or T2 FS) may give further information with regard to inflammatory changes, and a semi-coronal T1 FS sequence with regard to erosions (Fig. 19.8). Abnormalities at these screening sequences can be further characterised by assessing vascularised abnormalities using semi-coronal and/or semi-axial T1 FS after intravenous Gadolinium (Gd) injection (PUHAKKA et al. 2003; MUCHE et al. 2003) (Fig. 19.8). This should always be performed when there is suspicion of infectious sacroiliitis in order to diagnose or exclude abscess formation. Acute inflammatory activity presents with oedema in the joint space and/or bone marrow, which is known to be an early and non-specific sign of various abnormalities, and contrast enhancement caused by increased vascularisation. Erosions, sclerosis, and changes of joint width are signs of chronic disease, as well as fat deposition in the bone marrow, which can be regarded a sign of degeneration and healing (BRAUN et al. 2000; PUHAKKA et al. 2003) (Fig. 19.8).

There are few published proposals for grading/quantification of MR abnormalities (AHLSTRÖM et al. 1990; BRAUN et al. 2000; PUHAKKA et al. 2003). The first grading proposed by AHLSTRÖM et al. (1990) divided MR abnormalities into two types. Type I lesions were characterised by a low signal intensity on T1-weighted images and a high signal intensity on phase-contrast and/or T2-weighted

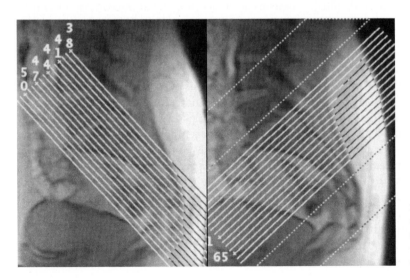

Fig. 19.7. Recommended MR slice orientations, including both semi-coronal slices parallel to a line joining the upper dorsal aspect of S1 and S3 and perpendicular semi-axial slices

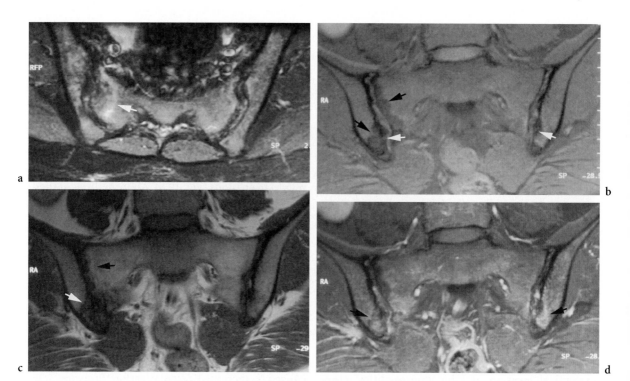

Fig. 19.8a–d. Recommended MR sequences: (**a**) semi-axial STIR and (**b**) semi-coronal T1 image, supplemented by (**c**) semi-coronal T1 FS image before and (**d**) after Gd in a 42-year-old woman with psoriasis and right-sided grade 2 changes at radiography. The STIR image displays definite increased signal intensity around the right joint (*arrow*). The T1 image shows decreased signal intensity corresponding to the inferior part of the joint, compatible with sclerosis (*white arrow*). There is accompanying joint space narrowing and slightly increased signal intensity in the sacrum corresponding to slight fatty marrow changes (*black arrow*). The T1 FS image (**c**) displays definite erosion at both SIJs, most pronounced at the right iliac joint facet (*white arrows*). The iliac area with sclerosis shows lower signal intensity than corresponding to the sacral areas of fatty marrow changes (*black arrows*). Enhancement in the subchondral bone, and also in both joint spaces is clearly seen on the post-contrast image (**d**, *arrows*)

images, being compatible with active inflammation. Type II lesions consisted of changes presenting with low signal intensity at all sequences, corresponding to chronic changes. This division does not take into account the frequent occurrence of fatty marrow changes in chronic disease (PUHAKKA et al. 2003). BRAUN et al. (2000) subsequently proposed a grading of disease activity based on quantitative evaluation of contrast enhancement at dynamic MR imaging divided in three stages and supplemented by the New York criteria for joint destruction. Only single section of the joint can be visualised by a dynamic post-contrast sequence and the evaluation of quantitative enhancement may be difficult. This grading has therefore not gained wide acceptance.

A semi-quantitative grading system has been elaborated and tested by PUHAKKA et al. (2003, 2004c). It was based on the following sequences: STIR, T1, and T1 FS before and after intravenous Gd contrast using both semi-coronal and semi-axial slice orientation. Abnormalities of the cartilaginous and ligamentous joint portion were scored sepa-

rately for the following sign of activity: bone marrow oedema and Gd contrast enhancement in the bone marrow, cartilaginous and ligamentous joint space, and at entheses outside the joint. Assessment of joint destruction/chronic changes was based on erosions, osseous sclerosis (low signal intensity at T1 and/or T1 FS), and fat accumulation in the bone marrow, joint space alteration and new bone formation at entheses. All parameters were scored 0–3, where 0=normal, 1=minimal, 2=moderate and 3=severe. Based on an analysis of 41 patients, it was concluded that parameters indicating disease activity can be monitored with a good intra-observer and relative good inter-observer agreement, whereas grading of chronic changes in the form of joint destruction, especially joint space narrowing, but also osseous sclerosis may be more difficult (Table 19.1). The grading has, however, been shown to have sensitivity to change in a 1-year follow-up study, being able to detect decreasing disease activity, but increasing chronic changes without concomitant clinical signs indicating this (PUHAKKA et al. 2004b,c).

Table 19.1. Inter- and intra-observer agreement for the most frequent disease parameters present at MR imaging based on 41 patients (82 SIJs) (PUHAKKA et al. 2003)

	Inter-observer analysis		Intra-observer analysis	
	Agreement (%)	Kappa value	Agreement (%)	Kappa value
Oedema bone	73	0.49	95	0.89
Enhancement bone	73	0.47	98	0.94
Enhancement joint space	82	0.64	98	0.94
Bone erosion	77	0.54	98	0.95
Osseous sclerosis	71	0.41	93	0.85
Fatty degeneration	84	0.67	93	0.84
Joint space alteration	59	0.18	95	0.90

Although the study by PUHAKKA et al. (2003) revealed a significant correlation between bone marrow oedema on STIR and contrast enhancement in the bone marrow, it has not been proved that post-contrast sequences are unnecessary. STIR has been reported to be less sensitive than post-contrast sequences with regard to joint space inflammation (MUCHE et al. 2003). It has to be determined whether or not post-contrast sequences are needed, and the semi-quantitative grading has to be modified taking into account the poor inter-observer agreement for joint space alteration.

19.3.4
Scintigraphy

Quantitative radioisotope scanning allows comparison of the SIJ uptake, the sacrum being used as a reference point. It may be used to diagnose early SpA without definite radiographic changes of the SIJ (SKAAR et al. 1992) (Fig. 19.9). It is a sensitive method, but its specificity is somewhat low, as it may be impossible to differentiate abnormalities due to sacroiliitis from other causes of low back pain such as degenerative joint disease and even normal joints (control persons) (VERLOOY et al. 1992). Once it was proved that MR imaging is superior to quantitative scintigraphy for the detection of sacroiliitis (BLUM et al. 1996; BATTAFARANO et al. 1993), the use of scintigraphy with its inherent radiation risk has declined and is usually limited to localisation of infectious axial lesions.

19.3.5
Ultrasound

Ultrasound has gained widespread acceptance in the diagnosis of inflammatory disorders, but

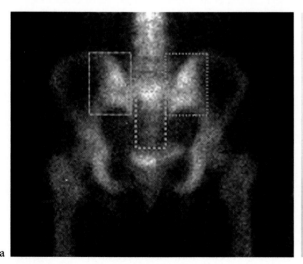
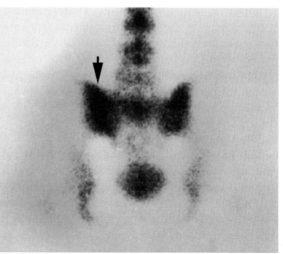

Fig. 19.9a,b. Quantitative scintigraphy. **a** Normal joints with drawing of the areas of measurements. **b** Left-sided sacroiliitis in a patient with normal radiograph. Posteroanterior view shows increased accumulation on the left (*arrow*) compared to the right side

mainly when located to peripheral joints. Ultrasound can only visualise the superficial part of the SIJs and the surrounding soft tissue structures, including the posterior stabilising ligaments (Fig. 19.10). Despite this, it has been reported possible to diagnose active sacroiliitis based on increased vascularisation in the posterior part of the joints (ARSLAN et al. 1999), and ultrasound has been used to demonstrate passive motion in the SIJ (LUND et al. 1996). In addition ultrasound can be used to guide corticosteroid injection, but only into the posterior part of the joint.

19.4
Inflammatory Disorders

The SIJs may be involved in most inflammatory disorders, but predominantly in the group of disorders defined as seronegative spondylarthropathies. Sacroiliitis can occur in rheumatoid arthritis and also in pustulotic arthro-osteitis, SAPHO (synovitis, acne, pustulosis, hyperostosis, osteitis) syndrome and chronic recurrent multifocal osteomyelitis, which today are regarded as atypical forms of SpA. Also other inflammatory disorders may involve the SIJ, but rarely.

19.4.1
Seronegative Spondylarthropathies (SpA)

The group of SpA as defined by The European Spondylarthropathy Study Group (ESSG) in 1991 (DOUGADOS et al. 1991) was divided into five entities: ankylosing spondylitis (AS), psoriatic arthritis, reactive arthritis, arthritis associated with inflammatory bowel diseases (enteropathic arthropathy), and undifferentiated SpA. The prevalence of SpA has been estimated at between 0.5% and 1.9%, which is similar to that of rheumatoid arthritis (SARAUX et al. 1999; BRAUN et al. 1998).

The ESSG classification is based on clinical findings and radiographic evidence of sacroiliitis. Radiographic sacroiliitis has a high specificity (97.8%), but a low sensitivity (54.4%) for SpA. This low sensitivity may contribute to the fact that a SpA diagnosis may be delayed several years (ZINK et al. 2000; BRAUN et al. 2000). As mainly young patients are affected by SpA (ZINK et al. 2000) an early diagnosis, especially of AS, is valuable with regard to therapy, prognosis, and evaluation of working capac-

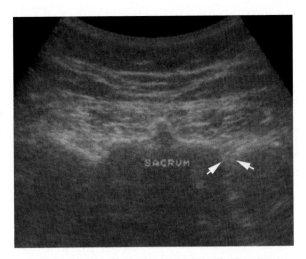

Fig. 19.10. Ultrasound, transverse section, showing the posterior border of the sacrum with the spinous process in the midline and the joint space on each side (*arrows*)

ity. Sacroiliitis is commonly the first manifestation of SpA, and the diagnosis of sacroiliitis by imaging is therefore important in order to detect early SpA. Since the establishment of the ESSG criteria in 1991 the diagnostic value of CT and MR imaging in the diagnosis of sacroiliitis has been proved and cross-sectional imaging has obtained an important role in identification of abnormalities of the SIJ in early SpA. Especially MR imaging has been found valuable for the early SpA diagnosis being able to detect joint inflammation before the occurrence of changes visible at CT, in addition to visualisation of chronic joint changes later on (BATTAFARANO et al. 1993; BLUM et al. 1996; YU et al. 1998; OOSTVEEN et al. 1999; BRAUN et al. 2000).

There is no well-established method for evaluation, localisation and characterisation of pathological MR findings of the SIJ in SpA, although the need for this is obvious. MR abnormalities in the different forms of SpA have mainly been described based on semi-coronal slices (MUCHE et al. 2003), which limit characterisation of changes in the ligamentous part of the joint. At the moment efforts are being put into the elaboration of a widely accepted method for classification of the different MR abnormalities, which will make it possible to include MR findings in future internationally accepted diagnostic criteria for the different forms of SpA. Verification of relatively specific MR signs justifying classification of the different forms of SpA demands several years of follow-up and is not jet published. The following stated MR features, which are based mainly on a cross-sectional analysis (MUCHE et al. 2003) and preliminary results of 5 years

MR follow-up at Aarhus University should therefore not be regarded as definite.

19.4.1.1
Ankylosing Spondylitis

AS is the most frequent form of SpA with a world wide prevalence ranging up to 0.9% (BRAUN et al. 1998). It is a chronic inflammatory disease, usually starting before the age of 40 years. There is a male predominance (ZINK et al. 2000) and a frequent association with the tissue type HLA B27. AS usually starts with inflammatory back pain due to sacroiliitis, which is considered a hallmark of AS, but spread to the spine occur during the course of the disease. Progression from inflammation to new bone formation and ankylosis is characteristic for the disease.

According to the modified New York criteria at least grade 2 sacroiliitis bilaterally or grade 3 unilaterally is necessary for the diagnosis of AS (VAN DER LINDEN et al. 1984) (Fig. 19.4). Several years of disease may pass before unequivocal changes are evident on radiographs. The early visible changes are blurring of the cortical margins, superficial erosions and subchondral sclerosis, sometimes with patchy periarticular osteoporosis. As erosion progresses, the joint space will for a period appear wider, but with further disease progression the erosions fill in with chondroid and fibrous material, which calcify, resulting in joint space narrowing and eventually joint fusion. This course corresponds to increasing grades according to the New York criteria (Fig. 19.4). Bilateral sacroiliitis is more frequent in AS than in the other forms of SpA (HELLIWELL et al. 1998) and is commonly seen at presentation, but the changes may be somewhat asymmetrical (MUCHE et al. 2003). During the course of the disease the joint changes usually became symmetric.

Joint space alteration, erosion and subchondral sclerosis are visualised earlier and better at CT and MR imaging than at radiography. MR imaging, in addition, visualises inflammatory changes, which usually are bilateral, but may be asymmetric regarding the extent. In early AS the MR findings include erosion of the cartilaginous joint facets with concomitant oedema and enhancement in the joint space and subchondral bone (Fig. 19.11). The changes are usually most pronounced at the iliac side of the joint, but sacral involvement may also occur, and is observed more frequently in AS than in other forms of SpA (MUCHE et al. 2003). During

the healing of inflammatory abnormalities, fatty marrow changes often supervene and are seen predominantly in AS patients, whereas they are rare in reactive arthritis and undifferentiated SpA, and also in psoriatic and enteropathic arthritis unless these progress to AS-like involvements (unpublished data). It may therefore be possible to predict the development of progressing AS relatively early based on sacral involvement and the presence of fatty marrow degeneration.

As the disease progress, joint space widening with variable inflammatory activity, and often pronounced subchondral sclerosis are seen at MR imaging (Fig. 19.12). A certain determination of the extent of osseous sclerosis may, however, be best obtained at CT, because the signals at MR imaging can vary. Sclerosis presents as regions of lower signal intensity on T1 FS than areas corresponding to regions with fatty marrow changes, but can on T1 images present either as low signal intensity areas or contain high signal intensity areas due to fatty marrow changes within the sclerotic bone (PUHAKKA et al. 2003).

More advanced AS changes are characterised by progressing ankylosis with variable inflammation and regression of the sclerosis which gradually disappear when the joints ankylosis.

MR imaging may not only be important in patients with early AS, but also in definite and advanced AS because commencement of therapy with biological agents demands disease activity, which may only be detectable and quantifiable at MR imaging (Fig. 19.12).

19.4.1.2
Psoriatic Arthritis

Although psoriatic arthritis (PsA) is classified as one of the SpAs it is predominantly a peripheral joint disorder, which may involve the SIJ and the spine. Sacroiliac joint involvement is therefore not uniformly present, and the reported prevalence of sacroiliitis in PsA has varied considerably with the highest value of radiographic sacroiliitis grade 2 or more being nearly 80% in patients with long lasting PsA, but without a significant relation to HLA B27 (BATTISTONE et al. 1999).

The radiographic features may vary. Manifest psoriatic changes of the SIJ visible at radiography can be either symmetrical or asymmetrical (HELLIWELL et al. 1998), and often involve both the cartilaginous and ligamentous part of the joint (Fig. 19.8). Slight changes detectable only at CT or MR imaging seems

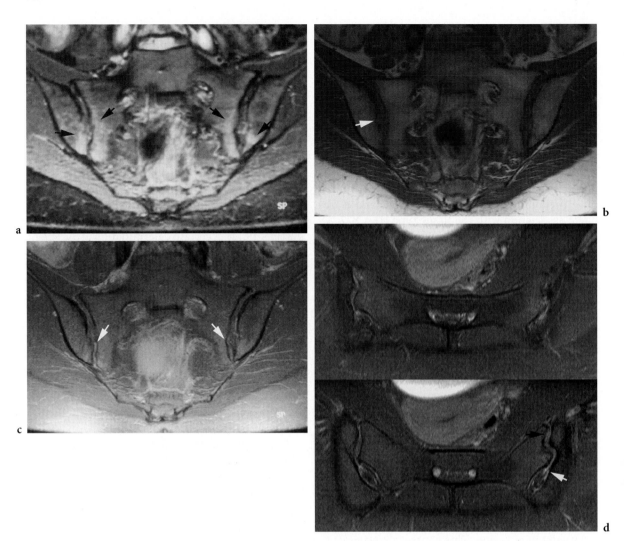

Fig. 19.11a–d. Early ankylosing spondylitis (AS), MR imaging in a patient with suspicious changes at radiography (Fig. 19.4b). (a) Semi-coronal STIR, (b) T1, and (c) post-contrast T1 FS, and (d) semi-axial post-contrast T1 FS. The semi-coronal images display nearly symmetrical oedema and enhancement in the subchondral bone (*black arrows*) and the joint space (*white arrows*). At axial images (d) the involvement is seen to occur both in the cartilaginous (*black arrow*) and the ligamentous part of the joint (*white arrow*). The T1 image (b) shows irregular joint space width with erosion of the iliac joint facet on the right side (*arrow*), but no fatty marrow changes

Fig. 19.12a–h. Later stage of AS. **a** Radiograph displaying bilateral grade 3 changes. **b** CT image showing erosion, especially of the iliac joint facets, with subchondral sclerosis (*arrows*). MR imaging, (c) semi-coronal STIR, (d) T1 and (e) T1 FS, and (f) semi-axial post-contrast T1 FS, demonstrating joint erosion and joint space irregularity with areas showing widening and areas with narrowing, but only scattered fatty marrow changes (d, *arrow*). There is sclerosis appearing as areas of low signal intensity at T1 FS (e, *arrows*). The semi-axial slices (f) reveal involvement of both the cartilaginous (*black arrow*) and the ligamentous part of the joint (*white arrow*). Follow-up MR examination after 1 year therapy, (g) semi-axial post-contrast T1 FS image and (h) semi-coronal T1 show markedly decreased inflammatory enhancement in the subchondral bone and the joint space, but a demarcated enhancing sacral erosion (g, *arrow*). Besides, moderate fatty marrow changes have supervened (h, *arrows*)

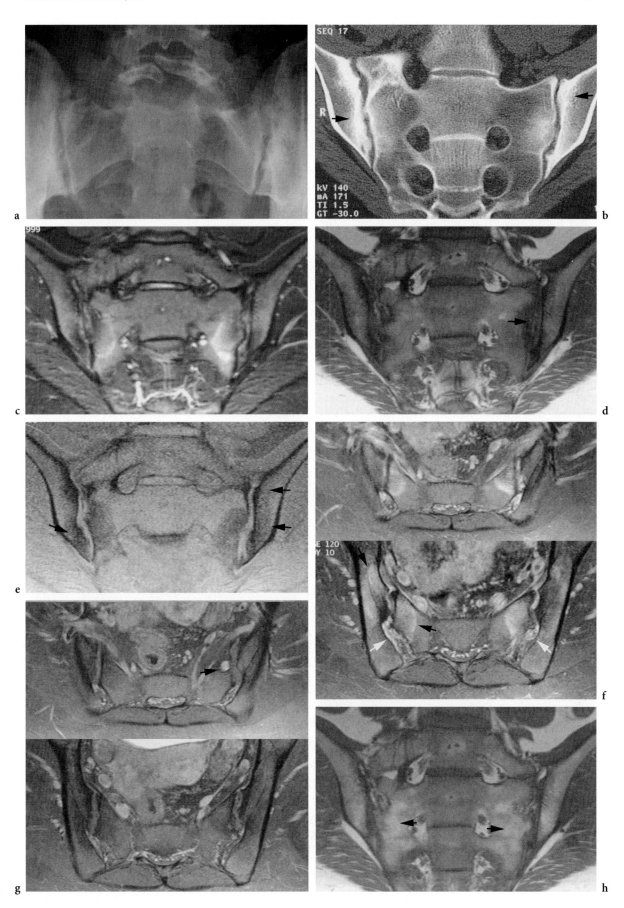

predominantly to involve the distal synovial part of the joint (Fig. 19.13).

19.4.1.3
Reactive Arthritis

Reactive arthritis (ReA) is an inflammatory joint disorder which occurs after a preceding infection of the urogenital tract or the gut. It may, like PsA, be a predominant peripheral disease, which typically presents as asymmetric oligo- or mono-arthritis in lower limb joints. In about half of the patients the disorder is associated with HLA B27. ReA is often transient, but a chronic course occurs in 20% of the patients (SIEPER et al. 2002). The prevalence of chronic ReA has been estimated to be about 0.1% (BRAUN et al. 1998). It may share features with AS including clinical signs of sacroiliitis, spondylitis and uveitis in addition to a frequent association with HLA B27, suggesting a relation between the two disorders. Manifest sacroiliitis visible at radiography is symmetrical in about half of the patients (HELLI-WELL et al. 1998), but slight SIJ changes in uncomplicated, non-chronic ReA, is often asymmetrical

and usually involve the distal synovial part of the joint and the entheses in the ligamentous part of the joint (Fig. 19.14).

19.4.1.4
Enteropathic Arthropathy

It is well known that the inflammatory bowel disorders, Crohn's disease and ulcerative colitis, can be accompanied by arthropathy. It can be classified as a SpA [enteropathic SpA (EnA)] in over 30% of patients and sacroiliitis may in addition occur without symptoms. The involvement of the SIJ is often bilateral, but is not as strongly associated with HLA B27 (DE VLAM et al. 2000). At radiography the sacroiliitis in EnA seems rather similar to that of AS (HELLIWELL et al. 1998), but using cross-sectional imaging it seems to be somewhat special, characterised by a more dominant involvement of the ligamentous part of the joint than seen in the other forms of SpA (MESTER et al. 2000). Entheseal and ligamentous mineralisation seems frequent and is best visualised by CT (see Fig. 19.6), whereas detection of inflammation at entheses demands MR imaging (Fig. 19.15).

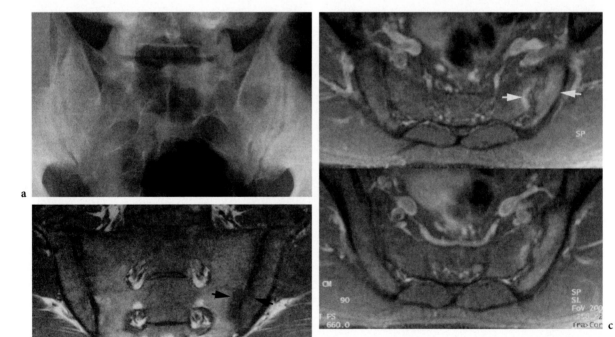

Fig. 19.13a–c. Psoriatic arthritis. Slight changes in a 40-year-old man. **a** Suspicious changes at radiography with slight blurring of the joint facets. MR imaging, (**b**) coronal T1 image show slightly decreased signal intensity in the subchondral bone on the left side (*arrows*); **c** Axial T1 FS images after Gd demonstrate moderate joint space and subchondral enhancement at the lower part of the left SIJ, most extensive on the iliac side (*arrows*)

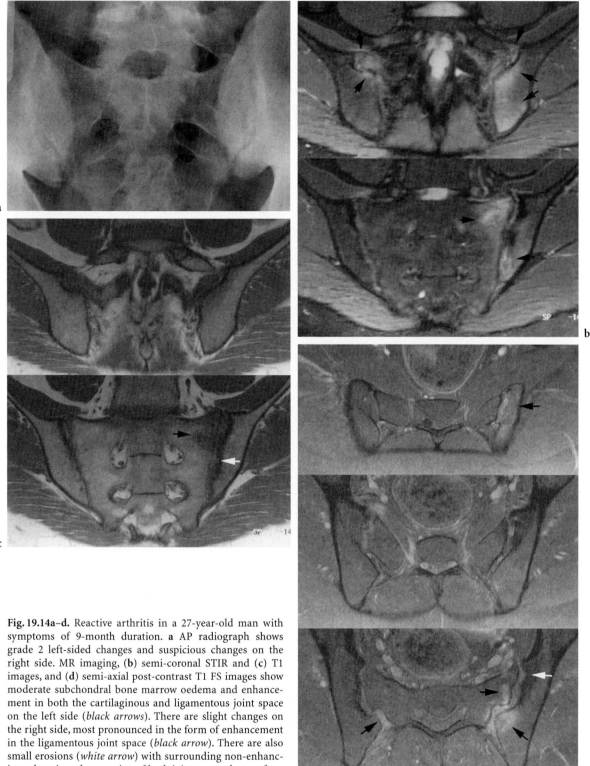

Fig. 19.14a–d. Reactive arthritis in a 27-year-old man with symptoms of 9-month duration. **a** AP radiograph shows grade 2 left-sided changes and suspicious changes on the right side. MR imaging, (**b**) semi-coronal STIR and (**c**) T1 images, and (**d**) semi-axial post-contrast T1 FS images show moderate subchondral bone marrow oedema and enhancement in both the cartilaginous and ligamentous joint space on the left side (*black arrows*). There are slight changes on the right side, most pronounced in the form of enhancement in the ligamentous joint space (*black arrow*). There are also small erosions (*white arrow*) with surrounding non-enhancing sclerosis and narrowing of both joint spaces, but no fatty marrow changes as often seen in AS

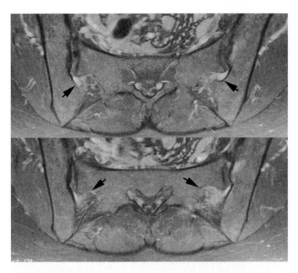

Fig. 19.15. Enteropathic arthropathy. MR imaging, semi-transverse post-contrast T1 FS images showing pronounced enhancement in the ligamentous part of the joint (*arrows*) and only slight enhancement corresponding to the cartilaginous part of the left joint

19.4.1.5
Undifferentiated SpA

In the ESSG classification patients with inflammatory arthropathy suggesting an early stage of SpA, but who do not meet the criteria for AS, PsA, ReA or EnA, were pooled under the term undifferentiated SpA (uSpA). Included under this term are patients with clinical, but not radiographic signs of sacroiliitis and/or relationship to HLA B27. The only thing which differentiates uSpA from AS is the lack of ≥ grade 2 bilateral or grade 3 unilateral sacroiliitis at radiography. The prevalence of uSpA has been estimated to be about 0.7% (BRAUN et al. 1998), but a 10-year follow-up analysis showed progression of uSpA to classified forms of SpA (mostly AS) in about half the patients (MAU et al. 1988). With the inclusion of MR abnormalities in the diagnostic criteria, the group of uSpA will probably diminish substantially.

19.4.2
Atypical forms of SpA

Sacroiliitis is not a specific feature of the above mentioned SpA forms because it occurs in other rheumatic diseases, including atypical forms of SpA. Pustulotic arthro-osteitis and SAPHO syndrome, and also chronic recurrent multifocal osteomyelitis are today regarded as forms of SpA.

19.4.2.1
Pustulotic Arthro-osteitis

The dermal disease pustulosis palmoplantaris (PPP) may be accompanied by arthro-osteitis which often involves the anterior chest wall, but involvement of the spine and sacroiliac joint may also occur (KAHN and CHAMOT 1992; EARWAKER and COTTEN 2003). The skeletal disorder should be termed pustulotic arthro-osteitis, but has also been grouped together with similar disorders under the term SAPHO syndrome. This term encompasses several disorders, which have in common a frequent occurrence of osteitis and hyperostotic osseous lesions associated with acne, PPP or other dermal diseases, including children who also fulfil the criteria for chronic recurrent multifocal osteomyelitis. The group of patients with SAPHO syndrome have many similarities with the classified forms of SpA and the included disorders can often be regarded as atypical forms of SpA (KAHN and CHAMOT 1992). Involvement in the region of the sacroiliac joint is not infrequent in SAPHO patient groups, but the radiographic features are best described for patients having involvement associated with PPP (JURIK et al. 1988). They usually have a characteristic radiographic feature in the form of a predominant osseous lesion adjacent to a joint facet, which may be eroded, whereas the other side of the joint is normal. Such characteristic lesions may be multifocal (Fig. 19.16). However, sacroiliitis with involvement of both sides of the SIJ, as seen in AS, has also been reported, but predominantly in patients who also have dermal changes outside the palmar and plantar area, and thereby a dermal disorder consistent with pustular psoriasis.

19.4.2.2
Chronic Recurrent Multifocal Osteomyelitis

Chronic recurrent multifocal osteomyelitis (CRMO) is a rare non-infectious inflammatory osseous lesion with a characteristic fluctuating clinical course. As the osseous lesions radiographically can simulate subacute or chronic osteitis, the diagnosis is based on exclusion of infection. CRMO lesions are frequently associated with dermal disorders, especially PPP, and there may be accompanying peripheral arthritis and sacroiliitis, especially when patients are followed into adulthood, linking the disease to SpA (HUBER et al. 2002; VITTECOQ et al. 2000). Involvement in the region of the SIJ in childhood will characteristically consist of a predominant osseous

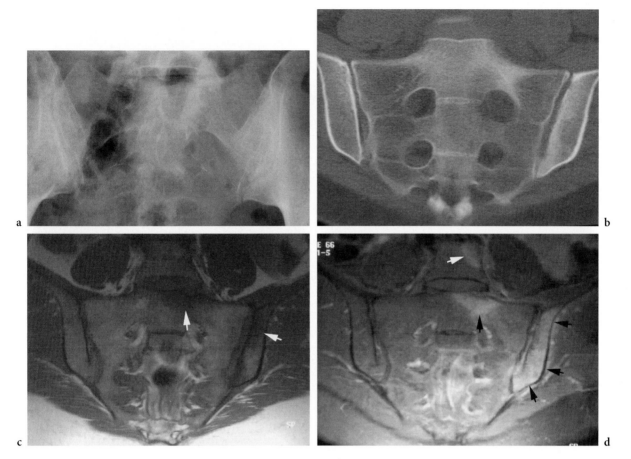

Fig. 19.16a–d. PAO changes in a 36-year-old woman. a Radiograph showing slight irregular iliac joint facet on the left side with subchondral sclerosis. b CT more clearly delineating the superficial erosion and revealing sclerosis involving at least 2 cm of the iliac bone. MR imaging, (c) semi-coronal T1 image show decreased signal intensity corresponding to the iliac subchondral bone and also at the upper part of the sacrum adjacent to the intervertebral space (*arrows*), but no fatty marrow changes. d Semi-coronal post-contrast T1 FS image demonstrates pronounced predominantly osseous enhancement of the left iliac bone and also of the upper part of the sacral bone adjacent to the intervertebral space (*black arrows*). An additional enhancing osseous lesion was seen in the 5th lumbar vertebra (*white arrow*), but the intervertebral disks were normal

sclerotic lesion adjacent to the joint facet with some degree of osseous hyperostosis, but without involvement of the other side of the joint. CT and MR will display a inflammatory osseous lesion without signs indicating infection such as abscess formation and sequestration (Fig. 19.17).

19.4.3
Juvenile Chronic Arthritis

SpA may start in childhood and is then often grouped together with other forms of arthritis under the term juvenile chronic arthritis. As with adult forms, juvenile SpA can be classified as AS, PsA, ReA, EnA and uSpA, but sacroiliitis is generally less common in children with SpA than in adults (ROSENBERG

2000). A juvenile SpA in children younger than 12 years rarely starts in the SIJ, probably due to a different blood supply in childhood. Also the radiographic features are different with not fully developed irregular joint facets being a normal finding in childhood. It can therefore be difficult to obtain evidence of sacroiliitis in children (Fig. 19.18), and the diagnosis of juvenile SpA is not always obtained in childhood. Radiographic evidence of sacroiliitis may, however, occur beyond childhood, reported to be present in 6% of a common group of patients with juvenile chronic arthritis after a mean follow-up of 14.9 years (FLATO et al. 2002).

MR imaging makes it possible to distinguish normal growth changes from active inflammatory disease and also to detect joint destruction (Fig. 19.18), which can establish the diagnose of

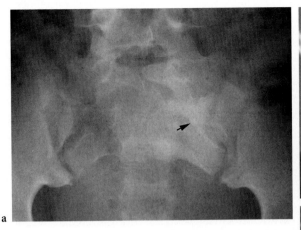

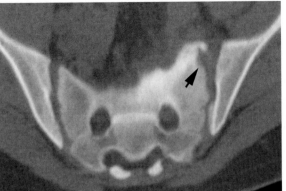

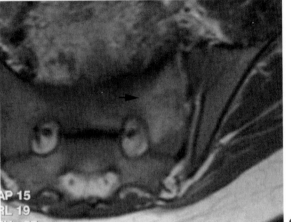

Fig. 19.17a–c. CRMO lesion. **a** AP radiograph showing irregular left-sided sacral joint facet with subchondral sclerosis (*arrow*). **b** Semi-coronal CT slice display erosion of the sacral joint facet (*arrow*) with subchondral sclerosis and hyperostosis. MR imaging, (**c**) post-contrast T1 image shows osseous enhancement of the sacral bone (*black arrow*), but no signs indicating infection

juvenile SpA. Sacroiliitis at MR imaging has been reported as present in 39 of 98 children with juvenile SpA, but detectable at radiography in only 18 (Bollow et al. 1998). The higher sensitivity of MR imaging is mainly due to the ability to document early erosive and acute changes (Fig. 19.18).

19.4.4
Rheumatoid Arthritis

Rheumatoid arthritis (RA) predominantly involves peripheral joints and the cervical spine, but may involve all joints, including the SIJ. The frequency of sacroiliitis at radiography increases with the disease duration and severity, reported to be present in more than 60% in patients with a duration > 2 years (de Carvalho and Graudal 1980). However, most changes reported were grade 2 or less (Fig. 19.19), and pronounced arthritis is rare, unless the patients also have features related to SpA such as HLA B27 (Jurik et al. 1987). Involvement of the SIJ as part of RA has, to the author's, knowledge not been systematically evaluated at CT or MR imaging.

19.4.5
Other Inflammatory Disorders

Crystal arthropathies such as gout (Fig. 19.20) and pseudo-gout occasionally involve the SIJ. Other systemic conditions reported to cause inflammatory involvement of the SIJ include systemic lupus erythematosus, Sjögren's syndrome, Whipple's and Behçet's disease, and sarcoidosis.

19.5
Infectious Arthritis

Septic arthritis of the SIJ is relatively rare and in most instances caused by staphylococci, but other microbes including tubercle bacilli also occur. The infection is usually hematogenous and often occurs in relatively young patients whereas it is rare in elderly (Zimmermann et al. 1996). A history of pelvic trauma may occur in children, but in adults the most common predisposing factors are intravenous drug use, infection of the skin and respira-

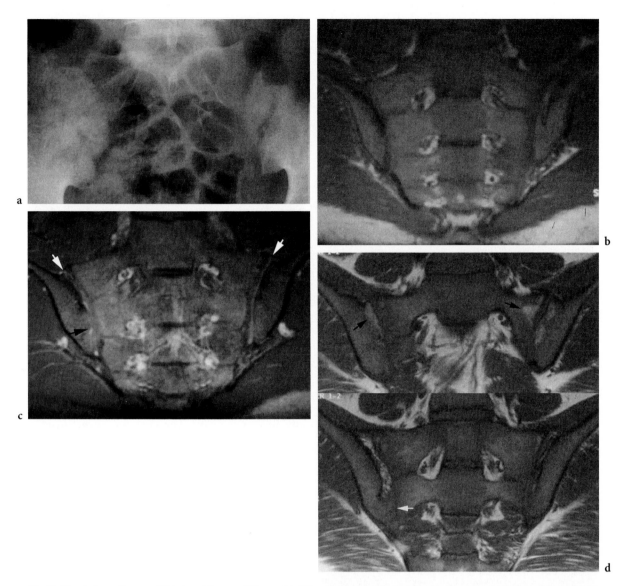

Fig. 19.18a–d. Juvenile sacroiliitis in a 14-year-old boy with SIJ pain of 8-month duration. **a** AP radiograph shows blurred joint facets bilaterally with asymmetric joint space width, narrowest on the right side. MR imaging, (**b**) semi-coronal T1 and (**c**) semi-coronal post-contrast T1 FS image show relative narrow joint space on the right side and enhancement in both joint spaces (*white arrows*) accompanied by slight subchondral enhancement most pronounced on the right side, where there is additionally enhancing erosion (*back arrow*). There are no fatty bone marrow changes. **d** At 3 years later, semi-coronal T1 images, demonstrating that partial ankylosis (*white arrow*) and fatty bone marrow changes (*black arrows*) have supervened

tory or urogenital tract. In drug addicts, the SIJ is more commonly affected by septic arthritis than any other joint (BRANCOS et al. 1991).

It is important to be aware that conventional radiographs are usually normal during the first 2–3 weeks. The initial radiographic changes consist of blurring of the joint facets and subchondral bone with gradual development of joint space widening due to osseous destruction (Fig. 19.21). Such joint and osseous changes can be visualised earlier and better at CT than at radiography, but MR imaging is superior in the early stages of infection, clearly displaying the extent of bone and soft tissue involvement, including possible abscess formation, in addition to joint destruction (SANDRASEGARAN et al. 1994) (Fig. 19.21). At MR imaging the features of acute infection consist of decreased signal intensity at T1 and increased intensity at STIR or T2 FS corresponding to the affected joint and bone areas, and adjacent muscles. A post-contrast sequence is necessary with regard to abscess formation (Fig. 19.21). MR imaging often reveals features specific of acute

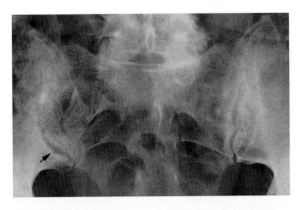

Fig. 19.19. Slight right-sided sacroiliitis in a patient with rheumatoid arthritis in the form of blurring and small erosion of the iliac joint facet (*arrow*)

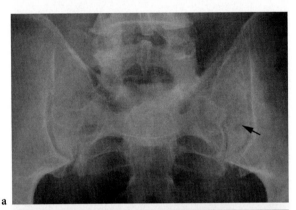

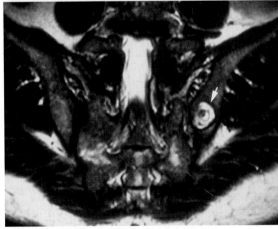

Fig. 19.20a,b. Tophaceous gout at the left SIJ displayed as a slight radiolucency at radiography (**a**, *arrow*) and as a round subchondral, intraosseous process with irregular high signal intensity on T2-weighted MR image (**b**, *arrow*)

septic sacroiliitis in the form of anterior and/or posterior trans-capsular infiltration of juxta-articular muscles, which are not seen in SpA (STÜRZEN-BECHER et al. 2000), but subacute infection often looks less aggressive (Fig. 19.22). Other characteris-

tic signs of infection are that the involvement is usually unilateral, and there may be bone sequestration (ZIMMERMANN et al. 1996).

CT can be valuable for detecting sequestration and for guidance of percutaneous needle arthrocentesis. Other imaging modalities such as scintigraphy are useful primarily in the initial evaluation of patients with non-specific presentation.

19.6
Differential Diagnosis Including Degenerative Changes

Degenerative and stress induced changes may cause low back pain with or without irradiation to the back of the thigh and there may be accompanying tenderness of the SIJ. Such changes may therefore be difficult to differentiate from sacroiliitis clinically. Degenerative changes of the SIJ seem frequent. They may present as osteoarthritis, which when looked for are relative common in patients with low back pain, found to be present in 75% of patients evaluated with CT and being associated with aging (HODGE and BESSETTE 1999). The changes consist of joint space narrowing, osteophyte formation and/or subchondral sclerosis, occasionally with intraarticular vacuum-phenomena, but no erosions (Fig. 19.23). Degenerative changes may also present as anterior para-articular bridging osteophytes or ligamentous calcification, which on frontal radiographs may resemble the true osseous fusion seen in AS (RESNICK et al. 1977), but can be delineated at CT. Degenerative changes have not been systematically evaluated by MR imaging.

Due to the great forces put upon the SIJ region, stress induced structural changes may occur, often in the form of osseous sclerosis of the iliac bone corresponding to the cartilaginous part of the joint. There is usually no concomitant joint space narrowing, or sacral changes (Fig. 19.24), and no signs of inflammation at MR imaging. Such changes may occur after pregnancies (osteitis condensans ilii) and can then gradually regress.

Metabolic disorders such as hyperparathyroidism may involve the SIJ region and simulate sacroiliitis. This is also the case for insufficiency fractures which, however, can be differentiated by MR imaging. Traumatic lesions of the SIJ are seen most commonly after violent injuries, and metastatic carcinoma or sarcoma may rarely mimic sacroiliitis and cause differential diagnostic problems.

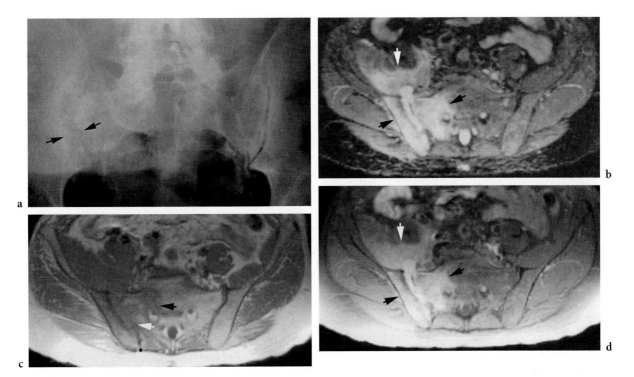

Fig. 19.21a–d. Acute infectious arthritis. **a** AP radiograph in a drug addict showing destruction of the joint facets with joint widening at the right side (*arrows*). MR imaging, (**b**) axial STIR, (**c**) T1 and (**d**) post-contrast T1 FS image show pronounced inflammation with increased signal intensity at STIR and enhancement corresponding to the joint space and subchondral bone (**b,d**, *black arrows*). The oedema and enhancement involve the adjacent voluminous muscles (**b,d**, *white arrows*), which have underlying enhancing joint extension. There are no non-enhancing areas suggesting abscess formation. The T1 image shows decreased signal intensity around the eroded joint, especially at the sacral side (**c**, *black arrow*), where the cartilaginous joint facet has disappeared (**c**, *white arrow*), but there is no visible sequestration

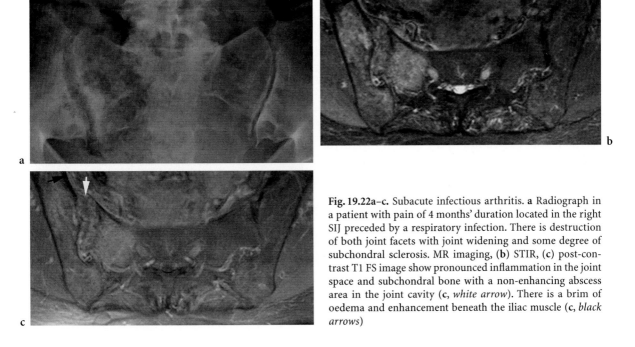

Fig. 19.22a–c. Subacute infectious arthritis. **a** Radiograph in a patient with pain of 4 months' duration located in the right SIJ preceded by a respiratory infection. There is destruction of both joint facets with joint widening and some degree of subchondral sclerosis. MR imaging, (**b**) STIR, (**c**) post-contrast T1 FS image show pronounced inflammation in the joint space and subchondral bone with a non-enhancing abscess area in the joint cavity (**c**, *white arrow*). There is a brim of oedema and enhancement beneath the iliac muscle (**c**, *black arrows*)

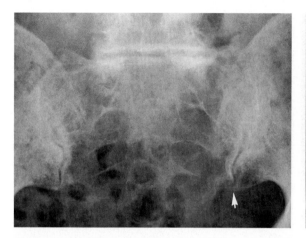

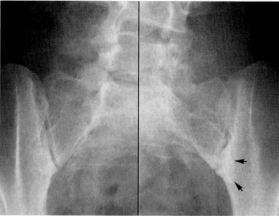

Fig. 19.23. Degenerative SIJ changes in a 64-year-old woman with low back pain. AP radiograph showing narrowing of the SIJs with osteophyte formation (*arrow*) and slight subchondral sclerosis contrasting against a general osteoporotic bone structure

Fig. 19.24. Stress induced changes in a 27-year-old woman with idiopathic scoliosis. Oblique projections of the SIJs show a triangular area of subchondral sclerosis in the iliac bone at the distal part of the left SIJ (*arrows*)

19.7
Conclusion

Anteroposterior (AP) or PA radiography of the SIJs is a widely used screening examination in patient's suspected of sacroiliitis. The sensitivity and specificity of radiography is relatively low, and the diagnosis of sacroiliitis may be delayed when based on radiography. Cross-sectional imaging therefore plays an important role in identification of abnormalities of the SIJs in early seronegative SpA.

MR imaging and CT have almost equal efficacy superior to radiography in staging joint destruction as part of sacroiliitis, but MR imaging in addition allows visualisation and grading of active inflammatory changes in the joint space, subchondral bone, and surrounding ligaments. MR imaging is therefore preferable diagnostically in the evaluation of sacroiliitis and is not associated with radiation.

There is not yet an established, widely accepted method for evaluation and quantification of MR abnormalities. It is therefore difficult at the moment to include MR findings in staging criteria for AS, and in the elaboration of diagnostic criteria for other forms of SpA. Proposals for grading MR abnormalities are currently under evaluation; hopefully resulting in future accepted diagnostic criteria. There is no doubt that the capability of MR imaging to distinguish between acute and chronic changes, and to estimate the degree of disease activity, can be beneficial with regard to classification of the different forms of SpA and for monitoring the disease course, including the effect of pharmacological treatment. Where possible, MR imaging should therefore be used for the evaluation of sacroiliitis in SpA, offering the advantage of being able to exclude infection, which is the most important differential diagnosis.

References

Ahlström H, Feltelius N, Nyman R et al (1990) Magnetic resonance imaging of sacroiliac joint inflammation. Arthritis Rheum 33:1763–1769

Arslan H, Sakarya ME, Adak B et al (1999) Duplex and color Doppler sonographic findings in active sacroiliitis. Am J Roentgenol 173:677–680

Battafarano DF, West SG, Rak KM et al (1993) Comparison of bone scan, computed tomography, and magnetic resonance imaging in the diagnosis of active sacroiliitis. Semin Arthritis Rheum 23:161–176

Battistone MJ, Manaster BJ, Reda DJ et al (1998) Radiographic diagnosis of sacroiliitis - are sacroiliac views really better? J Rheumatol 25:2395–2401

Battistone MJ, Manaster BJ, Reda DJ et al (1999) The prevalence of sacroiliitis in psoriatic arthritis: new perspectives from a large, multicenter cohort. A Department of Veterans Affairs Cooperative Study. Skeletal Radiol 28:196–201

Blum U, Buitrago-Tellez C, Mundinger A et al (1996) Magnetic resonance imaging (MRI) for detection of active sacroiliitis – a prospective study comparing conventional radiography, scintigraphy, and contrast enhanced MRI. J Rheumatol 23:2107–2115

Bollow M, Braun J, Biedermann T et al (1998) Use of contrast-enhanced MR imaging to detect sacroiliitis in children. Skeletal Radiol 27:606–616

Bowen V, Cassidy JD (1981) Macroscopic and microscopic

anatomy of the sacroiliac joint from embryonic life until the eighth decade. Spine 6:620–628

Brancos MA, Peris P, Miro JM et al (1991) Septic arthritis in heroin addicts. Semin Arthritis Rheum 21:81–87

Braun J, Bollow M, Remlinger G et al (1998) Prevalence of spondylarthropathies in HLA-B27 positive and negative blood donors. Arthritis Rheum 41:58–67

Braun J, Sieper J, Bollow M (2000) Imaging of sacroiliitis. Clin Rheumatol 19:51–57

Braun J, Brandt J, Listing J et al (2002) Treatment of active ankylosing spondylitis with infliximab: a randomised controlled multicentre trial. Lancet 359:1187–1193

Carrera GF, Foley WD, Kozin F et al (1981) CT of sacroiliitis. Am J Roentgenol 136:41–46

De Carvalho A, Graudal H (1980) Sacroiliac joint involvement in classical or definite rheumatoid arthritis. Acta Radiol Diagn (Stockh) 21:417–423

De Vlam K, Mielants H, Cuvelier C et al (2000) Spondyloarthropathy is underestimated in inflammatory bowel disease: prevalence and HLA association. J Rheumatol 27:2860–2865

Dougados M, van der Linden S, Juhlin R et al (1991) The European Spondylarthropathy Study Group preliminary criteria for the classification of spondylarthropathy. Arthritis Rheum 34:1218–1227

Earwaker JW, Cotten A (2003) SAPHO: syndrome or concept? Imaging findings. Skeletal Radiol 32:311–327

Elgafy H, Semaan HB, Ebraheim NA et al (2001) Computed tomography findings in patients with sacroiliac pain. Clin Orthop (382):112–118

Fam AG, Rubenstein JD, Chin-Sang H et al (1985) Computed tomography in the diagnosis of early ankylosing spondylitis. Arthritis Rheum 28:930–937

Flato B, Smerdel A, Johnston V et al (2002) The influence of patient characteristics, disease variables, and HLA alleles on the development of radiographically evident sacroiliitis in juvenile idiopathic arthritis. Arthritis Rheum 46:986–994

Francois RJ, Gardner DL, Degrave EJ et al (2000) Histopathologic evidence that sacroiliitis in ankylosing spondylitis is not merely enthesitis. Arthritis Rheum 43:2011–2024

Geijer M, Sihlbom H, Göthlin JH et al (1998) The role of CT in the diagnosis of sacroiliitis. Acta Radiol 39:265–268

Helliwell PS, Hickling P, Wright V (1998) Do the radiological changes of classic ankylosing spondylitis differ from the changes found in the spondylitis associated with inflammatory bowel disease, psoriasis, and reactive arthritis? Ann Rheum Dis 57:135–140

Hodge JC, Bessette B (1999) The incidence of sacroiliac joint disease in patients with low-back pain. Can Assoc Radiol J 50:321–323

Hollingsworth PN, Cheah PS, Dawkins RL et al (1983) Observer variation in grading sacroiliac radiographs in HLA-B27 positive individuals. J Rheumatol 10:247–254

Huber AM, Lam PY, Duffy CM et al (2002) Chronic recurrent multifocal osteomyelitis: clinical outcomes after more than five years of follow-up. J Pediatr 141:198–203

Jurik AG, de Carvalho A, Graudal H (1987) Radiographic visualisation of seropositive rheumatoid arthritis in carriers of HLA-B27. Fortschr Geb Rontgenstr Nuklearmed 147:14–20

Jurik AG, Helmig O, Graudal H (1988) Skeletal disease, arthroosteitis, in adult patients with pustulosis palmoplantaris.

Scand J Rheumatol [Suppl] 70:3–15

Jurik AG, Hansen J, Puhakka KB (2002) Effective radiation dose from semicoronal CT of the sacroiliac joints in comparison with axial CT and conventional radiography. Eur Radiol 12:2820–2825

Kahn MF, Chamot AM (1992) SAPHO syndrome. Rheum Dis Clin North Am 18:225–246

Lund PJ, Krupinski EA, Brooks WJ (1996) Ultrasound evaluation of sacroiliac motion in normal volunteers. Acad Radiol 3:192–196

Mau W, Zeidler H, Mau R et al (1988) Clinical features and prognosis of patients with possible ankylosing spondylitis. Results of a 10-year followup. J Rheumatol 15:1109–1114

Mester AR, Makó EK, Karlinger K et al (2000) Enteropathic arthritis in the sacroiliac joint. Imaging and differential diagnosis. Eur J Radiol 35:199–208

Muche B, Bollow M, Francois RJ et al (2003) Anatomic structures involved in early- and late-stage sacroiliitis in spondylarthritis: a detailed analysis by contrast-enhanced magnetic resonance imaging. Arthritis Rheum 48:1374–1384

Murphey MD, Wetzel LH, Bramble JM et al (1991) Sacroiliitis: MR imaging findings. Radiology 180:239–244

Oostveen J, Prevo R, den Boer J et al (1999) Early detection of sacroiliitis on magnetic resonance imaging and subsequent development of sacroiliitis on plain radiography. A prospective, longitudinal study. J Rheumatol 26:1953–1958

Puhakka KB, Jurik AG, Egund N et al (2003) Imaging of sacroiliitis in early seronegative spondylarthropathy. Assessment of abnormalities by MR in comparison with radiography and CT. Acta Radiol 44:218–229

Puhakka KB, Melsen F, Jurik AG et al (2004a) MR imaging of the normal sacroiliac joint with correlation to histology. Skeletal Radiol 33:15–28

Puhakka KB, Jurik AG, Schiøttz-Christensen B et al (2004b) MR imaging of early seronegative spondylarthropathy. Abnormalities associated to clinical and laboratory findings. Rheumatology 43:234–237

Puhakka KB, Jurik AG, Schiøttz-Christensen B et al (2004c) MRI abnormalities of the sacroiliac joints in early spondylarthropathy: a 1-year follow-up study. Acta Rheumatol 335:332–338

Resnick D, Niwayama G, Goergen TG (1977) Comparison of radiographic abnormalities of the sacroiliac joint in degenerative disease and ankylosing spondylitis. Am J Roentgenol 128:189–196

Rosenberg AM (2000) Juvenile onset spondyloarthropathies. Curr Opin Rheumatol 12:425–429

Sandrasegaran K, Saifuddin A, Coral A et al (1994) Magnetic resonance imaging of septic sacroiliitis. Skeletal Radiol 23:289–292

Sieper J, Rudwaleit M, Braun J et al (2002) Diagnosing reactive arthritis: role of clinical setting in the value of serologic and microbiologic assays. Arthritis Rheum 46:319–327

Saraux A, Guedes C, Allain J et al (1999) Prevalence of rheumatoid arthritis and spondyloarthropathy in Brittany, France. J Rheumatol 26:2622–2627

Skaar O, Dale K, Lindegaard MW et al (1992) Quantitative radio-isotope scanning of the sacroiliac joints in ankylosing spondylitis. Acta Radiol 33:169–171

Stürzenbecher A, Braun J, Paris S et al (2000) MR imaging of septic sacroiliitis. Skeletal Radiol 29:439–446

Van der Linden S, Valkenburg HA, Cats A (1984) Evaluation of diagnostic criteria for ankylosing spondylitis. A proposal for modification of the New York criteria. Arthritis Rheum 27:361–368

Van Tubergen A, Heuft-Dorenbosch L, Schulpen G et al (2003) Radiographic assessment of sacroiliitis by radiologists and rheumatologists: does training improve quality? Ann Rheum Dis 62:519–525

Verlooy H, Mortelmans L, Vleugels S, de Roo M (1992) Quantitative scintigraphy of the sacroiliac joints. Clin Imaging 16:230–233

Vittecoq O, Said LA, Michot C et al (2000) Evolution of chronic recurrent multifocal osteitis toward spondylarthropathy over the long term. Arthritis Rheum 43:109–119

Yu W, Feng F, Dion E et al (1998) Comparison of radiography, computed tomography and magnetic resonance imaging in the detection of sacroiliitis accompanying ankylosing spondylitis. Skeletal Radiol 27:311–320

Zimmermann B III, Mikolich DJ, Lally EV (1996) Septic sacroiliitis. Semin Arthritis Rheum 26:592–604

Zink A, Braun J, Listing J et al (2000) Disability and handicap in rheumatoid arthritis and ankylosing spondylitis – results from the German rheumatological database. German Collaborative Arthritis Centers. J Rheumatol 27:613–622

20 Bone and Soft Tissue Infection

A. Mark Davies and Richard William Whitehouse

CONTENTS

20.1
Introduction

Osteomyelitis is an infection of bone and bone marrow caused by blood-borne organisms, (haematogenous) spread from a contiguous source of infection or by direct inoculation from a penetrating injury or surgical wound. The term osteomyelitis also encompasses granulomatous infections such as tuberculosis (TB) or fungal infections. The morbidity associated with osteomyelitis has long been recognised. Each year, acute osteomyelitis affects approximately 10 of every 100000 people in the developed world (LIDGREN and LINDBERG 1972). Its incidence is related to socioeconomic factors and increases in hot and humid climates. The risk of developing chronic osteomyelitis is substantially reduced with modern antibiotic therapy. The commonest sites of bone infection in the pelvis are the

A. M. DAVIES, MD
Consultant Radiologist, The MRI Centre, Royal Orthopaedic Hospital, Birmingham, B31 2AP, UK
R. W. WHITEHOUSE, MD
Department of Clinical Radiology, Manchester Royal Infirmary, Oxford Road, Manchester, M13 9WL, UK

sacroiliac joints, hip joints and proximal femur. The first two are covered in Chaps. 10 and 19. The presentation and imaging features of osteomyelitis of the proximal femur are similar to that of any long bone and will not be discussed in this chapter nor will infections associated with sepsis from the intrapelvic organs. This chapter will concentrate on infections involving the pelvic bones and surrounding soft tissues.

20.2
Acute and Subacute Osteomyelitis

20.2.1
Incidence, Age and Sex

Osteomyelitis of the pelvic bones is rare with an estimated incidence of 1%–11% of all cases of haematogenous osteomyelitis (BEAUPRE and CARROLL 1979; EDWARD et al. 1978; EVANS et al. 1985; MORREY et al. 1978; WELD 1960; YOUNG 1934). As with all osteomyelitis this tends to be a disease of children with an average age between 8 and 14 years (HIGHLAND and LAMONT 1983; MAH et al. 1994; RAND et al. 1993; SUCATO and GILLESPIE 1997; DAVIDSON et al. 2003), although it is well recognised in infants and throughout adult life (CHOMA et al. 1994). There is an unexplained male preponderance of approximately two-thirds of cases (HIGHLAND and LAMONT 1983; MAH et al. 1994; RAND et al. 1993; SUCATO and GILLESPIE 1997; DAVIDSON et al. 2003).

20.2.2
Detection

Pelvic osteomyelitis can have very variable presenting features mimicking spinal, abdominal, sciatic and hip conditions (MORGAN and YATES 1966; HAMMOND and MACNICOL 2001; MACNICOL 2001; OUDJHANE and AZOUZ 2001; DAVIDSON et al. 2003). Only half the children with subsequently proven pelvic osteomyelitis are febrile at presentation (DAVIDSON et al. 2003). The onus is frequently, therefore, on imaging to first detect the focus of infection and then to suggest the correct diagnosis. The radiograph is routinely the first imaging investigation and, as with acute osteomyelitis at more common sites, is usually normal in the first 1 to 2 weeks (SAMMAK et al. 1999). Indeed, there is arguably a greater problem with pelvic osteomyelitis as DAVIDSON and co-workers (2003) reported normal initial radiographs in 84% cases (Fig. 20.1a). The subtle, early lesions in the pelvis are easily overlooked due to the curvature of the bones and may also be obscured by overlying soft tissues, bowel gas, faecal material and, in older patients, vascular calcifications. One of the cardinal signs of osteomyelitis, periosteal new bone formation, may be missed on the conventional anteroposterior (AP) radiograph of the pelvis unless it involves the inner or outer margins of the iliac bones or the superior or inferior margins of the pubic rami (Fig. 20.2a).

If there is a clinical suspicion of osteomyelitis, in the presence of normal radiographs, then further imaging is indicated. Ultrasound is virtually essential in the patient with suspected septic arthritis of the hip (see Chap. 10) but is of doubtful value

in pelvic osteomyelitis (MAH et al. 1994; DAVIDSON et al. 2003). However, an ultrasound of the hip is a quick and useful test if only to exclude a septic arthritis, which can have a similar presentation and tends to be a more rapidly progressive condition with potentially more serious sequelae. Bone scintigraphy using the most commonly available radioisotope, technetium 99m (Tc 99m) will usually demonstrate increased activity on all phases of a triple-phase bone scan within hours of the onset of infection (SAMMAK et al. 1999). Bone scintigraphy can be normal in up to 10% cases of pelvic osteomyelitis (HIGHLAND and LaMONT 1983; SUCATO and GILLESPIE 1997; DAVIDSON et al. 2003). Radioisotope activity in the bladder may obscure pubic or distal sacral lesions on the routine frontal and posterior projections (Fig. 20.1b). The conspicuity of pubic lesions can be improved by performing a "brim view". The sensitivity in the pelvis is likely to be increased with the use of single photon emission computed tomography (SPECT). Alternative agents include gallium-67, indium-111-labelled leukocytes and Tc-99m-labelled leukocytes. Although these may have some merits they require more laborious preparation, involve a greater radiation burden to the patients, can give false positive diagnoses and persistent red marrow activity can cause problems

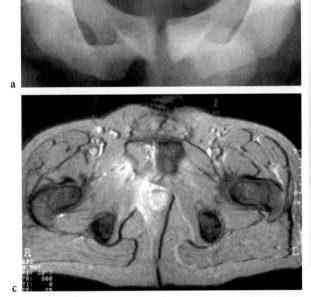

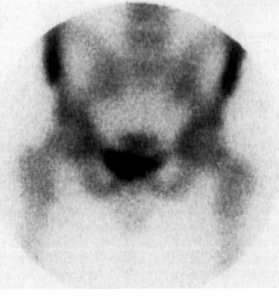

Fig. 20.1a–c. Acute osteomyelitis of the right pubis. **a** AP radiograph of the pubis shows a little rarefaction of the right pubis but is otherwise normal. **b** Anterior image from bone scintigraphy showing increased activity over the right pubis partially obscured by the bladder activity. **c** Axial T1-weighted fat suppressed contrast enhanced MR image showing a small area of destruction in the right pubis with florid surrounding marrow and soft tissue oedema. The small signal void within the lesion is likely to represent an early sequestrum

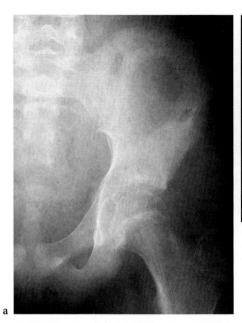

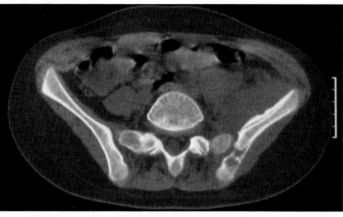

Fig. 20.2a,b. Acute osteomyelitis of the ilium initially thought to be a Ewing's sarcoma. **a** AP radiograph showing a lytic lesion within the blade of the ilium and a lamellar periosteal reaction along inner rim. Biopsy defect noted laterally. **b** The CT more clearly reveals the periosteal new bone formation anteriorly, bone destruction posteriorly and overlying soft tissue mass

with interpretation (WUKICH et al. 1978; SAMMAK et al. 1999). The ability of bone scintigraphy to image the entire skeleton is useful in suspected multifocal infection and in neonates and young children where there may be limited localising signs.

Computed tomography (CT) has in the past been reported to be useful in the detection of pelvic osteomyelitis and in defining the extent of the inflammatory process (Fig. 20.2b) (RAND et al. 1993; VIANI et al. 1999; DAVIDSON et al. 2003). This role, particularly in the early case, has been largely superseded by magnetic resonance (MR) imaging. CT can still be helpful in chronic osteomyelitis in confirming/excluding the presence of sequestra. Now that it is becoming increasingly available MR imaging is the investigation of choice in demonstrating acute and subacute osteomyelitis (Fig. 20.1c). It is more sensitive to marrow abnormalities than the other routinely available imaging techniques.

20.2.3
Site

Haematogenous spread of osteomyelitis typically begins in the metaphyseal equivalent areas which are the margins of the iliac blade, particularly adjacent to the sacroiliac joint, around the acetabulum (Fig. 20.3), and adjacent to the pubic symphysis (NIXON 1978; KRICUN 1993). The percentage incidence at different sites varies between studies, though this is undoubtedly influenced by many

reports including only a handful of cases. Compiling their data with previously reported cases in children, DAVIDSON and co-workers (2003) found the most commonly involved site was the ilium (35%) followed by the acetabulum (24%), the pubis (18%) and the ischium (17%).

20.2.4
Diagnosis

Establishing the diagnosis of osteomyelitis is based on a combination of appropriate clinical presentation, serological results, imaging findings and, where possible, microbiological proof. Many published reports detail the efficacy of MR imaging in identifying osteomyelitis (MORRISON et al. 1993; JARAMILLO et al. 1995). While the sensitivity of MR imaging in detecting marrow change is not in doubt the remarkably high sensitivity in the diagnosis of osteomyelitis is questionable. Simple detection of an abnormality is relatively straightforward. It depends on the acumen of the reporting radiologist as to whether osteomyelitis is diagnosed correctly or, as is often the case in reality, is only one of a relatively large differential diagnosis. It has long been recognised that osteomyelitis, notably subacute, may be misdiagnosed as a bone tumour, particularly in the age group where both infection and tumour are at their most common (GLEDHILL 1973; ROBERTS et al. 1982; BAXTER WILLIS and ROZENCWAIG 1996; RASOOL 2001a; OUDJHANE and

Azouz 2001). The pelvis is no exception with abscess cavities readily mistaken for an aneurysmal bone cyst or Langerhans cell histiocytosis (eosinophilic granuloma) and more aggressive appearing lesions with a malignant round cell tumour such as Ewing's sarcoma (Fig. 20.2a). Obviously, the converse may occur with potentially more serious consequences. In the adolescent on MR imaging, early osteomyelitis can mimic avulsion stress to the ischium as well as osteoid osteoma in a juxtaarticular origin and visa versa. Infection of the ischiopubic synchondrosis in children may mimic an osteochondritis (Van Neck phenomenon) (Iqbal et al. 2004).

Conventional radiographs of pelvic osteomyelitis can be relatively non-specific. In many cases MR imaging can help distinguish tumour from infection. Radiographic features of an aggressive lesion with cortical breaching and a *solid* soft tissue component on MR imaging favours a sarcoma. Bone abscesses typically exhibit a target-like appearance with four layers on MR imaging (Martí-Bonmati et al. 1993). A useful indicator of infection rather than tumour is the "penumbra sign" which refers to the relatively hyperintense granulation tissue lining on T1-weighted

images compared with the lower signal intensity with the lower signal intensity contents and surrounding oedema and reactive sclerosis of an intraosseous abscess (Fig. 20.3b) (Grey et al. 1998; Marui et al. 2002). The conspicuity of this granulation layer on MR imaging can be increased by the administration of a gadolinium chelate (Munk et al. 1993; Tehranzadeh et al. 1992). It should be noted that any cyst lining, regardless of the nature of the lesion, would also tend to show contrast enhancement. In the pelvis the penumbra sign is most frequently seen in cases arising around the acetabulum (Fig. 20.3b).

Biopsy and culture are fundamental to establishing a diagnosis. These are necessary to ensure that the diagnosis of infection is correct and that the appropriate antibiotic treatment instituted, which is important in countries where numerous different infective agents, not just staphylococcus aureus, are endemic. Image-guided biopsy is advised utilising an approach which would not prejudice subsequent surgery if a tumour were identified. CT-guided biopsy is probably preferable to fluoroscopy to ensure accurate needle positioning in deep-seated pelvic lesions (Fig. 20.4). Most units are not set up

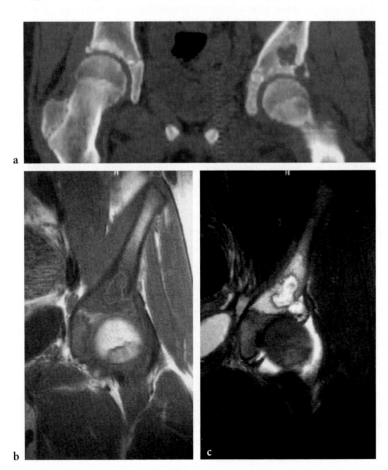

a

b   c

Fig. 20.3a–c. Subacute osteomyelitis. **a** Coronal CT reconstruction showing a multiloculated lytic lesion containing flecks of calcification arising in the roof of the acetabulum. **b** Coronal T1-weighted MR image showing low signal intensity marrow oedema. The relatively high intensity thin granulation tissue around the abscess cavity indicates a positive "penumbra sign". **c** Coronal short T1-inversion recovery (STIR) image allowing distinction of the central loculated abscess from the surrounding oedema. There is a reactive hip joint effusion

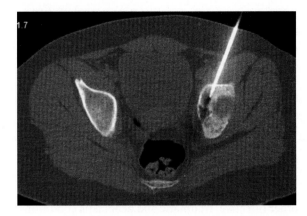

Fig. 20.4. CT-guided needle biopsy of a left acetabular lesion which was proven to be osteomyelitis on histology

to use MR for image-guided procedures. The pre-biopsy MR scan is helpful in showing the most suitable site for the biopsy.

20.3
Chronic Osteomyelitis and Chronic Recurrent Multifocal Osteomyelitis

Chronic osteomyelitis of the pelvic bones exhibiting the classic features of sequestrum, involucrum formation etc. is uncommon in the pelvis. The ilium is, however, a well recognised site for the sclerosing form of chronic osteomyelitis (STEINBACH 1966; JURIK et al. 1988). The radiographic features are those of dense sclerosis involving the blade of the ilium (Fig. 20.5a). The differential diagnosis in the younger patient includes osteosarcoma and in the elderly Paget's disease. Bone scintigraphy is useful as sclerosing osteomyelitis of the ilium is most frequently found in chronic recurrent multifocal osteomyelitis (CRMO) (Fig. 20.5b). CRMO is an inflammatory disease of unknown aetiology, which predominantly affects children and adolescents. It belongs to a variety of aseptic osteomyelitis-like conditions of bone, many of which are associated with dermatological lesions. These have been lumped together under the acronym SAPHO syndrome (synovitis, acne, pustulosis, hyperostosis and osteitis). Whether CRMO is a distinct clinical entity or part of the spectrum of diseases including SAPHO syndrome continues to be debated (EARWAKER and COTTEN 2003). The clavicle and long bones are more frequently involved than the pelvis. In the authors experience identification of bone-forming lesions arising concomitantly in the medial two thirds of the clavicle and the ilium almost invariable indicates CRMO (Fig. 20.5) Biopsy is advised to exclude other conditions but in CRMO typically just shows non-specific inflammatory changes and culture is usually negative. Monitoring disease activity in the presence of so much sclerosis can be difficult using radiographs. MR imaging will show increasing water content in active exacerbations. It has been sug-

Fig. 20.5a,b. Chronic recurrent multifocal osteomyelitis. **a** AP radiograph of the pelvis showing sclerosing osteomyelitis of the right ilium. **b** Anterior bone scintigraphy image showing involvement of the right ilium, left proximal femur, sternum, right clavicle and acromion

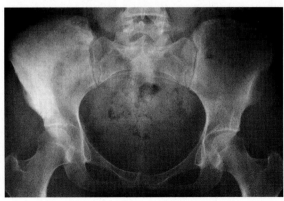

a

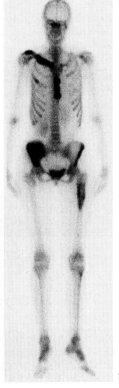

b

gested that positron emission scanning (PET) may have a role in future in assessing disease activity.

20.4
Tuberculosis

Tuberculosis (TB) remains a major cause of skeletal infection in many developing countries (RASOOL 2001b). The resurgence in some countries has been largely attributed to the acquired immunodeficiency syndrome (AIDS) (see Sect. 20.6), but is also due in part to inefficient immunisation programmes,

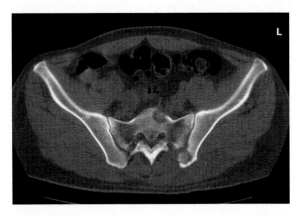

Fig. 20.6. Multifocal osseous lytic lesions with central sequestra, in the sacrum and left ilium. Left SI joint involvement is also evident, other lesions were present in the spine. Biopsy confirmed TB

increasing migration/travel and intravenous drug abuse. In the past the bone lesions of TB were frequently multifocal, though more recent series indicate a predominantly solitary presentation (RASOOL 2001b). In the experience of the authors, multifocal osseous TB is re-emerging, particularly in patients of Asian ethnicity (Fig. 20.6). The two most important aspects of the disease are that concomitant pulmonary disease occurs in only 12%–50% of patients and that the radiographic appearances are non-specific (Fig. 20.7) (WATTS and LIFESO 1996; ABD EL BAGI et al. 1999). It can frequently be mistaken for other infective, traumatic and neoplastic conditions (YAO and SARTORIS 1995; RASOOL 2001b). Late presentation with a history of symptoms extending back months or even years is typical. In the pelvis, TB characteristically involves the sacroiliac and hips joints with subsequent spread to the adjacent bones. Uncommonly the pubic bones and ischia may be involved (MOORE and RAFII 2001). One of the commoner manifestations of TB in the pelvis is extension of a spinal abscess down the iliopsoas muscles.

20.5
Soft Tissue Infection

Soft tissue infections of the pelvis may be primary or secondary to a joint infection. Again, they are commoner in immunocompromised patients (see Sect. 20.6). The advent of cross-sectional imaging

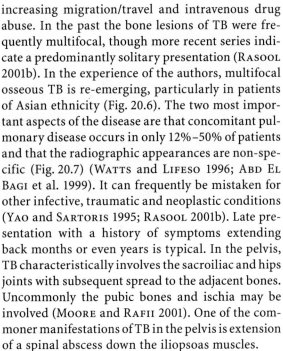

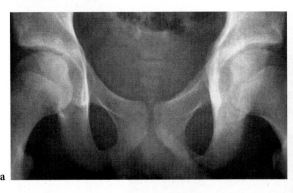

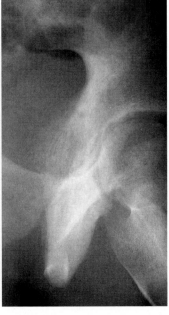

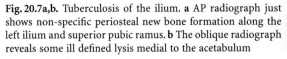

Fig. 20.7a,b. Tuberculosis of the ilium. **a** AP radiograph just shows non-specific periosteal new bone formation along the left ilium and superior pubic ramus. **b** The oblique radiograph reveals some ill defined lysis medial to the acetabulum

has dramatically improved our ability to detect and diagnose these infections (STRUK et al. 2001). Ultrasound will readily detect the predominantly cystic soft tissue abscesses. The degree of echogenicity can be very variable dependent on the quantity of debris and semisolid contents (STRUK et al. 2001). Colour or power Doppler will show absent blood flow within the abscess but hyperaemia in the wall and immediate surrounding soft tissues (BUREAU et al. 1999). Both CT and MR imaging will demonstrate the abscess to good effect (Fig. 20.8), as well as confirming/excluding the presence of adjacent bone or joint involvement. In the immobile or chronically debilitated patient pressure sores may result in decubitus ulcers over the ischia and greater trochanters with secondary infection of the bone. This can be identified on radiographs by the resorption of the cortex with varying degrees of bone destruction as well as gas within the soft tissues (Fig. 20.9).

The more diffuse form of muscle infection, pyomyositis, may be a particular diagnostic problem if affecting the intrapelvic muscles (ORLICEK et al. 2001; PECKETT et al. 2001). Pyomyositis is uncommon in temperate climates unless, as stated, the patient is immunocompromised. Pyomyositis of the iliacus and obturator internus muscles in children tend to have non-specific presenting features. MR imaging will show diffuse swelling and loss of definition of the muscle with or without discrete abscess formation (YUH et al. 1988; ORLICEK et al. 2001; PECKETT et al. 2001).

20.6
Immunodeficiency Associated Infections

The worldwide epidemic of acquired immunodeficiency syndrome (AIDS) due to infection with the human immunodeficiency virus (HIV) is now the commonest cause of severe musculoskeletal infections associated with immunocompromised states. Other conditions causing immunodeficiency, such as diabetes mellitus, may be commoner and also associated with an increased risk of infection, but is rarely life threatening. Septic arthritis of the knee and hip is the most prevalent form of musculoskeletal infection in HIV-positive patients (TEHRANZA-DEH et al. 1996; BARZILAI et al. 1999). Osteomyelitis is the second commonest infection in these patients with the femoral head the commonest site involving the pelvis. Unlike conventional osteomyelitis, HIV related osteomyelitis can be associated with a

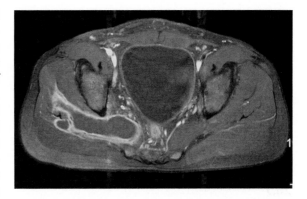

Fig. 20.8. Axial fat suppressed post-contrast T1 weighted image through the pelvis demonstrates a tuberculous abscess within piriformis muscle

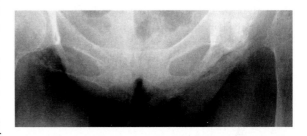

Fig. 20.9. AP radiograph in a paraplegic showing decubitus ulcers eroding both ischia and an old untreated left femoral neck fracture

mortality of up to 20% (TEHRANZADEH et al. 2004). Staphylococcus aureus is the commonest causative pathogen but many other more exotic organisms have been reported including mycobacterial species. A disease apparently unique to immunocompromised patients, particularly the HIV-infected population, is bacillary angiomatoid osteomyelitis due to gram negative Rickettsia-like bacilli (BUREAU and CARDINAL 2001; TEHRANZADEH et al. 2004). This is a multisystem infectious disease which involves bone in approximately a third of cases producing aggressive lytic bone lesions with surrounding soft tissue inflammation (BARON et al. 1990).

The AIDS epidemic has been largely responsible for the resurgence of mycobacterium tuberculosis infections in the developed world over the past two decades. The commonest sites of involvement in descending order are the spine, the hip and knee joints, the metaphyses of the long bones of the lower limb and the hands and feet (TEHRANZADEH et al. 2004). The commonest site in the pelvis is the sacroiliac joint (see Chap. 19). A point worthy of note is that AIDS-related skeletal TB may have a multicentric distribution in about 30% cases.

The incidence of skeletal muscle infection, pyomyositis, has also increased in the AIDS era. Prompt diagnosis is important otherwise the condition may be fatal. MR imaging is excellent in demonstrating the epicentre of infection, necessary when determining treatment by aspiration or surgical drainage (MAJOR and TEHRANZADEH 1997; STEINBACH et al. 1993).

20.7
Parasitic Infections

Parasitic infestations that may calcify or cause calcification and thereby be visible on radiographs of the pelvis include cysticercosis and guinea worm in the muscles and schistosomiasis in the urinary tract. The calcified dead cysts of cysticercosis are typically oval with a lucent centre, up to 1 cm in length, and oriented in the direction of the muscle fibres (Fig. 20.10a). The dead guinea worm is seen as long coiled or curled calcifications that in time can break up due to the action of the surrounding muscles (Fig. 20.10b).

The only parasitic infection to involve the bones of the pelvis is hydatid disease most commonly due to *Echinococcus granulosus*. Bone infection occurs in less than 5% of cases with the commonest sites, in descending order of incidence, being the spine, the epiphyses of long bones, the ilium, skull and posterior ribs (BEGGS 1985; MERKLE et al. 1997; ABD EL BAGI et al. 1999). The radiographic appearances are those of a multiloculated "soap bubble" lesion with marginal sclerosis usually arising in the ilium (ABD EL BAGI et al. 1999).

20.8
Conclusion

Musculoskeletal infections of the pelvis can present in a large variety of ways. Early diagnosis depends on a high index of clinical suspicion and early use of cross sectional imaging, particularly MR imaging (HAMMOND and MACNICOL 2001; MACNICOL 2001). In problem cases where the imaging features cannot clearly differentiate infection from tumour the old adage "Biopsy the infection and culture the tumour", cannot be overemphasized. Culture and sensitivity is important as many different organisms can give rise to similar imaging features in the pelvis.

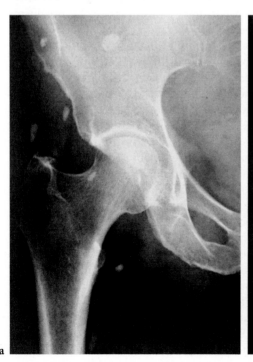 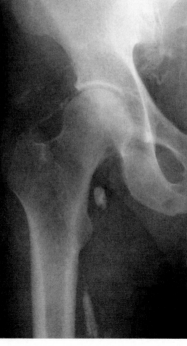

a   b

Fig. 20.10. a AP radiograph of the hip showing the oval calcifications of cysticercosis, aligned with the muscle fibres. **b** AP radiograph of the hip showing the linear and coiled calcifications of dead guinea worms

References

Abd El Bagi ME, Sammak BM, Al Shahed MS, Yousef BA, Demuren OA, Al Jared M, Al Thagafi MA (1999) Rare bone infections "excluding the spine": pictorial review. Eur Radiol 9:1078–1087

Baron AL, Steinbach LS, LeBoit PE (1990) Osteolytic lesions and bacillary angiomatosis in HIV infection: radiologic differentiation from AIDS-related Kaposi sarcoma. Radiology 177:77–81

Barzilai A, Varon D, Martinowitz U, Heim M, Schulman S (1999) Characteristics of septic arthritis in human immunodeficiency virus-infected haemophiliacs versus other risk groups. Rheumatology 38:139–142

Baxter Willis R, Rozencwaig R (1996) Pediatric osteomyelitis masquerading as skeletal neoplasia. Orthop Clin North Am 27:625–634

Beaupre A, Carroll N (1979) The three syndromes of iliac osteomyelitis in children. J Bone Joint Surg (Am) 61:1087–1092

Beggs I (1985) The radiology of hydatid disease. AJR 145:639–648

Bureau NJ, Cardinal E (2001) Imaging of musculoskeletal and spinal infections in AIDS. Radiol Clin North Am 39:343–355

Bureau NJ, Chhem RK, Cardinal E (1999) Musculoskeletal infections: ultrasound manifestations. RadioGraphics 19:1585–1592

Choma TJ, Davlin LB, Wagner JS (1994) Iliac osteomyelitis in the newborn presenting as non-specific musculoskeletal sepsis. Orthopedics 17:632–634

Davidson D, Letts M, Khoshhal K (2003) Pelvic osteomyelitis in children: a comparison of decades from 1980–1989 with 1990–2001. J Pediatr Orthop 23:514–521

Earwaker JWS, Cotton A (1993) SAPHO: syndrome or concept? Imaging findings. Skeletal Radiol 32:311–327

Edward SM, Baker CJ, Granberry WM, Barrett FF (1978) Pelvic osteomyelitis in children. Paediatr 61:62–67

Evans TW, Evely RS Morcos SK (1985) Asymptomatic osteomyelitis of the pubis. Postgrad Med J 61:267–268

Gledhill RB (1973) Subacute osteomyelitis in children. Clin Orthop 96:57–69

Grey AC, Davies AM, Mangham DC, Grimer RJ, Ritchie DA (1998) The Penumbra sign on T1-weighted MR imaging in subacute osteomyelitis: frequency, cause and significance. Clin Radiol 53:587–592

Hammond P, Macnicol MF (2001) Osteomyelitis of the pelvis and proximal femur: diagnostic difficulties. J Pediatr Orthop 10B:113–119

Highland TR, LaMont RL (1983) Osteomyelitis of the pelvis in children. J Bone Joint Surg (Am) 65:230–234

Iqbal A, McKenna D, Hayes R, O'Keefe D (2004) Osteomyelitis of the ischiopubic synchondrosis: imaging findings. Skeletal Radiol 33:176–180

Jaramillo D, Treves ST, Kasser JR, Harper M, Sundel R, Laor T (1995) Osteomyelitis and septic arthritis in children: appropriate use of imaging to guide treatment. AJR 165:399–403

Jurik AG, Moller SH, Mosekilde L (1988) Chronic sclerosing osteomyelitis of the iliac bone. Etiological possibilities. Skeletal Radiol 17:114–118

Kricun ME (1993) Imaging of bone tumors. Saunders, Philadelphia, pp 352–353

Lidgren L, Lindberg L (1972) Orthopedic infections during a 5 year period. Acta Orthop Scand 43:325–334

Macnicol MF (2001) Editorial: patterns of musculoskeletal infection in childhood. J Bone Joint Surg (Br) 83:1–2

Mah ET, LeQuesne GW, Gent RJ, Paterson DC (1994) Ultrasonic signs of pelvic osteomyelitis in children. Pediatr Radiol 24:484–487

Major NM, Tehranzadeh J (1997) Musculoskeletal manifestations of AIDS. Radiol Clin North Am 35:1167–1189

Martí-Bonmatí L, Aparisi F, Poyatos C, Vilar J (1993) Brodie abscess: MR imaging appearance in 10 patients. JMRI 3:543–546

Marui T, Yamamoto T, Akisue T, Nakatani T, Hitora T, Nagira K, Yoshiya S, Kurosaka M (2002) Subacute osteomyelitis of long bones: diagnostic usefulness of the penumbra sign on MRI. Clin Imag 26:314–318

Merkle E, Schulte M, Vogel J (1997) Musculoskeletal involvement in cystic echinococcosis: report of eight cases and review of the literature. AJR 168:1531–1534

Moore SL, Rafii M (2001) Imaging of musculoskeletal and spinal tuberculosis. Radiol Clin North Am 39:329–342

Morgan A, Yates AK (1966) The diagnosis of acute osteomyelitis of the pelvis. Postgrad Med J 42:74–78

Morrey BF, Bianco AJ, Rhodes KH (1978) Hematogenous osteomyelitis at uncommon sites in children. Mayo Clin Proc 53:707–713

Morrison WB, Schweitzer ME, Bock GW et al (1993) Diagnosis of osteomyelitis: utility of fat-suppressed contrast-enhanced MR imaging. Radiology 189:251–257

Munk PL, Vellet AD, Hilborn MD, Crues JV, Helms CA, Poon PY (1993) Musculoskeletal infection: findings on magnetic resonance imaging. Can Assoc Radiol 45:355–362

Nixon GW (1978) Hematogenous osteomyelitis of metaphyseal-equivalent locations. AJR 130:123–129

Orlicek SL, Abramson JS, Woods CR, Givner LB (2001) Obturator internus muscle abscess in children. J Pediatr Orthop 21:744–748

Oudjhane K, Azouz EM (2001) Imaging of osteomyelitis in children. Radiol Clin North Am 39:251–266

Peckett WRC, Butler-Manuel A, Apthorp LA (2001) Pyomyositis of the iliacus muscle in a child. J Bone Joint Surg (Br) 83B:103–105

Rand N, Mosheiff R, Matan Y et al (1993) Osteomyelitis of the pelvis. J Bone Joint Surg (Br) 75:731–733

Rasool MN (2001a) Primary subacute haematogenous osteomyelitis in children. J Bone Joint Surg (Br) 83B:93–98

Rasool MN (2001b) Osseous manifestations of tuberculosis in children. J Pediatr Orthop 21:749–755

Roberts JM, Drummond DS, Breed AL, Chesney J (1982) Subacute hematogenous osteomyelitis in children: a retrospective study. J Pediatr Orthop 2:249–254

Sammak B, El Bagi A, Al Shahed M, Hamilton D, Al Nabulsi J, Youseff B, Al Thagafi M (1999) Osteomyelitis: a review of currently used imaging techniques. Eur Radiol 9:894–900

Steinbach HL (1966) Infections of bones. Semin Roentgenol 1:337–369

Steinbach L, Tehranzadeh J, Fleckenstein JL et al (1993) Musculoskeletal manifestations of human immunodeficiency virus infection. Radiology 186:833–838

Struk DW, Munk PL, Lee MJ, Ho SGF, Worsley DF (2001)

Imaging of soft tissue infections. Radiol Clin North Am 39:277–303

Sucato DJ, Gillespie R (1997) Salmonella pelvic osteomyelitis in normal children: report of two cases and a review of the literature. J Pediatr Orthop 17:463–466

Tehranzadeh J, Wang F, Mesgarzadeh M (1992) Magnetic resonance imaging of osteomyelitis. Crit Rev Diagn Imaging 33:495–534

Tehranzadeh J, O'Malley P, Rafii M (1996) The spectrum of osteoarticular and soft tissue changes in patients with immunodeficiency virus (HIV) infection. Crit Rev Diagn Imaging 37:305–347

Tehranzadeh J, Ter-Oganesyan RR, Steinbach LS (2004) Musculoskeletal disorders associated with HIV infection and AIDS, part 1. Infectious musculoskeletal conditions. Skeletal Radiol 33:249–259

Viani RM, Bromberg K, Bradley JS (1999) Obturator internus muscle abscess in children: report of seven cases and review. Clin Infect Dis 28:117–122

Watts H, Lifeso R (1996) Tuberculosis of bones and joints. J Bone Joint Surg (Am) 76A:288–298

Weld PW (1960) Osteomyelitis of the ilium masquerading as acute appendicitis. JAMA 173:634–636

Wukich DK, Abreu SH, Callaghan JJ, van Nostrand D, Savory CG, Eggli DF, Garcia YE, Berrey BH (1978) Diagnosis of infection by preoperative scintigraphy with indium labelled white blood cells. J Bone Joint Surg (Br) 69B:1353–1360

Yao DC, Sartoris DJ (1995) Musculoskeletal tuberculosis. Radiol Clin North Am 33:679–689

Young F (1934) Acute osteomyelitis of the ilium. Surg Gynecol Obstet 58:986–994

Yuh WTC, Schreiber AE, Montgomery WJ, Ehara S (1988) MR imaging of pyomyositis. Skeletal Radiol 17:190–193

21 Metabolic and Endocrine Disorders

Judith E. Adams

J. E. Adams MBBS, FRCR, FRCP
Professor of Diagnostic Radiology, Imaging Science and Biomedical Engineering, The Medical School, Stopford Building, University of Manchester, Oxford Road, Manchester M13 9PT, UK

21.1
Introduction

Metabolic diseases of the skeleton affect bone as a tissue; all bones are involved histologically, although radiological features are not always evident. Such diseases can be caused by genetic, endocrine, nutritional or biochemical disorders. Knowledge of bone structure, development and physiology is essential to the understanding of the effects that metabolic bone disorders have on the skeleton, and in interpreting the abnormal features which they cause on radiographs and other imaging techniques (Adams 2005a).

21.1.1
Bone Structure and Physiology

Bone is normally present in anatomical bones in two forms:
- compact (cortical) bone which forms the outer cortex of bones
- trabecular, or cancellous, bone which is found within the cortical envelope and mainly in vertebral bodies, the pelvis and the ends of long bones.

All bones contain both types of bony tissue, although the relative amounts of each vary, and both contribute to bone strength. Bone is a specialised tissue made up of a matrix of collagen fibres and mucopolysaccharides (35% by weight) and inorganic crystalline mineral matrix (calcium hydroxyapatite) which is distributed along the length of the collagen fibres. This inorganic component accounts for 65% of osseous tissue by weight. Despite its hardness, bone remains a metabolically active tissue throughout life, being constantly resorbed and accreted by bone cells, the activity of which can be modified by many factors (Mundy 1999a). As a consequence, bones remodel from birth to maturity maintaining their basic shape, repair following fracture and respond to physical forces (i.e. mechanical stresses related to bone deformity) throughout life. The strength of bone is related not only to its hardness and other physical properties, but also to size and the architectural arrangement of the compact and trabecular bone. The skeleton contains 99% of the total body calcium and therefore plays a vital role in the maintenance of calcium homeostasis.

21.1.2
Bone Turnover

Bone formation (osteoblastic activity) and bone resorption (osteoclastic activity) constitutes bone turnover, a process which takes place on bone surfaces and continues throughout life (PARFITT 1988). Trabecular bone has a greater surface to volume area than compact bone, and is consequently some eight times more metabolically active. Bone formation and bone resorption are linked in a consistent sequence under normal circumstances. Precursor bone cells are activated at a particular skeletal site to form osteoclasts which erode a fairly constant amount of bone. After a period of time the bone resorption ceases and osteoblasts are recruited to fill the eroded space with new bone tissue. This coupling of osteo-blastic and osteoclastic activity constitutes the Basal Multi-cellular Unit (BMU) of bone, and normally are in balance, with the amount of bone eroded being replaced with the same amount of new bone. The amount of bone in the skeleton at any moment in time depends on peak bone mass attained during puberty and adolescence, and the balance between bone resorption and formation in later life. If the process of bone turnover becomes uncoupled, excessive osteoclastic resorption or defective osteoblastic function result in a net loss of bone (osteoporosis). If there is increase in both bone resorption and bone formation this constitutes increased bone turnover. Woven, immature bone, instead of mature lamellar bone, is laid down, as occurs in Paget's disease of bone. Increased activation frequency of resorption units also results in high bone turnover state (hyperparathyroidism, postmenopausal bone loss). Bisphosphonate therapy reduces the activation of resorption units by inhibiting osteoclasts, and reversal in the mineral deficit contributes to increase in bone mineral density (BMD).

Bones grow in length by enchondral ossification and remodel by periosteal apposition and endosteal resorption in the shaft, and osteoclastic resorption along the periosteal surface of the metaphysic to maintain their normal shape as the bone grows in length. Defective osteoclastic function prevents this normal resorption of bone which is essential to maintain bone health by continual slow renewal throughout life. Defective osteoclastic function (MUNDY 1999b) in some diseases (i.e. osteopetrosis) can result in abnormal bone modelling and sclerosis on radiographs. Bone resorption by osteoclasts is a single stage process in which collagen and mineral are removed together. Bone formation is a two-stage process: osteoblasts lay down osteoid, which subsequently becomes mineralised. Pre-requisites for normal mineralisation are vitamin D (1,25 [OH]$_2$ D$_3$), normal levels of phosphorus and alkaline phosphatase and a normal pH. Defects in the mineralization process will result in rickets or osteomalacia.

The most common metabolic disorders of bone are:
- hyperparathyroidism, in which a tumour or hyperplasia of the parathyroid glands causes increase in parathormone production and stimulation of osteoclasts and consequent bone resorption,
- rickets and osteomalacia in which there is a defective mineralisation of osteoid due to vitamin D deficiency, hypophosphataemia, lack of alkaline phosphatase (hypophosphatasia) or severe acidaemia;
- osteoporosis, in which there is a deficiency of bone mass leading to insufficiency (low trauma) fractures.

Other metabolic bone disorders include osteogenesis imperfecta, hyperphosphatasia, hyperphosphataemia and osteopetrosis.

21.2
Parathyroid Disorders

Most parathyroid tumours are functionally active and result in the clinical syndrome of primary hyperparathyroidism. This is the most common endocrine disorder after diabetes and thyroid disease, with an incidence within the population of approximately 1 in 1000 (0.1%). The incidence is higher in the elderly than those under 40, and is most common in women aged 60 or older. Over the past 50 years the prevalence of the condition has increased some tenfold; this increase is due principally to the detection, by chance, of hypercalcaemia in patients, many of whom are asymptomatic, through routine use of multi-channel autoanalysis of serum samples since the 1970's.

21.2.1
Hyperparathyroidism

21.2.1.1
Primary Hyperparathyroidism

The majority (80%) of patients with primary hyperparathyroidism (HAYES and CONWAY 1991) have a single adenoma. Multiple parathyroid adenomas may occur in 4% of cases. Chief cell hyperplasia of all glands occurs in 15–20% of patients; the histological diagnosis depends on the finding that more than one parathyroid gland is affected histologically. Genetic factors are relevant in a proportion of these patients (familial hyperplasia, multiple endocrine neoplasia (MEN) syndromes).

Carcinoma of the parathyroid is an infrequent cause of primary hyperparathyroidism (0.5%) (WYNNE et al 1992). The malignant tumour is slow growing but locally invasive. Cure may be obtained by adequate surgical excision and there is a 50% or greater 5 year survival rate. Recurrence is common (30%) and metastases to regional lymph nodes, lung, liver and bones occur late in 30% of cases. Biochemical remission may rarely occur spontaneously, presumably due to infarction of the tumour, but this is extremely rare, since the parathyroid glands have a very rich blood supply from both the inferior and superior thyroid arteries. Metastases, when solitary, may be resected with benefit.

21.2.1.2
Secondary Hyperparathyroidism

Secondary hyperparathyroidism is induced by any condition or circumstance which causes the serum calcium to fall. This occurs in vitamin D deficiency, intestinal malabsorption of calcium and in chronic renal failure (through lack of the active metabolite of vitamin D, $1,25(OH)_2$ D, and retention of phosphorus. If this secondary hyperparathyroidism is of sufficiently long standing, an autonomous adenoma may develop in the hyperplastic parathyroid glands, a condition referred to as tertiary hyperparathyroidism. This condition is usually associated with chronic renal disease but it has also been observed in patients with long standing vitamin D deficiency and osteomalacia from other causes.

21.2.2
Clinical Presentation

Most patients with primary hyperparathyroidism have mild disease and commonly have no symptoms, the diagnosis being made by the finding of asymptomatic hypercalcaemia. The most common clinical presentations, particularly in younger patients, are related to renal stones and nephrocalcinosis (25–35%), high blood pressure (40–60%), acute arthropathy (pseudogout), caused by calcium pyrophosphate dihydrate deposition (chondrocalcinosis), osteoporosis, peptic ulcer and acute pancreatitis, depression, confusional states, proximal muscle weakness and mild non-specific symptoms such as lethargy, arthralgia and difficulties with mental concentration.

21.2.3
Treatment

Surgical removal of the overactive parathyroid tissue is generally recommended. In experienced hands surgical excision is successful in curing the condition in over 90% of patients (KAPLAN et al. 1992). The decision to operate, particularly in the elderly and those with asymptomatic disease, requires careful assessment (CONSENSUS DEVELOPMENT CONFERENCE PANEL 1991). Conservative treatment may be judged to be the management of choice with monitoring of the serum calcium, renal function, blood pressure and bone density at regular intervals (DAVIES 1992; DAVIES et al 2002).

21.2.4
Radiological Findings

With the increased number of patients with primary hyperparathyroidism being diagnosed with asymptomatic hypercalcaemia, the majority (95%) of patients will have no radiological abnormalities.

Sub-periosteal erosions - of cortical bone is pathognomonic of hyperparathyroidism (HAYES and CONWAY 1991, GENANT et al 1973). The most sensitive site to identify this early sub-periosteal erosion is along the radial aspects of the middle phalanges of the index and middle fingers. In the pelvis they may be seen in the symphysis pubis, the sacroiliac joints (predominating at the iliac side of the joint) and along the femoral neck. (Fig. 21.1a) However, if no subperiosteal erosions are identified

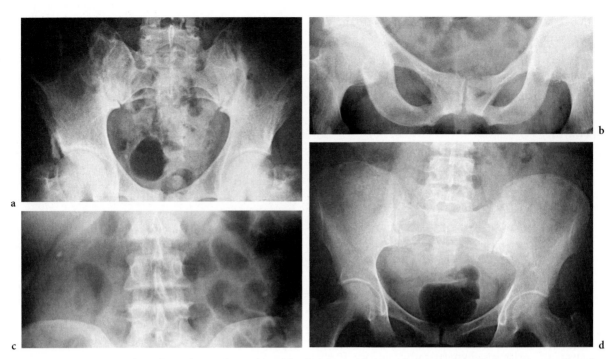

Fig. 21.1a–d. Hyperparathyroidism. **a)** AP pelvic radiograph of patient with severe hyperparathyroidism showing erosion of both sacro-iliac joints, predominantly involving the iliac side of the joint, and multiple cysts (brown 'tumours') in the iliac wings (image courtesy Dr R Whitehouse, Manchester Royal Infirmary, UK). **b)** Coned AP view of the pelvis in a patient with primary hyperparathyroidism showing chondrocalcinosis in the symphysis pubis and the right hip joint and **c)** coned view of the kidneys showing nephocalcinosis. These features would be diagnostic of hyperparathyroidism. **d)** AP view of the pelvis in a woman with hyperparathyroidism with cysts (brown tumours) in the right iliac wing and right ischium (image courtesy Dr R Whitehouse, Manchester Royal Infirmary, UK)

in the phalanges, they are unlikely to be identified radiographically elsewhere in the skeleton. Subperiosteal erosions in sites other than the phalanges indicate more severe and long standing hyperparathyroidism, such as may be found secondary to chronic renal impairment.

21.2.4.1
Chondrocalcinosis

The deposition of calcium pyrophosphate dihydrate (CPPD) causes articular cartilage and fibrocartilage to become visible on radiographs (DODDS and STEINBACK 1968). This is most likely to be identified on radiographs of the hand (triangular ligament), the knees (articular cartilage and menisci) and in the pelvis in the symphysis pubis and hip joints (Fig. 21.1b). Clinically patients may present with acute pain resembling gout, but on joint aspiration pyrophosphate crystals, rather than urate crystals, are found. Affected joints may be asymptomatic, and chondrocalcinosis noted radiographically might bring the diagnosis of hyperparathyroidism

to light in an asymptomatic patient. The combination of chondrocalcinosis in the symphysis pubis and nephrocalcinosis on an abdominal radiograph is diagnostic of hyperparathyroidism (Fig. 21.1c). Chondrocalcinosis is a feature of primary disease, rather than that secondary to chronic renal impairment.

Brown tumours (osteitis fibrosa cystica) are cystic lesions within bone in which there has been excessive osteoclastic resorption. Histologically the cavities are filled with fibrous tissue and osteoclasts, with necrosis and haemorrhagic liquefaction. Radiographically, brown tumours appear as low density, multi-loculated cysts that can occur in any skeletal site and may cause expansion of bones (Fig. 21.1d). They are now rarely seen.

21.2.4.2
Osteosclerosis

Osteosclerosis occurs uncommonly in primary hyperparathyroidism (GENANT et al 1975) but is a common feature of disease secondary to chronic renal impairment (SUNDARAM 1989). In primary disease, with normal renal function, it results from an exaggerated osteoblastic response following bone resorption. In secondary causes of hyperparathyroidism it results from excessive accumulation of poorly mineralised osteoid, which appears denser radiographically than normal bone. The increase in bone density affects particularly the axial skeleton. In the vertebral bodies the vertebral end plates are preferentially involved, giving bands of dense bones adjacent to the end plates with a central band of lower normal bone density. These alternating bands give a striped pattern described as a "rugger jersey" spine, and may be evident on a pelvic radiograph (Fig. 21.2a).

21.2.4.3
Osteoporosis

With excessive bone resorption the bones may appear reduced in density in some patients, particularly in postmenopausal women and the elderly. This can be confirmed by bone densitometry, which is an integral component in the evaluation of hyperparathyroidism. In primary hyperparathyroidism there is a pattern of skeletal involvement that preferentially affects the cortical, as opposed to the trabecular, bone. BMD measurements made in sites in which cortical bone predominates, e.g. in the distal forearm, may show the most marked reduction (WISHART et al 1990). Bone density increases after parathyroidectomy in primary hyperparathyroidism (SILVERBERG et al 1995).

21.2.4.4
Intracortical Bone Resorption

Results from increased osteoclastic activity in haversian canals. Radiographically this causes linear translucencies within the cortex (cortical "tunnelling"). This feature is not specific for hyperparathyroidism, and can be found in other conditions in which bone turnover is increased (e.g. Normal childhood, Paget's disease of bone).

21.2.4.5
Metastatic Calcification

Soft tissue calcification, other than in articular cartilage and fibrocartilage, does not occur in primary hyperparathyroidism, unless there is associ-

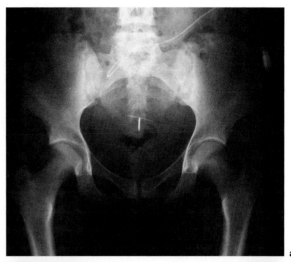

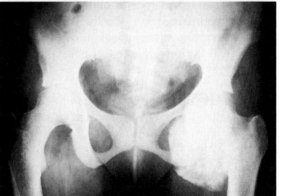

Fig. 21.2a,b. Azotaemic (renal) osteodystrophy. **a)** Pelvic radiograph of a woman of 38 years with chronic renal impairment and on ambulatory peritoneal dialysis. Tenchkoff catheter (and IUCD) visible in the pelvis. Erosions (of the iliac margins) of the sacro-iliac joints and the symphysis pubis due to secondary hyperparathyroidism. There is also some endplate sclerosis of the lumbar vertebrae ('rugger jersey' spine). **b)** Patient with chronic renal failure with maetastic calcification in the soft tissue adjacent to the left hip joint. This occurs as a result of phosphate retention due to glomerular insufficiency combined with secondary hyperparathyroidism causing the calcium X phosphate product to be elevated

ated reduced glomerular function resulting in phosphate retention. The latter causes an increase in the calcium x phosphate product, and consequently amorphous calcium phosphate is precipitated in organs and soft tissues (PARFITT 1969). If there are features of hyperparathyroidism i.e. sub-periosteal erosions, and additionally vascular or soft tissue calcifications e.g. around joints and in vessels, this implies impaired renal function in association with hyperparathyroidism. In the pelvis this soft tissue calcification can be seen in arteries, around the hip joints and ischium (Fig. 21.2b).

21.2.5
Hypoparathyroidism

Hypoparathyroidism can result from reduced or absent parathyroid hormone production or from end organ (kidney, bone or both) resistance. This may be the result of the parathyroid glands failing to develop, the glands being damaged or removed, the function of the glands being reduced by altered regulation, or the action of PTH being impaired (DIMICH et al 1967). The biochemical abnormality which results is hypocalcaemia; this can clinically cause neuromuscular symptoms and signs such as tetany and fits. Acquired hypoparathyroidism can result from surgical removal of the parathyroid glands or from autoimmune disorders. Post-surgical hypoparathyroidism is more common, and occurs in approximately 13% of patients following neck surgery. Idiopathic hypoparathyroidism usually presents during childhood, is more common in girls and rare in black races. It may be associated with pernicious anaemia and Addison's disease, and there may be antibodies to a number of endocrine glands as part of a generalised autoimmune disorder.

21.2.5.1
Radiological Abnormalities

There may be localised (23%) or generalised (9%) osteosclerosis in affected patients. Metastatic calcification may be present in the basal ganglia or in

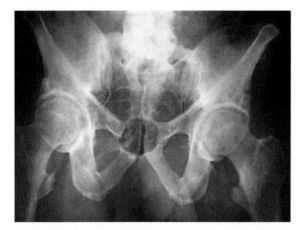

Fig. 21.3. Hypoparathyroidism. Pelvic radiograph of a man with hypoparathyroidism showing ligamentous ossification (enthesopathy), a rare but recognised complication of hypoparathyroidism (Reproduced with permission from ADAMS and DAVIES (1977)

the subcutaneous tissue, particularly about the hips and shoulders (STEINBACH and WALDRON 1952). A rare but recognised complication of hypoparathyroidism is an enthesopathy with extraskeletal ossification in a paraspinal distribution and elsewhere, including around the pelvis and hips. In the spine this skeletal hyperostosis resembles most closely that described by FORESTIER as "senile" hyperostosis (STEINBACH and WALDRON 1952; SALVESEN and BOE 1953; ADAMS and DAVIES 1977) (Fig. 21.3). Differentiating features from ankylosing spondylitis are that there is no erosive arthropathy and the sacroiliac joints appear normal. Clinically the patients may have pain and stiffness in the back with limitation of movement. Extra-skeletal ossification may be present around the pelvis, hip and in the inter-osseous membranes and tendinous insertions elsewhere.

21.2.6
Pseudohypoparathyroidism and Pseudo-pseudohypoparathyroidism

Pseudohypoparathyroidism (PHP) describes a group of genetic disorders characterised by hypocalcaemia, hyperphosphataemia, raised PTH and target tissue unresponsiveness to PTH, first described by ALBRIGHT et al. in 1942 (ALBRIGHT et al 1942). Affected patients are short in stature, have reduced intellect, rounded faces, and shortened metacarpals, particularly the fourth and fifth. Metastatic calcification, bowing of long bones and exostoses can occur. There is usually absence of the normal caudal widening of the lumbar inter-pedicular distances. Cord compression has been reported occasionally, resulting from lumbar or cervical spinal stenosis or ossifications of the paravertebral ligaments (OKADA et al 1994). In the pelvis the capital femoral epiphyses are small with a reduced height and slipping of the capital femoral epiphysis, coxa vara and valga have been described. Bony exostoses may occur (STEINBACH and YOUNG 1966).

Clinical features include tetany, cataracts, and nail dystrophy. Some of the clinical and radiological features of PHP may resemble those in other hereditary syndromes, including Turner's syndrome, acrodysostosis, Prader-Willi syndrome, fibrodysplasia ossificans progressiva and multiple hereditary exostosis.

In PHP there is end-organ unresponsiveness to parathyroid hormone since the parathyroid glands are normal and produce PTH. This usually involves unresponsiveness of both bone and kidneys. However, there is a rare variation of PHP in which the kidneys are unresponsive to PTH, but the osseous response to the hormone is normal (KOLB and STEINBACH 1962). The condition is referred to as pseudo-hypohyperparathyroidism, and has the histologic and radiological features resemble those of azotaemic osteodystrophy.

Radiographic abnormalities may not be evident at birth but subsequently there develops premature epiphyseal fusion, calvarial thickening, bone exostoses, and calcification in the basal ganglia and in the soft tissue. Metacarpal shortening is present, particularly affecting the fourth and fifth digits. Soft tissue calcification occurs in a plaque like distribution in the subcutaneous area. Rarely, soft tissue ossification can occur in a peri-articular distribution, usually involving the hands and feet.

In induviduals with pseudo-pseudohypoparathyroidism (PPHP) the dysplastic and other features are the same as PHP, but there are no associated parathyroid or other biochemical abnormalities. The abnormalities of metacarpal and metatarsal shortening, calvarial thickening, exostoses, soft tissue calcification and ossification are best identified on radiographs. Bone density may be normal, reduced or increased.

21.3
Rickets and Osteomalacia

21.3.1
Introduction

The mineralization of bone matrix depends on adequate supplies of 1,25 di-hydroxy vitamin D (1,25 $(OH)_2D$), calcium, phosphorus and alkaline phosphatase, and on a normal body pH. If there is a deficiency of any of these substances, or if there is severe systemic acidosis, mineralization of bone will be defective. This results in a qualitative abnormality of bone, with a reduction in the mineral to osteoid ratio, resulting in rickets in children and osteomalacia in adults. Rickets and osteomalacia are therefore synonymous, and represent the same disease process, but are the manifestation in the growing, or the mature, skeleton respectively. In the immature skeleton the radiographic abnormalities predominate at the growing ends of the bones where enchondral ossification is occurring, giving the classic appearance of rickets. At skeletal maturity, when

the process of enchondral ossification has ceased, the defective mineralization of osteoid is evident radiographically as Looser's zones (pseudofractures, Milkman's fracture), which are pathognomonic of osteomalacia (PITT 1981; ADAMS 2005b).

21.3.2
Causes of Vitamin D Deficiency

Deficiency of vitamin D may occur as a consequence of simple dietary deficiency, lack of sunlight (as 7-dehydrocholesterol is converted to vitamin D3 in the skin by the ultraviolet light of the sun), malabsorption states (vitamin D is fat soluble and absorbed in the small bowel), chronic liver disease (which affects hydroxylation at the 25 position) and chronic renal disease (in which the active metabolite 1,25 dihydroxy D is not produced). Consequently, a wide variety of diseases may result in vitamin D deficiency and the radiological features will be similar, being those of rickets or osteomalacia. This similarity of radiological features, but variation in response to treatment, contributed to some early confusion before the metabolism of vitamin D was unravelled in the 1970s. Rickets due to nutritional deprivation was cured by ultraviolet light or physiological doses of vitamin D (400 IU per day), but that associated with chronic renal disease was not, except if very large pharmacological doses (up to 300,000 IU per day) were used. This led to the terms "refractory rickets" and "vitamin D resistant rickets" being used for these conditions. Within these terms were included the diseases that cause the clinical and radiological features of rickets, but were related to phosphate, not vitamin D, deficiency (X-linked hypophosphataemia, and genetic disorders involving defects in 1-alpha hydroxylase and the vitamin D receptor).

21.3.2.1
Genetic Disorders of Vitamin D Metabolism

PRADER et al (PRADER et al 1961) described the condition in which rickets occurred within the first year of life and was characterised by severe hypocalcaemia, dental enamel hypoplasia and which responded to large amounts of vitamin D. The term "vitamin D dependency" was used for this syndrome. It is now recognised that this disease is due to an inborn error of metabolism in which there is deficient hydroxylation of 25(OH)D in the kidney due to defective activity of the renal 25(OH)D 1-alpha hydroxylase. The preferred term for this condition is pseudo vitamin D deficiency rickets (PDDR) and it is inherited as an autosomal recessive trait (GLORIEUX and ST-ARNAUD 2005)

Another in-born error of vitamin D metabolism was described in 1978 (BROOKS et al. 1978), which clinically resembled pseudo-vitamin D deficiency rickets but with high circulating concentrations of $1,25(OH)_2D$. This condition results from a spectrum of mutations which affect the vitamin D receptor (VDR) in target tissues causing resistance to the action of $1,25(OH)_2D$ (end organ resistance). Affected patients have complete alopecia.

21.3.3
Radiological Appearances

21.3.3.1
Rickets

In the immature skeleton the effect of vitamin D deficiency and the consequent defective mineralisation of osteoid is seen principally at the growing ends of bones (PITT 1993; ADAMS 2005). In the early stage there is apparent widening of the growth plate which is the translucent "unmineralised" gap between the mineralised metaphysis and epiphysis. More severe change produces "cupping" of the metaphysis, with irregular and poor mineralisation. There may be a thin "ghost-like" rim or mineralisation at the periphery of the metaphysis, as this mineralisation occurs by membranous ossification at the periosteum. The margin of the epiphysis appears indistinct as enchondral ossification at this site is also defective. These changes predominate at the sites of bones which are growing most actively, which are around the knee, the wrist (particularly the ulna), the anterior ends of the middle ribs, the proximal femur and the distal tibia, and depend on the age of the child. If rickets is suspected it is these anatomical sites which are most likely to show radiographic abnormality.

Rachitic bone is soft and bends and this results in genu valgum or genu varum, deformity of the hips (coxa valga or more commonly coxa vara) (Fig. 21.4a), in-drawing of the ribs at the insertion of the diaphragm (Harrison's sulcus) and protrusio acetabuli and triradiate deformity of the pelvis, which can cause problems with subsequent parturition. In very severe rickets, when little skeletal growth is taking place (i.e. owing to nutritional deprivation or chronic ill health), paradoxically radiological features of

rickets may not be evident at the growth plate. In rickets of prematurity little abnormality may be present at the metaphysis since no skeletal growth is taking place in the premature infant. However, the bones are osteopenic and prone to fractures. In mild vitamin D deficiency the radiographic features of rickets may only become apparent at puberty during the growth spurt, and the metaphyseal abnormalities predominate at the knee.

With appropriate treatment of vitamin D deficiency the radiographic features of healing lag behind the improvement in biochemical parameters (two weeks) and clinical symptoms. With treatment, the zone of provisional calcification will mineralise. This mineralised zone is initially separated by translucent osteoid from the shaft of the bone, and be mistaken for a metaphyseal fracture of child abuse (BRILL et al 1998). Reduced bone density and poor definition of epiphyses are helpful distinguishing features for rickets. The section of abnormal bone following healing of rickets may be visible for a period of time, and give some indication as to the age of onset and duration of the period of rickets. Eventually this zone will become indistinguishable from normal bone with remodelling over a period of three to four months. The zone of provisional calcification which was present at the onset of the disturbance to enchondral ossification may remain (HARRIS growth arrest line) (HARRIS 1933) as a marker of the age of skeletal maturity at which the rickets occurred. However, this is not specific for rickets and can occur in any condition (i.e. period of ill health, lead poisoning) that inhibits normal enchondral ossification. There will be evidence of retarded growth and development in rickets, but in my experience, this tends to be more marked when the vitamin D deficiency is associated with chronic diseases that reduce calorie intake, general well-being and activity (i.e. malabsorption, chronic renal disease) than with simple nutritional vitamin D deficiency.

Vitamin D deficiency is associated with hypocalcaemia. In an attempt to maintain calcium homeostasis the parathyroid glands are stimulated to secrete PTH. This results in another important feature of vitamin D deficiency rickets. Evidence of secondary hyperparathyroidism, with increased osteoclastic resorption, will be evident histologically, although not always radiographically.

Metaphyseal chondrodysplasias encompass a variety of inherited bone dysplasias in which there are metaphyseal abnormalities which may range from mild (Schmit Type) to severe (Jansen) (TAYBI

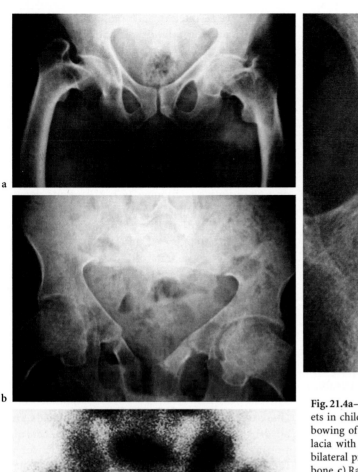

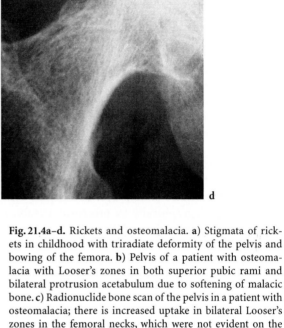

Fig. 21.4a–d. Rickets and osteomalacia. **a)** Stigmata of rickets in childhood with triradiate deformity of the pelvis and bowing of the femora. **b)** Pelvis of a patient with osteomalacia with Looser's zones in both superior pubic rami and bilateral protrusion acetabulum due to softening of malacic bone. **c)** Radionuclide bone scan of the pelvis in a patient with osteomalacia; there is increased uptake in bilateral Looser's zones in the femoral necks, which were not evident on the pelvic radiograph. **d)** Amyloid deposition disease: accumulation of beta-2-microglobulin results in juxta-articular, well corticated cysts in the around the large joints, as seen in the acetabular margin of the right hip

and LACHMAN 1996). Normal serum biochemistry serve to differentiate these dysplasias from other rachitic disorders the radiographic abnormalities at the metaphyses may simulate.

21.3.3.2
Osteomalacia:

At skeletal maturity the epiphysis fuses to the metaphysis with obliteration of the growth plate and cessation of longitudinal bone growth. However, bone turnover continues throughout life to maintain the tensile integrity of the skeleton. Vitamin D deficiency in the adult skeleton results in osteomalacia, the pathognomonic radiographic feature of which is the Looser's zone, named after E

Looser who described them in 1908 (LOOSER 1920). Looser's zones (pseudo-fractures, Milkman's fractures) (MILKMAN 1930) are translucent areas in the bone that are composed of unmineralised osteoid (Fig. 21.4b). They are typically bilateral and symmetrical. Radiographically they appear as radiolucent lines that are perpendicular to the bone cortex, do not usually extend across the entire bone shaft and characteristically have a slightly sclerotic margin. Looser's zones can occur in any bone, but most typically are found in the medial aspect of the femoral neck, the pubic rami, the lateral border of the scapula and the ribs (Fig. 21.4a) and less commonly the ilium. They may not always be visible on radiographs; radionuclide bone scans are more sensitive in identifying radiographic occult Looser's zones (HAIN and FOGELMAN 2002) (Fig. 21.4c).

Looser's zones must be differentiated from insufficiency fractures that can occur in osteoporotic bone, particularly in the pubic rami, sacrum and calcaneus. Such insufficiency fractures consist of multiple micro-fractures in brittle, osteoporotic bone and often show florid callus formation, serving to differentiate them from Looser's zones (DESMET and NEFF 1985; MCKENNA et al 1987). Incremental fractures occur in Paget's disease of bone and resemble Looser's zones in appearance, but tend to occur on the convexity of the cortex of the bone involved (MILGRAM 1977; WHITEHOUSE 2002), rather than medially, as in osteomalacia. The other typical features of Paget's disease (sclerosis, disorganised trabecular pattern and enlarged bone) serve as distinguishing radiological features.

Complete fractures can occur through Looser's zones, but with no evidence of callus formation until the osteomalacia is treated with vitamin D. Then there will be quite florid callus formation around fractures and healing of fractures and Looser's zones, with little residual deformity. However, as in rickets, osteomalacic bone is soft and bends. This is evident radiographically by protrusio acetabuli, in which the femoral head deforms the acetabular margin so that the normal 'teardrop' outline is lost (Fig. 21.4b). There may be bowing of the long bones of the legs and a tri-radiate deformity of the pelvis (Fig. 21.4a and 21.4b), particularly if the cause of the vitamin D deficiency has persisted since childhood, and has been inadequately treated or untreated.

In osteomalacia, as in rickets, hypocalcaemia acts as stimulus to secondary hyperparathyroidism. This may be manifested radiographically as subperiosteal erosion, particularly in the phalanges but other sites (sacroiliac joints, symphysis pubis, proximal tibia, outer ends of the clavicle, skull vault – "pepperpot" skull) may be involved, depending on the intensity and duration of the hyperparathyroidism. There may also be cortical tunnelling and a hazy trabecular pattern. Generalised osteopenia may occur and vertebral bodies may have biconcave endplates, due to deformation of the malacic bone by the cartilaginous intervertebral disc ("cod fish" deformity) (RESNICK 1982).

Azotaemic (renal) osteodystrophy: The bone disease associated with chronic renal impairment is complex and multi-factorial, and has changed over past decades (SUNDARAM 1989; ADAMS 2002). Whereas originally features of vitamin D deficiency (rickets/osteomalacia) and secondary hyperparathyroidism (erosions, osteosclerosis, brown cysts) predominated, improvement in management and therapy have resulted in such radiographic features being present in a minority of patients. Metastatic calcification (Fig. 21.2b) and "adynamic" bone develop as a complication of disease (phosphate retention) and treatment (phosphate binders). New complications (amyloid deposition, non-infective spondyloarthropathy, osteonecrosis) are now seen in long-term hemodialysis and/or renal transplantation (Fig. 21.4d) (SARGENT et al 1989; THEODOROU et al 2002). Radiographs remain the most important imaging techniques, but occasionally other imaging and quantitative techniques (CT, MRI, bone densitometry) are relevant to diagnosis and management.

In extreme cases of soft tissue calcification there may be ischaemic necrosis of the skin, muscle and subcutaneous tissue, referred to as "calciphylaxis". This condition can occur in patients with advanced renal disease, in those on regular dialysis and also those with functioning renal allografts (GIPSTEIN et al 1976).

21.3.4
Renal Tubular Defects

Glucose, inorganic phosphate and amino acids are absorbed in the proximal renal tubule; concentration and acidification of urine in exchange for a fixed base occur in the distal renal tubule. Renal tubular disorders may involve either the proximal or the distal tubule, or both. Such disorders will result in a spectrum of biochemical disturbances that may result in loss of phosphate, glucose, or amino acids alone, or in combination, with additional defects in urine acidification and concentration. Such defects of tubular function may be inherited and present from birth (Toni-Fanconi syndrome, cystinosis, X-linked hypophosphataemia), or later in life (e.g. tubular function being compromised by deposition of copper in Wilson's disease, hereditary tyrosinaemia), or be acquired by tubular dysfunction being induced by the effects of toxins or therapies (paraquat, lysol burns, toluene "glue sniffing" inhalation, ifosfamide, gentamicin, streptozotocin, valproic acid), deposition of heavy metals or other substances (multiple myeloma, cadmium, lead, mercury), related to immunological disorders (interstitial nephritis, renal transplantation), or with the production of a humoral substance in tumour induced osteomalacia (TIO), also know as "oncogenic rickets" (RYAN and REISS 1984; LAWSON 2002). In these renal tubular disorders rickets or osteomalacia can be caused by multiple factors, including hyperphosphaturia, hypophosphataemia, and reduced 1 alpha hydroxylation of 25(OH)D. Where the serum calcium is generally normal, secondary hyperparathyroidism does not occur.

21.3.4.1
X-linked Hypophosphataemia

X-linked hypophosphataemia (XLH) is a genetic disorder transmitted as an X-linked dominant trait (WEISMAN and HOCHBERG 1994). Sporadic cases also occur through spontaneous mutations. The incidence is approximately 1 in 25,000, and XLH is now the most common cause of genetically induced rickets. The disease is characterised by phosphaturia throughout life, hypophosphataemia, rickets and osteomalacia. Clinically affected individuals may be short in stature, principally due to defective growth in the legs, which are bowed; the trunk is usually normal (STEENDIJK and HAUSPIE 1992). Rickets becomes clinically evident at about 6–12 months of age or older. Treatment with phosphate supple-

ments and large pharmacological doses of vitamin D (hence the term "vitamin D-resistant rickets") could heal the radiological features of rickets, and also increase longitudinal growth (GLORIEUX et al 1980). The radiological features of XLH are characteristic (MILGRAM and COMPERE 1981). There is defective mineralisation of the metaphysis and widening of the growth plate (rickets). The metaphyseal margin tends to be less indistinct than in nutritional rickets and the affected metaphysis is not as wide. Changes are most marked at the knee, wrist, ankle and proximal femur (Fig. 21.5a). Healing can be induced with appropriate treatment (phosphate supplements, 1,25(OH)$_2$D) (GLORIEUX et al 1980). The growth plates fuse normally at skeletal maturation. The bones are often short and under-tubulated (shaft wide in relation to bone length) with bowing of the femur and tibia which may be marked. Following skeletal maturation, Looser's zones appear and persist in patients with XLH. They tend to be in sites which are different from those which occur in nutritional osteomalacia, and often affect the outer cortex of the bowed femur, although they do occur along the medial cortex of the shaft also. Looser's zones

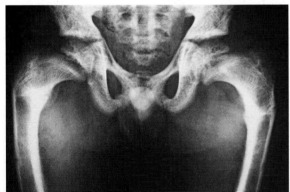

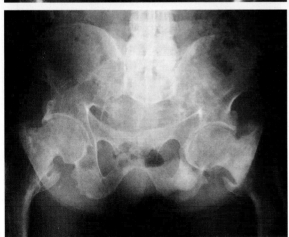

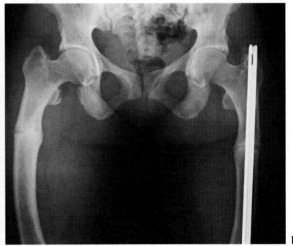

Fig. 21.5a–c. X-linked hypophosphataemic osteomalacia (XLH). **a)** Pelvic radiograph of an affected child showing rachitic changes at the metaphyses of the proximal femora, which are bowed. There is a coarse and dense trabecular pattern which is a feature of the condition. **b)** There are chronic Looser's zones in both femoral shafts with an intra-medullary nail in the left femur. The femora are bowed and there is evidence of early ligamentous ossification (enthesopathy) at the lesser trochanters. Note that in contrast to ankylosing spondylitis the sacro-iliac joints are normal. **c)** Pelvic radiograph of an older affected patient with tri-radiate deformity of the pelvis, bowing of the femora and ligamentous ossification around the pelvis

in the ribs and pelvis are rare. Although Looser's zones may heal with appropriate treatment, those that have been present for many years persist radiographically and are presumably filled with fibrous tissue (Fig. 21.5b).

Although there is defective mineralisation of osteoid in XLH, the bones are commonly and characteristically increased in density, with a coarse and prominent trabecular pattern (Fig. 21.5a). This is a feature of the disease, and is not related to treatment with vitamin D and phosphate supplements, as it is present in those who have not received treatment.

X-linked hypophosphataemia is characterised by an enthesopathy, in which there is inflammation in the junctional area between bone and tendon insertion that heals by ossification at affected sites (POLISSON et al 1985). As a result ectopic bone forms around the pelvis and spine (Fig. 21.5c). This may result in complete ankylosis of the spine, resembling ankylosing spondylitis, and clinically limiting mobility. However, the absence of inflammatory arthritis, with normal sacroiliac joints, serves to differentiate XLH from ankylosing spondylitis. Ossification can occur in the inter-osseous membrane of the forearm and in the leg between the tibia and the fibula. Separate, small ossicles can occur around the joints of the hands and ossification of tendon insertions in the hands cause "whiskering" of bone margins.

A rare complication of XLH is spinal cord compression caused by a combination of ossification of the ligamentum flavum, thickening of the laminae, and hyperostosis around the apophyseal joints (ADAMS and DAVIES 1986). It is important to be aware of this rare complication of the disease since surgical decompression by laminectomy is curative, and is best performed as an elective procedure by an experienced surgeon rather than as an emergency. Computed tomography (CT) is a useful imaging technique for demonstrating the extent of intraspinal ossification.

Extra skeletal ossification is uncommon in patients with XLH before the age of 40 years. The extent to which radiographic abnormalities of rickets and osteomalacia, osteosclerosis, abnormalities of bone modelling and extra skeletal ossification are present varies between affected individuals (HARDY et al 1989). In some, all the features are present and so are diagnostic of the condition. In others, there may only be minor abnormalities and the diagnosis of X-linked hypophosphataemic rickets may be overlooked (ECONS et al 1994).

21.3.4.2
Tumour Induced "Oncogenic" Rickets/Osteomalacia

Tumour induced osteomalacia (TIO) or "oncogenic" rickets and osteomalacia was first reported in 1947 (MCCANCE 1947). The condition is characterised by phosphaturia and hypophosphataemia induced by a factor ('phosphatonin') produced by the tumour which has various effects (inhibiting production of $1,25(OH)_2D$; direct effect on the renal tubule), and is associated with the clinical and radiographic features of rickets or osteomalacia (Fig. 21.4a and 21.6). Such features may precede identification of the causative tumour by long periods (1–16 years). The tumours are usually small, benign and of vascular origin (e.g. haemangiopericytoma), but there are now known to be a wide spectrum of tumours that may result in this syndrome, some of which may be malignant (EDMINSTER and SUNDARAM 2002). The causative lesions may originate in the skeleton and occur in neurofibromatosis. The biochemical abnormalities will be cured, and the rickets/osteomalacia will heal, with surgical removal of the tumour. Often the tumours are extremely small and elude detection for many years. It is important that the affected patient is vigilant about self examination, and reports any small palpable lump or skin lesion. More sophisticated imaging (CT, MRI) may be helpful in localising deep-seated lesions (EDMINSTER and SUNDARAM 2002) (Fig. 21.6).

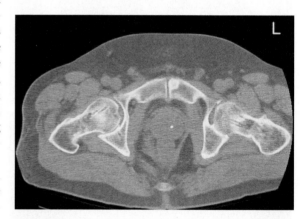

Fig. 21.6. Oncogenic (tumour induced) osteomalacia. Computed tomography scan of pubic rami in a man who has had acquired hypophophataemic osteomalacia for some 16 years. There is a sclerotic lesion in the left pubic ramus which was active on a octreotide scan and could represent the causative tumour, but this cannot be confirmed as the patient currently does not wish to have the lesion removed. (Image courtesy of Dr R Whitehouse, Manchester Royal Infirmary, UK; case report reference from MORAN and PAUL (2002) with permission)

21.3.5
Other Causes of Rickets and Osteomalacia Not Related to Vitamin D Deficiency or Hypophosphataemia

21.3.5.1
Hypophosphatasia

Hypophosphatasia is a rare disorder which was first described by RATHBUN in 1948 (RATHBUN et al 1961). It is generally transmitted as an autosomal recessive trait, but autosomal dominant inheritance has also been reported. The disease is characterised by reduced levels of serum alkaline phosphatase (both bone and liver iso-enzymes), with raised levels of phospho-ethanolamine in both the blood and the urine. Serum calcium and phosphorus levels are not reduced; in peri-natal and infantile disease there can be hypercalciuria and hypercalcaemia attributed to the imbalance between calcium absorption from the gut and defective growth and mineralisation of the skeleton. The latter results in rickets in childhood and osteomalacia in adults. The severity of the condition varies greatly, being diagnosed either in the peri-natal period, in infancy or childhood, but in some patients only becoming apparent in adult life (WEINSTEIN and WHYTE 1981). The condition can wax and wane and tends to be more severe in children than when it becomes apparent in later life. In severely affected neonates there is little, if any, evidence of mineralisation of the skeleton; in extreme cases there may be such poor mineralisation that only the skull base is visualised radiographically. Death ensues soon after birth since there is inadequate bony support for the thorax or brain. Less severely affected children survive with rachitic metaphyseal changes appearing soon after birth as growth proceeds. The abnormalities at the growth plates resemble nutritional vitamin D deficiency rickets, but in hypophosphatasia larger, irregular lucent defects often extend into the metaphyses and diaphyses. There may be generalised reduction in bone density with a coarse trabecular pattern. The long bones, particularly those in the lower limbs, become bowed, fractures may occur and be the presenting feature. Such fractures may or may not heal; when they do unite, it is through subperiosteal new bone formation. In severe disease, multiple fractures may cause deformity and limb shortening.

In adult onset of the disease the presenting clinical feature is usually a fracture, occurring after relatively minor trauma, particularly in the metatarsals. Fracture healing is slow or absent with little callus formation, but will occur following intramedullary nailing (ANDERTON 1979). The features of osteomalacia may be present with Looser's zones, a coarse trabecular pattern and bowing deformities of the limbs. Chondrocalcinosis and extraskeletal ossification of tendinous and ligamentous insertions to bone may occur (CHUCK et al 1989). The diagnosis is confirmed by the biochemical changes of reduced alkaline phosphatase and raised blood and urine phosphoethanolamine. As there is no effective treatment for hypophosphatasia, severely affected patients can prove a challenge to orthopaedic management (ANDERTON 1979).

21.4
Osteoporosis

21.4.1
Introduction

Osteoporosis is the most common metabolic bone disease, and affects 1 in 2 postmenopausal women and 1 in 5 men in their lifetime (VAN STAA et al 2001). The disease is characterised by reduced bone mass and deterioration in trabecular structure. The clinical consequence is low trauma fractures, particularly in the spine, wrist and hip (MAYO-SMITH and ROSENTHAL 1991; QUEK and PEH 2002). All may be associated with pain and deformity, and hip fractures cause significant mortality. In the past there was little effective preventative or bone enhancing therapy, but now this is not the case. Supplementary calcium and vitamin D, bisphosphonates and selective oestrogen receptor modulators (SERMs) and bone enhancing therapy (teriparatide, strontium ranelate) increase bone density and reduce future fracture risk (EASTELL 1998). It is therefore relevant to identify patients at risk, preferably before fractures occur. Radiologists have an important role to play in this objective. There are features on radiographs that should be recognised and reported clearly; if present it should be suggested that the patient be referred to a clinician with a special interest in osteoporosis management and that bone densitometry be performed to confirm the diagnosis (KANIS and GLÜER 2000). Imaging techniques also play a role in identifying fractures that are related to pathologies other than osteoporosis (metastases, myeloma) (BAUR et al 1998).

21.4.1.1
Causes of Osteoporosis

Osteoporosis may be generalized or regional (QUEK and PEH 2002).
- Generalised: the most common cause is the bone loss that occurs with ageing (senile) and in women after the menopause (postmenopausal). Osteoporosis can be associated with endocrine disorders (Cushing's disease, thyrotoxicosis, hyperparathyroidism), medications (glucocorticoid therapy, heparin), deficiency states (scurvy, malnutrition), osteogenesis imperfecta (RAUCH and GLORIEUX 2004) and other miscellaneous conditions (excess alcohol consumption, coeliac disease, cystic fibrosis).
- Regional: this can occur in a limb with disuse (e.g following a fracture or stroke) and around joints in inflammatory diseases (rheumatoid arthritis). There are also specific conditions which include reflex sympathetic osteodystrophy (Sudeck's atrophy) and transient osteoporosis of the hip.

21.4.2
Radiographic Features

With loss of bone mass the bones appear more radiolucent (osteopenic). The cortex of bones becomes thinned and the number of trabeculae is reduced. In the vertebrae the horizontal trabeculae are the first to be lost with preservation of the primary vertical trabeculae. This results in a prominent vertical striated appearance in the spine. In the proximal femur there is accentuation of the principal compressive and tensile trabeculae with reduction in trabecular number in Ward's area.

- Fractures: fractures occur in sites rich in trabecular bone, particularly the wrist, vertebrae and hip. All are associated with significant morbidity, and hip fractures with mortality. Vertebral fractures are the most common osteoporotic fracture; 30% may be asymptomatic. They are defined as wedge, endplate or crush (FERRAR et al 2005, JIANG et al 2004; GENANT et al 1993). They are powerful predictors of future fracture (hip X2; vertebral X5). It is therefore extremely important that if they are present they are accurately reported by radiologists. There is currently a joint initiative between the International Osteoporosis Foundation (IOF), the European Society of Skeletal Radiology (Osteoporosis Group – Chairman Professor JE Adams) to improve the sensitivity and accuracy of reporting of vertebral fractures by European radiologists and an interactive teaching CD is available (www.osteofound.org).

- Micro-fractures can occur, particularly in the sacral alar, pubic rami and calcaneus (PEH 1996) (Fig. 21.7a and 21.7b). There may be profuse callus formation mimicking other pathologies. These micro-fractures may be difficult to identify on radiographs due to superimposition of other structures (e.g. bowel overlying sacrum), and radionuclide bone scans (RNS), CT and MR imaging may be required ('Honda' sign of sacral fractures) for identification (HAIN and FOGELMAN 2002) (Fig. 21.7b). These imaging methods are also relevant to differentiating osteoporotic fractures from fractures due to other pathologies (metastases, myeloma) (JERGAS 2003).

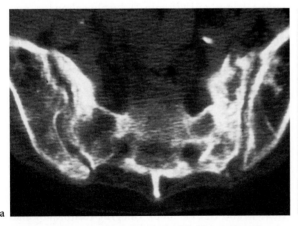
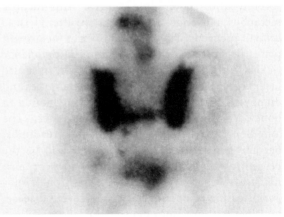

a
b

Fig. 21.7a,b. Osteoporosis. **a)** Computed tomography scan of the sacrum showing insufficiency fractures of the sacral ala which could not be identified on the pelvic radiograph due to overlying bowel gas. **b)** Corresponding radionuclide scan showing increase uptake in the sacral ala giving the characteristic 'Honda' sign

21.4.3
Bone Densitometry

If low trauma fractures are present with the other radiographic features (thin cortex, reduced trabeculae) the diagnosis of osteoporosis is not difficult to make. However, if no fractures are present, judging bone density from radiographs is imprecise. As there are effective bone-preserving/enhancing therapies now available it is important to identify patients at risk of fracture, and before fractures occur. This is the role of bone densitometry techniques. Several methods for measuring bone mineral density (BMD) are available, including dual energy X-ray absorptiometry (DXA) and quantitative computed tomography (QCT), which can be applied to axial and peripheral skeletal sites. Quantitative ultrasound (QUS) can only be applied to peripheral sites, most commonly the calcaneus, and although it predicts fracture risk in postmenopausal women, the method does not measure BMD (HANS et al 2003). QCT provides separate measures of cortical and trabecular bone, giving true volumetric density (mg/cm^3). Also in the limbs it can measure cross-sectional area of muscle and bone, from which can be derived biomechanical parameters [stress-strain index and moment from inertia]) (RAUCH and SCHOENAU 2001), which gives it an important role in research studies, but it involves a higher radiation dose than DXA in axial sites (approximately 90 microsieverts in lumbar spine) and the World Health Organisation definition of osteoporosis in terms of BMD (T score below –2.5) is not applicable (GUGLIELMI and LANG 2002). DXA is the most widely used technique and has advantages (fast scanning [less than 1 min], low radiation dose [1–6 microsieverts- less than one day's natural background radiation] and is applicable to multiple sites [lumbar spine, hip, radius and whole body, from which total and regional BMD and body composition – lean muscle and fat mass can be derived]) (ADAMS 2003). There are some limitations which include measures of integral (cortical and trabecular) bone and an areal (g/cm^2), rather than a volumetric BMD. The latter results in DXA measures being size dependent, causing under-estimate of BMD in small individuals and over-estimated BMD in large individuals. This is a particular problem in growing children (MUGHAL et al 2005; NATIONAL OSTEOPOROSIS SOCIETY 2004).

Bone mineral density BMD) predicts about 70% of bone strength; BMD methods are therefore predictors of fracture (MARSHALL et al 1996, KANIS 2002; CUMMINGS et al 2002, BLAKE and FOGELMAN 2004).

Site specific BMD is the best predictor of fractures; DXA femoral neck BMD is the optimum method for predicting hip fractures (KANIS and GLÜER 2000). DXA of the hip is therefore currently the 'reference standard' for the diagnosis of osteoporosis by bone density (WHO definition T score below –2.5) (WORLD HEALTH ORGANISATION 1994). When performing DXA-BMD of the proximal femur the leg is positioned with slight abduction and internal rotation, and secure on a positioner provided by the scanner manufacturer (Fig. 21.8a). This is to ensure the femoral neck is parallel to the scanner table; any external rotation (evident by prominence of the lesser trochanter) will result in foreshortening of the femoral neck, and false elevation of BMD (same amount of calcium in smaller area). Different positions of the femur can result in variations of BMD of 1.7–4.1% (WILSON et al 1991) (Fig. 21.8d). In the hip scan the area of analysis varies between scanner manufacturers. BMD is provided for four sites: femoral neck, trochanter, Ward's area and total hip (Fig. 21.8b and 21.8c). Diagnosis is generally based on femoral neck and total hip BMD. The precision (reproducibility) with skilled and experienced technical staff should a coefficient of variation (CV) of 1% or less in these sites. Interpretation of results requires appropriate sex- and ethnic-reference database for comparison; those provided by the scanner manufacturer are generally used. The current favoured method of interpretation is to calculate the standard deviation (SD) of the patient's result in relation to mean BMD of young normals (T score) or age-matched individuals (Z score) (NATIONAL OSTEOPOROSIS SOCIETY 2002; WATTS 2004). Images must be scrutinised for abnormalities that can result in errors in DXA measurements (osteophytes in the lumbar spine or hip; Paget's disease) and for identifying vertebral fractures and other pathologies on DXA images (ADAMS 2003). Hip axis length (HAL) can be measured on some DXA scanners (a line drawn along middle of femoral neck from the inner border of pelvis to the lateral margin of the femur) and has been found to be related to hip fracture in postmenopausal women, the risk being higher the longer the HAL (FAULKNER et al 1994).

To overcome the problems of the size dependency of DXA methods have been devised to calculate bone volume from the 2D DXA scans, to obtain bone mineral apparent density (BMAD) (NATIONAL OSTEOPOROSIS SOCIETY 2004). In the spine the vertebrae are assumed to be either cubes (CARTER et al 1992) or cylinders (KROGER et al 1992). In the proximal femur the femoral neck is assumed to be a cylinder

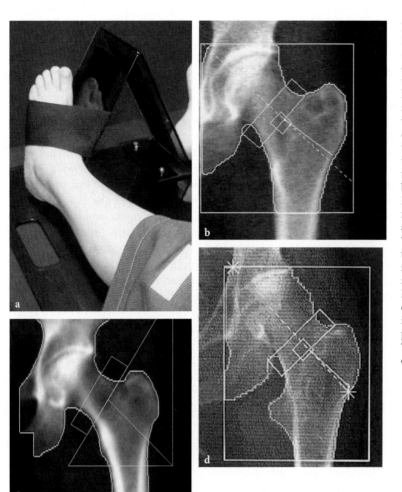

Fig. 21.8a–d. Bone densitometry. **a)** Dual energy X-ray absorptiometry (DXA) of the proximal femur is the optimum technique for predicting fracture risk in the hip. To scan the hip the leg is slightly abducted and internally rotated, and fixed on a positioner provided by the scanner manufacturer, to ensure that the femoral neck is parallel to the scanner table to avoid false elevation of bone mineral density (BMD) due to foreshortening of the femoral neck. **b)** DXA hip scan on Hologic and **c)** GE Lunar scanners. The sites measure are femoral neck, trochanter, Ward's area and total hip and BMD is given as an 'areal' density (g/cm^2), and interpretation is generally made on the femoral neck and total hip results. The sites are not identical between manufacturers. **d)** DXA of the hip with poor positioning of the femoral neck due to some external rotation of the leg, as evident by the prominence of the lesser trochanter. This will cause over-estimation of BMD due to foreshortening of the femoral

(Lu et al 1996). Methods have also been devised to extract biomechanical parameters from the proximal femur scans (Wang et al 2005).

21.5
Other Metabolic Bone Disorders

21.5.1
Introduction

A number of congenital and familial disorders can be associated with increased bone density (osteosclerosis) and abnormal bone modelling. These include osteopetrosis, pyknodysostosis, metaphyseal dysplasia (Pyle's disease), craniometaphyseal dysplasia, frontometaphyseal dysplasia, osteodysplasty (Melnick-Needles syndrome), progressive diaphysial dysplasia (Camurati-Engelmann disease), hereditary multiple diaphysial sclerosis (Ribbing's disease),

craniodiaphysial dysplasia, endosteal hyperostosis (Worth and Van Buchem types), dysosteosclerosis, tubular stenosis and occulodento-osseous dysplasia (Greenspan 1991). All are rare and have different natural histories, genetic transmission, complications and radiographic features. Many are dysplasias rather than metabolic bone disorders. The only condition to be considered in this chapter is osteopetrosis.

21.5.2
Osteopetrosis

In this condition there is defective osteoclastic resorption of the primary spongiosa of bone. Osteoclasts in affected bone are usually devoid of the ruffled borders by which osteoclasts adhere to the bone surface and through which their resorptive activity is expressed. In the presence of continued bone formation, there is generalised osteosclerosis and abnormalities of metaphyseal modelling. There have been reports of reversal of the osteosclerosis following successful bone marrow transplantation.

Osteopetrosis was first described by ALBERS-SCHONBERG in 1904, and is sometimes referred to as marble bone disease, osteosclerosis fragilis generalisata and osteopetrosis generalisata (STOKER 2002). There are two main clinical forms::

- The lethal form of osteopetrosis with precocious manifestations and an autosomal recessive transmission and benign osteopetrosis with late manifestations inherited by autosomal dominant transmission.

- There is also a more rare autosomal recessive (intermediate) form which presents during childhood, with the signs and symptoms of the lethal form, but the outcome on life expectancy is not known. The syndrome previously described as osteopetrosis with renal tubular acidosis and cerebral calcification, is now recognised as an inborn error of metabolism, carbonic anhydrase II deficiency. Neuronal storage disease with malignant osteopetrosis has been described, as has the rare lethal, transient infantile and post infectious form of the disorder.

In individuals affected by the autosomal recessive lethal type there is obliteration of the marrow cavity leading to anaemia, thrombocytopaenia and recurrent infection. Clinically there is hepatosplenomegaly, hydrocephalus and cranial nerve involvement resulting in blindness and deafness. Radiographically all the bones are dense with lack of cortico-medullary differentiation. Modelling of affected bones is abnormal with expansion of the metaphyseal region and undertubulation of bone. This is most evident in the long bones, particularly the distal femur and proximal humerus. Although the bones are dense, they are brittle and horizontal pathological fractures are common. Sclerosis of endplates of the vertebral bodies produces a "sandwich" appearance. MR imaging may assist in monitoring those with severe disease who undergo marrow transplantation, since success will be indicated by expansion of the marrow cavity.

There is an intermediate recessive form of the disease which is milder than that seen in infants and distinct from the less severe autosomal dominant disease. Affected individuals suffer pathological fracture and anaemia and are of short stature, with hepatomegaly. The radiographic features include diffuse osteosclerosis, abnormal bone modelling and a "bone within a bone" appearance.

Benign, autosomal dominant type of osteopetrosis (Albers-Schonberg disease) is often asymptomatic, and the diagnosis may come to light either incidentally, or through the occurrence of a pathological fracture. Other presentations include anaemia and facial palsy or deafness from cranial nerve compression. Problems may occur after tooth extraction, as there is an increased incidence of osteomyelitis, particularly of the mandible. Radiographic features are similar to those of the autosomal recessive form of the disease, but less severe. The bones are diffusely sclerotic, with thickened cortices and defective modelling (Fig. 21.9). There may be alternating sclerotic and radiolucent bands at the ends of diaphyses, a "bone within a bone" appearance and the vertebral endplates appear sclerotic. In 1987, ANDERSEN and BOLLERSLEV classified this form of the disease into two distinct radiological types. In Type I fractures are unusual, in contrast to Type II in which fractures are common. Transverse bands in the metaphyses are more commonly a feature in Type II disease, as is a raised serum acid phosphatase.

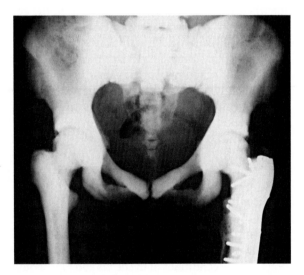

Fig. 21.9. Osteopetrosis. There is generalised sclerosis of the bones of the pelvis with a treated fracture of the left femur

21.5.3
Hyperphosphatasia

Hyperphosphatasia is a rare genetic disorder resulting from mutations in osteoprotegerin (OPG), and is characterised by markedly elevated serum alkaline phosphatase levels (CUNDY 2002).Affected children have episodes of fever, bone pain and progressive enlargement of the skull, with bowing of the long bones and associated pathological fractures. Radiographically the features resemble Paget's disease of bone, and it is sometimes referred to as "juvenile" Paget's disease, osteitis deformans in children or hyperostosis corticalis. There is an increased rate of bone turnover, with woven bone failing to mature into lamellar bone. Radiographically, this increased rate of bone turnover is evidenced by decreased bone density with coarsening and disorganisation of the trabecular pattern. In the skull the diploic space is widened and there is patchy sclerosis. The diaphyses of the long bones become expanded with cortical thickening along their concave aspects. The long bones may be bowed, resulting in coxa vara and protrusio acetabuli. The vertebral bodies are reduced in density, reduced in height and biconcave. The bowing of the limbs cause affected individuals to be short in height. There is often premature loss of dentition due to resorption of dentine with replacement of the pulp by osteoid.

The radiographic features closely resemble those of Paget's disease, but are diagnostic as they involve the whole skeleton and affect children from the age of 2 years. In contrast, Paget's disease is rare before the age of 40 years and skeletal involvement is either monostotic or asymmetrically polyostotic. On radionuclide scanning there is generalised increase in uptake giving a "super scan", due to excessive osteoblastic activity, with absence of evidence of renal uptake.

21.6
Conclusion

Metabolic and endocrine diseases affect the entire skeleton. Recognition of the radiological manifestations of these conditions in the pelvis and hips should therefore stimulate inquiry into the relevant biochemical status of the patient and may also precipitate further radiological investigation as appropriate

References

Adams JE (2002) Dialysis bone disease. Semin Dial 15:277–289

Adams JE (2003) Dual energy X-ray absorptiometry. In: Grampp S (ed) Radiology of osteoporosis. Springer Berlin Heidelberg pp 87–100

Adams JE (2005) Metabolic bone disease. In: Hodler J, Von Schulthess GK, Zollikofer ChL (eds) Musculoskeletal diseases – diagnostic and interventional techniques. Springer-Verlag Italia, pp 89–105

Adams JE (2005) Radiology of rickets and osteomalacia. In: Feldman D, Pike JW, Glorieux FH (eds) Vitamin D (2nd edition). Elsevier, San Diego, California and London, volume 2, pp 967–994

Adams JE, Davies M (1977) Paravertebral and peripheral ligamentous ossification: an unusual association of hypoparathyroidism. Postgrad Med J 53:167–172

Adams JE, Davies M (1986) Intra-spinal new bone formation and spinal cord compression in familial hypophosphataemic vitamin D resistant osteomalacia. Q J Med 61:1117–1129

Albright F, Burnett CH, Smith PH et al (1942) Pseudohypoparathyroidism - an example of "Seabright-Bantam Syndrome." Report of 3 cases. Endocrinol 30:922–932

Anderton JM (1979) Orthopaedic problems in adult hypophosphatasia: a report of two cases. J Bone Joint Surg Br 61:82–84

Baur A, Stäbler A, Brüning R, Bartl R, Krödel A, Reiser M, Deimling M (1998) Diffusion-weighted MR imaging of bone marrow: differentiation of benign versus pathologic compression fractures. Radiology 207:349–356

Blake GM, Fogelman I (2004) Bone densitometry and fracture risk prediction. Eur J Nucl Med Mol Imaging 31:785–786

Brill PW, Winchester P, Kleinman PK (1998) Differential diagnosis 1: diseases simulating abuse. In: Kleinman PK (ed) Diagnostic imaging of child abuse (2nd edn). Mosby, Inc. St. Louis, Missouri, pp 178–196

Brooks MH, Bell NH, Love L, Stern PH, Orfei E, Queener SF, Hamstra AJ, DeLuca HF (1978) Vitamin-D-dependent rickets type II. Resistance of target organs to 1,25-dihydroxyvitamin D. N Engl J Med 298:996–999

Carter DR, Bouxsein ML, Marcus R (1992) New approaches for interpreting projected bone densitometry data. J Bone Miner Res 7:137–145

Chuck AJ, Pattrick MG, Hamilton E, Wilson R, Doherty M (1989) Crystal deposition in hypophosphatasia: a reappraisal. Ann Rheum Dis 48:571–576

Consensus Development Conference Panel: Diagnosis and management of asymptomatic primary hyperparathyroidism: Consensus Development Conference Statement (1991) Ann Int Med 114:593–397

Cummings SR, Bates D, Black D (2002) Clinical use of bone densitometry. JAMA 288(15):1889–1897

Cundy T (2002) Idiopathic hyperphosphatasia. Semin Musculoskelet Radiol 6:307–312

Davies M (1992) Primary hyperparathyroidism: aggressive or conservative treatment? Clin Endocrinol (Oxf) 36:325–332

Davies M, Fraser WD, Hosking DJ (2002) The management of primary hyperparathyroidism. Clin Endocrinol (Oxf) 57:145–155

DeSmet AA, Neff JR (1985) Pubic and sacral insufficiency fractures: clinical course and radiological findings. Am J Roentgenol 145:601–606

Dimich A, Bedrossian PB, Wallach S (1967) Hypoparathyroidism. Arch Intern Med 120:449–458

Dodds WJ, Steinbach HL (1968) Primary hyperparathyroidism and articular cartilage calcification. Am J Roentgenol Radium Ther Nucl Med 104:884–892

Eastell R (1998) Treatment of postmenopausal osteoporosis. N Engl J Med 338:736–746

Econs MJ, Samsa GP, Monger M, Drezner MK, Feussner JR (1994) X-Linked hypophosphatemic rickets: a disease often unknown to affected patients. Bone Miner 24:17–24

Edminster KA, Sundaram M (2002) Oncogenic osteomalacia. Semin Musculoskelet Radiol 6:191–196

Faulkner KG, McClung M, Cummings SR (1994) Automated evaluation of hip axis length for predicting hip fracture. J Bone Miner Res 9:1065–1070

Ferrar L, Jiang G, Adams J, Eastell R (2005) Identification of vertebral fractures: an update. Osteoporos Int 16:717–728

Genant HK, Heck LL, Lanzl LH, Rossmann K, Horst JV, Paloyan E (1973) Primary hyperparathyroidism. A comprehensive study of clinical, biochemical and radiographic manifestations. Radiology 109:513–524

Genant HK, Baron JM, Straus FH, Paloyan E, Jowsey J (1975) Osteosclerosis in primary hyperparathyroidism. Am J Med 59:104–113

Genant HK, Wu CY, van Kuijk C, Nevitt MC (1993) Vertebral fracture assessment using a semiquantitative technique. J Bone Miner Res 8:1137–1148

Gipstein RM, Coburn JW, Adams DA, Lee DB, Parsa KP, Sellers A, Suki WN, Massry SG (1976) Calciphylaxis in man. A syndrome of tissue necrosis and vascular calcification in 11 patients with chronic renal failure. Arch Intern Med 136:1273–1280

Glorieux FH, St-Arnaud R (2005) Vitamin D Pseudo-deficiency. In:Eds. D. Feldman, F.H. Glorieux and J.W. Pike. Vitamin D, Volume 2, Academic Press, San Diego, California, pp 1197–1205

Glorieux FH, Marie PJ, Pettifor JM, Delvin EE (1980) Bone response to phosphate salts, ergocalciferol, and calcitriol in hypophosphatemic vitamin D-resistant rickets. N Engl J Med 303:1023–1031

Greenspan A (1991) Sclerosing bone dysplasias--a target-site approach. Skeletal Radiol 20:561–583

Guglielmi G, Lang TF (2002) Quantitative computed tomography. Semin Musculoskelet Radiol 6:219–227

Hain SF, Fogelman I (2002) Nuclear medicine studies inmetabolic disease. Semin Musculoskelet Radiol 6:323–329

Hans D, Genton L, Allaoua S, Pichard C, Slosman DO (2003) Hip fracture discrimination study: QUS of the radius and the calcaneum. J Clin Densitom 6:163–172

Hardy DC, Murphy WA, Siegel BA, Reid IR, Whyte MP (1989) X-linked hypophosphatemia in adults: prevalence of skeletal radiographic and scintigraphic features. Radiology 171:403–414

Harris HA (1933) Rickets. In:Bone growth in health and disease. Oxford Medical Publications, Oxford University Press, London, p 87

Hayes CW, Conway WF (1991) Hyperparathyroidism. Radiol Clin North Am 29:85–96

Jiang G, Eastell R, Barrington NA, Ferrar L (2004) Comparison of methods for the visual identification of prevalent vertebral fracture in osteoporosis. Osteoporos Int 15:887–896

Kanis J (2002) Diagnosis of osteoporosis and assessment of fracture risk. Lancet 359:1929–1936

Kanis JA, Glüer CC (2000) An update on the diagnosis and assessment of osteoporosis with densitometry. Committee of Scientific Advisors, International Osteoporosis Foundation. Osteoporos Int 11:192–202

Kaplan EL, Yoshiro Y, Salti G (1992) Primary hyperparathyroidism in the 1990s. Ann Surg 215:300–315

Kolb FO, Steinbach HL (1962) Pseudohypoparathyroidism with secondary hyperparathyroidism and osteitis fibrosa. J Clin Endocrinol Metab 22:59–70

Kröger H, Kotaniemi A, Vainio P, Alhava E (1992) Bone densitometry of the spine and femur in children by dual-energy x-ray absorptiometry. Bone Miner 17:75–85

Lawson J (2002) Drug-induced metabolic bone disorders. Semin Musculoskel Radiol 6:285–297

Looser E (1920) Uber spatrachitis und osteomalacie Klinishe ront-genologische und pathologischanatomische Untersuchungen. Drsch Z Chir 152:210–357

Lu PW, Cowell Lloyd-Jones CTSA et al (1996) Volumetric bone mineral density in normal subjects, aged 5–27 years. J Clin Endocrinol Metab 81:1586–1590

Marshall D, Johnell O, Wedel H (1996) Meta-analysis of how well measures of bone mineral density predict occurrence of osteoporotic fractures. BMJ 312:1254–1259

Mayo-Smith W, Rosenthal DI (1991) Radiographic appearances of osteopenia. Radiol Clin North Am 29:37–47

McCance RA (1947) Osteomalacia with Looser's nodes (Milkman's syndrome) due to raised resistance to vitamin D acquired about the age of 15 years. Q J Med16:33–47

McKenna MJ, Kleerekoper M, Ellis BI, Rao DS, Parfitt AM, Frame B (1987) Atypical insufficiency fractures confused with Looser zones of osteomalacia. Bone 8:71–78

Milgram JW (1977) Radiographical and pathological assessment of the activity of Paget's disease of bone. Clin Orthop 127:63–69

Milgram JW, Compere CL (1981) Hypophosphatemic vitamin D refractory osteomalacia with bilateral femoral pseudofractures. Clin Orthop Relat Res null:78–85

Milkman LA (1930) Pseudofractures (hunger osteopathy, late rickets, osteomalacia). Am J Roentgenol 24:29–37

Mughal MZ, Ward K, Adams J (2005) Assessmant of Bone status inchildren by densitometric and quantitative ultrasound techniques. In: Imaging in Children 2nd Edition. Eds Carty H, Brunelle F, Stringer DA, Kao SC. Elsevier Ltd volume 1:pp 477–486

Mundy GR (1999) Bone remodelling and its disorders (2nd edn) Martin Dunitz, London, pp 1–82

Mundy GR (1999) Osteopetrosis, in Bone remodelling and its disorders (2nd edn) Martin Dunitz, London, pp193–199

National Osteoporosis Society (2002) Position statement on the reporting of dual energy X-ray absorptiometry (DXA) bone mineral density scans. National Osteoporosis Society, Camerton, Bath BA2 0PJ. www.nos.org.uk

National Osteoporosis Society (2004) A practical guide to bone densitometry in children. National Osteoporosis Society, Camerton, Bath BA2 0PJ www.nos.org.uk

Okada K, Iida K, Sakusabe N, Saitoh H, Abe E, Sato K (1994) Pseudohypoparathyroidism-associated spinal stenosis. Spine 19:1186–1189

Parfitt AM (1969) Soft-tissue calcification in uremia. Arch Intern Med 124:544–556

Parfitt AM (1988) Bone remodelling: Relationship to the amount and structure of bone, and the pathogenesis and prevention of fracture, in Osteoporosis – Etiology, Diagnosis and Management, (Eds B. L. Riggs and L.J. Melton), Raven Press, New York, pp 45–93

Peh WC, Khong PL, Yin Y, Ho WY, Evans NS, Gilula LA, Yeung HW, Davies AM (1996) Imaging of pelvic insufficiency fractures. Radiographics 16:335–348

Pitt MJ (1981) Rachitic and osteomalacic syndromes. Radiol Clin North Am 19:581–599

Pitt MJ (1993) Rickets and osteomalacia are still around. Radiol Clin North Am 29:97–118

Polisson RP, Martinez S, Khoury M, Harrell RM, Lyles KW, Friedman N, Harrelson JM, Reisner E, Drezner MK (1985) Calcification of entheses associated with X-linked hypophosphatemic osteomalacia. N Engl J Med 313:1–6

Quek ST, Peh WC (2002) Radiology of osteoporosis. Semin Musculoskel Radiol 6:197–206

Rathbun JC, MacDonald JW, Robinson HM, Wanklin JM (1961) Hypophosphatasia: a genetic study. Arch Dis Child 36:540–542

Rauch F, Schoenau E (2001) Changes in bone density during childhood and adolescence: an approach based on bone's biological organization. J Bone Miner Res 16:597–604

Rauch F, Glorieux FH (2004) Osteogenesis imperfecta Lancet 363:1377–1385

Resnick DL (1982) Fish vertebrae. Arthritis Rheum 25:1073–1077

Ryan EA, Reiss E (1984) Oncogenous osteomalacia. Review of the world literature of 42 cases and report of two new cases. Am J Med 77:501–512

Salvesen HA, Boe J (1953) Idiopathic hypoparathyroidism. Acta Endocinol 14:214–226

Sargent MA, Fleming SJ, Chattopadhyay C, Ackrill P, Sambrook P (1989) Bone cysts and haemodialysis-related amyloidosis. Clin Radiol 40:277–281

Silverberg SJ, Gartenberg F, Jacobs TP et al (1995) Increased bone density after parathyroidectomy in primary hyperparathyroidism J Clin Endocrinol Metab 80:729–734

Steendijk R, Hauspie RC (1992) The pattern of growth and growth retardation of patients with hypophosphataemic vitamin D-resistant rickets: a longitudinal study. Eur J Pediatr 151:422–427

Steinbach H, Waldron BR (1952) Idiopathic hypoparathyroidism: analysis of 52 cases, including report of new case. Medicine 31:133–154

Steinbach HL, Young DA (1966) The roentgen appearance of pseudohypoparathyroidism (PH) and pseudo-pseudohypoparathyroidism (PPH). Differentiation from other syndromes associated with short metacarpals, metatarsals, and phalanges. Am J Roentgenol Radium Ther Nucl Med 97:49–66

Stoker DJ (2002) Osteopetrosis. Semin Musculoskelet Radiol 6:299–305

Study Group on assessment of fracture risk and its application to screening for postmenopausal osteoporosis WHO (1994) Technical report 843, World Health Organisation, Geneva, Switzerland, pp 5

Sundaram M (1989) Renal osteodystrophy. Skelet Radiol, 18:415–426

Taybi H, Lachman R (1996) Radiology of syndromes, metabolic disorders and skeletal dysplasias. 4th edn. Mosby Year Book, St. Louis, Missouri

Theodorou DJ, Theodorou SJ, Resnick D (2002) Imaging in dialysis spondyloarthropathy. Semin Dial 15:290–296

van Staa TP, Dennison EM, Leufkens HG, Cooper C (2001) Epidemiology of fractures in England and Wales. Bone 29:517–522

Wang XF, Duan Y, Beck TJ, Seeman E (2005) Varying contributions of growth and ageing to racial and sex differences in femoral neck structure and strength in old age. Bone 36:978–986

Watts NB (2004) Fundamentals and pitfalls of bone densitometry using dual-energy X-ray absorptiometry (DXA) Osteoporos Int 15:847–854

Weinstein RS, Whyte MP (1981) Heterogeneity of adult hypophosphatasia. Report of severe and mild cases. Arch Intern Med 141:727–731

Weisman Y, Hochberg Z (1994) Genetic rickets and osteomalacia. Curr Ther Endocrinol Metab 5:492–495

Whitehouse RW (2002) Paget's disease of bone. Semin Musculoskel Radiol 6(4):313–322

Wilson CR, Fogelman I, Blake GM, Rodin A (1991) The effect of positioning on dual energy X-ray bone densitometry of the proximal femur. Bone Miner 13:69–76

Wilson LC, Hall CM (2002) Albright's osteodystrophy and pseudohypoparathyroidism Semin Musculoskel Radiol 6:273–283

Wishart J, Horowitz M, Need A, Nordin BE (1990) Relationship between forearm and vertebral mineral density in postmenopausal women with primary hyperparathyroidism. Arch Intern Med 150:1329–1331

Wynne AG, van Heerden J, Carney JA, Fitzpatrick LA (1992) Parathyroid carcinoma: clinical and pathologic features in 43 patients. Medicine (Baltimore) 71:197–205

22 Tumours and Tumour-Like Lesions

DAVID RITCHIE, A. MARK DAVIES and DANIEL VANEL

CONTENTS

22.1
Introduction

In recent years, the management of tumours and tumour-like lesions of the bony pelvis, hip, groin and buttocks has improved due in part to advances in imaging. Cross-sectional imaging, particularly magnetic resonance (MR) imaging has had a major impact in tumour imaging particularly in surgical staging. This chapter discusses the role of imaging in tumours and tumour-like conditions around the bony pelvis and hips and is followed by a review of the more common bone and soft tissue lesions.

21.2
Epidemiology

There are several series analysing tumours around the bony pelvis, hip, groin and buttocks but most are affected to an extent by tertiary referral patterns that skew the true incidence. The incidence data quoted have been calculated by combining several authoritative texts on the subject (KRANSDORF 1995a,b; CAMPANACCI 1999; UNNI 1996). In this chapter, the bony pelvis and hip includes the ilium, ischium, pubis, sacrum and proximal femur. The soft tissues include the groin, buttocks and para and intraarticular regions of the hip but does not include the thigh or pelvic viscera.

The most common malignant bone tumours around the bony pelvis and hip are metastatic lesions and myeloma but the true incidence is unknown as many metastatic and myelomatous lesions do not present to specialised centres and may not be biopsied. Excluding metastatic disease and myeloma and combining the remaining primary malignant bone tumours from UNNI (1996) and CAMPANACCI (1999) (Table 22.1), 39% occurred in the ilium, 31% in the proximal femur, 19% in the sacrum, 7% in the pubis and 3% in the ischium. Chondrosarcoma is the most common primary malignant bone tumour with the majority in the ilium and proximal femur. Of the benign bone tumours in two large series, 60% occurred in the proximal femur, 17% in the ilium, 14% in the sacrum, 4% in the pubis and 3% in the ischium. Osteoid osteoma and osteochondroma accounted for more than 50% of benign bone tumours and were most commonly found in the proximal femur. In Campanacci's series of tumour-like lesions of bone around the pelvis and hip, excluding brown tumours, 67% were located in the

D. RITCHIE, MD
Department of Radiology, Royal Liverpool University Hospital, Prescot Street, Liverpool, L7 8XP, UK
A. M. DAVIES, MD
Consultant Radiologist, The MRI Centre, Royal Orthopaedic Hospital, Birmingham, B31 2AP, UK
D. VANEL, MD
Professor, Department of Radiology, Institut Gustave Roussy, 39 rue Camille Desmoulins, 94805 Villejuif, France

Table 22.1. Incidence of primary bone tumours around the pelvis and hips in descending order of incidence. Figures obtained by combining the results of UNNI (1996) and CAMPANACCI (1999). In the benign group, the figures for osteochondroma and chondroma are an underestimate as only the symptomatic lesions have been included. In the malignant group, metastases and myeloma have been excluded and the "lymphomas" contains patients with primary and generalised lymphoma. Note in the pelvis, chordoma is only found in the sacrum

Benign bone tumours (n=923)	%	Primary malignant bone tumour (n=2508)	%
Osteoid osteoma	33	Chondrosarcoma	28
Osteochondroma	22	Osteosarcoma	21
Giant cell tumour	19	Ewing's sarcoma	18
Chondroblastoma	7	Lymphoma	15
Osteoblastoma	6	Chordoma	10
Chondroma	5	Fibrosarcoma	4
Chondromyxoid fibroma	2	Malignant fibrous histiocytoma	2
Haemangioma	2	Malignant vascular tumour	2

proximal femur and 26% in the ilium. Of the femoral lesions, 71% were due to simple bone cyst, 17% Langerhans cell histiocytosis and 11% aneurysmal bone cyst. Langerhans cell histiocytosis (eosinophilic granuloma) was more common than simple or aneurysmal bone cyst in the ilium.

In Kransdorf 's series of 12,370 cases of soft tissue sarcoma, 7.5% were located around the hip, groin and buttocks (KRANSDORF 1995b; Table 22.2). Malignant fibrous histiocytoma (25.3%) and liposarcoma (19.2%) were the most common soft tissue sarcomas over 25 years. Infantile fibrosarcoma, angiomatoid malignant fibrous histiocytoma and rhabdomyosarcoma were the most soft tissue sarcomas under 15 years and synovial sarcoma between 16–25 years. In Kransdorf's series of 18,677 benign soft tissue tumours (including some tumour-like lesions; KRANSDORF 1995a), 50% were located around the hip, groin and buttocks. Lipoma accounted for 17.8% of all lesions and was the most common tumour over 26 years of age. Lipoblastoma, fibrous hamartoma of infancy and nodular fasciitis were the most common lesions under 15 years and neurofibroma, fibromatosis and benign fibrous histiocytoma between 16–25 years.

22.3
Detection

Patients with musculoskeletal tumours often present with pain and/or swelling. Delay in the diagnosis of pelvic tumours is not uncommon and is often

Table 22.2. Incidence of soft tissue tumours around the hip and buttocks in descending order of incidence (KRANSDORF 1995a,b)

Benign soft tissue tumours (n=935)	%	Malignant soft tissue tumours (n=930)	%
Lipoma	18	Malignant fibrous histiocytoma	25
Benign fibrous histiocytoma	9	Liposarcoma	19
Neurofibroma	9	Leiomyosarcoma	10
Myxoma	9	Dermatofibrosarcoma protuberans	8
Nodular/proliferative fasciitis	9	MPNST	6
Deep fibromatosis	8	Synovial sarcoma	6
Haemangiopericytoma	6	Fibrosarcoma	5
Schwannoma	6	Extraskeletal chondrosarcoma	3
Haemangioma	5	Angiosarcoma/haemangioendothelioma	3

MPNST, malignant peripheral nerve sheath tumour.

due to misdiagnosis (Wurtz et al. 1999). Despite newer imaging techniques, the radiograph remains the initial imaging investigation of choice although detection depends to a certain extent on radiographic technique, size and location and aggressiveness of the lesion. If the radiograph is under or overexposed or if the positioning is suboptimal, then a lesion may easily be overlooked. Lesions in the pubis or ischium are more easily detected since they contain less cancellous bone whereas lesions arising in thick cancellous bone such as the ilium may remain occult until there is sufficient destruction of the trabecular bone or evidence of cortical involvement (Fig. 22.1). Some aggressive tumours, including round cell tumours, typically show a permeative pattern of bone destruction and little or no apparent cortical destruction. However, in such cases, close inspection of the radiograph may reveal subtle intracortical lucencies as well as a periosteal reaction. The prominence of the overlying soft tissues and viscera around the pelvis means that some lesions, particularly those arising in the ilium or sacrum may be obscured until they reach a large size. Soft tissue lesions will only be seen if they display mass effect, bone or joint involvement or mineralisation.

The main role of bone scintigraphy (99mTc-methylene diphosphonate) is in the detection of metastatic disease although it also plays an important role in the detection of osteoid osteomas. Ultrasound (US) is useful for evaluating soft tissue lesions, guides biopsy and allows assessment of vascular lesions using colour flow Doppler techniques. Computed tomography (CT) is superior to MR

imaging at detecting matrix and periosteal mineralisation and cortical involvement and in selected cases both modalities may be complementary. However, for most bone and more complex soft tissue tumours, MR imaging is required for pre-operative staging, and imaging of suspected recurrence. As the anatomical site is large, adequate coverage will often require a body coil but the resolution is compromised. Alternatively, for localised lesions a dedicated hip, a flexible wrap round or phased-array pelvic coil can offer improved resolution with adequate coverage. Protocols vary with anatomical site and lesion extent (see Sect. 22.5).

22.4
Diagnosis

Before assessing the imaging studies, it is important to have relevant clinical information including symptoms, patient age, multiplicity, ethnic origin and family history. In general, benign bone tumours are more common than malignant bone tumours in childhood and young adults, whereas in older adults the reverse is true. Although age is important, the incidence of tumours in different age groups should also be taken into account. Metastases are by far the most common malignant bone tumours affecting the pelvis and hip over the age of 40 years whereas a malignant bone tumour in the second decade is likely to be due to an osteosarcoma or Ewing's sarcoma. Multiplicity of lesions in an older adult usu-

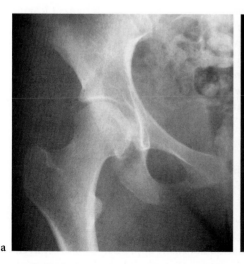 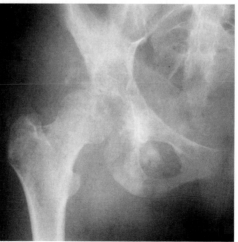

a   b

Fig. 22.1a,b. Osteosarcoma. **a** AP radiograph. The subtle lysis of the medial acetabulum was initially overlooked. **b** AP radiograph 5 months later when the diagnosis was first made. There is mixed lysis and sclerosis within the acetabulum and ischium with a large soft tissue mass containing amorphous tumour mineralization. The tumour mass is causing subluxation of the hip

ally indicates metastatic disease, multiple myeloma or lymphoma. In childhood, multiple lesions are more likely to be benign and the differential includes polyostotic fibrous dysplasia, Langerhans cell histiocytosis (Fig. 22.2), multiple enchondromatosis (Ollier's disease) and multiple exostoses (diaphyseal aclasis). Multiple lesions in the soft tissues include lipomas, fibromatosis, neurofibromatosis and arteriovenous malformations.

22.4.1
Location

Some bone tumours have a predilection for a particular bone. Osteoid osteomas and simple bone cysts are commonly found in the femoral neck and chordoma in the sacrum. In the growing skeleton, most primary neoplasms, both benign and malignant, occur in the vascular metaphysis whereas relatively few arise in the epiphysis. In children, a lesion in the femoral capital epiphysis should suggest either chondroblastoma (Fig. 22.3) or abscess. In adults, the differential for subarticular lesions includes metastasis, intraosseous ganglion, giant cell tumour and rarely, clear cell chondrosarcoma. Cartilaginous lesions are more frequently found in the region of the triradiate cartilage but chondroblastoma can also be found in the iliac crest at the site of the apophysis. Marrow-related lesions including myeloma, metastases, lymphoma predominate in the ilium due to the abundance of red marrow. Transarticular spread across joints of limited mobility, such as the sacroiliac joints is suggestive of a malignant lesion or locally aggressive lesions such as giant cell tumour (ABDELWAHAB et al. 1991).

Most soft tissue lesions do not have a predilection for a particular site around the bony pelvis, hip and groin but ganglion cysts are relatively common anterior to the hip and lesions in the path of a nerve such as the sciatic nerve should raise the possibility of a neural tumour.

22.4.2
Radiographic Features

22.4.2.1
Patterns of Bone Destruction

There may be difficulty in detecting early bone destruction in the sacrum and iliac bones due to their broad curved shape, large marrow space and

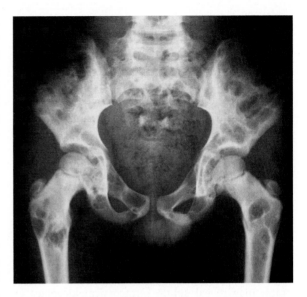

Fig. 22.2. Langerhans cell histiocytosis. AP radiograph showing multiple well defined lytic lesions

superimposition of bowel gas, faecal residue and vascular calcifications. Lesions involving the remaining pelvic bones and hip are usually easier to detect. Three basic patterns of bone destruction have been described and to a certain extent reflect the rate of tumour growth: geographic, moth-eaten and permeative. Geographic bone destruction is the slowest rate of growth and is depicted by well defined lytic lesion with a narrow zone of transition with or without a sclerotic rim (Fig. 22.4). A moth-eaten pattern with a wider zone of transition indicates a moderately aggressive lesion of intermediate growth rate and a permeative pattern with a wide zone of transition indicates a locally aggressive lesion with a rapid rate of growth (Fig. 22.5). Malignant lesions tend to have an aggressive (moth-eaten/permeative) pattern and benign lesions an indolent (geographic) pattern. However, there can be overlap between benign and malignant lesions and some tumours may show more than one pattern due to variable growth rate.

22.4.2.2
Tumour matrix

Bone and cartilage forming tumours often exhibit typical mineralisation patterns. In complex anatomical areas, such as the pelvis, CT will reveal mineralisation not easily appreciated on the conventional radiograph. Organised bone is characteristic of benign bone forming lesions such as an osteoblastoma whereas malignant osteoid is described

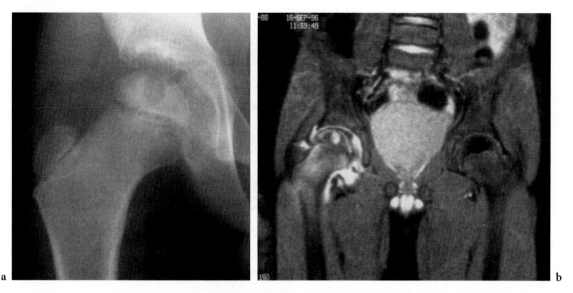

Fig. 22.3a,b. Chondroblastoma. **a** AP radiograph showing a well defined lytic lesion in the proximal femoral epiphysis. **b** Coronal T2-weighted image with fat suppression revealing the epiphyseal lesion with surrounding marrow oedema and a large joint effusion

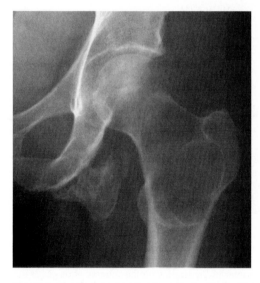

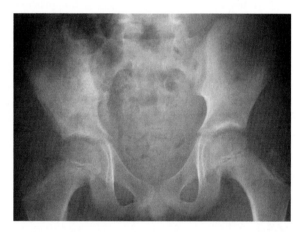

Fig. 22.5. Ewing's sarcoma. AP radiograph showing permeative bone destruction in the ilium with a lamellar periosteal reaction laterally

Fig. 22.4. Simple bone cyst. AP radiograph showing a well defined lytic lesion arising in the proximal femur with a thin sclerotic rim. There is an incidental chronic avulsion injury of the ischial apophysis that should not be mistaken for a bone-forming tumour

as fluffy, ill-defined, amorphous and cloud-like densities and indicates an aggressive bone lesion such as osteosarcoma (Fig. 22.1). Mineralised cartilage is variously described as flocculent, stippled, annular, comma shaped or pop corn calcification (Fig. 22.6). Identification of mineralised cartilage identifies the histological origin but does not distinguish between a benign or malignant tumour.

Mineralisation may also occur in various tumour and tumour-like lesions of the soft tissues, including malignant lesions such as synovial sarcoma and soft tissue chondrosarcoma and benign conditions such as haemangiomas (phleboliths).

22.4.2.3
Host Bone Response and Periosteal Reaction

The host response to a tumour can be assessed to a certain extent by its effect on the bony cortex.

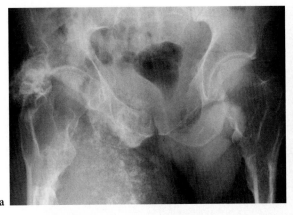
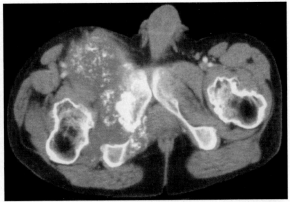

a   b

Fig. 22.6a,b. Diaphyseal aclasis with malignant transformation. **a** AP radiograph and (**b**) CT showing multiple osteochondromas with a large peripheral chondrosarcoma arising from the right pubis

Aggressive lesions tend to penetrate the cortex whereas the cortex may be an effective barrier to more indolent lesions. Slow growing intramedullary lesions tend to cause endosteal scalloping and may be associated with a smooth periosteal reaction. If the lesion continues to grow, the process of endosteal resorption and periosteal reaction will be repeated, resulting in an expansile lesion with a "cortical shell" (Fig. 22.7) or lamellar periosteal reaction (onion-skin) (Fig. 22.5). A more aggressive, complex, interrupted periosteal reaction may result in a "Codman's triangle", commonly found with primary bone sarcomas such as osteosarcoma although rarely seen in the pelvis. Other patterns such as the "sunburst" or "hair on end" patterns are also found. In intraarticular osteoid osteoma of the hip, the periosteal reaction is often limited.

22.4.3
Cross-Sectional Imaging

Scintigraphy using gallium-67 citrate and more recently fluorine-18 fluorodeoxyglucose (FDG) PET scanning have been helpful in distinguishing benign from malignant nerve sheath tumours and may be useful in patients with neurofibromatosis (Levine et al. 1987; Cardona et al. 2003). However, uptake of FDG can been shown in various histiocytic, fibroblastic and some neurogenic lesions regardless of whether they are benign or malignant. Therefore, for many musculoskeletal tumours, FDG PET scanning cannot be used to differentiate benign from malignant lesions, and it would appear that, as yet, FDG-PET scanning has a limited role in grading, staging, and monitoring of musculoskeletal sarcomas (Aoki et al. 2003).

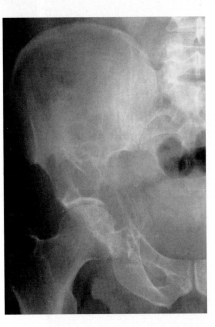

Fig. 22.7. Plasmacytoma. AP radiograph showing an expansile multiloculated lesion. The differential diagnosis in the middle aged and elderly would include metastases from renal and thyroid primaries. Depending on the country of origin of the patient, hydatid disease would also be have to be considered

Ultrasound has high accuracy in diagnosing the most common soft tissue lesions including lipomas and ganglion cysts and may obviate the need for further imaging. Lipomas are compressible, usually hyperechoic (relative to adjacent muscle or subcutaneous fat) and typically contain echogenic lines. Ganglion cysts are typically transonic with acoustic enhancement posteriorly and a well defined lobulated outline.

Whilst CT and MR imaging are equally good at detecting lipomatous and fluid containing lesions, CT is superior to MR imaging in demonstrating intralesional gas, mineralisation and cortical destruction

(Fig. 22.6b). CT is especially useful in the diagnosis of osteoid osteoma and the peripheral mineralisation of myositis ossificans (Fig. 22.8). On MR imaging, tissue characterisation based on signal intensities alone is not usually possible as most lesions display non-specific low to intermediate signal intensity (similar to muscle) on T1-weighting and high signal intensity on T2-weighting. The appearances will also vary with the type of tumour matrix and presence of mineralisation, necrosis and haemorrhage. Therefore, the same type of tumour may have different MR appearances. However, some lesions or parts of lesions may have more characteristics findings that may reduce the differential diagnosis.

For soft tissue tumours, the signs with the greatest specificity for malignancy included tumour necrosis, bone or neurovascular involvement and a mean diameter of more than 5 cm. For bone and soft tissue tumours, dynamic contrast-enhanced MR imaging using gadopentetate dimeglumine (Gd-DTPA) has been used to differentiate benign from malignant bone lesions (VERSTRAETE and LANG 2000; VAN RIJSWIJK et al. 2004). In general, malignant lesions tend to show more and a greater rate of enhancement than benign lesions but there is considerable overlap and the technique is of limited practical value in most cases. For example highly vascularised or perfused lesions such as ABC, Langerhans cell histiocytosis, osteoid osteoma, acute osteomyelitis and immature myositis ossificans may all show values in the malignant tumour range. However, dynamic imaging may be useful in differentiating benign from malignant myxoid tumours and "inactive" from an "active" cartilaginous tumours.

22.5
Staging

The objective of surgical staging is to define the tumour in terms of histological grade and anatomical extent. This guides local and adjuvant treatment and allows prediction of prognosis and possible recurrence and metastatic disease. It also allows comparative studies of different treatment regimens for similar groups of patients. Of the staging systems, the Enneking system is the most popular and has been adopted by the Musculoskeletal Tumour Society (ENNEKING et al. 1980). The Enneking system is applicable to mesenchymal tumours including osteosarcoma and chondrosarcoma but not round cell tumours such as Ewing's sarcoma and lymphoma.

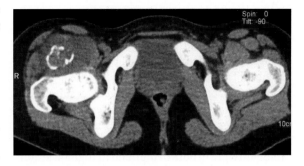

Fig. 22.8. Myositis ossificans. CT showing typical peripheral mineralization

Stage I lesions are classified as histologically low-grade lesions whereas stage II lesions are high grade. The stages are subdivided into A and B depending on whether the lesion is intra- (A) or extracompartmental (B) and is based on imaging findings. Patients with metastases at presentation are classified as stage III, irrespective of histological grade. Therefore, two of the three staging components, namely compartment status and metastatic spread rely entirely on imaging. For local staging, MR imaging is undoubtedly superior to CT at defining the intraosseous, soft tissue and extracompartmental spread of tumours and is the imaging method of choice (BLOEM et al. 1988; DE BEUCKELEER et al. 1996). However, in the pelvis, cortical involvement and periosteal reaction may be difficult to assess and in certain cases both techniques may be complementary. For indeterminate and aggressive lesions requiring biopsy, Gd-DTPA enhanced, fat-suppressed T1-weighted images are helpful in increasing lesion conspicuity and differentiating viable from necrotic tumour. A dynamic Gd-DTPA sequence may be useful as a baseline study prior to subsequent assessment of the tumour response to chemotherapy, especially for patients with osteosarcoma, Ewing's sarcoma or lymphoma. It is important that the local staging should precede biopsy as post-biopsy oedema/haemorrhage might exaggerate the size and extent of the tumour. Local staging requires accurate evaluation of bone and soft tissue extent, assessment of neurovascular and joint involvement and exclusion of skip metastases and lymphadenopathy, and this is discussed further in the following section.

22.5.1.1
Extent in Bone

For pelvic and proximal femoral lesions, MR sequences in all three planes may be required for an adequate assessment. Furthermore, where a primary bone sarcoma in the proximal femur is suspected, a large field of view T1-weighted sequence of the femur is required to exclude skip metastases. The field of view should include the adjacent joint for measurement purposes. T1-weighted, fat suppressed T2-weighted or STIR sequences all demonstrate contrast between osseous tumour and normal marrow although peri-tumoral oedema may obscure the true tumour margin in both benign and malignant lesions (Fig. 22.9). Indeed, benign lesions such as Langerhans cell histiocytosis, chondroblastoma, osteoid osteoma all cause extensive surrounding inflammatory response that can lead to confusion with a more aggressive process (Fig. 22.3b). Some authorities advocate a dynamic MR study to distinguish tumour from peri-tumoral oedema. The enhancement pattern is early with tumour and delayed with peritumoral oedema. However, this technique does not exclude isolated nests of tumour cells and it is prudent to include all abnormal marrow signal as suggestive of tumour for measurement purposes (SHAPEERO and VANEL 2000). Most of the oedema will resolve following chemotherapy and this can be verified on the re-staging MR scan prior to definitive surgery.

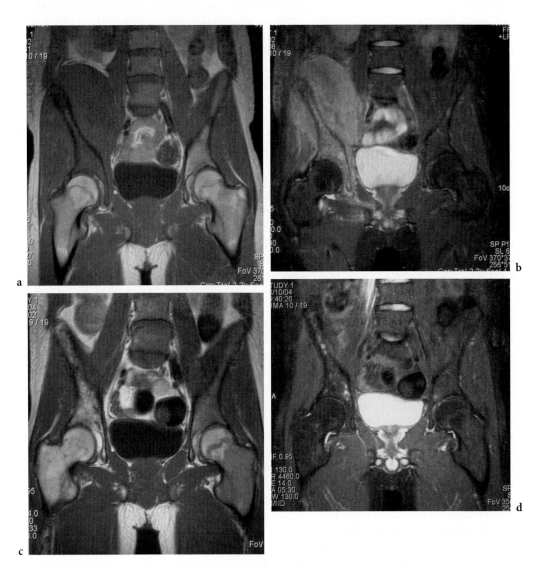

Fig. 22.9a–d. Ewing's sarcoma. **a** Coronal T1-weighted and (**b**) Coronal STIR images pre-treatment showing a massive tumour arising from the right ilium with soft tissue extension. **c** Coronal T1-weighted and (**d**) Coronal STIR images after treatment with chemotherapy and radiotherapy. There was an excellent response with almost complete regression of the tumour. Only a few foci of abnormal intraosseous signal remain. The fatty marrow on the right appears slightly hyperintense due to the radiotherapy effect

22.5.1.2
Extent in Soft Tissue

A lesion confined to a single bone or muscle within the pelvis is considered intracompartmental, but many lesions often show extracompartmental spread at presentation. In the upper thigh, there are three compartments: anterior, posterior and medial. The anterior compartment contains the tensor fascia lata and the quadriceps musculature. The posterior compartment contains the hamstring muscles and the sciatic nerve and the medial compartment contains the gracilis and adductor muscles. The groin and inguinal region including the neurovascular bundle are extracompartmental (ANDERSON et al. 1999). Typically, most bone and soft tissue tumours are isointense with muscle on T1-weighted images and optimal demonstration of soft tissue extent requires STIR or fat suppressed T2-weighted sequences (Fig. 22.9b). As with bone, distinguishing tumour from peri-neoplastic oedema may be problematic. For bone tumours that have spread into para-osseous soft tissues, the normal low SI cortex will typically display increased SI due to tumour replacement. With some aggressive tumours such as Ewing's sarcoma, the cortical destruction may be subtle but close inspection of the cortex will often reveal diffuse infiltration.

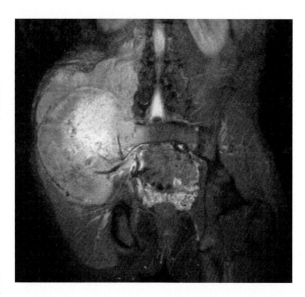

Fig. 22.10. Ewing's sarcoma. Coronal STIR image showing a massive tumour arising from the right ilium, extending across the sacroiliac joint into the sacrum and up the paravertebral muscles

the joint was found in around half the patients with chondrosarcoma or osteosarcoma and in only 4% of patients with Ewing's sarcoma (OZAKI et al. 2003). Most of the tumours infiltrated through the posterior part of the joint (Fig. 22.10b).

22.5.1.3
Joint Involvement

In primary bone sarcomas, assessment of joint involvement determines the need for articular resection. Pathological fracture into the joint can be taken as unequivocal evidence of joint involvement but the presence of a joint effusion by itself is an unreliable sign of joint involvement. However, the absence of an effusion has a high negative predictive value for joint invasion (SCHIMA et al. 1994). In a series of 67 patients with primary bone sarcomas around the hip, involvement of the hip joint was suspected by pre-operative imaging in 29 cases and confirmed histologically in 15 cases (OZAKI et al. 2002). Intraarticular involvement was found in 39% of chondrosarcomas, 12.5% of osteosarcomas and in none of the Ewing's sarcomas. The presence of cartilage disruption or mass inside the joint were more specific for intraarticular involvement than diffuse signal change or joint effusion. Most tumours infiltrated the joint through spread along the ligamentum teres. In another series by the same author analysing peri-articular primary bone sarcomas around the sacroiliac joint, infiltration of

22.5.1.4
Neurovascular Involvement

Encasement of the neurovascular bundle usually contraindicates limb salvage surgery. Tumours that involve the femoral triangle and medial pelvis predispose to iliac/femoral neurovascular involvement and lesions around the lateral sacrum, ischial tuberosity and posterior upper thigh to involvement of the sciatic nerve. Fortunately the prevalence of neurovascular involvement in musculoskeletal sarcomas is low (PANICEK et al. 1997). MR imaging can demonstrate whether the tumour is in close contact or encasing the neurovascular bundle but cannot distinguish mere contact from adherence or early invasion (Fig. 22.11). Optimal contrast between neurovascular bundle and other tissues including tumour is best achieved on T1-weighted fat sat post Gad DTPA or proton density (PD) fat-suppressed sequences (SAIFUDDIN et al. 2000). MR angiography adequately depicts the major vascular anatomy of suspected tumours and may be helpful in pre-operative planning but is not usually required in the work-up of most musculoskeletal tumours (LANG et

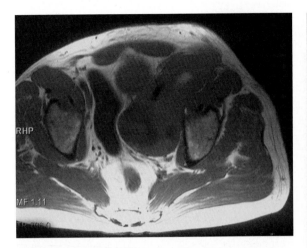

Fig. 22.11. Synovial sarcoma. Axial T1-weighted image showing a large intrapelvic mass encasing the left iliac vessels

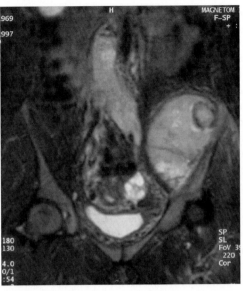

Fig. 22.12. Osteosarcoma. Coronal STIR image showing a large osteosarcoma arising from the left ilium. There is extension of the tumour up the inferior vena cava

al. 1995). Occasionally, large pelvic sarcomas may invade and extend along the pelvic veins and inferior vena cava (Fig. 22.12).

22.5.1.5
Lymphadenopathy

Lymph node spread is uncommon and usually a sign of late disease. There may be difficulty in distinguishing metastasis from reactive hyperplasia with the exception of the enlarged mineralised node due to spread from osteosarcoma (BEARCROFT and DAVIES 1999).

22.5.1.6
Distant Metastases

For detection of distant metastases, CT is the best technique at present for detecting early pulmonary metastases and should be performed routinely in the initial staging of bone and soft tissue sarcomas. Bone scintigraphy is of little value in assessing the primary lesion but is essential in the exclusion of multifocal disease in bone sarcomas. Alternatively, whole-body MR imaging may be performed for this purpose.

22.6
Biopsy

Musculoskeletal biopsy is best performed in the institution where definitive treatment is planned

and should only take place after the local staging has been completed. Close liaison among the radiologist, pathologist and orthopaedic surgeon is important in choosing the biopsy site. The biopsy may be a relatively minor procedure but the consequences of a poorly performed procedure may be significant. Complications resulting in alterations in treatment plan and outcome tend to be more common with open rather than percutaneous biopsy (MANKIN et al. 1996). The biopsy should be made within a single compartment avoiding neurovascular structures through an approach that can be resected at the definitive surgical procedure. It should be taken from the most aggressive and viable part of the lesion as determined by imaging. Many authorities now accept percutaneous biopsy as the technique of choice. The technique is quick, safe and has a low risk of complications and tumour seeding. Percutaneous biopsy has an accuracy rate of around 90% in most series (DUPUY et al. 1998). For soft tissue lesions, biopsy is usually performed with a Tru-Cut needle (Boston Scientific, Natick, MA) under ultrasound guidance, whereas a trephine bone-cutting needle under fluoroscopic or CT control is usually required for bony lesions. With the introduction of open configuration MR systems and MR compatible instruments, MR guided musculoskeletal biopsy has been shown to have a high success rate (GENANT et al. 2002). Dynamic contrast enhanced MR imaging is helpful in revealing regions with the fastest contrast enhancement, knowledge occasionally that may be useful when selecting the optimal biopsy site. MR guided biopsy is also likely to be useful for lesions that may be occult on other imaging guidance techniques such as an intramedullary lesions that have not breached the cortex. However, at the present time, MR guidance is more expensive and more time consuming than other imaging guided techniques and currently ultrasound, CT and fluoroscopic guidance remain the preferred imaging modalities.

22.7
Follow-Up

Follow-up cross-sectional imaging is often required both in the short-term for monitoring pre-operative chemotherapy and/or radiotherapy and long-term for suspected recurrence. Neoadjuvant chemotherapy is routinely used in almost all bone sarcomas with the exception of chondrosarcoma and chordoma and is increasingly being used in the management of some soft tissue sarcomas. Monitoring preoperative chemotherapy is important as the response to chemotherapy is one of the most reliable predictors of outcome. Pre-operative evaluation may have an impact on treatment protocols, post-operative chemotherapy, timing of surgery and planning radiotherapy. Doppler ultrasound has been used to assess the response of chemotherapy if there is a significant extraosseous component but the technique is operator dependent and reproducibility may be questionable on sequential scans (van der Woude et al. 1995). Conventional imaging techniques including static MR imaging are of limited value in differentiating good and poor responders. However, obliteration of the extraosseous component in Ewing's sarcoma usually indicates a good response and increased or unchanged tumour volume and increased peritumoral oedema suggests a poor response. On the other hand, it is worth noting that an increase in tumour volume may also be due to intralesional haemorrhage in a responsive tumour rather than due to a poor response (Fig. 22.9) (van der Woude et al. 1998). Standard contrast-enhanced MR imaging is also of limited value as viable tumour, revascularised necrotic tissue and reactive hyperaemia may all enhance. Consequently, much work has focused on dynamic contrast enhanced MR imaging. The alterations in time-intensity curves before and after chemotherapy have been shown to correlate well with tumour response. Foci of tumour that enhance within 3–6 s of the arterial phase correlate with viable tumour whereas late or gradual enhancement corresponds correlate with tumour necrosis, oedema or granulation tissue. A simple dynamic contrast enhanced technique with post-processing (subtraction, colour-encoding and time intensity curves) has been developed that can be used on standard MR consoles (Shapeero and Vanel 2000). One of the limiting factors is the failure of the technique to detect scattered tumour cells without nodule formation particularly in Ewing's sarcoma as they do not enhance sufficiently to be resolved on MR images. In osteosarcoma, this is not usually a problem as diffuse residual disease tends to persist as nodular islands. It should also be noted that the chondroblastic components of osteosarcoma typically show low vascularity mimicking tumour necrosis but knowledge of the pre-chemotherapy appearances should avoid this pitfall. Caution should also be shown if scanning is performed after the first cycle of chemotherapy as young granulation tissue replacing tumour necrosis may mimic viable tumour. Therefore, the final decision as to whether the patient is a responder or not should be delayed until the last pre-operative MR study.

In the long term, patients should be monitored to exclude tumour recurrence, metastatic disease and complications of treatment. Local recurrence is common if resection margins have not been wide and patients present with pain and or swelling. Radiographs may show bone destruction or a soft tissue mass close to the site of previous surgery and may be easier to detect if mineralised. Ultrasound is useful in excluding suspected soft tissue recurrences but the complex anatomy of the pelvis and depth of the tissues may make adequate assessment more difficult. Therefore, MR imaging is the technique of choice in the detection of early recurrence when local control may still be surgically achievable (Davies and Vanel 1998). Problems may be encountered in assessing the pelvis after hindquarter amputation due to major changes in the anatomy (Fig. 22.13) (Fowler et al. 1992). Diffuse high signal intensity on T2-weighting is frequently seen after surgery and can be prolonged following radiotherapy. Most recurrent tumours present with a mass that displays high signal intensity on T2-weighting although knowledge of the pre-operative MR characteristics is important as some lesions display low or intermediate signal intensity SI on T2-weighting (Vanel et al. 1994). Static intravenous contrast enhanced MR images are useful in distinguishing enhancing tumour from non-

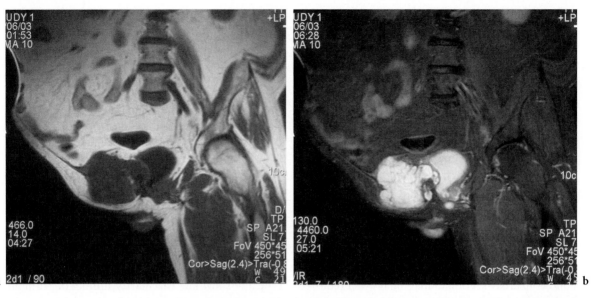

Fig. 22.13a,b. Recurrent chondrosarcoma. **a** Coronal T1-weighted and (**b**) coronal STIR images following hindquarter amputation. There is loss of the normal symmetrical soft tissue planes with recurrent tumour invading the bladder

enhancing seromas but healing granulation tissue will also enhance (Fig. 22.14) (DAVIES et al. 2004). A pitfall to the unwary is the soft tissue expander which may be inserted into the pelvis to displace small bowel from a radiation field. This will appear on follow-up MR imaging as a well defined mass hypointense on T1 and hyperintense on T2-weighted images and as a low attenuation mass with a hyperintense rim on CT (Fig. 22.15) (SAUNDERS et al. 1998). Where there is doubt in differentiating recurrent tumour from post-treatment changes then dynamic contrast enhanced MR imaging may again be useful. However, it should noted that within the first 6 months of radiotherapy young reactive granulation tissue may mimic recurrent tumour. Diffusion-weighted MR imaging may be helpful (BAUR et al. 2001). FDG PET scanning has shown promising results in the patients with suspected recurrence and equivocal MR findings (BREDELLA et al. 2002).

The vast majority of musculoskeletal sarcomas metastasise to the lungs. Routine follow-up chest radiographs are performed every 3 months for 2 years and every 6 months thereafter up to 5 years. If there is suspicion of metastatic disease in the chest then a CT scan is performed but routine CT scans of the lungs are not recommended. Osseous metastases may occur with bone sarcomas and may occur in the absence of pulmonary metastases. However, bone scintigraphy is not recommended unless the patient has local recurrence, lung metastases or bone pain. A pitfall to the unwary on MR imaging are the foci

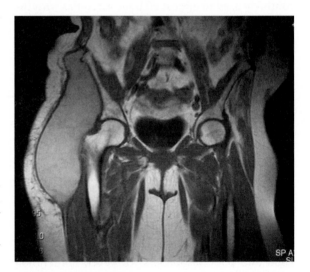

Fig. 22.14. Postoperative seroma. Coronal T1-weighted image showing a well defined mass lying adjacent to the right ilium and greater trochanter at the site of previous excision of a sarcoma. The hyperintense contents indicate either subacute haemorrhage or highly proteinaceous material

of marrow conversion due to granulocyte-stimulating therapy which may mimic disseminated disease (HARTMAN et al. 2004).

The treatment of musculoskeletal sarcoma is often protracted and complications are not uncommon. These include infections associated with immunosuppressive and toxic effects of chemotherapy, mechanical loosening and infective complications of prostheses. In the long term, pain or loss of function

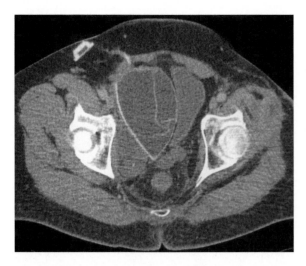

Fig. 22.15. Soft tissue expander. The CT shows the expander as an intrapelvic soft tissue mass with a hyperintense rim overlying the recurrent soft tissue sarcoma lying on the right iliacus muscle. The entry portal to the expander is visible in the anterior subcutaneous tissues

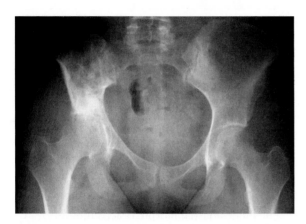

Fig. 22.16. Radiation induced osteosarcoma following treatment of a Wilms' tumour in childhood. AP radiograph showing the sarcoma in the right ilium. There is also radiation induced hypoplasia of the right hemipelvis

in a radiation field should raise the possibility of bone necrosis or radiation induced sarcoma (Fig. 22.16). Metastases to lymph nodes are uncommon. However, groin lymphadenopathy may be due to other causes including a foreign body reaction to lymphatic uptake of metal shed by the prosthesis (DAVIES et al. 2001). In patients treated with above knee amputation, posttraumatic neuromas in the thigh may mimic lymphadenopathy (BOUTIN et al. 1998).

22.8
Bone Tumours

22.8.1
Benign Bone Tumours

Osteoid osteoma accounts for 33% of benign bone tumours of the pelvis and hip but 94% of these arise in the femoral neck and involvement of the pelvis is uncommon. There a male predominance (3:1) and most present in the second. Radiographs of cortical lesions usually reveal a lucent or mineralised nidus with surrounding sclerosis. However, with intraarticular lesions, often found in the femoral neck, the surrounding sclerosis may be absent and the nidus occult (Fig. 22.17). In such cases, the reactive changes are more likely to result in a synovitis and joint effusion and lesions may mimic a monoarthropathy. Bone scintigraphy is useful in identifying the location and may reveal the "double density sign" where the central nidus shows greater uptake than the inflammatory response in the surrounding bone. CT is usually required for precise localisation and helps plan for arthroscopic or percutaneous resection or CT-guided radiofrequency thermoablation (Fig. 22.17c). On MR imaging, appearances can be confusing as there is typically extensive marrow oedema and surrounding inflammatory changes that may obscure the nidus or suggest another process such as infection, trauma or tumour. The nidus may have variable signal intensity depending on the amount of fibrovascular tissue and mineralisation (DAVIES et al. 2002). Non-mineralised nidi typically show homogeneous enhancement whereas enhancement in mineralised lesions results in the ring enhancement sign (YOUSEFF et al. 1996). Osteoblastoma is histologically similar to osteoid osteoma and also has a predisposition for the femoral neck. The radiological appearances may also be similar but osteoid osteomas tend to be less than 1 cm in size and osteoblastomas larger than 2 cm. Radiologically, sub-periosteal lesions are often associated with a soft tissue mass and matrix mineralisation Occasionally, some lesions display aggressive features with cortical destruction and infiltration of adjacent structures mimicking an osteosarcoma. The term "aggressive osteoblastoma" is controversial (CHEUNG et al. 1997).

Chondroblastoma is a relatively uncommon benign bone but has a predilection for the proximal femur accounting for 22% of all chondroblastomas. Approximately 60% of cases present in the second decade with a slight male predominance. The lesion

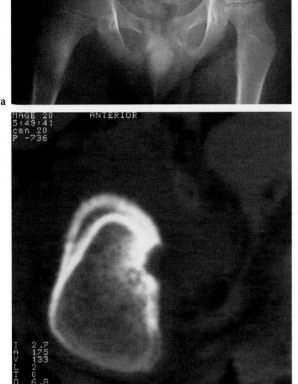

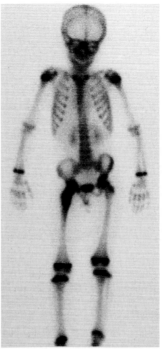

Fig. 22.17a–c. Osteoid osteoma. **a** AP radiograph showing osteopenia of the right proximal femur with faint sclerosis along the medial aspect of the femoral neck. **b** Bone scintigraphy showing non-specific increased activity in the right proximal femur. **c** CT showing the typical nidus medially and mild lamellar periosteal reaction anteriorly. The surrounding soft tissue swelling is due to the associated joint effusion

favours an epiphyseal or apophyseal location and accounts for the high incidence in the femoral head or capital epiphysis and greater trochanter. Less commonly it develops in the acetabulum in the region of the tri-radiate cartilage. Radiographs typically show a well defined lytic lesion with or without sclerotic margins (Fig. 22.3a). Mineralisation is common but is often subtle and more easily detected on CT. Expansion should raise the possibility of a secondary aneurysmal bone cyst. On MR imaging, T2-weighted images typically show variable amounts of intermediate/low SI tissue that are due to haemosiderin, calcifications and chondroblast hypercellularity as well as fluid-fluid levels in cases with secondary ABC components. A reactive inflammatory response is common and results in surrounding bone marrow oedema and often joint effusion (Fig. 22.3b). Similar imaging appearances may be seen with clear cell chondrosarcoma but chondroblastoma occurs in younger patients, is smaller than clear cell chondrosarcoma and is more confined to the epiphysis (COLLINS et al. 2003).

Uncommonly, chondroblastoma may follow a more aggressive course and metastatic disease has been described (RAMAPPA et al. 2000).

Enchondroma (chondroma) accounts for 5% of benign bone tumours around the pelvis and hip but 75% of these lesions occur in the proximal femur and involvement of the pelvis is uncommon. Radiologically, enchondromas are usually less than 5 cm in size and are characterised by a well-defined lytic lesion that may contain punctate or stippled calcifications. Differentiation from a low grade chondrosarcoma may be difficult both radiologically and histologically and this is discussed further in the section on chondrosarcoma. The risk of malignant transformation in enchondroma is controversial. Some authors argue that the risk of malignant transformation in a solitary enchondroma greater than 8 cm in size is 5%, whereas others maintain that such lesions were chondrosarcomas from their inception. However, in Ollier's disease (multiple enchondromas or enchondromatosis), the overall risk of sarcomatous transformation is 25% and much higher in Maffucci's syndrome (enchondromatosis and soft tissue haemangiomas).

Osteochondroma (exostosis) is a common benign bone tumour that accounts for 22% of benign bone tumours around the pelvis and hip. It is a growth plate aberration rather than a true tumour but is classified with benign chondrogenic tumours. It most commonly occurs in the proximal femur (53%) and most cases in the pelvis arise in the iliac bone (38%). Radiographically, lesions appear as a sessile or pedunculated exophytic outgrowth from the bone surface that shows continuity with the marrow cavity and cortex (Fig. 22.18). The cartilage cap may be calcified. A painful lesion or continued growth after maturity should raise the possibility of sarcomatous degeneration in the cartilage cap although this is rare in solitary lesions. A cap thickness of greater than 2 cm is suggestive of malignant transformation. The cartilage cap displays low signal intensity on T1-weighted and very high SI on T2-weighted and STIR images due to its high water content and is easily distinguished from adjacent muscle and ossific stalk (Fig. 22.18b). MR imaging is also helpful in excluding other complications including bursitis and pressure effects on adjacent structures. In hereditary multiple exostoses (diaphyseal aclasis), 9% of the lesions occur in the pelvis and hip. Sarcomatous degeneration has a reported incidence of between 1.5%–10% but the true incidence is probably less than 1% (Fig. 22.6) (PETERSON 1989).

Giant cell tumour is a locally aggressive tumour that accounts for 19% of benign bone tumours around the pelvis and hip. It has a predilection for the sacrum and accounts for 57% of all benign sacral tumours. Radiographically, lesions are typically osteolytic and expansile and usually have a geographic pattern of bone destruction with a well defined margin (Fig. 22.19). However, in up to 15% of cases, a more aggressive appearance may be seen with ill-defined margins and soft tissue infiltration. On MR imaging, lesions are inhomogeneous with variable signal intensity and often fluid-fluid levels due to secondary aneurysmal bone cyst formation. Foci of low or intermediate signal intensity on T2-weighted images are usually present and are likely to be due to collagen deposition, high cellularity and haemosiderin from previous haemorrhage. Peritumoral oedema is uncommon in the absence of a fracture. There is inhomogeneous enhancement in the solid areas of the tumour and peripherally about the cystic regions. Sacral lesions are often difficult to manage and standard treatments are associated with significant complica-

tions and recurrence rates. Arterial embolization either alone or in conjunction with other therapy seems to be of value (LIN et al. 2002). Giant cell tumour may rarely develop in pagetoid bone.

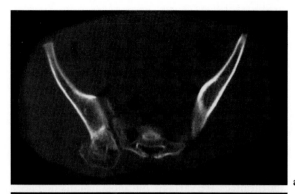

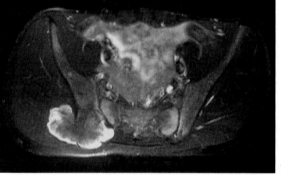

Fig. 22.18a,b. Osteochondroma. **a** CT showing the osteochondroma to be arising from the posterior ilium. The trabeculae are continuous with the underlying medullary bone. **b** Axial T2-weighted image with fat suppression showing a thin hyperintense cartilage cap

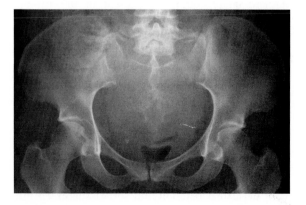

Fig. 22.19. Giant cell tumour. AP radiograph showing almost complete destruction of the sacrum

22.8.2
Malignant Bone Tumours

Osteosarcoma is the second most common primary bony malignancy of the pelvis and hip accounting for 21% of all primary malignancies excluding myeloma. The majority arise in the second decade and are more common in males (Fig. 22.1). Lesions occurring in older patients are often due to secondary degeneration of a pre-existing condition. Approximately 37% of all Paget's osteosarcomas and 29% of all radiation osteosarcomas occurred in the pelvis in one series (Fig. 22.16) (UNNI 1996). Primary lesions are most commonly found in the ilium (45%) or proximal femur (35%) and most are high grade. It is generally accepted that micrometastases are present in most patients at presentation although only 27% may be demonstrable by imaging techniques (BIELACK et al. 2002). The radiological appearances are variable but most lesions display a mixed lytic/sclerotic appearance with a moth-eaten or permeative pattern of bone destruction and soft tissue extension is common (Fig. 22.1). Matrix mineralisation appears as cloud-like or fluffy densities and helps to differentiate from other sarcomas including Ewing's sarcoma. Periosteal reaction is common but more difficult to detect in the ilium. On MR imaging, lesions typically display low to intermediate signal intensity on T1-weighting and inhomogeneous high signal intensity on T2-weighting. Mineralised foci often display low signal on all sequences.

Chondrosarcoma is the most common primary bone sarcoma around the pelvis and hip. Lesions of the pelvis and hip account for approximately 39% of all chondrosarcomas and 28% of all primary bony malignancies excluding myeloma. The majority involve the ilium (40%) and proximal femur (38%). Patients more commonly present in the 4th–6th decades with non-mechanical pain. Central intramedullary lesions are more common than peripheral lesions, which typically occur in the cap of a pre-existing osteochondroma. In the pelvic bones, lesions may attain a large size before being detected as the cancellous infiltration and mineralisation may be occult on initial radiographs. A poorer prognosis is associated with large, high grade lesions in the pelvis. The imaging appearances are variable and reflect tumour grade. High grade lesions typically have a permeative pattern of bone destruction with periosteal reaction and soft tissue extension. Low grade lesions often have a less aggressive geographic pattern that results in endosteal scalloping

and cortical expansion. However, enchondromas can have similar appearances both radiologically and histologically resulting in a diagnostic dilemma. Some argue that the a size greater than 5 cm is a reliable predictor of malignancy whereas others place more importance on the depth of cortical involvement. Cortical scalloping of greater than two-thirds of the cortical thickness should raise the possibility of chondrosarcoma (MURPHEY et al. 1998). Bone scintigraphy and dynamic contrast enhanced MR scanning also have their proponents but there is still controversy. However, in the pelvic bones, as enchondromas are uncommon, chondrosarcoma is much more likely than enchondroma, particularly if the lesion is greater than 5 cm in size and the patient is over 30 years of age. CT is the most sensitive technique for detecting mineralisation and will detect mineralisation in over 90% of cases. On MR imaging, the non-mineralised chondroid matrix displays high signal intensity on T2-weighting and separated into lobules by low signal fibrovascular septa (Fig. 22.13). Mineralised components will display low signal intensity on all sequences although low signal intensity can also be found in dedifferentiated chondrosarcoma (SAIFUDDIN et al. 2004). Soft tissue infiltration and transarticular spread extension are best assessed by MR. Of the rarer sub-groups, clear cell chondrosarcoma has a predilection for the epimetaphyseal region of the proximal femur and carries a better prognosis (COLLINS et al. 2003).

Although malignant fibrous histiocytoma (MFH) and fibrosarcoma are different pathological entities, they are discussed together as they have similar imaging appearances. Together, they account for 6% of malignant bone tumours around the pelvis and hip. Approximately 23% of all MFH/fibrosarcomas arise in the pelvis and most of these occur in the ilium or proximal femur. Both lesions may arise secondarily to previous irradiation, Paget's disease or de-differentiation of a chondrosarcoma. MFH may also arise in a previous bone infarct. Radiographs typically show a lytic lesions with an aggressive moth-eaten pattern of bone destruction. Dystrophic mineralisation is occasionally present but periosteal reactions and expansive growth are rarely seen (LINK et al. 1998). On MR imaging, the signal characteristics are non-specific but lesions may display an inhomogeneous, nodular signal pattern with peripheral enhancement. If the collagen content is high then a lower signal intensity on T2-weighting may be obtained. Foci of haemorrhage and necrosis may be present and extraosseous tumour spread is frequent.

Fig. 22.20a,b. Chordoma. **a** Lateral radiograph which shows subtle destruction of the posterior aspect of S1. **b** Sagittal T2-weighted image showing the tumour extending posteriorly into the spinal canal

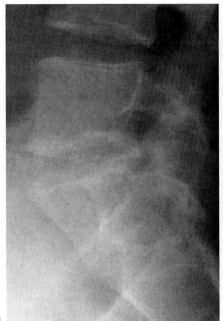

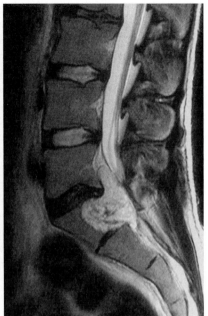

a

b

Chordoma is a slow growing, low grade, malignant neoplasm (arising from notochordal remnants) that is most common primary malignant tumour of the sacrum. Sacral lesions account for approximately 50% of all chordomas and 50% of all primary sacral malignancies excluding myeloma. It is more common in males and the majority occur in the 6th and 7th decades. Lesions typically arise centrally in the lower sacral segments and may attain a large size as they usually grow anteriorly into the posterior pelvic cavity. Lesions may be difficult to detect but approximately 80% of chordomas are visible on conventional radiographs (Fig. 22.20). Lesions are usually slow growing and often show geographic destruction with a sclerotic margin in up to 45% of cases. Intralesional mineralisation can be seen in up to 70% of cases on radiographs and in 90% of cases by CT. On CT, the non-mineralised portions typically show low attenuation due to the myxoid nature of the tissue. On MR imaging, the non-mineralised portions display low to intermediate signal intensity on T1-weighting and very high signal intensity on T2-weighting whereas the mineralised portions display low signal intensity on all sequences. Inhomogeneous enhancement is typically seen on post-contrast sequences. Accurate staging with MR imaging and a wide resection are required as many recurrences are thought to be due to residual tumour in the gluteal muscles (BRUNEL et al. 2002; BARATTI et al. 2003).

Ewing's sarcoma is an aggressive round cell tumour with a predilection for the pelvis and hip. Lesions of the pelvis and hip account for 35% of all Ewing's sarcomas and approximately of 18% of all primary malignant bone tumours around the pelvis and hip excluding myeloma. Presentation is usually in the second decade with a painful swelling and slight male predominance. Lesions are most commonly found in the ilium (45%) and proximal femur (24%) (see Figs. 22.5, 22.9). Poor prognostic factors include pelvic location, size > 8 cm, age > 17 years and metastatic disease at presentation. Radiographs show an aggressive lytic lesion with a moth-eaten or permeative pattern of bone destruction and lamellated periosteal reaction that may be difficult to detect in the pelvis. Although lesions do not produce a mineralised matrix, reactive sclerotic components may occur and are more common in the pelvis. On MR imaging, lesions are usually hypo- or isointense with muscle on T1-weighting but are of variable signal intensity on T2-weighting. Components displaying low or intermediate signal intensity on T2-weighting are probably due to high cellularity. Haemorrhage and necrosis may also be present.

Multiple myeloma is the most common primary malignancy of bone around the pelvis and hip and most commonly presents in the 6th and 7th decades. Approximately 33% of lesions occur around the pelvis and hip, most commonly in the ilium and proximal femur. The ilium is a common site for solitary plasmacytoma but conventional imaging may underestimate the disease extent as 33% of patients with newly diagnosed solitary plasmacytoma by routine criteria in one study had additional lesions detected on MR imaging of the dorsolumbar spine (MOULOPOULOS et al. 1995). Radiographically, most lesions show a moth-eaten pattern with focal punched out lesions but myeloma may also display a diffuse osteoporosis. Plasmacytomas typically present as expansile geographic lesions (Fig. 22.7). Occasionally myeloma can have a sclerosing appearance.

Metastatic lymphoma is common around the pelvis and hip whereas primary lymphoma of bone is rare. At least 33% of lymphomas involve the pelvis and 80% of those involve the ilium or the proximal femur. Involvement is usually by haematogenous spread and less commonly direct extension from affected lymph nodes and adjacent soft tissues. Radiographically, all lymphomas show a predominantly lytic aggressive moth-eaten or permeative pattern of bone destruction although a sclerotic or mixed appearance is not uncommon with Hodgkin's disease. Periosteal reaction, cortical destruction and soft tissue extension are common and sequestra may also be present. On MR imaging, there is often a large para-osseous soft tissue component without obvious frank destruction but close inspection of the axial MR images will usually reveal subtle permeation in the cortex (KRISHNAN et al. 2003). Most lesions are iso- or hypointense to skeletal muscle on T1-weighting and inhomogeneous and variable signal on T2-weighting (WHITE et al. 1998).

Metastases are the most common tumours around the pelvis and hip. In a large series of bone metastases, 16% occurred in proximal femur, 12% in ilium (CAMPANACCI 1999). The majority of metastases are from lung, breast, prostate, colon, kidney and bladder primaries. Radiographically, the majority have a moth-eaten pattern of bone destruction without a periosteal reaction. Occasionally, metastases have an expansile appearance indicating a slower rate of growth and often a renal or thyroid primary site. Prostatic metastases are usually sclerotic and breast, bladder and gastrointestinal primaries may be lytic, sclerotic or mixed (Fig. 22.21). The MR imaging features are non-specific. Osteoblastic metastases display low signal intensity on all sequences.

22.8.3
Tumour-Like Lesions of Bone

There are several lesions that may mimic bone tumours. Gout, infection, Paget's disease, stress fractures and chronic avulsion injuries are discussed in other chapters (see Fig. 22.4).

Fibrous dysplasia is a relatively common developmental anomaly that commonly affects the bony pelvis and hip in both monostotic and polyostotic forms. Polyostotic disease tends to present in the first decade with pain or pathological fracture or with endocrine problems (Albright's syndrome). Monostotic disease more commonly presents in the second decade as an incidental finding or after innocuous trauma. Radiographs show a well defined, intramedullary, expansile lesion often with endosteal scalloping and sclerotic margin of variable thickness. The matrix is variable ranging from lucent to sclerotic. In the proximal femur, the abnormal modelling may result in marked varus deformity, often referred to as the "Shepherd's crook" deformity (Fig. 22.22). MR imaging shows a hypo or isointense signal intensity compared with muscle on T1-weighting and a variable signal intensity on T2-weighting depending on the cellularity and fibrous and mineralised components.

Langerhans cell histiocytosis (LCH) is a relatively uncommon spectrum of diseases but does have a predilection for the pelvis and hip. In one series, 20% of all lesions occurred in the ilium and 15% in the proximal femur (CAMPANACCI 1999). Its localised form, eosinophilic granuloma, accounts for 70% of cases and heals spontaneously. In the early phase, radiographs and MR imaging typically demonstrate an aggressive pattern of bone destruction with ill-defined margins and lamellated periosteal reaction simulating Ewing's sarcoma (Fig. 22.23). However, in the later healing phase, they have well defined sclerotic margins simulating a benign bone tumour.

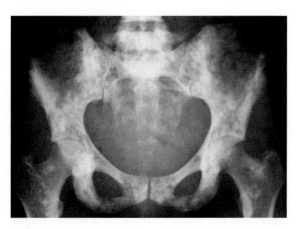

Fig. 22.21. Metastases. AP radiograph showing disseminated sclerotic breast metastases

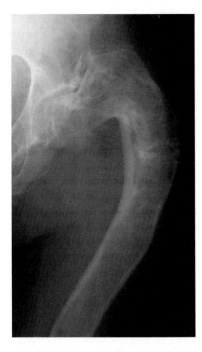

Fig. 22.22. Polyostotic fibrous dysplasia. AP radiograph showing the disease affecting the ilium and femur. A combination of bone softening and previous fractures has resulted in the "shepherd's crook" appearance of the proximal femur

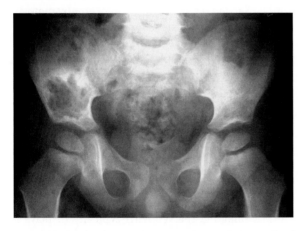

Fig. 22.23. Langerhans cell histiocytosis. AP radiograph of solitary lesion (eosinophilic granuloma) arising in the right ilium. There is some surrounding sclerosis and lamellar periosteal reaction laterally

The simple (unicameral) bone cyst (SBC) has a predisposition for the proximal femur accounting for 25% of all simple bone cysts and 71% of tumour-like lesions in the proximal femur (Fig. 22.4) (CAMPANACCI 1999). Lesions in the pelvis are uncommon and usually found in the ilium. Radiographs reveal a well-defined lytic lesion often with a sclerotic rim. On CT and MR imaging, lesions typically display fluid characteristics although the density on CT

and signal intensity on T1-weighted MR imaging may be greater than water due to high protein content. Fluid-fluid levels and solid areas representing reparative tissue may be seen in SBC complicated by fracture.

Aneurysmal bone cyst (ABC) is a benign expansile lesion characterised by multiple blood-filled cystic cavities. It is relatively uncommon in the pelvis and hips with approximately 7% of all ABCs found in the proximal femur, 6% in the ilium and 2% in the sacrum, pubis and ischium. 80% of lesions occur between 5–15 years of age and most are primary lesions. ABC like features can be found with other precursor lesions including giant cell tumour, chondroblastoma and telangiectatic osteosarcoma and are termed secondary lesions. For primary lesions, the imaging appearances mirror its evolution through various stages. In the early phase, radiographs show a markedly expansile lytic lesion that may have a "blown out" appearance (Fig. 22.24). The periosteal new bone may be barely perceptible due to the rapid rate of growth and mimic an aggressive sarcoma (CAMPANACCI 1999). In the stabilisation phase, the periosteal bone matures resulting in a surrounding mineralised shell and in the healing phase, there is consolidation of the lesion with further thickening and maturation of the periosteal bone. Cross-sectional imaging is also useful (MAHNKEN et al. 2003). In the early phase, the thin rim of intact periosteal tissue gives a low signal on all MR sequences and CT may reveal subtle periosteal mineralisation that is radiographically occult. MR imaging is more sensitive than CT at detecting fluid-fluid levels that result from the sedimentation effect of blood products within the cystic spaces (Fig. 22.24b). In primary lesions, intravenous contrast confirms rim and septal enhancement, whereas in secondary lesions the enhancement pattern depends on the extent and nature of the underlying lesion. It is worth stressing that telangiectatic osteosarcoma may resemble ABC both on imaging and histology.

22.9
Joint Tumours

Primary synovial osteochondromatosis is an uncommon condition that results in synovial metaplasia and multiple round intrasynovial cartilaginous nodules that may ossify. After the knee, the hip is the second most common site of involvement accounting for approximately 17.3% of all cases

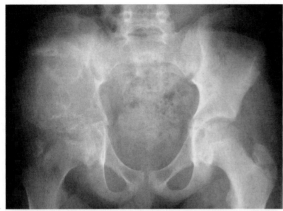

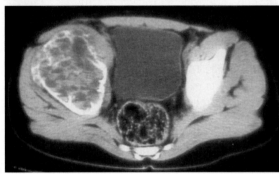

a

b

Fig. 22.24a,b. Aneurysmal bone cyst. **a** AP radiograph showing a large multiloculated lesion arising in the right ilium. **b** CT showing expansion with multiple fluid-fluid levels

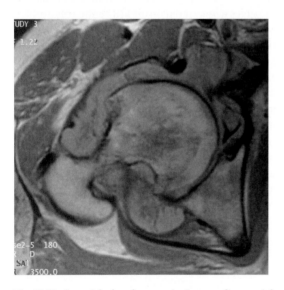

Fig. 22.25. Synovial chondromatosis. Intermediate weighted image showing a large hip joint effusion containing some signal voids due to calcification. There is concentric erosion of the femoral neck – "apple core sign"

(CAMPANACCI 1999). It has a male preference and presents in the 3rd–5th decades with joint stiffness and variable pain. As the disease progresses, secondary osteoarthritis is common. The radiographic appearances varies with the extent and duration of the condition. Nodule mineralisation is common and may vary from small punctate to larger denser calcifications and less commonly ossifications. Well defined bony erosions are also common in a tight joint such as the hip. Erosion of the femoral neck may produce the so-called "apple core sign" and result in a fracture (Fig. 22.25). The mineralised nodules are often of similar size although a dominant nodule may be present. On MR imaging, unmineralised lesions are less common than mineralised lesions but give an intermediate signal intensity on T1-weighting and a very high signal intensity on T2-weighting (KRAMER et al. 1993). However, the majority of cases contain foci of low/intermediate signal intensity on both T1-weighting and T2-weighting due to calcification of cartilaginous nodules. Nodules typically show peripheral enhancement following intravenous gadolinium administration. Chondrosarcomatous degeneration is very rare but has been reported (WITTKOP et al. 2002). Secondary synovial osteochondromatosis due to pre-existing osteochondroma has also been also been recorded around hip (PEH et al. 1999).

Pigmented villonodular synovitis is a term given to a proliferative tumour-like disorder of synovium of joints or tendon sheaths. After the knee, the hip is the second most commonly involved joint accounting for 17% of all cases (CAMPANNACCI 1999). It usually presents in young or middle aged adults with a painful effusion. Radiographs may show an effusion but there is preservation of joint space and bone density. Well-defined erosions are commonly found on both sides of the joint due to the tight hip capsule. On MR imaging, the synovitis typically displays a characteristic low/intermediate signal intensity on both T1-weighted and T2-weighted sequences. This is due to the paramagnetic effect of haemosiderin-laden synovial tissue that has results from recurrent intraarticular bleeding (CHENG et al. 2004). On gradient echo (GRE) sequences, the effect is exaggerated due to increased magnetic susceptibility. This results in areas of very low signal intensity and "blooming" artefact on T2-weighted GRE sequences. Typically, lesions show marked enhancement following intravenous contrast.

22.10
Soft Tissue Tumours

22.10.1
Benign Soft Tissue Tumours

Benign fibrous histiocytoma is a common benign tumour accounting for 9.4% of benign tumours around the hip, groin and buttocks. It usually presents as a nodular skin mass and imaging is usually only required in the uncommon deep variety as they may mimic a more aggressive process. On MR imaging, the signal characteristics are non-specific.

Nodular fasciitis [pseudosarcomatous fibromatosis (fasciitis)] is a benign soft tissue lesion that accounts for 8% of benign soft tissue lesions around the hip, groin and buttocks. On MR imaging, lesions are usually well-defined but can be irregular. Histologic findings reflect the different signal intensity characteristics and enhancement pattern on MR imaging. Of the subtypes, myxoid lesions tend to have characteristic findings with homogeneous signal intensity comparable with muscle on T1-weighted images, high signal intensity on T2-weighted image and homogeneous enhancement (WANG et al. 2002). The fibrous and cellular lesions display more variable appearances.

Fibromatosis (extraabdominal desmoid tumour) accounts for 6.7% of benign soft tissue tumours around the hip, groin and buttocks. The majority of lesions occur in young adults with a peak incidence between 25 and 35 years. Lesions are usually solitary but synchronous, multicentric lesions have been recorded in up to 15% of cases. On MR imaging, in the proliferative phase, much of the lesion shows increased signal intensity on T2-weighting reflecting the cellular predominance whereas in the involutional or residual phase low signal intensity predominates due to the high collagen content. Enhancement is variable and more marked in the proliferative phase. Recurrence is common where the resection margins have not been wide.

Lipomas are common benign lesions that accounted for 16.1% of benign tumours around the hip, groin and buttocks in Kransdorf's (KRANSDORF 1995a,b) series but this is likely to be an underestimate as lesions are often found incidentally. Superficial lesions are much more common than deep lesions and may blend in with subcutaneous fat. Most present with a painless slow growing soft tissue mass although pressure effects on adjacent structures including peripheral nerves and bones is not uncommon (Fig. 22.26). Radiographically, lipo-

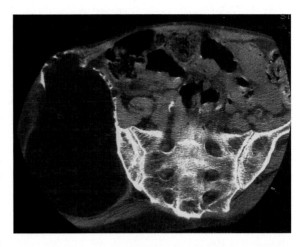

Fig. 22.26. Lipoma. CT showing a massive low attenuation lipoma arising in the right buttock causing erosion of the underlying ilium

mas may appear as a soft tissue mass of low (fatty) density. Ultrasound typically shows a compressible elliptical mass of variable echogenicity that often contains linear echogenic lines at right angles to the ultrasound beam. On CT and MR imaging, lesions are homogeneous, do not enhance and have similar density and signal characteristics to subcutaneous fat (Fig. 22.26). However, simple lipomas containing various connective tissue elements, spindle cell and pleomorphic variants of lipoma may contain foci of non-lipomatous tissue that may be indistinguishable from atypical lipoma (well-differentiated liposarcoma). Mineralisation due to cartilaginous or osseous metaplasia may be seen in large lipomas or lesions that have been present for some time.

Haemangioma is a relatively common soft tissue lesion but only accounted for 4.7% of benign soft tissue tumours around the hip, groin and buttocks in Kransdorf's series (KRANSDORF 1995a,b). However, this is likely to be an underestimate as many lesions are superficial and do not require imaging or intervention. Lesions usually present in first four decades with a painless mass that may vary in size. Deep lesions (usually cavernous) may require imaging. Phleboliths are common in haemangiomas and may be detected on radiographs. However, phleboliths are also common incidental findings in the lower pelvic cavity due to thrombosed iliac veins. Where embolotherapy is being considered, angiography is helpful in confirming the type and extent of the lesion (MITTY et al. 1991). Ultrasound displays an inhomogeneous mixed echo pattern and phleboliths may cause acoustic shadowing (DERCHI et al. 1989). Doppler shows high flow in arteriovenous malformations and slow flow in cavernous lesions.

On MR imaging, lesions are inhomogeneous and often poorly marginated but usually have a characteristic appearance. Lesions often contain reactive fatty tissue that displays high signal intensity on T1-weighting (Fig. 22.27). The slow flowing blood in the anomalous vessels of a cavernous or venous haemangioma often displays very high signal intensity on T2-weighting whereas the fast flowing blood of an arteriovenous malformation results in flow voids on all sequences. In cavernous haemangiomas, rounded foci of low signal intensity may be due to phleboliths. Intermediate and malignant vasoformative tumours are much less common than haemangiomas and more common in the soft tissues than bone. Haemangioendothelioma and haemangiopericytoma are usually of intermediate aggressiveness and may be benign whereas angiosarcoma is an aggressive malignant tumour with a poor prognosis. On MR imaging, there may be difficulty in distinguishing benign from malignant vascular soft tissue lesions but fatty overgrowth is common in haemangiomas and lacking in intermediate and malignant vasoformative tumours.

Benign nerve sheath tumours are relatively common around the hip, groin and buttocks with neurofibroma accounting for 8.3% and schwannoma for 5.0% of benign soft tissue tumours around the hip, groin and buttocks. Schwannomas (neurolemmomas) are well-encapsulated tumours arising from the nerve sheath that displace the nerve fibres eccentrically whereas neurofibromas are non-encapsulated lesions that separate the nerve fibres and cause fusiform enlargement of the nerve. Patients usually present with a painless mass of less than 5 cm although neurofibromas of large nerves are more likely to present with neurological symptoms. Schwannomas tend to occur in an older age group (20–50 years) than neurofibroma (20–30 years). Plexiform neurofibromas are pathognomonic of neurofibromatosis (NF) type 1. On ultrasound, small neurofibromas (< 2 cm) tend to have a homogeneous hypoechoic appearance whereas lesions equal to or larger than 2 cm often show a characteristic "target" pattern. This reflects the internal architecture with a central hyperechoic fibrous component and peripheral hypoechoic myxoid component. It may not be possible to differentiate neurofibroma from schwannoma although an eccentric location favours schwannoma. Although ultrasound is adequate for superficial or small neurofibromas, MR imaging is the imaging technique of choice for staging large or deep lesions or plexiform neurofibromas. On MR imaging, in lesions arising from larger nerves, the

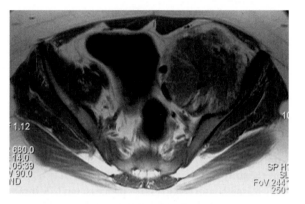

Fig. 22.27. Haemangioma. Axial T1-weighted image showing a lobulated mass arising within the pelvis and containing fatty elements

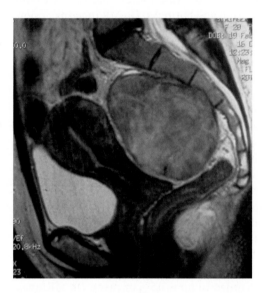

Fig. 22.28. Giant presacral schwannoma. Sagittal T2-weighted image showing a large rounded presacral mass attached to the anterior surface of the sacrum

nerve can often be seen entering and exiting the fusiform mass as a tubular structure. However, differentiation between neurofibroma and schwannoma is not always possible. Both lesions are homogeneous and iso- or slightly hyperintense to muscle on T1-weighting, inhomogeneous and mainly hyperintense on T2-weighting and enhance strongly with intravenous Gad-DTPA. The MR equivalent of the ultrasound "target" sign is often present on T2-weighted images, more commonly in neurofibroma than schwannoma. The fibrous central component displays low signal intensity and the peripheral myxoid component high signal intensity. A fibrous pseudocapsule, cystic change, necrosis and haemorrhage are all more common in schwannoma than neurofibroma. A large round soft tissue mass arising on the anterior surface of the sacrum is typical of a giant presacral schwannoma (Fig. 22.28) (Popuri and Davies 2002).

Myxomas are more commonly found in the thigh than the hip, groin and buttocks but account for 9% of benign soft tissue tumours around the hip, groin and buttocks. Patients present with a slowly enlarging mass most commonly in the 5th–7th decades. The lesion resembles a cyst on both CT and MR imaging due to the high water content of mucin and in one series the true solid nature of these lesions was best appreciated on ultrasound and contrast enhanced MR imaging (Murphey et al. 2002).

22.10.2
Malignant Soft Tissue Tumours

Dermatofibrosarcoma protuberans is a slow growing intermediate grade malignancy most commonly seen in the 3rd–5th decades that originates in the dermal layer of the skin and accounts for 8.4% of soft tissue sarcomas around the hip, groin and buttocks. Most lesions are small and superficial and imaging is usually only required for rare large lesions that infiltrate deeper structures (Kransdorf and Meis-Kindblom 1994). The MR appearances are non-specific but the cutaneous components and lobular architecture of most lesions should suggest the diagnosis.

Malignant fibrous histiocytoma (MFH) is the most common soft tissue sarcoma accounting for 25.3% of lesions around the hip, groin and buttocks.

Lesions are more common in males with a peak incidence in the 5th–7th decades. On MR imaging, lesions are typically inhomogeneous and lobulated, often with relatively well defined margins and a reactive pseudocapsule (Fig. 22.29). Lesions display variable signal intensity depending on the different components. Foci of myxoid change and necrosis give low signal intensity on T1-weighting and high signal intensity on T2-weighting. Dense fibrous tissue and mineralised components tend to give low or intermediate signal intensity on all sequences. Haemorrhage is common and the signal characteristics will vary with age of the haematoma (Fig. 22.29). Inhomogeneous enhancement is typical.

Liposarcoma is the second most common soft tissue sarcoma after MFH and accounts for 19.2% of soft tissue sarcomas around the hip, groin and buttocks. Patients present most commonly in the 5th and 6th decades with an enlarging mass that can occasionally be painful. The majority (80%) are due to low grade well-differentiated or low/intermediate grade myxoid subtypes that carry a better prognosis than the more aggressive high grade round cell, pleomorphic and dedifferentiated subtypes. Plain radiography may detect mineralisations in up to 10%. On MR imaging, well-differentiated lesions always contain a predominance of demonstrable fat (usually > 75%), as well as a smaller amount of linear or nodular non-adipose tissue that display non-specific signal intensities. A total of 50% of the remainder (mainly myxoid liposarcoma) contain demonstrable fat but this is often less than 25% of the tumour volume. The non-adipose components often show enhancement.

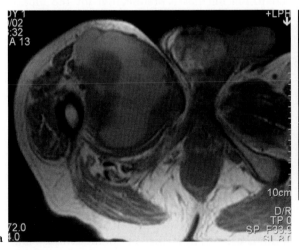
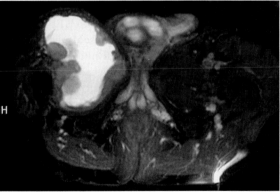

Fig. 22.29a,b. High grade spindle cell sarcoma. **a** Axial T1-weighted and (**b**) Axial T2-weighted image with fat suppression showing a large necrotic tumour within the adductor compartment. The hyperintense areas on the T1-weighted image indicate subacute haemorrhage

Synovial sarcoma is an aggressive sarcoma that accounts for 5.7% of soft tissue sarcomas around the hip, groin and buttocks. It is most common from 6–45 years and sex incidence is equal. Metastatic disease is mainly pulmonary (90%) and 25% have metastases at presentation. The prognosis is guarded with an overall 10-year survival rate of 51% (Deshmukh et al. 2004). Patients with lesions of less than 5 cm in longest diameter had a 10-year survival of 88% compared with a 10-year survival of 38% and 8% for patients with sarcomas 5–10 cm and greater than 10 cm in longest diameter, respectively. Calcifications are found in up to 30% of cases but may be difficult to detect in pelvic lesions without CT. On MR imaging, small lesions may have a homogeneous appearance but most lesions show a well defined lobulated inhomogeneous mass. On T1-weighting, lesions usually display low/intermediate signal intensity although foci of high signal intensity due to intratumoral haemorrhage (methaemoglobin) may be seen in up to 40% of cases (Fig. 22.11). On T2-weighting, a markedly inhomogeneous pattern of variable signal intensity is found in most lesions. Inhomogeneous enhancement is typical. Osseous involvement is not uncommon if site of origin is close to bone.

Malignant peripheral nerve sheath tumours (MPNST) are generally high grade sarcomas and account for 6.2% of all soft tissue sarcomas around the hip, groin and buttocks. Between 25%–70% are associated with neurofibromatosis type 1. Between 3%–13% of patients with neurofibromatosis will develop a malignant peripheral nerve sheath tumour whereas malignant transformation in a solitary neurofibroma is rare and schwannoma extremely rare. Patients most commonly present between 20–50 years but patients with NF1 are more commonly male and tend to present earlier than in patients without NF1. Most, if not all, MPNST in NF1 patients arise from pre-existing neurofibromas and therefore, sudden enlargement of a pre-existing neurofibroma is an ominous finding. The prognosis is guarded with a 5-year survival rate of only 43.7% (Wanebo et al. 1993). Worsened prognosis is associated with older patient age, larger tumour size, more central location of the tumour, and positive margins after resection. Patients present with a soft tissue mass often with neurological symptoms in the affected nerve. Any peripheral nerve may be affected although major nerve trunks sciatic nerve or sacral plexus most commonly involved. Imaging features may be non-specific and differentiation from benign nerve sheath tumours may be difficult.

Ultrasound and CT show irregular inhomogeneous masses with necrotic and cystic foci and occasionally calcification. Scintigraphy using gallium-67 citrate and more recently PET (FDG-PET) scanning has been helpful in distinguishing benign from malignant nerve sheath tumours and may be useful in the follow-up of patients with NF1 (Levine et al. 1987; Cardona et al. 2003). On MR imaging, MPNST are often large (> 5 cm) and irregular and may have a fusiform shape with tapered ends that merge into a parent nerve. Lesions are typically inhomogeneous, particularly on T2-weighting due in part to haemorrhage, necrosis, cystic change and mineralisation. The "target" sign, commonly seen in neurofibromas, is uncommon in MPNST. Irregular, nodular, peripheral enhancement with central necrosis is typical of MPNST although central necrosis can also be seen in ancient schwannomas.

Leiomyosarcoma is the third most common sarcoma accounting for 10.3% of soft tissue sarcomas around the hip, groin and buttocks. Patients most commonly present with a painless slow growing mass in the 5th–6th decades. The prognosis is guarded with a 50% mortality at 3 years in a recent study (Mankin et al. 2004). MR imaging typically shows a non-specific, inhomogeneous, enhancing mass with necrosis although more superficial lesions tend to be small, well-defined and homogeneous.

22.10.3
Tumour-Like Lesions of Soft Tissues

Idiopathic tumoral calcinosis is a relatively rare condition but has a predilection for the hips. It mainly affects blacks and usually presents in the first two decades with a slow growing peri-articular soft tissue mass that may ulcerate and drain chalky-like material. A family history is present in 30%–40% of cases. Similar appearances may be found in metabolic disease including chronic renal failure. Radiographs reveal well defined, juxta-articular, lobulated calcific masses containing lucent fibrous septations. On CT, the masses may be uniformly calcified or cystic with calcific walls and fluid-fluid levels. The MR appearances are also variable with low signal intensity on all sequences in calcified lesions and diffuse or focal areas of high signal intensity on T2-weighting if the lesions are inflammatory or contain fluid. Fluid-fluid levels are also demonstrated on MR imaging and are due to the sedimentation of calcium within the masses (Smeets et al. 1996).

Cystic lesions are not uncommon around the hip and include iliopsoas and trochanteric bursae and para-labral cysts. The iliopsoas bursa is located beneath the musculotendinous part of the iliopsoas muscle, anterior to the hip joint capsule and communicates with the hip in 15% of patients. Iliopsoas bursitis often presents as an inguinal mass that may be difficult to distinguish from other groin masses including hernia, lymphadenopathy, femoral artery aneurysm, and various other benign and malignant soft tissue masses. The condition primarily affects patients over the range of 50 years with pre-existing hip disease, usually of long duration. Compression of the femoral neurovascular bundle is common and large lesions may extend above the inguinal ligament into the pelvis. Cross-sectional imaging typically shows a well-defined, thin-walled cystic mass although the bursal contents may include solid components. Ultrasound is the simplest, quickest and most cost effective means of demonstrating the hip joint effusion and contents and extent of the bursa, but MR imaging provides a better appreciation of the regional anatomy and underlying hip disease (WUNDERBALDINGER et al. 2002).

The greater trochanteric bursa complex is situated between the greater trochanter with the attachment of the gluteus medius tendon and the tensor fascia lata. Tears of the gluteus medius tendon have a strong association with bursitis superior to the greater trochanter (submedialis bursa) and a weaker association with bursitis lateral to the trochanter (trochanteric bursitis) (CVITANIC et al. 2004). Clinicians are now becoming increasingly aware that tears of the abductor tendons, as opposed to trochanteric bursitis, may be the leading cause of greater trochanteric pain syndrome.

As in the shoulder, paralabral cysts are not uncommon around the hip. They are related to labral tears and there is an increased incidence in developmental dysplasia of the hip. These cysts are typically extraarticular in location and may erode into the adjacent bone. They may or may not fill with contrast material at the time of MR arthrography. Identification of a cyst around the hip joint should raise the possibility of an underlying acetabular-labral tear (PETERSILGE 2000). MR arthrography is considerably more accurate in the detection of acetabular labral lesions compared with MR imaging.

Myositis ossificans is a benign, mineralising, intramuscular mass that is usually post-traumatic and relatively common around the hip and pelvis. Initially a painful non-specific mass, by 3–4 weeks,

flocculated densities appear within the lesion. The lesion demonstrates a centrifugal pattern of maturation with the periphery demarcated by initial immature bone about a cellular centre - "zone phenomenon". Ultrasound is useful in demonstrating this zonal phenomenon before the typical peripheral ossification is detected radiographically at 6–8 weeks. On MR imaging, early lesions display intermediate SI on T1-weighted images and inhomogeneous high SI on T2-weighted images but the margins are ill-defined and often difficult to distinguish from the diffuse surrounding oedema. Within 2–3 weeks, peripheral, curvilinear hypointense structures corresponding to peripheral mineralisation begin to appear and can be confirmed by CT (Fig. 22.8). This pattern of maturation differentiates the lesion from soft tissue or parosteal osteosarcoma where the mineralisation tends to be central. By 5–6 months, the lesion tends to reduce in size as it ossifies and reaches maturity. MR imaging now shows an inhomogeneous mass containing fatty marrow and dense ossification.

References

Abdelwahab IF, Miller TT, Hermann G et al (1991) Transarticular invasion of joints by bone tumors: hypothesis. Skeletal Radiol 20:279–283

Anderson MW, ThomasTemple H, Dussault RG et al (1999) Compartment anatomy: relevance to staging and biopsy of musculoskeletal tumours. Am J Roentgenol 173:1663–1671

Aoki J, Endo K, Watanabe H et al (2003) FDG-PET for evaluating musculoskeletal tumors: a review. J Orthop Sci 8:435–441

Baratti D, Gronchi A, Pennacchioli E et al (2003) Chordoma: natural history and results in 28 patients treated at a single institution. Ann Surg Oncol 10:291–296

Baur A, Huber A, Arbogast S, Durr HR, Zysk S, Wendtner C, Deimling M, Reiser M. (2001) Diffusion-weighted imaging of tumor recurrencies and posttherapeutical soft-tissue changes in humans. Eur Radiol 11:828–833

Bearcroft PWP, Davies AM (1999) Follow-up of musculo-skeletal tumors 2: metastatic disease. Eur Radiol 9:192–200

Bielack SS, Kempf-Bielack B, Delling G et al (2002) Prognostic factors in high-grade osteosarcoma of the extremities or trunk: an analysis of 1,702 patients treated on neoadjuvant cooperative osteosarcoma study group protocols. J Clin Oncol 20:776–790

Bloem JL, Taminiau AHM, Eulderink F et al (1988) Radiologic staging of primary bone sarcoma: MR imaging, scintigraphy, angiography, and CT correlated with pathologic examination. Radiology 169:805–810

Boutin RD, Pathria MN, Resnick D (1998) Disorders in the stumps of amputee patients: MR imaging. AJR 171:497–501

Bredella MA, Caputo GR, Steinbach LS (2002) Value of FDP positron emission tomography in conjunction with MR imaging for evaluating therapy response in patients with musculoskeletal sarcomas. Am J Roentgenol 179:1145–1150

Brunel H, Peretti-Viton P, Benguigui-Charmeau V et al (2002) MRI: an essential examen for the management of sacrococcygeal chordromas J Neuroradiol 29:15–22

Campanacci M (1999) Bone and soft tissue tumours: clinical features, imaging, pathology and treatment, 2nd edn. Springer, Vienna New York

Cardona S, Schwarzbach M, Hinz U et al (2003) Evaluation of F18-deoxyglucose positron emission tomography (FDG-PET) to assess the nature of neurogenic tumours. Eur J Surg Oncol 29:536–541

Cheng XG, You YH, Liu W et al (2004) MRI features of pigmented villonodular synovitis (PVNS). Clin Rheumatol 23:31–34

Cheung FM, Wu WC, Lam CK et al (1997) Diagnostic criteria for pseudomalignant osteoblastoma. Histopathology 31:196–200

Collins MS, Koyama T, Swee RG et al (2003) Clear cell chondrosarcoma: radiographic, computed tomographic, and magnetic resonance findings in 34 patients with pathologic correlation. Skeletal Radiol 32:687–94

Cvitanic O, Henzie G, Skezas N et al (2004) MRI diagnosis of tears of the hip abductor tendons (gluteus medius and gluteus minimus). Am J Roentgenol 182:137–143

Davies AM, Vanel D (1998) Follow-up of musculoskeletal tumors. 1. Local recurrence. Eur Radiol 8:791–799

Davies AM, Cooper SA, Mangham DC et al (2001) Metal-containing lymph nodes following prosthetic replacement of osseous malignancy: potential role of MR imaging in characterization. Eur Radiol 11:841–844

Davies AM, Hall AD, Strouhal PD, Evans N, Grimer RJ (2004) The MR imaging appearances and natural history of seromas following excision of soft tissue tumours. Eur Radiol 14:1196–1202

Davies M, Cassar-Pullicino VN, Davies AM, McCall IW, Tyrell PNM (2002) The diagnostic accuracy of MRI in osteoid osteoma. Skeletal Radiol 31:559–569

De Beuckeleer LH, de Schepper AM, Ramon F (1996) Magnetic resonance imaging of pelvic bone tumors. J Belge Radiol 79:11–30

Derchi LE, Balconi G, de Flaviis L et al (1989) Sonographic appearances of hemangiomas of skeletal muscle. J Ultrasound Med 8:263–267

Deshmukh R, Mankin HJ, Singer S (2004) Synovial sarcoma: the importance of size and location for survival. Clin Orthop 419:155–161

Dupuy DE, Rosenberg AE, Punyaratabandhu T et al (1998) Accuracy of CT-guided needle biopsy of musculoskeletal neoplasms. Am J Roentgenol 171:759–762

Enneking WF, Spanier SS, Goodman MA (1980) A system for the surgical staging of musculoskeletal sarcoma. Clin Orthop 153:106–120

Fowler J, Davies AM, Carter SR, Grimer RJ (1992) CT appearances of the pelvis following hindquarter amputation. BJR 65:1093–1096

Genant JW, Vandevenne JE, Bergman AG et al (2002) Interventional musculoskeletal procedures performed by using MR imaging guidance with a vertically open MR unit: assessment of techniques and applicability. Radiology 223:127–136

Hartman RP, Sundaram M, Okuno SH, Sim FH (2004) Effect of granulocyte-stimulating factors on marrow of adult patients with musculoskeletal malignancies: incidence and MRI findings. AJR 183:645–653

Kramer J, Recht M, Deely DM et al (1993) MRI appearance of idiopathic synovial osteochondromatosis. J Comput Assist Tomogr 17:772–776

Kransdorf MJ (1995a) Benign soft-tissue tumors in a large referral population: distribution of diagnoses by age, sex, and location. Am J Roentgenol 164:395–402

Kransdorf MJ (1995b) Malignant soft-tissue tumors in a large referral population: distribution of diagnoses by age, sex, and location. Am J Roentgenol 164:129–134

Kransdorf MJ, Meis-Kindblom JM (1994) Dermatofibrosarcoma protuberans: radiologic appearance. Am J Roentgenol 163:391–394

Krishnan A, Shirkhoda A, Tehranzadeh J et al (2003) Primary bone lymphoma: radiographic-MR imaging correlation. Radiographics 23:1371–1383

Lang P, Grampp S, Vahlensieck M et al (1995) Primary bone tumours: value of MR angiography for pre-operative planning and monitoring response to chemotherapy. Am J Roentgenol 165:135–142

Levine E, Huntrakoon M, Wetzel LH (1987) Malignant nerve-sheath neoplasms in neurofibromatosis: distinction from benign tumors by using imaging techniques. Am J Roentgenol 149:1059–1064

Lin PP, Guzel VB, Moura MF et al (2002) Long-term follow-up of patients with giant cell tumour of the sacrum treated with selective embolisation. Cancer 95:1317–1325

Link TM, Haeussler MD, Poppek S et al (1998) Malignant fibrous histiocytoma of bone: conventional X-ray and MR imaging features. Skeletal Radiol 27:552–558

Mahnken AH, Nolte-Ernsting CC, Wildberger JE et al (2003) Aneurysmal bone cyst: value of MR imaging and conventional radiography. Eur Radiol 13:1118–1124

Mankin HJ, Mankin CJ, Simon MA (1996) The hazards of biopsy, revisited. Members of the musculoskeletal tumor society. J Bone Joint Surg Am 78(A):656

Mankin HJ, Casas-Ganem J, Kim JI et al (2004) Leiomyosarcoma of somatic soft tissues. Clin Orthop 421:225–231

Mitty HA, Hermann G, Abdelwahab IF et al (1991) Role of angiography in limb-tumor surgery. Radiographics 11:1029–1044

Moulopoulos LA, Dimopoulos MA, Smith TL et al (1995) Prognostic significance of magnetic resonance imaging in patients with asymptomatic myeloma. J Clin Oncol 13:251–256

Murphey MD, Fleming DJ, Boyea SR et al (1998) From the archives of the AFIP. Enchondroma versus chondrosarcoma in the appendicular skeleton: differentiating features. Radiographics 18:1213–1237

Murphey MD, McRae GA, Fanburg-Smith JC et al (2002) Imaging of soft-tissue myxoma with emphasis on CT and MR and comparison of radiologic and pathologic findings. Radiology 225:215–224

Ozaki T, Putzke M, Burger H et al (2002) Infiltration of sarcomas into the hip joint. Acta Orthop Scand 73:220–226

Ozaki T, Rodl R, Gosheger G et al (2003) Sacral infiltration in pelvic sarcomas: joint infiltration analysis II. Clin Orthop 407:152–158

Panicek DM, Hilton S, Schwartz LH (1997) Assessment of

neurovascular involvement by malignant musculoskeletal tumors. Sarcoma 1:281–283

Peh WC, Shek TW, Davies AM, et al. (1999) Osteochondroma and secondary synovial osteochondromatosis. Skeletal Radiol 28:169–174

Petersilge CA (2000) From the RSNA refresher courses. Radiological Society of North America. Chronic adult hip pain: MR arthrography of the hip. Radiographics 20:S43–S52

Peterson HA (1989) Multiple hereditary osteochondromata. Clin Orthop 239:222–230

Popuri R, Davies AM (2002) MR imaging features of giant pre-sacral schwannomas: a report of 4 cases. Eur Radiol 12:2365–2369

Ramappa AJ, Lee FY, Tang P et al (2000) Chondroblastoma of bone. J Bone Joint Surg Am 82-A:1140–1145

Saifuddin A, Twin P, Emanuel R et al (2000) An audit of MRI for bone and soft tissue tumours performed at referral centres. Clin Radiol 55:537–541

Saifuddin A, Mann BS, Mahroof S et al (2004) Dedifferentiated chondrosarcoma: use of MRI to guide needle biopsy. Clin Radiol 59:268–272

Saunders A, Davies AM, Grimer RJ (1998) MR imaging of soft tissue expanders used in the management of musculoskeletal sarcomas. Br J Radiol 71:926–929

Schima W, Amann G, Stiglbauer R et al (1994) Preoperative staging of osteosarcoma: efficacy on MR imaging in detecting joint involvement. Am J Roentgenol 63:1171–1175

Shapeero LG, Vanel D (2000) Imaging evaluation of the response of high-grade osteosarcoma and Ewing sarcoma to chemotherapy with emphasis on dynamic contrast-enhanced MR imaging. Semin Musculoskeletal Radiol 4:137–146

Smeets HGW, Lamers RJS, Sastrowijoto SH (1996) Tumoral calcinosis. AJR 167:818–819

Unni KK (1996) Dahlin's bone tumors: general aspects and data on 11,087 cases, 5th edn. Lippincott-Raven, Philadelphia

Van der Woude HJ, Bloem JL, Oostayen JA et al (1995) Treatment of high-grade bone sarcomas with neo-adjuvant chemotherapy: the utility of sequential color Doppler sonography in predicting histopathologic response. Am J Roentgenol 165:125–133

Van der Woude HJ, Bloem JL, Hogendoorn PC (1998) Preoperative evaluation and monitoring chemotherapy in patients with high-grade osteogenic and Ewing's sarcoma: review of current imaging modalities. Skeletal Radiol 27:57–71

Vanel D, Shapeero LG, de Baere T et al (1994) MR imaging in the follow-up of malignant and aggressive soft tissue tumours: results of 511 examinations. Radiology 190:263–268

Van Rijswijk CSP, Geirnaerdt MJA, Hogendoorn PCW, Taminiau AHM, van Coevorden F, Zwinderman AH, Pope TL, Bloem JL (2004) Soft-tissue tumors: value of static and dynamic gadopentetate dimeglumine enhanced MR imaging in prediction of malignancy. Radiology 233:493–502

Verstraete KL, Lang P (2000) Benign and soft tissue tumours: the role of contrast agents for MR imaging. Eur Radiol 34:229–246

Wanebo JE, Malik JM, VandenBerg SR et al (1993) Malignant peripheral nerve sheath tumors. A clinicopathologic study of 28 cases. Cancer 71:1247–1253

Wang XL, de Schepper AM, Vanhoenacker F et al (2002) Nodular fasciitis: correlation of MRI findings and histopathology. Skeletal Radiol 31:155–161

White LM, Schweitzer ME, Khalili K et al (1998) MR imaging of primary lymphoma of bone: variability of T2-weighted signal intensity. Am J Roentgenol 170:1243–1247

Wittkop B, Davies AM, Mangham DC (2002) Primary synovial chondromatosis and synovial chondrosarcoma: a pictorial review. Eur Radiol 12:2112–2119

Wunderbaldinger P, Bremer C, Schellenberger E et al (2002) Imaging features of iliopsoas bursitis. Eur Radiol 12:409–415

Wurtz LD, Peabody TD, Simon MA (1999) Delay in the diagnosis and treatment of primary bone sarcoma of the pelvis. J Bone Joint Surg Am 81:317–325

Youssef BA, Haddad MC, Zahrani A et al (1996) Osteoid osteoma and osteoblastoma: MRI appearances and the significance of ring enhancement. Eur Radiol 6:291–296

23 Paget's Disease of Bone

RICHARD WILLIAMS WHITEHOUSE and A. MARK DAVIES

CONTENTS

23.1
Introduction

Paget's disease of bone, named after the nineteenth century British surgeon Sir James Paget, remains a condition of disputed aetiology, with virus infection and genetic susceptibility both implicated. Although sporadic and seemingly random in the sites and extent of bone involvement in individuals, because markedly altered bone turnover and cellular activity are histologically and biochemically characteristic of the condition, it is often placed with metabolic bone diseases.

The pelvis, sacral and lumbar spine and femora are the commonest locations for this condition, with the pelvis (including the sacrum) involved in about two thirds of cases.

R. W. WHITEHOUSE, MD
Department of Clinical Radiology, Manchester Royal Infirmary, Oxford Road, Manchester, M13 9WL, UK
A. M. DAVIES, MD
Consultant Radiologist, The MRI Centre, Royal Orthopaedic Hospital, Birmingham, B31 2AP, UK

Paget's disease of bone has been considered a common disorder affecting approximately 3%–4% of the population over 40 years of age. Consequently it is the second commonest bone pathology of "metabolic" origin, after osteoporosis. However, the prevalence of Paget's disease varies considerably around the world, being rare in the Far East and commonest in the north west of England. Since the 1980's, studies and reports from around the world have suggested a marked reduction in the incidence of new cases of Paget's disease of bone. In addition the age at first presentation appears to be increasing whilst both the severity and extent of bone involvement in new cases is decreasing. If substantiated and continued, these trends will result in the condition becoming rare. There has not, as yet been any report of a reduction in the incidence of the serious complications of Paget's disease, in particular the development of bone sarcoma.

23.2
Aetiology

Paget's disease remains of uncertain and disputed aetiology. The two main theories are of "slow" virus infection and genetic abnormality. Ownership of dogs not vaccinated against canine distemper virus appears to increase the risk of developing Paget's disease, but so does ownership of cats or birds (KHAN et al. 1996) or a history of measles (RENIER et al. 1996b). Contact with cattle, ingestion of meat from sick livestock and frequent ingestion of brains or bovid viscera during youth are also risk factors (LÓPEZ et al. 1997). There are regional variations in the significance of these risk factors. These observations support one or more transmissible agents as aetiological in Paget's disease.

On electron microscopy, the nuclei of osteoclasts from pagetic bone contain lesions similar to "viral inclusion bodies" seen in other virally mediated conditions. In some centres, in-situ hybridisation techniques have demonstrated messenger RNA (mRNA) transcripts derived from various paramyxoviruses in bone cells from pagetic lesions, with measles and canine distemper virus being the most often found. The findings of these studies have proved difficult to replicate in other centres (HELFRICH et al. 2000; OOI et al. 2000). Recently, in one study using an in-situ reverse transcriptase polymerase chain reaction technique, canine distemper virus mRNA has been found in 100% of material from pagetic bone (MEE et al. 1998). It has however been claimed that measles virus is only found in laboratories that support a measles virus aetiology and canine distemper virus in laboratories that support the latter virus as the causative agent (RALSTON and HELFRICH 1999). Osteoclast precursors transduced with measles virus genes can produce osteoclast like cells with features similar to Pagetic osteoclasts (KURIHARA et al. 2000; REDDY et al. 2001). An infectious virus has never been isolated from pagetic bone but a full length viral gene has now been sequenced from pagetic bone (FRIEDRICHS et al. 2002). Difficulties of contamination and reproducibility of these tests have dogged interpretation of the results of these viral gene studies.

Genetic studies have also been inconsistent (GOOD et al. 2001; NANCE et al. 2000). Paget's disease is commoner than expected in first degree relatives of patients with the condition. However, there are both familial and sporadic forms of Paget's disease with different genetic abnormalities. At least six mutations in the ubiquitin-associated domain of the SQSTM1 (p62-sequestosome 1) gene have been identified in patients with familial Paget's disease and a proportion, but not all of sporadic cases (HOCK-ING et al. 2002; EEKHOFF et al. 2004; JOHNSON et al. 2003). Familial Paget's disease has an earlier age of onset and greater fracture rate than sporadic forms. In an American study, familial cases were less likely to record the US or Canada as their grandparents' birthplace, strengthening a case for genetic rather than local environmental factors in the development of the disease (SETON et al. 2003). Mutations in the TNFRSF11A gene causing early onset Paget like disease have also been described (NAKATSUKA et al. 2003). Differences in the genetic polymorphism of the oestrogen receptor-alpha gene and the calcium sensing receptor gene between pagetic and non-pagetic patients have also been detected, which may contribute to genetic susceptibility to the disease (DONÁTH et al. 2004).

Hyperphosphatasemia (Juvenile Paget's disease) is genetically distinct from Paget's disease and asso-ciated with osteoprotegerin deficiency caused by homozygous deletion of the gene encoding osteo-protegerin (TNFRSF11B) (WHYTE et al. 2002).

Other environmental causes for Paget's disease have been suggested, for example calcium arsenate (LEVER 2002), a pesticide used in the cotton industry has been suggested as a possible cause of the marked variation in prevalence of Paget's disease in Lanca-shire. Oral bacterial flora have also been suggested as causative agents (DICKINSON 1999). Evidence for these hypotheses is extremely limited.

23.3
Epidemiology

Paget's disease varies widely in prevalence both within and between countries (ARMAS et al. 2002). It has been historically commonest in the North West of England, rare in the Far East (YIP et al. 1996) and commoner in other countries with high proportions of Caucasians, particularly of Western European origin. A high prevalence of the disease is found in Buenos Aires, for example, where 95% of patients were of European descent, particularly Ital-ian and Russian (GÓMEZ and MAUTALEN 2001). An archaeological study of 2770 skeletons from Humber in England dating from 900 to 1850 AD showed a prevalence of 2.1% in those aged over 40 years, with a non-significant increase from 1.7% to 3.1% pre- and post-1500 AD (ROGERS et al. 2002). More recently, comparative surveys of pelvic radiographs and biochemical tests from many studies around the world have suggested a marked reduction in inci-dence of new cases of Paget's disease (CUNDY et al. 1997, 1999; COOPER et al. 1999; DOYLE et al. 2002), reduced severity and number of sites involved in new cases (MORALES et al. 2002)and an older age at presentation over the last 25 years (RAPADO et al. 1999; CUNDY et al. 1997), typically finding a halv-ing of incidence over this period (VAN STAA et al. 2002). The condition is slightly commoner in men and is also slightly commoner in the right side of the body.

23.4
Imaging Appearances

Both the incidental demonstration of Paget's dis-ease and its diagnosis is most often accomplished by radiography. Biochemically, Paget's disease may be suspected, or activity of known disease monitored by measurement of urinary hydroxyproline and serum total alkaline phosphatase (FRASER 1997). Further evaluation of biochemically suspected Paget's disease and the identification of extent and severity of disease is usually by radiographs and bone scintigraphy. The imaging appearances of Paget's disease are consequently primarily by reference to those modalities (HOFFMAN 1998).

Paget's disease is described as passing through three phases, as demonstrated on conventional radiography. An initial lytic phase, a mixed phase and a sclerotic phase. The lytic phase is infrequently seen, being most often identified in the skull (because it may persist in this location, known as osteoporosis circumscripta) and in long bones. It is usually of short duration, rapidly progressing to the mixed phase. In this second phase abnormally coarsened and disorganised new bone is formed, resulting in thickening and heterogeneous density of the bone cortex and coarsening of the trabecular bone. These changes in both the cortex and medullary bone results in loss of definition of the margin between cortical and trabecular bone. The affected bone enlarges and distorts as if softened and has a spongy textural appearance on imaging (Fig. 23.1). Histologically, haversian systems in cortical bone are destroyed and the new bone formed to replace them is in irregular plates creating a mosaic appearance.

The final, sclerotic phase represents reduction in the previously overactive osteoclastic bone resorption present in the first two phases, whilst osteoblast activity continues, resulting in increasing bone density and "filling in" of previously lytic areas, with a resultant more amorphous appearance to the bone (Fig. 23.2) (SMITH et al. 2002). Eventually the disease becomes quiescent.

The bone marrow may be involved in active disease, with increased bone vascularity and development of a fibro-vascular stroma which replaces the usually fatty marrow. More often, marrow appears uninvolved, particularly in the later stages of the disease, with fat attenuation on CT scanning (Fig. 23.3) and fat equivalent signal characteristics on MR scanning in the interstices between coarsened trabeculae (WHITEHOUSE 2002).

In long bones, such as the femur, Paget's disease characteristically involves a bone end (subarticular region) and extends in a confluent fashion for a variable distance along the shaft. Pagetic lesions most commonly arise in the proximal ends of long bones, in the cancellous part of an epiphysis or metaphysis

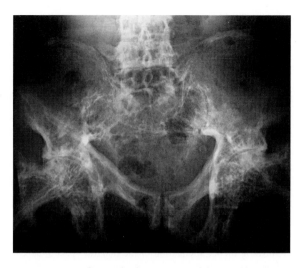

Fig. 23.1. AP radiograph showing mixed lytic and sclerotic Paget's disease involving the entire pelvis, both femora and lower lumbar spine

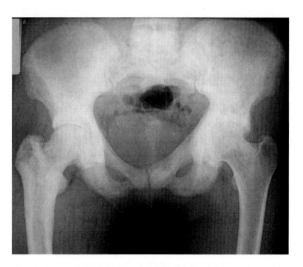

Fig. 23.2. AP radiograph showing sclerotic Paget's disease of the pelvis, right femur and lower lumbar spine. There is a mild left sided pelvic deformity

(RENIER et al. 1996). The involved region ends with a "V" shaped zone of transition to normal bone. This "V" or flame shaped end gives the impression of a progressing lesion growing along the bone, though the speed of progression of this edge on serial films is often disproportionately slow compared to the length of bone already involved and apparent duration of the disease. Typical rate of progression in the femur is about 9 mm/year (RENIER and AUDRAN 1997a). This has led to the suggestion that Paget's disease has an earlier age of onset than generally appreciated, possibly in the second or third decade. Although Paget's disease is considered rare

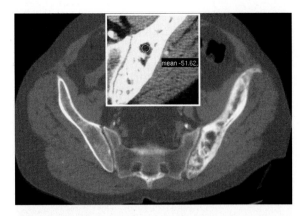

Fig. 23.3. CT of the pelvis demonstrating mixed Paget's disease of the left ilium. The inset is a soft tissue window of the ilium, confirming the fat attenuation of the marrow space (–51 CT units)

in patients under 40 years of age, approximately 10% of patients with Paget's disease were under 40 in one series (CHOMA et al. 2004). It may be that the rate of progress of Paget's disease through bone is not linear, being very rapid initially and slower, or even halted, by the time of diagnosis. Alternatively, Paget's disease may progress in a series of waves (RENIER and AUDRAN 1997b). Treatment with bisphosphonates also halts progression of the disease, making prospective study of the progression of disease problematic. The flame edge is lytic but changes to mixed disease towards the articular surface of "origin" of the pagetic bone.

Pelvic involvement is usually seen as mixed or sclerotic disease. Bilateral skeletal involvement in Paget's disease is usually asymmetrical, the pelvis being the only site likely to be involved bilaterally in an individual patient with polyostotic disease (RENIER and AUDRAN 1997b). Progression of disease through the pelvis is slow, typically taking 13 years to spread to all the bones around the obturator foramen and 30 years to spread through the entire pelvis. The generic radiographic changes described above are seen as loss of trabeculae with coarsening of those remaining and thickening and splitting of the iliopectineal line and teardrop. Enlargement of the ilium is particularly noticeable if the other ilium is unaffected. The bone softening results in pelvic deformity, particularly protrusio acetabuli.

At diagnosis Paget's disease may be monostotic or polyostotic and subsequent development of new sites of disease seems uncommon, though it does occur. Progression of disease from one bone to an adjacent bone is also unusual unless the intervening joint is already bridged by ankylosis or osteophytes, although again, this has been described. Paget's dis-

ease *causing* ankylosis and extension of disease over several spinal segments has also been described.

Bone scintigraphy is routinely used to demonstrate extent and distribution of Paget's disease as markedly increased activity is seen in active disease and can be used to quantify disease activity and response to treatment (HAIN and FOGELMAN 2002). Occasionally activity may be low in lytic disease and is also less impressive, though higher than normal, in quiescent disease. The typical distribution of pagetic disease in long bones, including the flame edge, is clearly demonstrated on bone scans. In the spine, characteristically the whole vertebra, including the posterior elements is involved, giving rise to an isotope bone scan appearance described as a "clover", "heart" (ROTÉS et al. 2004) or "mouse's face" shape (Fig. 23.4) (C.K KIM et al. 1997). PET scanning may also show increased metabolic activity in Pagetic bone (COOK et al. 2002), even when biochemically inactive with normal alkaline phosphatase and alanine amino transferase levels (SPIETH et al. 2003).

Computed tomography (CT) of the abdomen and pelvis may demonstrate incidental Paget's disease. CT can be useful in early, difficult or unusual Pagetic lesions and may demonstrate altered trabecular patterns characteristic of Paget's disease (CHRÉTIEN 1995). Large intertrabecular spaces may allow the marrow CT number to be measured, the confirmation of fatty marrow density being useful to exclude a marrow infiltrate (Fig. 23.3). CT can also be used to guide biopsy, needles of 14–17 G providing ade-

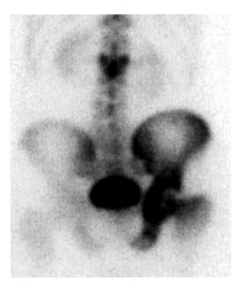

Fig. 23.4. Bone scintigraphy demonstrating increased activity in the left hemipelvis and L2 vertebra, from Paget's disease. Note the uniform involvement of the spinous process and pedicles, giving rise to the "mouse's face" shaped activity

quate specimens for bone diseases including Paget's disease (JELINEK et al. 1996).

Magnetic resonance imaging in uncomplicated Paget's disease usually demonstrates a normal marrow signal on all sequences, whilst the small size of the images and low spatial resolution may render the coarsened trabecular pattern and thickened cortex inconspicuous (Fig. 23.5). In active Paget's disease marrow signal abnormality may be present, due to increased vascularity and cellularity, particularly in paratrabecular and endosteal areas. Consequently bones with high trabecular content such as the pelvis and spine may show marked and complex marrow signal alterations during the active phase of the disease (VANDE-BERG et al. 2001). Recognition of the appearances of Paget's disease on MR and correlation with other imaging is important so as not to mistake it for more sinister pathology (WHITTEN and SAIFUDDIN 2003). Complications of Paget's disease, in particular tumour development and spinal neurological compromise are in particular best evaluated by MR imaging (BOUTIN et al. 1998).

The results of bone mineral densitometry will be significantly influenced if Paget's disease of bone is present in the measurement region. With respect to the pelvis and hips, this is particularly relevant to dual energy X-ray absorptiometry (DXA) of the hip. Typically, pagetic bone is 25%–35% denser than non-pagetic bone, on DXA measurement. Bisphosphonate treatment results in a small further increase in pagetic bone density, but a reduction in normal bone

density (LAROCHE et al. 1999). High DXA values may therefore alert to the possibility of Paget's disease but may result in underestimation of the fracture risk if Paget's disease is not appreciated.

23.5
Complications

23.5.1
Fracture and Deformity

Lytic pagetic bone is prone to fracture, particularly after biopsy, resulting in the recommendation that biopsy be avoided if the diagnosis is secure. This complication is however rarely seen due to the transient nature of lytic Paget's disease. Pagetic bone in the later stages is also more prone to insufficiency-type stress fracture than the bone density would suggest. Incremental incomplete fractures develop on the convexity of bowed pagetic bones, in particular the femur or tibia, and may be multiple. These may complete to transverse fractures of the shaft. Transverse fractures also occur without preceding incremental fracture. These fractures are more common in women and healing is poorer than in normal bone. Described sites of Pagetic pathological fracture include the tibia/fibula, vertebrae, femur and less commonly the pelvis, humerus and skull (Fig. 23.6). With the exception of vertebral and rib

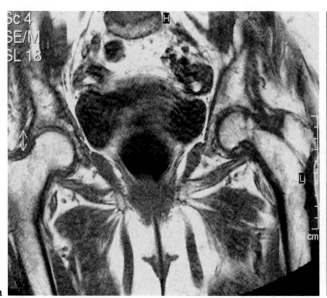
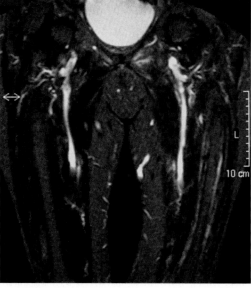

a   b

Fig. 23.5. a Coronal T1-weighted image demonstrating normal fatty marrow signal but thickened cortex in Paget's disease of the pelvis and both femora. b coronal STIR image demonstrating subtle increased signal within the cortex of the left femur due to active lytic Paget's disease. [Reproduced with permission from WHITEHOUSE (2002)]

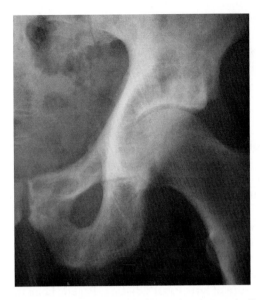

Fig. 23.6. AP radiograph showing sclerotic Paget's disease of the hemipelvis with an undisplaced insufficiency fracture of the ischium

fracture, the risk of fractures in non-pagetic bone of patients with Paget's disease is not increased. Whilst this may be a surveillance effect, it does suggest that patients with Paget's disease may be at increased risk of vertebral fracture and should be managed accordingly (MELTON et al. 2000). Long term bisphosphonate treatment may reduce bone density in non-pagetic parts of the skeleton, with consequent increase in the risk of fracture in non-pagetic bones (GUTTERIDGE et al. 2003).

There is a case report of a minor fracture of a pagetic coccyx causing a cauda equina syndrome from local haemorrhage (DAVIS et al. 1999), more commonly vertebral fractures or pagetic vertebral bone hypertrophy at higher levels would carry this risk (PONCELET 1999).

The deformity caused by enlargement of the bone and plastic deformation results in lateral bowing of the femur and protrusio acetabuli in the pelvis.

23.5.2
Arthritis

Altered load-bearing and deformity of sub-articular bone surfaces by Paget's disease are mechanisms by which arthritis may develop secondary to Paget's disease. Being most often involved by Paget's disease and also a major weight bearing joint, the hip is a prime site for pagetic arthritis. One study of arthritis and Paget's disease in the hip demonstrated slightly reduced articular cartilage thickness in pagetic hips compared to non-pagetic hips (mean 3 mm compared to 4 mm) but no significant difference in other osteoarthritic features (cysts, sclerosis or osteophytes), though the latter may be obscured by the Paget's disease. Significant osteoarthritis (Kellgren and Lawrence grade 2+) was commoner in non-pagetic hips (19 of 352 hips) than pagetic hips (5 of 129 hips) (HELLIWELL and PORTER 1999). Pagetic coxarthropathy may therefore be a secondary chondropathy, with progression to significant osteoarthritis being dependent on factors other than Paget's disease. A smaller study of rheumatology patients found Paget's disease adjacent to 100 joints in 69 patients with Paget's disease, 86 being hips, with osteoarthritic changes more severe on the pagetic side, though severity grading of arthritis in the pagetic joints was dependent on the presence of osteoarthritis elsewhere in the same patient (HELLIWELL 1995). Thus Paget's disease and hip osteoarthritis may be largely co-incidental rather than causal (Fig. 23.7). Despite this, pain is the commonest symptom of Paget's disease and osteoarthritis appears to be the commonest cause of pain in patients with Paget's disease (ALTMAN 1999). A survey of patients with Paget's disease gave deafness and bowed limbs as the commonest complications that patients complained of (30%–40%), whilst arthritis, described as a co-morbidity, was present in 64% (GOLD et al. 1996). Careful identification of the features of both conditions is therefore a relevant radiological challenge. The treatment of hip arthritis by joint replacement is technically more challenging in the presence of Paget's disease, with a higher failure rate for some prostheses but the outcome is still usually good.

When the sacroiliac joint is involved by Paget's disease, confluent pagetic bone may be present across the joint. There is evidence that Paget's disease can cross joints, but the sacroiliac joint is frequently ankylosed giving bone continuity when involved by Paget's disease. This may be due to pre-existing osteophytic bridges or ankylosing spondylitis or by cartilage loss secondary to the adjacent Paget's disease. The presence of pre-existing ankylosing spondylitis may allow more extensive Paget's disease of bone throughout confluent bone from the pelvis, sacrum and lumbar spine (PEEL et al. 1996). In addition, chondrocalcinosis has been demonstrated in the sacroiliac joints in some cases (BEZZA et al. 1999). In uncomplicated Paget's disease in the spine and around the sacroiliac joints, MR imaging does not contribute additional information to radiographic evaluation (OOSTVEEN and VAN DELAAR 2000).

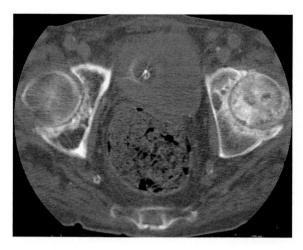

Fig. 23.7. CT scan through the hips demonstrating Paget's disease of the right acetabulum and osteoarthritis of the left hip. disease (Reproduced with permission from WHITEHOUSE (2002)]

23.5.3
Demineralisation

Demineralisation of bone is the earliest radiographic feature of Paget's disease, producing the "lytic" phase of the disease. Even after this has progressed to mixed disease, immobilisation can induce a rapid and severe demineralisation of Pagetic bone (WALLACE et al. 1996). This may be seen after immobilisation for fracture treatment or other surgical procedure such as hip joint replacement. Subsequent pathological fracture through the osteopenic pagetic bone is common. The radiographic appearances of immobilisation osteolysis, with or without pathological fracture, can be mistaken for bone destruction and malignant transformation. MR imaging is particularly valuable in distinguishing osteolysis in Paget's disease from more sinister complications, the demonstration of high signal (fatty) marrow on T1 weighted imaging being reassuring (Fig. 23.8), whilst areas of low signal may represent malignant degeneration (SUNDARAM et al. 2001). Occasionally, the use of bisphosphonates in Paget's disease may lead to osteomalacia. The radiographic appearances of osteomalacia superimposed on Paget's disease, may simulate marrow infiltration with malignancy (López et al. 2003).

23.5.4
Tumour (Primary and Secondary)

The development of primary bone sarcoma in pre-existing Paget's disease of bone is well recognised,

albeit rare (FENTON and RESNICK 1991). It is estimated to occur in less than 1% of patients with Paget's disease and is most common in the elderly, those with long duration Paget's disease and those with polyostotic Paget's disease. Exceptions will occur and sarcoma has been described in monostotic disease. The most commonly affected bones in descending order of frequency are the femur, pelvis and humerus. Pagetic sarcoma is often histologically heterogeneous but classified according to the most aggressive component; consequently most are osteosarcomas. Late presentation and histologically aggressive tumours in an elderly population may be factors contributing to the extremely poor prognosis for pagetic sarcoma, median survival being 9 months (GRIMER et al. 2003). Pagetic osteogenic sarcoma may rarely be multifocal at presentation (VUILLEMIN et al. 2000).

The majority of Paget's sarcomas are predominantly lytic on radiographs (65%) (Fig. 23.9a). The lysis usually appears ill-defined or permeative within a pre-existing area of Paget's disease. It may arise within the lytic, sclerotic or mixed phases of the underlying disease. Cortical destruction in three quarters of cases and a soft tissue mass in over half are the cardinal features that should suggest the diagnosis of malignancy, albeit not necessarily a sarcoma (López et al. 2003). Periosteal new bone formation and dense tumour mineralization is uncommon (Fig. 23.9b). Unlike most sarcomas of bone Paget's sarcoma may appear paradoxically photopenic on bone scintigraphy. MR imaging of Paget's sarcoma shows replacement of marrow fat with intermediate or low signal intensity tumour tissue on T1-weighted images with correspondingly high signal intensity on T2-weighted and short tau inversion recovery (STIR) images. The exception is seen if the tumour is particularly densely mineralised.

The involvement of Pagetic bone by metastatic disease is well documented, but whether Pagetic bone is a preferential site for bone metastases or the opposite remains controversial. Multiple myeloma (NEITZSCHMAN 1997) and lymphoma (YU et al. 1997) have rarely occurred in Pagetic bone and one family with Kaposi's sarcoma and Paget's disease has also been described (HALE and KELLY 1998). As the imaging features of these different malignancies occurring in association with Paget's disease cannot be distinguished biopsy diagnosis is mandatory as management and prognosis can vary (Fig. 23.10).

Giant cell tumours have been described in Paget's disease of bone (Fig. 23.11). These are most often in the facial skeleton and also seem to be familial in

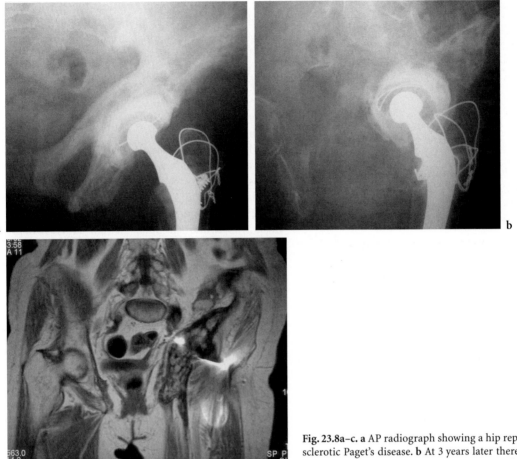

Fig. 23.8a–c. a AP radiograph showing a hip replacement and sclerotic Paget's disease. **b** At 3 years later there is migration of the prosthesis into a region of massive osteolysis. **c** Coronal T1-weighted image confirms pagetic bone with fatty marrow and no soft tissue mass

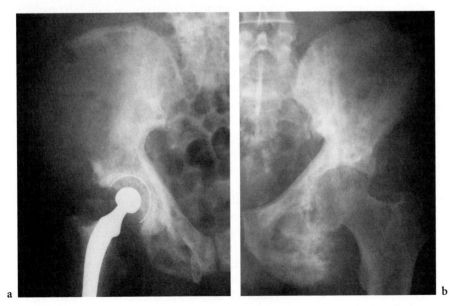

Fig. 23.9a,b. Two cases of osteosarcoma arising in Paget's disease. **a** Lytic tumour in the right ilium. **b** Mineralised tumour in the left ischium

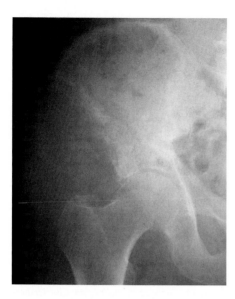

Fig. 23.10. Lymphoma arising in Paget's disease. Note the similarity to the osteosarcoma in Fig. 23.9a

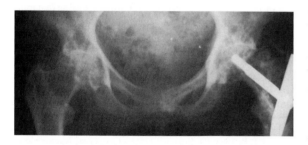

Fig. 23.11. Extensive Paget's disease. The lytic lesion in the right femoral neck proved to be a giant cell tumour. (Case courtesy of Dr D Ritchie)

an Italian population (RENDINA et al. 2004), and familial with facial and pelvic locations in a Korean family (G.S. KIM et al. 1997). Pseudosarcoma, a mass of non-mineralised pagetic osteoid, may develop in Paget's disease, usually in a paracortical location on a long bone in a lower limb (TINS et al. 2001; McNAIRN et al. 2001). A pelvic location for this complication has not been described. The MR appearances can be mixed, with both high and low signal areas on T1 weighted imaging (DONÁTH et al. 2000), consequently differentiation from a true sarcoma can be difficult and biopsy proof is usually required. Another cause of a para-osseous soft tissue mass in Paget's disease is extramedullary haematopoiesis. This is extremely rare and usually paraspinal in location, with only seven cases reported up to 1999 (RELEA et al. 1999).

23.6
Treatment

23.6.1
Medical

The medical treatment of Paget's disease is now predominantly by bisphosphonates. The more recently developed highly potent bisphosphonates are preferred (DRAKE et al. 2001). Adequate treatment appears to halt progression of the disease and alleviates the pain associated with active disease (SIRIS 1999). The hope that other complications of Paget's disease may be also be averted by bisphosphonate therapy has not yet been proven. Chronic bisphosphonate treatment may be detrimental to the rest of the skeleton, with an increased risk of osteoporotic fracture at other sites. This risk may be reduced by concomitant treatment with calcium and calcitriol (STEWART et al. 1999). Paget's disease resistant to one bisphosphonate is uncommon and may respond to an alternative formulation (JOSHUA et al. 2003). Other causes of pain in Paget's disease should be considered, particularly arthritis (being common), as treatment response to bisphosphonates will be poor if the cause is arthritis (VASIREDDY et al. 2003).

23.6.2
Surgical

Surgical treatment of Paget's disease in the pelvis and femora includes fracture management, osteotomy for correction of femoral bowing deformity and hip replacement for arthropathy or femoral neck fracture. Fracture healing is slower and poorer in Pagetic bone but is usually achieved (SHARDLOW et al. 1999) and there is the risk of immobilisation osteolysis after surgery (OAKLEY and MATHESON 2003).

Although osteotomy corrects deformity, the indication for femoral osteotomy in Paget's disease is usually pain with associated deformity. Average time to union of osteotomy is 6 months in Pagetic bone, with greater delay for diaphyseal osteotomy. Non-union appears commoner in femoral osteotomy fixed by intramedullary nail (PARVIZI et al. 2003).

Hip arthroplasties may be cemented or uncemented, both appear satisfactory in patients with Paget's disease (PARVIZI et al. 2002; CALDERONI et al. 2002; SOCHART and PORTER 2000). Following hip arthroplasty in Paget's disease, the risk of heterotopic ossification is moderately raised, but can be reduced by pre- or immediate post-operative irradiation (IORIO and HEALY 2002).

Osteomyelitis has been described as a complication in Paget's disease but there is little literature to support an increased risk of osteomyelitis in Pagetic bone after surgical intervention. The loosening or early failure of hip prostheses has been described in Paget's disease. Despite these considerations, surgical management with appropriate prostheses usually has a satisfactory outcome.

23.7
Differential Diagnosis

The radiographic appearances of Paget's disease are usually pathognomonic. Where sclerosis is marked and bone expansion minimal, the differential may include sclerotic malignant diseases such as osteosarcoma, metastatic prostate, breast or lung cancers, lymphoma and carcinoid (BASARIA et al. 2000). Rare diseases which more closely resemble Paget's disease both histologically or biochemically as well as on imaging are familial expansile osteolysis and hyperphosphatasaemia. The former, autosomal dominant condition most commonly affects the appendicular skeleton with focal pagetoid lesions (HUGHES et al. 2000). The latter condition is usually an inherited autosomal recessive condition, with pagetic manifestations throughout the skeleton presenting in early childhood, thus sometimes called juvenile Paget's disease (BONAKDARPOUR et al. 2000).

23.8
Conclusions

Paget's disease of bone may be disappearing. Complications of Paget's disease remain common in the elderly and may require medical and/or surgical management. Recognition of the disease, its severity and extent on isotope bone scanning, CT and MR, as well as conventional radiography remain important. Recognition of the complications of Paget's disease may require additional imaging.

References

Altman RD (1999) Paget's disease of bone: rheumatologic complications. Bone 24 [Suppl 5]:47S–48S

Armas JB, Pimentel F, Guyer PB et al (2002) Evidence of geographic variation in the occurrence of Paget's disease. Bone 30:649–650

Basaria S, McCarthy EF, Belzberg AJ, Ball DW (2000) Case of an ivory vertebra. J Endocrinol Invest 23:533–535

Bezza A, Lechevalier D, Monréal M et al (1999) L'atteinte sacro-iliaque au cours de la maladie de Paget. 6 observations. Presse Med 28:1157–1159

Bonakdarpour A, Maldjian C, Weiss S et al (2000) Hyperphosphatasemia: report of three cases. Eur J Radiol 35:54–58

Boutin RD, Spitz DJ, Newman JS et al (1998) Complications in Paget disease at MR imaging. Radiology 209:641–651

Calderoni P, Ferruzzi A, Andreoli I, Gualtieri G (2002) Hip arthroplasty in coxarthrosis secondary to Paget's disease. Chir Organi Mov 87:43–48

Choma TJ, Kuklo TR, Islinger RB et al (2004) Paget's disease of bone in patients younger than 40 years. Clin Orthop 418:202–204

Chrétien J. (1995) Etude des localisations vertébrales de la maladie de Paget. Ann Radiol (Paris) 38:169–176

Cook GJR, Blake GM, Marsden PK et al (2002) Quantification of skeletal kinetic indices in Paget's disease using dynamic 18F-fluoride positron emission tomography. J Bone Miner Res 17:854–859

Cooper C, Schafheutle K, Dennison E et al (1999) The epidemiology of Paget's disease in Britain: is the prevalence decreasing? J Bone Miner Res 14:192–197

Cundy T, McAnulty K, Wattie D et al (1997) Evidence for secular change in Paget's disease. Bone 20:69–71

Cundy T, Wattie D, Busch S et al (1999) Paget's disease in New Zealand: is it changing? Bone 24 [Suppl 5]:7S–9S

Davis DP, Bruffey JD, Rosen P (1999) Coccygeal fracture and Paget's disease presenting as acute cauda equina syndrome. J Emerg Med 17:251–254

Dickinson CJ (1999) Mouth bacteria as the cause of Paget's disease of bone. Med Hypotheses 52:209–212

Donáth J, Szilágyi M, Fornet B et al (2000) Pseudosarcoma in Paget's disease. Eur Radiol 10:1664–1668

Donáth J, Speer G, Poór G et al (2004) Vitamin D receptor, oestrogen receptor-alpha and calcium-sensing receptor genotypes, bone mineral density and biochemical markers in Paget's disease of bone. Rheumatology (Oxf) 43:692–695

Doyle T, Gunn J, Anderson G et al (2002) Paget's disease in New Zealand: evidence for declining prevalence. Bone 31:616–619

Drake WM, Kendler DL, Brown JP (2001) Consensus statement on the modern therapy of Paget's disease of bone from a Western Osteoporosis Alliance symposium. Clin Ther 23:620–626

Eekhoff EWM, Karperien M, Houtsma D et al (2004) Familial Paget's disease in The Netherlands: occurrence, identification of new mutations in the sequestosome 1 gene, and their clinical associations. Arthritis Rheum 50:1650–1654

Fenton P, Resnick D (1991) Metastases to bone affected by Paget's disease. A report of three cases. Int Orthop 15:397–399

Fraser WD (1997) Paget's disease of bone. Curr Opin Rheumatol 9:347–354

Friedrichs WE, Reddy SV, Bruder JM et al (2002) Sequence analysis of measles virus nucleocapsid transcripts in patients with Paget's disease. J Bone Miner Res 17:145–151

Gold DT, Boisture J, Shipp KM et al (1996) Paget's disease of bone and quality of life. J Bone Miner Res 11:1897–1904

Gómez AC, Mautalen CA (2001) European origin of patients with Paget's disease of bone in the Buenos Aires area. Eur J Epidemiol 17:409–411

Good D, Busfield F, Duffy D et al (2001) Familial Paget's disease of bone: nonlinkage to the PDB1 and PDB2 loci on chromosomes 6p and 18q in a large pedigree. J Bone Miner Res 16:33–38

Grimer RJ, Cannon SR, Taminiau AM et al (2003) Osteosarcoma over the age of forty. Eur J Cancer 39:157–163

Gutteridge DH, Retallack RW, Ward LC et al (2003) Bone density changes in Paget's disease 2 years after iv pamidronate: profound, sustained increases in pagetic bone with severity-related loss in forearm nonpagetic cortical bone. Bone 32:56–61

Hain SF, Fogelman I (2002) Nuclear medicine studies in metabolic bone disease. Semin Musculoskelet Radiol 6:323–329

Hale LR, Kelly JW (1998) Familial Kaposi's sarcoma and Paget's disease of bone. Australas J Dermatol 39:241–243

Helfrich MH, Hobson RP, Grabowski PS et al (2000) A negative search for a paramyxoviral etiology of Paget's disease of bone: molecular, immunological, and ultrastructural studies in UK patients. J Bone Miner Res 15:2315–2329

Helliwell PS (1995) Osteoarthritis and Paget's disease. Br J Rheumatol 34:1061–1063

Helliwell PS, Porter G (1999) Controlled study of the prevalence of radiological osteoarthritis in clinically unrecognised juxta-articular Paget's disease. Ann Rheum Dis 58:762–765

Hocking LJ, Lucas GJA, Daroszewska A et al (2002) Domain-specific mutations in sequestosome 1 (SQSTM1) cause familial and sporadic Paget's disease. Hum Mol Genet 11:2735–2739

Hoffman GS (1998) Radiographic findings in Paget's disease of bone. Cleve Clin J Med 65:273

Hughes AE, Ralston SH, Marken J et al (2000) Mutations in TNFRSF11A, affecting the signal peptide of RANK, cause familial expansile osteolysis. Nat Genet 24:45–48

Iorio R, Healy WL (2002) Heterotopic ossification after hip and knee arthroplasty: risk factors, prevention, and treatment. J Am Acad Orthop Surg 10:409–416

Jelinek JS, Kransdorf MJ, Gray R et al (1996) Percutaneous transpedicular biopsy of vertebral body lesions. Spine 21:2035–2040

Johnson PTL, Wisdom JH, Weldon KS et al (2003) Three novel mutations in SQSTM1 identified in familial Paget's disease of bone. J Bone Miner Res 18:1748–1753

Joshua F, Epstein M, Major G (2003) Bisphosphonate resistance in Paget's disease of bone. Arthritis Rheum 48:2321–2323

Khan SA, Brennan P, Newman J et al (1996) Paget's disease of bone and unvaccinated dogs. Bone 19:47–50

Kim GS, Kim SH, Cho JK et al (1997) Paget bone disease involving young adults in 3 generations of a Korean family. Medicine (Baltimore) 76:157–169

Kim CK, Estrada WN, Lorberboym M et al (1997) The 'mouse face' appearance of the vertebrae in Paget's disease. Clin Nucl Med 22:104–108

Kurihara N, Reddy SV, Menaa C et al (2000) Osteoclasts expressing the measles virus nucleocapsid gene display a pagetic phenotype. J Clin Invest 105:607–614

Laroche M, Delpech B, Bernard J et al (1999) Measurement of bone mineral density by dual X-ray absorptiometry in Paget's disease before and after pamidronate treatment. Calcif Tissue Int 65:188–191

Lever JH (2002) Paget's disease of bone in Lancashire and arsenic pesticide in cotton mill wastewater: a speculative hypothesis. Bone 31:434–436

López AG, Morales PA, Elena IA et al (1997) Cattle, pets, and Paget's disease of bone. Epidemiology 8:247–251

López C, Thomas DV, Davies AM (2003) Neoplastic transformation and tumour-like lesions in Paget's disease of bone: a pictorial review. Eur Radiol 13:L151–L163

McNairn JD, Damron TA, Landas SK, Ambrose JL (2001) Benign tumefactive soft tissue extension from Paget's disease of bone simulating malignancy. Skeletal Radiol 30:157–160

Mee AP, Dixon JA, Hoyland JA et al (1998) Detection of canine distemper virus in 100% of Paget's disease samples by in situ-reverse transcriptase-polymerase chain reaction. Bone 23:171–175

Melton LJ 3rd, Tiegs RD, Atkinson EJ et al (2000) Fracture risk among patients with Paget's disease: a population-based cohort study. J Bone Miner Res 15:2123–2128

Morales PAA, Bachiller CFJ, Abraira V et al (2002) Is clinical expressiveness of Paget's disease of bone decreasing? Bone 30:399–403

Nakatsuka K, Nishizawa Y, Ralston SH (2003) Phenotypic characterization of early onset Paget's disease of bone caused by a 27-bp duplication in the TNFRSF11A gene. J Bone Miner Res 18:1381–1385

Nance MA, Nuttall FQ, Econs MJ et al (2000) Heterogeneity in Paget disease of the bone. Am J Med Genet 92:303–307

Neitzschman HR (1997) Radiology case of the month. Paget's disease with onset of increasing bone pain. Paget's disease with coexisting multiple myeloma. J La State Med Soc 149:109–110

Oakley AP, Matheson JA (2003) Rapid osteolysis after revision hip arthroplasty in Paget's disease. J Arthroplasty 18:204–207

Ooi CG, Walsh CA, Gallagher JA et al (2000) Absence of measles virus and canine distemper virus transcripts in long-term bone marrow cultures from patients with Paget's disease of bone. Bone 27:417–421

Oostveen JC, van deLaar MA (2000) Magnetic resonance imaging in rheumatic disorders of the spine and sacroiliac joints. Semin Arthritis Rheum 30:52–69

Parvizi J, Schall DM, Lewallen DG, Sim FH (2002) Outcome of uncemented hip arthroplasty components in patients with Paget's disease. Clin Orthop 403:127–134

Parvizi J, Frankle MA, Tiegs RD et al (2003) Corrective osteotomy for deformity in Paget disease. J Bone Joint Surg Am 85-A:697–702

Peel NF, Barrington NA, Austin CA, Eastell R (1996) Paget's disease in a patient with ankylosing spondylitis - a diagnostic dilemma. Br J Rheumatol 35:1011–1014

Poncelet A (1999) The neurologic complications of Paget's disease. J Bone Miner Res 14 [Suppl 2]:88–91

Ralston SH, Helfrich MH (1999) Are paramyxoviruses involved in Paget's disease? A negative view. Bone 24 [Suppl 5]:17S–18S

Rapado A, Jiménez J, Morales A et al (1999) Patterns of diagnosis of Paget's disease in Spain. J Bone Miner Res 14 [Suppl 2]:96–98

Reddy SV, Kurihara N, Menaa C et al (2001) Osteoclasts formed by measles virus-infected osteoclast precursors from hCD46 transgenic mice express characteristics of pagetic osteoclasts. Endocrinology 142:2898–2905

Relea A, García-Urbón MV, Arboleya L, Zamora T (1999) Extramedullary hematopoiesis related to Paget's disease. Eur Radiol 9:205–207

Rendina D, Mossetti G, Soscia E et al (2004) Giant cell tumor and Paget's disease of bone in one family: geographic clustering. Clin Orthop 421:218–224

Renier JC, Audran M (1997a) Progression in length and width of pagetic lesions, and estimation of age at disease onset. Rev Rhum Engl Ed 64:35–43

Renier JC, Audran M (1997b) Polyostotic Paget's disease. A search for lesions of different durations and for new lesions. Rev Rhum Engl Ed 64:233–242

Renier JC, Leroy E, Audran M (1996a) The initial site of bone lesions in Paget's disease. A review of two hundred cases. Rev Rhum Engl Ed 63:823–829

Renier JC, Fanello S, Bos C et al (1996b) An etiologic study of Paget's disease. Rev Rhum Engl Ed 63:606–611

Rogers J, Jeffrey DR, Watt I (2002) Paget's disease in an archeological population. J Bone Miner Res 17:1127–1134

Rotés SD, Monfort J, Solano A et al (2004) The clover and heart signs in vertebral scintigraphic images are highly specific of Paget's disease of bone. Bone 34:605–608

Seton M, Choi HK, Hansen MF et al (2003) Analysis of environmental factors in familial versus sporadic Paget's disease of bone - the New England Registry for Paget's Disease of Bone. J Bone Miner Res 18:1519–1524

Shardlow DL, Giannoudis PV, Matthews SJ et al (1999) Stabilisation of acute femoral fractures in Paget's disease. Int Orthop 23:283–285

Siris ES (1999) Goals of treatment for Paget's disease of bone. J Bone Miner Res 14 [Suppl 2]:49–52

Smith SE, Murphey MD, Motamedi K et al (2002) From the archives of the AFIP. Radiologic spectrum of Paget disease of bone and its complications with pathologic correlation. Radiographics 22:1191–1216

Sochart DH, Porter ML (2000) Charnley low-friction arthroplasty for Paget's disease of the hip. J Arthroplasty 15:210–219

Spieth ME, Kasner DL, Manor WF (2003) Positron emission tomography and Paget disease: hot is not necessarily malignant. Clin Nucl Med 28:773–774

Stewart GO, Gutteridge DH, Price RI et al (1999) Prevention of appendicular bone loss in Paget's disease following treatment with intravenous pamidronate disodium. Bone 24:139–144

Sundaram M, Khanna G, El Khoury GY (2001) T1-weighted MR imaging for distinguishing large osteolysis of Paget's disease from sarcomatous degeneration. Skeletal Radiol 30:378–383

Tins BJ, Davies AM, Mangham DC (2001) MR imaging of pseudosarcoma in Paget's disease of bone: a report of two cases. Skeletal Radiol 30:161–165

Vande-Berg BC, Malghem J, Lecouvet FE et al (2001) Magnetic resonance appearance of uncomplicated Paget's disease of bone. Semin Musculoskelet Radiol 5:69–77

Van Staa TP, Selby P, Leufkens HGM et al (2002) Incidence and natural history of Paget's disease of bone in England and Wales. J Bone Miner Res 17:465–471

Vasireddy S, Talwalkar A, Miller H et al (2003) Patterns of pain in Paget's disease of bone and their outcomes on treatment with pamidronate. Clin Rheumatol 22:376–380

Vuillemin BV, Parlier CC, Cywiner GC et al (2000) Multifocal osteogenic sarcoma in Paget's disease. Skeletal Radiol 29:349–353

Wallace K, Haddad JG, Gannon FH et al (1996) Skeletal response to immobilization in Paget's disease of bone: a case report. Clin Orthop 328:236–240

Whitehouse RW (2002) Paget's disease of bone. Semin Musculoskelet Radiol 6:313–322

Whitten CR, Saifuddin A (2003) MRI of Paget's disease of bone. Clin Radiol 58:763–769

Whyte MP, Obrecht SE, Finnegan PM et al (2002) Osteoprotegerin deficiency and juvenile Paget's disease. N Engl J Med 347:175–184

Yip KM, Lee YL, Kumta SM et al (1996) The second case of Paget's disease (osteitis deformans) in a Chinese lady. Singapore Med J 37:665–667

Yu T, Squires F, Mammone J, DiMarcangelo M (1997) Lymphoma arising in Paget's disease. Skeletal Radiol 26:729–731

24 Hip Prosthesis

Stephen Eustace and Patricia Cunningham

CONTENTS

S. Eustace, MD; P. Cunningham, MD
Department of Radiology, Mater Misericordiae and Cappagh National Orthopaedic Hospital, Finglas, Dublin 11, Ireland

24.1
Introduction

Imaging of hip prostheses using conventional and newer techniques will be reviewed in this chapter. Conventional modalities, radiographs, arthrograms and scintigraphy remain useful methods of evaluating primary complications of hardware fixation (loosening and infection), but developments in technology, particularly techniques to reduce metal-induced artefact, allow detailed evaluation of adjacent soft tissues with both CT scan and MR imaging.

24.2
Anatomy and Definition of Terms

A total hip arthroplasty has both femoral and acetabular components.

The acetabular component includes a fixation cup made of either metal or plastic within which lies a polyethylene liner.

The femoral component includes a stem composed of metal and of a femoral head and neck component being composed of either metal or ceramic. The femoral component articulates with the polyethylene liner held within the cup of the acetabular component. Cemented and noncemented fixation methods are employed at either site. Cement fixation employs methylmethacrylate cement, while uncemented approaches employ bonding by either bone ingrowth to beads coating the prostheses surfaces or by direct chemical bonding induced by hydroxyapatite coating of the prostheses surfaces.

More recently a modification in total hip arthroplasty has been introduced termed "resurfacing" in which the surfaces of the femoral head and of the acetabulum are replaced by metallic components (Fig. 24.1). In this setting the metal coated femoral head articulates with a metal cup lining the acetabulum. Such metal-on-metal articulation is thought to increase release of metallic particles to the blood-

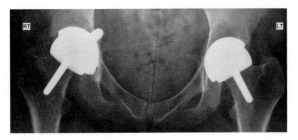

Fig. 24.1. AP radiograph showing bilateral metal-on-metal resurfacing prostheses. There is loosening of the acetabular component on the right

stream. At the time of writing it remains unclear whether such an effect has long term health implications for the patient but early results are promising (DANIEL et al. 2004). In a hemiarthroplasty the native acetabulum is not altered by surgery. The femoral head alone is replaced by a prosthetic device. Two forms of hemiarthroplasty are recognized and marketed termed unipolar and bipolar prostheses. In a unipolar prosthesis the head of the prosthesis articulates with the native acetabulum alone, in a bipolar prosthesis there are two articulations between the head of the prosthesis and the native acetabulum and between the head of the prosthesis and the neck of the prosthesis. Such a design minimises motion between the head of the prosthesis and the native acetabulum and preserves native articular cartilage. Bipolar hemiarthroplasty, although being considerably more expensive, is recommended when the femoral head of a high level ambulator is to be replaced.

Metal type selected for the prosthesis is dictated by mechanical needs, balancing requirements for elasticity with the requirement for durability and resistance. The biocompatibility of metallic alloys – stainless steel, cobalt chrome, and titanium alloy – is based on the presence of a constituent alloy that has the ability to form an adherent oxide coating that is stable, chemically inert, and hence biocompatible. The type of metal used in orthopaedic fixation devices has traditionally been dictated by the availability of the metal, cost, and mechanical qualities, which include the yield strength (the amount of elastic strain that may be applied to the metal before producing a permanent deformation), the fatigue strength (the ability of the metal to resist axial loading), and the modulus of the metal (the inherent mechanical property of the metal). Although stainless steel is frequently used for fixation, its low yield stress, rapid metal fatigue, and low modulus, leading to plate and prosthesis failure, have promoted the development of other alloys. In this regard, cobalt

chrome is favoured if tensile and fatigue strength are required, titanium is favoured if load sharing with adjacent bone (uncemented prostheses) is required (titanium has a similar modulus to cortical bone). In relation to MR imaging, titanium alloys are less ferromagnetic than both cobalt chrome and steel, induce less susceptibility artefact, and result in less marked image degradation (EUSTACE 1999).

24.3
Conventional Imaging

Loosening, which can complicate either cemented or noncemented fixation, represents the commonest cause of hardware failure, most commonly complicating total hip replacement.

24.3.1
Cement Fixation

Polymethylmethacrylate (PMMA) cement provides immediate stable fixation of both metal and non-metal components and functions to distribute load more evenly to bone. It does not have adhesive qualities and so fixation is achieved by physical interdigitations with an uneven surface rather than by chemical bonding.

Improvements in cementing, component design, and canal preparation [irrigation and removal of debris, creation of several small anchoring holes, and preservation of subchondral bone (nonreamed technique)] have decreased loosening rates particularly of the femoral component of total hip replacements. Although loosening occurs more rapidly in high-level ambulators, refinement in technique has resulted in a decrease in femoral component loosening from 30% to 60% at 5–10 years to 1.7% in one study (CHANDLER et al. 1991; WEISSMAN 1990). A similar but less marked reduction in loosening of the acetabular component from 41% to 16.7% has been observed using metal-backed components (HARRIS and PENENBERG 1987; WEISSMAN 1990).

24.3.2
Radiographic Appearances of Cement Component Loosening

Loosening of the femoral component of a total hip replacement is indicated by breakdown at the cement–bone interface to produce a linear lucent zone of 2 mm or greater, change in the position of the component by 4 mm or greater, and any progressive lucency or cement fracture (WEISSMAN 1990). The probability of loosening increases if lucency is wide and extensive. Loosening is confirmed if actual component migration is documented (Fig. 24.2).

Criteria indicating loosening of the acetabular component vary in differing series. Migration or change in position of the component by greater than 4 mm or 4° confirms loosening (YODER et al. 1988). Although documentation of acetabular position has been markedly simplified by the use of templates that permit direct measurement of superior or medial acetabular migration from the pelvic radiograph, several radiographic techniques have been described and may be used with equal effect (GOODMAN et al. 1988). Acetabular inclination that represents the tilt of the acetabular component with relation to the horizontal is measured as the angle between a line drawn along the long axis of the marker wire of the acetabular component and a line drawn between both ischial tuberosities, the bi-ischial line, or between the teardrops, the inter-teardrop line. The cup is positioned in such a way as to provide maximum range of motion without significant risk of dislocation (40–50° usually). Abnormal inclination immediately post surgery usually reflects surgical technique (a failure to shell out native acetabular floor or to recognise a dysplastic acetabulum); an acquired change in inclinations an indication of postoperative loosening.

Acetabular anteversion describes the relative anterior tilt of the acetabular component in the lateral plane, derived by measuring the angle between a line drawn along the long axis of the marker wire and the horizontal plane. It may be derived on the anteroposterior (AP) radiograph by dividing the maximum diameter of the marker wire by the minimum diameter and comparing the derived value with a table of previously derived values (the greater the anterior tilt, the more the marker wire assumes the shape of a circle in the AP plane). Measurement in the AP projection alone does not allow differentiation of retroversion from anteversion because both have the same appearance in this plane. In addition, perceived degree of anterior tilt may vary depending on where the radiograph is centred (GOODMAN et al. 1988). HARRIS and PENENBERG (1987) have described three stages of acetabular loosening: (1) evolving loosening indicated by discontinuous lucency at the cement–bone interface, (2) impending loosening indicated by continuous cement-bone

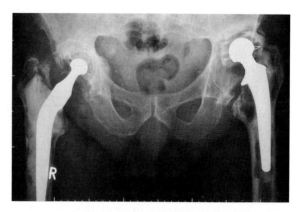

Fig. 24.2. Bilateral total hip replacements with cement fixation of femoral and acetabular components bilaterally. On the left side there is osteolysis surrounding the femoral and acetabular components with subsidence of the femoral component and rotation of the acetabular component secondary to gross loosening

lucency and (3) definite loosening indicated by documented component migration.

24.4
Arthrography in Cemented Component Loosening

Suspected loosening may be confirmed by the actual demonstration of contrast interdigitating between cement and bone at high-pressure arthrography. Arthrographic diagnosis may be enhanced by using either photographic or digital subtraction if available, radionuclide arthrography, and by imaging both pre-exercise and post exercise (ANDERSON and STAPLE 1973; BASSETT et al. 1985; FIROOZNIA et al. 1974; HENDRIX et al. 1983).Developments in CT scan, specifically reformatting techniques, suggest that CT arthrography may now be of considerable value in this setting, although this has not been scientifically evaluated to date (EUSTACE et al. 1998b). Injection of contrast under high pressure to the pseudojoint space has considerably reduced the false-negative rate at arthrography, although in a minority with surgically proven loosening, movement of contrast is limited by adhesions. HENDRIX et al. (1983), using high injection pressures, noted a 3% false-negative and a 5% false-positive rate at arthrography; however, such high pressures may be difficult to achieve in patients with lax pseudocapsules or communicating bursae following antecedent component dislocation. HARDY et al. (1988) documented improved diagnostic sensitivity in patients in whom arthrograms were reviewed following exercise, features of loosening being more marked in 42% of cases. The addition of technetium 99m sulphur colloid to water-soluble contrast at the time of injection may also improve diagnostic accuracy. It is felt that because radiopharmaceutical is less viscous than radiographic contrast, it is more likely to interdigitate at sites of loosening. RESNIK et al. (1986) found that the combined technique yielded 100% diagnostic sensitivity and specificity, justifying the additional time, effort and cost of such a practice.

The identification of contrast material at the cement–bone interface suggests component loosening (Fig. 24.3); however, in up to 40% of patients this may not be symptomatic and its identification requires correlation with other clinical parameters to determine its true significance (HARDY et al. 1988). Generally, arthrography tends to produce false-positive results for acetabular loosening and false-negative results for femoral loosening.

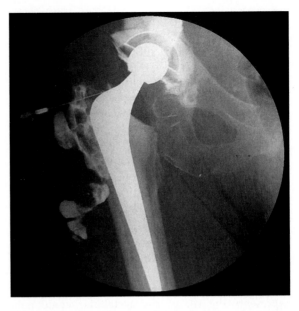

Fig. 24.3. Contrast arthrogram showing leakage and extension of contrast medium along the proximal shaft of the femoral component and into an adjacent blind ending sinus secondary to prosthesis infection

24.4.1
Technetium-99m Methylene Diphosphonate Bone Scanning in the Detection of Cemented Component Loosening

Concentration of technetium-99m methylene diphosphonate (MDP) following intravenous injection essentially reflects vascular perfusion to an area and osteoblastic activity (hydroxyapatite production) at that site. Following cemented prosthesis placement, marginal osteoblastic activity returns to normal at approximately 6 months in the majority of cases (CAMPEAU et al. 1976). In a minority, activity persists, most frequently at the tip of the prosthesis and in these patients scanning may be misleading (CAMPEAU et al. 1976). Similarly, because a loose prosthesis does not always induce marginal osteoblastic activity, the sensitivity of the test may be as low as 67% (ALIABIDI et al. 1989). Most patients have normal bone scintigraphy approximately 1 year after surgery, 20% have marginally increased activity for more than 1 year and 10% have persistent activity at the tip of the femoral stem and at the greater trochanter (Fig. 24.4) (CAMPEAU et al. 1976).

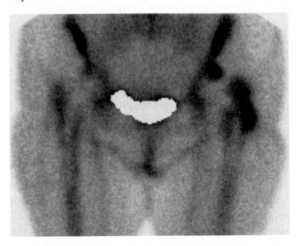

Fig. 24.4. Technetium 99m methylene diphosphonate bone scan on a patient with bilateral hip prostheses. There is concentration of the radionuclide in the roof of the left acetabulum and adjacent to the proximal shaft of the femoral component secondary to osteolysis and loosening

24.5
Noncemented Techniques

In an attempt to improve prosthesis stability, two forms of biologic fixation have been developed and are now widely used, particularly in young patients in whom preservation of bone stock facilitates potential revision in old age. Bone ingrowth components achieve fixation by fibrous and bony ingrowth (6 weeks to 1 year) between metallic beads coating the surface of the component. Hydroxyapatite components achieve fixation by forming chemical bonds at the metal–bone interface (no fibrous membrane is formed) within 6 weeks. In both cases, bonding is enhanced by drilling a conservative femoral canal resulting in a tight interface between component and native bone. Following initial ingrowth, remodelling occurs for up to 2 years. In most cases, bony ingrowth fills the spaces between the metallic beads; in a minority fibrous ingrowth occurs and a fibrous membrane is formed around the component (Fig. 24.5).

24.5.1
Radiographic Evaluation of Loosening in Noncemented Components

The determination of loosening in bone ingrowth components may be difficult because the development of fibrous union, which may be stable, results in the development of a worrisome lucent line at the metal-bone interface. Like cemented components, definite loosening is indicated by actual component migration. Progression in the diameter of the lucent line around the prosthesis, especially after 2 years, or an increase in the number of free metal beads at the metal–bone interface, dislodged by motion, suggest component loosening (ENGH and BOBYN 1988; ENGH and MASSIN 1989). Transfer of stresses of weight bearing to the metal component and away from the femoral neck may lead to bone loss in the medial femoral cortex as mature bonding occurs. Such transfer of stress may lead to the development of asymptomatic cortical thickening at the tip of the component and adjacent to the distal stem (ENGH and MASSIN 1989; KAPLAN et al. 1988).

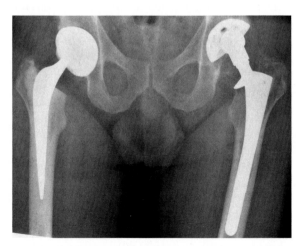

Fig. 24.5. Radiograph of a patient with bilateral total hip replacements, on the right with cement fixation of the femoral component and uncemented fixation of the acetabular component, on the left, with uncemented fixation of both the acetabular and femoral components

24.5.2
Technetium-99m MDP Scintigraphy in the Evaluation of Noncemented Component Loosening

Remodelling that occurs with bone ingrowth components results in increased uptake of radiopharmaceuticals and varies with the design of the component. The evaluation of loosening is therefore difficult and may only confidently be made by observing temporal changes in activity (WEISSMAN 1990).

24.5.3
Arthrography in the Evaluation of Noncemented Component Loosening

Incomplete ingrowth of bone around the porous surface of a bone ingrowth prosthesis creates channels for contrast to penetrate and may lead to the erroneous diagnosis of prosthesis loosening. As such, arthrography in uncemented bone ingrowth prostheses may lead to false-positive results (ANDERSON and STAPLE 1973; BASSETT et al. 1985; FIROOZNIA et al. 1974; HENDRIX et al. 1983). Like cemented components, false-negative results may occur secondary to underfilling of the joint with contrast.

24.6
The Evaluation of Prosthesis Infection

Infection is now considerably less common than aseptic component loosening, reflecting improved intraoperative technique and sterility. When infection does occur, detection may be difficult. Radiographic signs are unreliable, lack specificity and may be absent. When present, the identification of a rapidly developing cement–bone lucency with poorly defined margins, loculation and periosteal reaction are most suggestive of underlying infection (ALIABIDI et al. 1989; BERGSTROM et al. 1974).

24.6.1
Arthrographic Appearance and Aspiration Arthrography

Infection is suggested when contrast injected at arthrography outlines an irregular joint capsule, reflecting marginal inflammatory changes, and when it fills nonbursal cavities, sinus tracts and abscesses. Joint aspiration is routinely undertaken at the time of arthrography, and although one may assume that such a technique represents the gold standard, false-positive results are commonly encountered (positive predictive value, 54.2%) (skin commensals). False-negative results are considerably less frequent (negative predictive value, 99.2%) (Fig. 24.3) (Weissman 1990).

24.6.2
Scintigraphy

Scintigraphy is frequently undertaken in patients with suspected orthopaedic hardware infection. Despite initial enthusiasm for the technique and despite developments of tomographic scintigraphic imaging or single photon emission computed tomography (SPECT), studies evaluating sensitivity of scintigraphy have been unconvincing (Datz and Thorne 1986; Johnson et al. 1988; Streule et al. 1988).

Increased uptake of radiopharmaceutical may be seen in normal prostheses for up to 1 year following surgery, reflecting induced marginal osteoblastic activity. In such a way, it is only after 1 year that concentration of radiopharmaceutical may be considered abnormal, and that scintigraphy may be used effectively to indicate loosening or infection. Focal uptake of radiopharmaceutical is more commonly observed in patients with loose components, whereas diffuse uptake is more commonly observed in infection. These patterns, however, are merely trends and are not absolutely specific (Datz and Thorne 1986).

Attempts to improve the specificity of scintigraphy have seen the evaluation of both gallium and indium-labelled white cells. Gallium-67 is limited by low sensitivity (37%) (Aliabidi et al. 1989); however, a positive study or focal accumulation strongly suggests infection. Indium is felt to be more sensitive; however, interpretation of increased uptake must take account of increased marrow uptake of labelled white cells that occurs because of marrow displacement incurred at the time of surgery. Indium uptake is demonstrated diffusely adjacent to bone ingrowth components in 80% at up to 2 years following surgery, although the uptake is less marked than is seen on technetium bone scintigraphy. Similarly, increased uptake of indium has been previously observed in aseptic granulation tissue surrounding loose prostheses. Johnson et al. (1988) found the sensitivity of indium imaging to be 88% and the specificity to

be 90% when combined with technetium-99m MDP bone scintigraphy (subtraction technique). Indium imaging combined with marrow labelling technetium sulphur colloid also improves both the sensitivity and specificity of the technique.

Emerging data now suggests a potential role for PET (positron emission tomography) in the assessment of lower limb prosthesis infection. PET scanning employs positron emitting fluorine labelled to glucose which is taken up by actively metabolising cells via glut 1 receptors and overexpression of hexokinase in inflammatory and malignant cells. Preliminary reports suggest that PET sensitivity for detecting infection is more accurate in hip than in knee prostheses with a sensitivity of 90%, and specificity of 89.3% (Zhuang et al. 2000).

24.7
Specific Complications of Joint Prostheses

24.7.1
Acetabular Liner Wear

Wear of the polyethylene cup lining the acetabular component of hip replacements is a significant cause of morbidity, and after loosening represents the commonest cause of mechanical component failure. Rarely, particularly in young men, liner breaks down acutely and fracture or remodelling occurs within 1 year of surgery. More commonly, polyethylene liner breaks down gradually over years, reflecting chronic friction at the articular surface (Fig. 24.6).

Two radiographic methods are used to quantify the amount of wear, grossly indicated by the development of an eccentric position of the femoral head within the acetabular cup. The first involves measuring the width of the narrowest part of the socket in the weight-bearing area and subtracting it from the width of the widest part in the non-weight-bearing area, and the result halved. Liner wear is detected by serial measurements. The second method involves measuring the thickness of the acetabular component on the latest radiograph and comparing this with the thickness measured on the immediate postoperative radiograph (average wear is reported as 1.5 mm per year). A considerably less frequent cause of acetabular component failure (press fit mechanism) is loosening between the liner and the metal-backed component resulting in liner subluxation and even dislocation (Fig. 24.7).

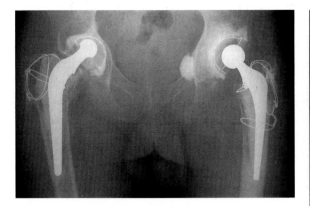

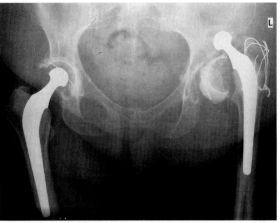

Fig. 24.6. Radiograph of a patient with bilateral total hip replacements complaining of pain on the right. There is eccentric migration of the right femoral component secondary to liner wear now complicated by the development of a giant cell granuloma in the acetabular roof

Fig. 24.7. Radiograph of a patient with bilateral total hip replacements complaining of pain on the left. There is rotation of the left acetabular component secondary to gross loosening now complicated by posterior dislocation of the femoral component

24.7.2
Giant Cell Granulomatous Reaction to Cement or Polyethylene Particles

Liberation of small (1–4 μm) polyethylene or polymethylmethacrylate (PMMA) particles to the pseudojoint space and adjacent tissues following acetabular liner wear or cement fragmentation may trigger an inflammatory cascade leading to lysis and cystic change in adjacent bone. Released polyethylene or cement particles trigger the local release of intracellular debris and inflammatory mediators. Local accumulation of inflammatory mediators produces a localised giant cell reaction and bony osteolysis, occasionally in the form of a mildly expanded pseudotumour. Radiographs in affected patients show evidence of liner wear accompanying well circumscribed often mildly expanded lytic bone lesions surrounding either the femoral or acetabular components (Figs. 24.8, 24.9). At scintigraphy sites of giant cell reaction show concentration of radiotracer on Tc99m MDP scans. MR images, when undertaken show high signal cystic lesions at the site of the giant cell reaction.

24.7.3
Heterotopic Bone

Mesenchymal cells in soft tissues adjacent to a hip prosthesis may differentiate and become osteoblastic following surgical trauma. Such differentiation to osteoblasts results in the formation of bone matrix and subsequently mineralised mature bone within the para-articular soft tissues (Fig. 24.10). Such devel-

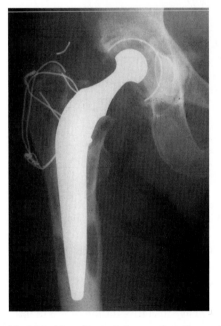

Fig. 24.8. AP radiograph in a patient 5 years following total hip replacement now complaining of right thigh pain. There is eccentric migration of the femoral head due to polyethylene liner wear in association with a mildly expansile lucent lesion encasing the distal femoral stem secondary to giant cell granulomatous reaction

opment of heterotopic bone occurs most frequently in patients with seronegative arthritis, Paget's and Forestier's disease and in paraplegics. In many patients, small amounts of heterotopic bone have little impact on function. In a minority, large amounts or seams of heterotopic bone produce mechanical effects and hinder hip mobility. In such cases surgical resection

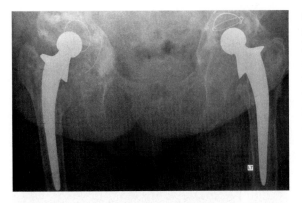

Fig. 24.9. Frontal radiograph of a patient with bilateral total hip replacements shows gross expansile osteolysis surrounding the acetabular components bilaterally, worse on the right secondary to granulomatous reactions

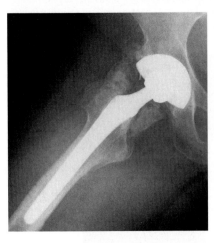

Fig. 24.10. Uncemented total hip replacement with gross mature heterotopic bone formation limiting hip mobility

of the heterotopic bone is undertaken. In this setting it is critical to prove that the heterotopic bone is mature Radiographs are employed to assess heterotopic bone formation prior undertaking surgical resection. No change in configuration over 3 months is considered a marker of maturity. Similar uptake of Tc99m in the heterotopic bone as in native bone indicates maturity. Resolution of oedema indicates maturity at MRI (Eustace 1999).

24.7.4
Dislocation

Dislocation is an uncommon complication of hip arthroplasty with most cases occurring in the first few weeks postoperatively. Dislocation is usually posteriorly with anterior dislocation being very rare. It most frequently occurs secondary to a posterior

approach for joint replacement, with trochanteric avulsion and deviation from the optimal acetabular orientation angles predisposing to subluxation and dislocation. Chronic dislocation in long standing prostheses occurs superimposed on liner wear where there is alteration in the biomechanical integrity of the prosthesis cup allowing posterior subluxation and dislocation (Fig. 24.7).

24.7.5
Abductor Avulsion

An anterolateral approach for total hip arthroplasty is favoured to avoid the complications of nonunion of the greater trochanteric osteotomy and separation of the trochanter. This approach involves the incision of the gluteus medius, vastus lateralis and gluteus minimus to gain access to the joint capsule without the need for trochanteric osteotomy. These muscles are then reattached at their trochanteric insertion with postoperative restoration of abductor muscle function and gait. However, patients occasionally present with prosthesis failure for which no cause can be found by traditional investigations. MRI is the investigation of choice in patients with clinically suspected abductor muscle avulsion as it cannot be diagnosed by radiography, arthrography, scintigraphy or CT. MRI in patients who have undergone joint replacement may be limited by susceptibility-induced loss of signal adjacent to the metal prosthesis. Satisfactory reduction in susceptibility artefact, allowing assessment of soft tissues adjacent to prostheses, may now be achieved by appropriate orientation of slice-select and frequency-encoded gradients, in conjunction with tissue excitation using RARE-based sequences (Twair et al. 2003; Eustace et al. 1998b; White et al. 2000). Artefact reduction is particularly effective when prostheses are cobalt chrome- or titanium-based rather than steel-based. Using these techniques allows clear identification of abductor muscle avulsion from the greater trochanteric attachments (Fig. 24.11).

24.8
Ultrasound

Ultrasound is particularly useful for visualising periprosthetic fluid collections. In the setting of infection it can be used to evaluate for soft tissue abscess and other extra-articular collections includ-

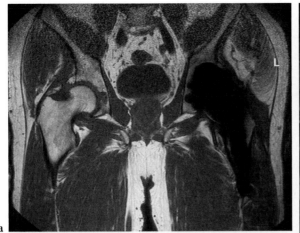

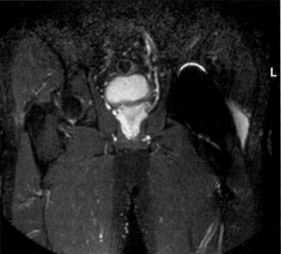

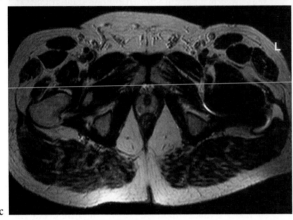

Fig. 24.11a–c. Coronal T1-weighted (**a**), coronal inversion recovery (**b**), and axial T2-weighted (**c**) images showing loculated fluid over the left greater trochanter following total hip replacement at the site of retraction of buttock abductors, indicating abductor avulsion

ing haematoma (VAN HOLSBEECK et al. 1994). Ultrasound may be useful in guiding percutaneous needle aspiration of a joint or a soft tissue collection.

24.9
Computed Tomography

Evaluation of hip prosthesis is limited due to the artefact produced which may obscure soft tissue abnormalities immediately adjacent to the prosthesis. Soft tissue and bone abnormalities distant to the prosthesis in the pelvis may still be visualised. The main method for artefact production is by missing projection data. Iterative deblurring reconstruction is less sensitive to missing projection than filtered backprojection and CT software can be used to exploit this. Using iterative methods of reconstruction artefact can be reduced sufficiently to evaluate the soft tissues adjacent to the prosthesis and allow bone edge detection (ROBERTSON et al. 1997)

Further improvement in CT image quality is possible with multidetector-row CT (HU et al. 2000).

The ability to image with very thin slices reduces artefacts produced by averaging partial volume and allows detailed reconstruction in any plane. Continuing investigations evaluating the bone-metal interface show that MDCT produces a decrease in metal artefact (PURI et al. 2002). A recent study has reported the value of CT in assessing focal osteolysis in total hip replacement (PARK et al. 2004).

24.10
Magnetic Resonance Imaging

Traditionally the use of MRI in assessing hip prosthesis has been limited by the susceptibility-induced loss of signal adjacent to the metallic prosthesis. Satisfactory reduction in artefact may be achieved by optimising the sequences used and the gradients applied. Appropriate orientation of slice-select and frequency-encoded gradients to manipulate artefact away from the tissue of interest allows assessment of the soft tissues adjacent to the metallic prosthesis. Fast spin-echo techniques use a 180° refocusing radiofrequency pulse, which corrects for signal loss due to static magnetic field homogeneities, such as those induced by metal prosthesis. Diffusion related signal loss may be reduced by increasing the echo train length and decreasing the interecho spacing (TARTAGLINO et al. 1994; EUSTACE et al. 1998a; SUH et al. 1998). MRI can be used to diagnose complications such as loosening, infection and giant cell reaction but these can all be identified using conventional methods. However, abductor muscle avulsion as a cause of failed hip prosthesis can only be diagnosed using MRI as described above (TWAIR et al. 2003).

References

Aliabidi P, Tumeh SS, Weissman BN et al (1989) Cemented total hip prosthesis: Radiographic and scintigraphic evaluation. Radiology 173:203–206

Anderson LS, Staple TW (1973) Arthrography of total hip replacement using subtraction technique. Techn Notes 109:470–471

Bassett LW, Loftus AA, Mankovich NJ (1985) Computer-processed subtraction arthrography. Radiology 157:821

Bergstrom B, Lidgren L, Lindberg L (1974) Radiographic abnormalities caused by postoperative infection following total hip arthroplasty. Clin Orthop 99:95–102

Campeau RJ, Hall MF, Miale A Jr (1976) Detection of total hip arthroplasty complications with Tc-99m pyrophosphate. J Nucl Med 17:526

Chandler HP, Reineck FT, Wixson RL et al (1981) Total hip replacements in patients younger than 30 years old. J Bone Joint Surg 65A:1426–1434

Daniel J, Pynsent PB, McMinn DJW (2004) Metal-on-metal resurfacing of the hip in patients under the age of 55 years with osteoarthritis. JBJS (Br) 86B:177–184

Datz FL, Thorne DA (1986) Effect of chronicity of infection on the sensitivity of the In-111-labeled leucocyte scan. AJR Am J Roentgenol 147:809–812

Engh CA, Bobyn JD (1988) The influence of stem size and extent of porous coating on femoral bone resorption after primary cementless hip arthroplasty. Clin Orthop 231:7–28

Engh CA, Massin P (1989) Cementless total hip arthroplasty using the anatomic medullary locking stem: results using survivorship analysis. Clin Orthop 249:141–158

Eustace SJ (1999) Magnetic resonance imaging of orthopaedic trauma, 1st edn. Lippincott, Williams and Wilkins, Philadelphia

Eustace S, Jara H, Goldberg R et al (1998a) A comparison of conventional spin-echo and turbo spin-echo imaging of soft tissue adjacent to orthopaedic hardware. AJR Am J Roentgenol 170:455–458

Eustace S, Shah B, Mason M (1998b) Imaging orthopaedic hardware with an emphasis on hip prostheses. Orthop Clin North Am 29:67–84

Firooznia H, Baruch H, Seliger G et al (1974) The value of subtraction in hip arthrography after total hip replacement. Bull Hosp Jt Dis 35:36–41

Goodman SB, Adler SJ, Fyhrie DP et al (1988) The acetabular
teardrop and its relevance to acetabular migration. Clin Orthop 236:199–204

Hardy DC, Reinus WR, Trotty WG et al (1988) Arthrography after total hip arthroplasty: utility of post ambulation radiographs. Skeletal Radiol 17:20–23

Harris WH, Penenberg BL (1987) Further follow up on socket fixation using a metal backed acetabular component for total hip replacement: a minimum 10 year follow up study. J Bone Joint Surg 69A:1140–1143

Hendrix RW, Wixson RL, Rana NA et al (1983) Arthrography after total hip arthroplasty: a modified technique used in the diagnosis of pain. Radiology 148:647–652

Hu H, He HD, Foley WD et al (2000) Four multidetector-row helical CT: image quality and volume coverage speed. Radiology 215:55–62

Johnson JA, Christie MJ, Sandler MP et al (1988) Detection of occult infection following total joint arthroplasty using sequential technetium-99m HDP bone scintigraphy and indium-111 WBC imaging. J Nucl Med 29:1347–1353

Kaplan PA, Montesi SA, Jardon OM et al (1988) Bone ingrowth hip prostheses in asymptomatic patients: radiographic features. Radiology 169:221–227

Park JS, Ryu KN, Hong HP, Park YK, Chun YS, Yoo MC (2004) Focal osteolysis in total hip replacement. Skeletal Radiol 33:632–640

Puri L, Wixson RL, Stern SH et al (2002) Use of helical computed tomography for the assessment of acetabular osteolysis after total hip arthroplasty. J Bone Joint Surg Am 84A:609–614

Resnik CS, Fratkin MJ, Cardea A (1986) Arthroscintigraphic evaluation of the painful total hip prosthesis. Clin Nucl Med 11:242–244

Robertson DD, Yuan J, Wang G et al (1997) Total Hip Prosthesis metal-artifact suppression usinh iterative deblurring reconstruction. J Comput Assist Tomogr 21:293–298

Streule K, De Schrijver M, Fridrich R (1988) 99Tcm-labeled HAS-nanocolloid versus 111-In oxine-labeled granulocytes in detecting skeletal septic process. Nucl Med Commun 9:59–67

Suh JS, Jeong EK, Shin KH et al (1998) Minimizing artifacts caused by metallic implants at MR imaging: experimental and clinical studies. AJR Am J Roentgenol 171:1207–1213

Tartaglino LM, Flanders AE, Vinitski S et al (1994) Metallic artifacts on MR images of the postoperative spine: reduction with fast spin-echo techniques. Radiology 190:565–569

Twair A, Ryan M, O'Connell M et al (2003) MRI of failed total hip replacement caused by abductor muscle avulsion. AJR Am J Roentgenol 181:1547–1550

Van Holsbeeck MT, Eyler WR, Sherman LS et al (1994) Detection of infection in loosened hip prostheses: efficacy of sonography. AJR Am J Roentgenol 163:381–384

Weissman BN (1990) Current topics in the radiology of joint replacement surgery. Radiol Clin North Am 28:1111–1134

White MW, Kim JK, Mehta M et al (2000) Complications of total hip arthroplasty: MR imaging – initial experience. Radiology 215:254–262

Yoder SA, Brand RA, Pederson DR et al (1988) Total hip acetabular component position affects component loosening rates. Clin Orthop 220:79–87

Zhuang H, Duarte PS, Pourdehnad M et al (2000) Excluion of chronic osteomyelitis with F-18 fluorodeoxyglucose positron emission tomographic imagimg. Clin Nucl Med 25:281–284

Subject Index

List of Contributors

Judith E. Adams, MBBS, FRCR, FRCP
Professor of Diagnostic Radiology
Imaging Science and Biomedical Engineering
The Medical School
Stopford Building
The University of Manchester
Oxford Road
Manchester M13 9PT
UK

Houman Alizadeh, MD
Department of Radiology B
University Hospital of Strasbourg
Pavillon Clovis Vincent BP 426
67091 Strasbourg
France

Antoni Basille, MD
Department of Radiology B
University Hospital of Strasbourg
Pavillon Clovis Vincent BP 426
67091 Strasbourg
France

Thomas H. Berquist, MD, FACR
Department of Radiology
Mayo Clinic
4500 San Pablo Road
Jacksonville, FL 32224-3899
USA

Guillaume Bierry, MD
Department of Radiology B
University Hospital of Strasbourg
Pavillon Clovis Vincent BP 426
67091 Strasbourg
France

Stefano Bianchi, MD
Institut de Radiologie
Clinique des Grangettes
7 Chemin des Grangettes
1224 Chêne-Bougeries
Switzerland

Xavier Buy, MD
Department of Radiology B
University Hospital of Strasbourg
Pavillon Clovis Vincent BP 426
67091 Strasbourg
France

Victor N. Cassar-Pullicino, MD, FRCR
Consultant and Clinical Director
Department of Diagnostic Radiology
Robert Jones & Agnes Hunt Orthopaedic Hospital
Oswestry, Shropshire SY10 7AG
UK

David Connell, MD
Consultant Musculoskeletal Radiologist
Royal National Orthopaedic Hospital
Stanmore HA7 4LP
UK

Patricia Cunningham, MD
Department of Radiology
Mater Misericordiae and
Cappagh National Orthopaedic Hospital
Finglas
Dublin 11
Ireland

Juan Cupelli, MD
Department of Radiology B
University Hospital of Strasbourg
Pavillon Clovis Vincent BP 426
67091 Strasbourg
France

Christian Czerny, MD
General Hospital, University Medical School Vienna
Währinger Gürtel 18–20
1090 Vienna
Austria

A. Mark Davies, MBChB, FRCR
Department of Radiology
The MRI Centre
Royal Orthopaedic Hospital
Birmingham B31 2AP
UK

Stephen Eustace, MD
Department of Radiology
Mater Misericordiae and
Cappagh National Orthopaedic Hospital
Finglas
Dublin 11
Ireland

IGNAC FOGELMAN, MD
Kings College and
Guys 'Hospital and
St. Thomas' NHS Trust
St. Thomas St
London, SE1 9 RT
UK

AFSHIN GANGI, MD, PhD
Professor, Department of Radiology B
University Hospital of Strasbourg
Pavillon Clovis Vincent BP 426
67091 Strasbourg
France

AMILCARE GENTILI, MD
Professor, Department of Radiology
University of California, San Diego
9300 Campus Point Drive
La Jolla, CA 92037
USA

SHARON F. HAIN, MD
The Institute of Nuclear Medicine
The Middlesex Hospital, UCH
London, UK
and
Charing Cross Hospital
Hammersmith Hospitals NHS Trust
London, UK

PHILIP HUGHES, MD
Consultant Radiologist
X-Ray Department West
Derriford Hospital
Derriford Road
Plymouth PL6 8DH
UK

HERWIG IMHOF, MD
Professor, Department of Radiology
AKH Vienna
Waehringer Guertel 18–20
1090 Vienna
Austria

KARL J. JOHNSON, MD
Department of Radiology
Princess of Wales
Birmingham Children's Hospital
Steelhouse Lane
Birmingham B4 6NH
UK

ANNE GRETHE JURIK, MD, DMSc
Associate Professor, Department of Radiology
Aarhus University Hospital
Noerrebrogade 44
8000 Aarhus C
Denmark

JOSEF KRAMER, MD, PhD
Röntgeninstitut am Schillerpark
Reanerstrasse 6–8
4020 Linz
Austria

GEORGE KOULOURIS, MD
MRI Fellow
The Alfred Hospital
Commercial Road
Melbourne Victoria 3004
Australia

GERHARD LAUB, PhD
Siemens Cardiovascular Center
Peter V. Ueberroth Bldg. Suite 3371
Los Angeles, CA, 90095-7206
USA

FREDERIC E. LECOUVET, MD
Department of Radiology and Medical Imaging
Université Catholique de Louvain
University Hospital St. Luc
10 Avenue Hippocrate
1200 Brussels
Belgium

BAUDOUIN MALDAGUE, MD
Department of Radiology and Medical Imaging
Université Catholique de Louvain
University Hospital St. Luc
10 Avenue Hippocrate
1200 Brussels
Belgium

JACQUES MALGHEM, MD
Department of Radiology and Medical Imaging
Université Catholique de Louvain
University Hospital St. Luc
10 Avenue Hippocrate
1200 Brussels
Belgium

CARLO MARTINOLI, MD
Professor of Radiology
Istituto di Radiologia
Università di Genova
Largo Rosanna Benzi 1
16100 Genova
Italy

WILFRED C. G. PEH, MD, MBBS, FRCP, FRCR
Clinical Professor and Senior Consultant Radiologist
Programme Office, Singapore Health Services
7 Hospital Drive #02-09
Singapore 169611
Republic of Singapore

JEFFREY J. PETERSON, MD
Department of Radiology
Mayo Clinic
4500 San Pablo Road
Jacksonville, FL 32224 -3899
USA

MICHAEL P. RECHT, MD
The Cleveland Clinic Foundation
Diagnostic Radiology/Musculoskeletal Section
95 Euclid Avenue
Cleveland, OH 44195-5145
USA

DAVID RITCHIE, MD
Department of Radiology
Royal Liverpool University Hospital
Prescot Street
Liverpool L7 8XP
UK

UGNE JULIA SKRIPKUS, MD
Musculoskeletal Radiology Fellow
University of California, San Diego
200 West Arbor Drive
San Diego, CA 92075
USA

JAMES TEH, MD
Department of Radiology
Nuffield Orthopaedic Centre
Windmill Road
Headington
Oxford OX3 7LD
UK

KAJ TALLROTH, MD
Associate Professor
Orton Orthopedic Hospital
Tenalavagen 10
00280 Helsinki
Finland

BERNHARD J. TINS, MD
Department of Diagnostic Radiology
Robert Jones & Agnes Hunt Orthopaedic Hospital
Oswestry, Shropshire SY10 7AG
UK

BRUNO C. VANDE BERG, MD, PhD
Department of Radiology and Medical Imaging
Université Catholique de Louvain
University Hospital St. Luc
10 Avenue Hippocrate
1200 Brussels
Belgium

DANIEL VANEL, MD
Professor, Department of Radiology
Institut Gustave Roussy
39 rue Camille Desmoulins
94805 Villejuif
France

RICHARD WILLIAM WHITEHOUSE, MD
Department of Clinical Radiology
Manchester Royal Infirmary
Oxford Road
Manchester, M13 9WL
UK

HELEN WILLIAMS, MD
Department of Radiology
Princess of Wales
Birmingham Children's Hospital
Steelhouse Lane
Birmingham, B4 6NH
UK

DAVID WILSON, MD
Department of Radiology
Nuffield Orthopaedic Centre
NHS Trust
Windmill Road, Headington
Oxford OX3 7LD
UK

NEVILLE B. WRIGHT, MB, ChB, DMRD, FRCR
Department of Paediatric Radiology
Royal Manchester Children's Hospital
Central Manchester &
Manchester Children's University Hospitals NHS Trust
Hospital Road
Pendlebury M27 4HA
UK

MEDICAL RADIOLOGY Diagnostic Imaging and Radiation Oncology

Titles in the series already published

DIAGNOSTIC IMAGING

MEDICAL RADIOLOGY Diagnostic Imaging and Radiation Oncology

Titles in the series already published

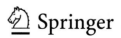 Springer

MEDICAL RADIOLOGY Diagnostic Imaging and Radiation Oncology

Titles in the series already published

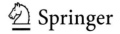 Springer